EGFR Signaling Networks in Cancer Therapy

CANCER DRUG DISCOVERY AND DEVELOPMENT
Beverly A. Teicher, SERIES EDITOR

Checkpoint Responses in Cancer Therapy, edited by Wei Dai, 2008

Cancer Proteomics: From Bench to Bedside, edited by Sayed S. Daoud, 2008

Transforming Growth Factor-b in Cancer Therapy, Volume II: Cancer Treatment and Therapy, edited by Sonia Jakowlew, 2008

Transforming Growth Factor-b in Cancer Therapy, Volume 1: Basic and Clinical Biology, edited by Sonia Jakowlew, 2008

Microtubule Targets in Cancer Therapy, edited by Antonio T. Fojo, 2008

Antiangiogenic Agents in Cancer Therapy, Second Edition, edited by Beverly A. Teicher and Lee M. Ellis, 2007

Apoptosis and Senescence in Cancer Chemotherapy and Radiotherapy, Second Edition, edited by David A. Gerwitz, Shawn Edan Holtz, and Steven Grant, 2007

Molecular Targeting in Oncology, edited by Howard L. Kaufman, Scott Wadler, and Karen Antman, 2007

In Vivo Imaging of Cancer Therapy, edited by Anthony F. Shields and Patricia Price, 2007

Cytokines in the Genesis and Treatment of Cancer, edited by Michael A. Caligiuri, Michael T. Lotze, and Frances R. Balkwill, 2007

Regional Cancer Therapy, edited by Peter M. Schlag and Ulrike Stein, 2007

Gene Therapy for Cancer, edited by Kelly K. Hunt, Stephan A. Vorburger, and Stephen G. Swisher, 2007

Deoxynucleoside Analogs in Cancer Therapy, edited by Godefridus J. Peters, 2006

Cancer Drug Resistance, edited by Beverly A. Teicher, 2006

Histone Deacetylases: Transcriptional Regulation and Other Cellular Functions, edited by Eric Verdin, 2006

Immunotherapy of Cancer, edited by Mary L. Disis, 2006

Biomarkers in Breast Cancer: Molecular Diagnostics for Predicting and Monitoring Therapeutic Effect, edited by Giampietro Gasparini and Daniel F. Hayes, 2006

Protein Tyrosine Kinases: From Inhibitors to Useful Drugs, edited by Doriana Fabbro and Frank McCormick, 2005

Bone Metastasis: Experimental and Clinical Therapeutics, edited by Gurmit Singh and Shafaat A. Rabbani, 2005

The Oncogenomics Handbook, edited by William J. LaRochelle and Richard A. Shimkets, 2005

Camptothecins in Cancer Therapy, edited by Thomas G. Burke and Val R. Adams, 2005

Combination Cancer Therapy: Modulators and Potentiators, edited by Gary K. Schwartz, 2005

Cancer Chemoprevention, Volume 2: Strategies for Cancer Chemoprevention, edited by Gary J. Kelloff, Ernest T. Hawk, and Caroline C. Sigman, 2005

Death Receptors in Cancer Therapy, edited by Wafik S. El-Deiry, 2005

Cancer Chemoprevention, Volume 1: Promising Cancer Chemopreventive Agents, edited by Gary J. Kelloff, Ernest T. Hawk, and Caroline C. Sigman, 2004

Proteasome Inhibitors in Cancer Therapy, edited by Julian Adams, 2004

Nucleic Acid Therapeutics in Cancer, edited by Alan M. Gewirtz, 2004

DNA Repair in Cancer Therapy, edited by Lawrence C. Panasci and Moulay A. Alaoui-Jamali, 2004

Hematopoietic Growth Factors in Oncology: Basic Science and Clinical Therapeutics, edited by George Morstyn, MaryAnn Foote, and Graham J. Lieschke, 2004

Handbook of Anticancer Pharmacokinetics and Pharmacodynamics, edited by William D. Figg and Howard L. McLeod, 2004

Anticancer Drug Development Guide: Preclinical Screening, Clinical Trials, and Approval, Second Edition, edited by Beverly A. Teicher and Paul A. Andrews, 2004

Handbook of Cancer Vaccines, edited by Michael A. Morse, Timothy M. Clay, and Kim H. Lyerly, 2004

Drug Delivery Systems in Cancer Therapy, edited by Dennis M. Brown, 2003

Oncogene-Directed Therapies, edited by Janusz Rak, 2003

Cell Cycle Inhibitors in Cancer Therapy: Current Strategies, edited by Antonio Giordano and Kenneth J. Soprano, 2003

Chemoradiation in Cancer Therapy, edited by Hak Choy, 2003

Fluoropyrimidines in Cancer Therapy, edited by Youcef M. Rustum, 2003

Targets for Cancer Chemotherapy: Transcription Factors and Other Nuclear Proteins, edited by Nicholas B. La Thangue and Lan R. Bandara, 2002

Tumor Targeting in Cancer Therapy, edited by Michel Pagé, 2002

Hormone Therapy in Breast and Prostate Cancer, edited by V. Craig Jordan and Barrington J. A. Furr, 2002

Tumor Models in Cancer Research, edited by Beverly A. Teicher, 2002

Tumor Suppressor Genes in Human Cancer, edited by David E. Fisher, 2001

Matrix Metalloproteinase Inhibitors in Cancer Therapy, edited by Neil J. Clendeninn and Krzysztof Appelt, 2001

Farnesyltransferase Inhibitors in Cancer, edited by Saïd M. Sebti and Andrew D. Hamilton, 2001

EGFR Signaling Networks in Cancer Therapy

Edited by

John D. Haley, PhD
OSI Pharmaceuticals, Farmingdale, New York, USA

William John Gullick, PhD
University of Kent, Canterbury, UK

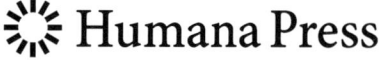

Editors
John D. Haley
OSI Pharmaceuticals
Farmingdale, NY 11735
USA
jhaley@osip.com

William John Gullick
University of Kent
Department of Biosciences
Canterbury, Kent
UK CT2 7NJ
w.j.gullick@ukc.ac.uk

Series Editor
Beverly A. Teicher
Vice President, Oncology Research
Genzyme Corporation
49 New York Avenue
Framingham, MA 01701

ISBN 978-1-58829-948-2   e-ISBN 978-1-59745-356-1
DOI: 10.1007/978-1-59745-356-1

Library of Congress Control Number: 2008923173

© 2008 Humana Press, a part of Springer Science+Business Media, LLC
All rights reserved. This work may not be translated or copied in whole or in part without the written permission of the publisher (Humana Press, c/o Springer Science+Business Media, LLC, 233 Spring Street, New York, NY 10013, USA), except for brief excerpts in connection with reviews or scholarly analysis. Use in connection with any form of information storage and retrieval, electronic adaptation, computer software, or by similar or dissimilar methodology now known or hereafter developed is forbidden.

The use in this publication of trade names, trademarks, service marks, and similar terms, even if they are not identified as such, is not to be taken as an expression of opinion as to whether or not they are subject to proprietary rights.

While the advice and information in this book are believed to be true and accurate at the date of going to press, neither the authors nor the editors nor the publisher can accept any legal responsibility for any errors or omissions that may be made. The publisher makes no warranty, express or implied, with respect to the material contained herein.

Printed on acid-free paper

9 8 7 6 5 4 3 2 1

springer.com

Preface

The epidermal growth factor (EGF) receptor and its downstream signal transduction networks have been implicated in the ontology and maintenance of tumor tissues, which has motivated the discovery and development of molecularly targeted anti-EGF receptor therapies. Over decades of study, the EGF receptor structure, its ligand binding domains, the physical biochemistry underlying its intrinsic tyrosine kinase catalytic function and the modular interactions with SH2, PTB, and SH3 domain containing signaling adaptor proteins required for signal transduction, have been extensively dissected. Not only is the EGF receptor the nexus of many streams of information, but it also forms one part of a calculating device by forming dimers and oligomers with the other three receptors in its family in response to at least eleven ligands (some of which are expressed in multiple forms with overlapping or quite distinct functions). This phenomenon, while recruiting to the inner surface of the cell membrane and activating multiple second messenger proteins, also allows the possibility of cross talk between these systems, permitting a further layer of information to be exchanged.

Less well described are the cross regulation of the EGF receptor and other anti-apoptotic, mitogenic and metabolic signaling systems. The study of these systems has yielded new surprises. One hurdle in these efforts has been that signal transduction pathways have frequently been defined in the generic absence of their tissue-specific or cell-interaction specific context. It is worth recalling, however, that despite these many "known and unknown, unknowns" much progress has been achieved in the last fifty years of research on this system. As opposed to many other cell surface signaling proteins or protein families, we now have a wealth of knowledge, and, importantly, many vitally useful reagents such as antibodies and experimental models *in silico, in vitro,* and *in vivo,* all of which will assist in improving our understanding.

The volume is separated into two sections. The first section probes the molecular pathways and the intersection of signaling networks that are frequently deregulated in human cancers. Our aim here is to describe the EGF receptor in a tumor tissue-specific context. The second section illustrates the many ways in which the EGF receptor contributes to abnormal survival and migration signaling in cancer cells and to epithelial and mesenchymal transition and metastasis.

In this volume we describe the mitogenic, survival, adhesive, and migratory pathways within a framework of interacting subsystems that contribute to the activity and physiological regulation of the receptor in normal and neoplastic tissues. Recent work has clearly shown that epithelial tumor cells are capable of transdifferentiation to a more mesenchymal phenotype, a process resembling an epithelial to mesenchymal transition (EMT). Similarly, it has been shown that epithelial tumors can promote genetic alterations and loss of heterozygosity in surrounding stromal cells leading to hyperproliferation of activated stromal cells and tumor migration. These cellular transitions and cellular interactions have profound consequences for the EGF receptor signaling networks and for the dependence of carcinoma cells on those signals for survival. The interactions of the EGF receptor signaling with other cellular subsystems regulating survival, mitogenic and migration cues thus have medical meaning as we try to identify and develop treatments that not only cause apoptosis of tumor cells directly but also have impact on the altered cell populations from whence cancer recurrence occurs.

The importance of this EGF receptor and its family as a target in cancer drug development is manifest in the level of interest and investment in academic research and in pharmaceutical development. There have been mixed results and rewards to date. It can now be accepted that interdiction with agents such as antibodies or small molecule drugs does work, and in fact works quite well in some patients. We do, however, face frustration when we do not know the full potential of these targets. Current needs include better methods of patient selection, better surrogate markers, and especially better drugs. Although progress to these ends is continuous and indeed often exciting and encouraging, the only rational basis on which to found this enterprise is substantial increases in our knowledge of how the system works and how this knowledge may vary in the context of the living, differentiated cell. It is unlikely that acquisition of this knowledge will be an easy or a short task, but it is a good bet that it will be a productive one. Along with the contributors to this volume and those involved in exploring this fascinating system, we still have much to learn.

"Now this is not the end. It is not even the beginning of the end. But it is, perhaps, the end of the beginning." **Winston Churchill, Mansion House, November 1942.**

John D. Haley
William John Gullick

TABLE OF CONTENTS

Preface v

Contributors ix

SECTION I: EGFR SIGNALING NETWORKS

1   EGF Receptor Family Extracellular Domain Structures and Functions 3
    Antony W. Burgess and Thomas P.J. Garrett

2   EGFR Family Heterodimers in Cancer Pathogenesis and Treatment 15
    Howard M. Stern

3   Structure-function of EGFR Kinase Domain and Its Inhibitors 31
    Charles Eigenbrot

4   Internalization and Degradation of the EGF Receptor 47
    Alexander Sorkin

5   Differential Dependence of EGFR and ErbB2 on the Molecular Chaperone Hsp90 63
    Wanping Xu, Len Neckers

6   Activation of STATs 3 and 5 Through the EGFR Signaling Axis 73
    Priya Koppikar and Jennifer Rubin Grandis

7   The Intersection of EGFR and the Ras Signaling Pathway 89
    Marie Wislez and Jonathan M. Kurie

8   Phosphoinositide 3-Kinase Enzymes as Downstream Targets of the EGF Receptor 97
    Jan Domin

9   Convergence of EGF Receptor and Src Family Signaling Networks in Cancer 119
    Jessica E. Pritchard, Allison B. Jablonski, and Sarah J. Parsons

10 A Molecular Crosstalk between E-cadherin and EGFR Signaling Networks 139
    Julie Gavard and J. Silvio Gutkind

11 Crosstalk Between Insulin-like Growth Factor (IGF) and Epidermal Growth Factor (EGF) Receptors 155
    Marc A. Becker and Douglas Yee

12 Negative Regulation of Signaling by the EGFR Family 169
    Kermit L. Carraway, III, Lily Yen, Ellen Ingalla, and Colleen Sweeney

13 Nuclear ErbB Receptors: Pathways and Functions 187
    Hong-Jun Liao and Graham Carpenter

14 Temporal Dynamics of EGF Receptor Signaling by Quantitative
    Proteomics **199**
    Blagoy Blagoev, Irina Kratchmarova, Jesper V. Olsen and Matthias Mann

15 Computational and Mathematical Modeling of the EGF
    Receptor System **209**
    Colin G. Johnson, Emmet McIntyre, and William Gullick

SECTION II: EGFR IN TUMORIGENESIS AND EGFR TYROSINE KINASE
INHIBITORS IN CANCER THERAPY

16 Expression and Prognostic Significance of the EGFR
    in Solid Tumors **221**
    *Nicola Normanno, Caterina Bianco, Antonella De Luca, Luigi Strizzi,
    Marianna Gallo, Mario Mancino and David S. Salomon*

17 Signaling by the EGF Receptor in Human Cancers: Accentuate
    the Positive, Eliminate the Negative **235**
    *Haley L. Bennett, Tilman Brummer, Paul Timpson, Kate I. Patterson
    and Roger J. Daly*

18 EGFR Signaling in Invasion, Angiogenesis
    and Metastasis **257**
    Carol Box, Joanna Peak, Susanne Rogers, and Suzanne Eccles

19 Constitutive Activation of Truncated EGF Receptors
    in Glioblastoma **277**
    Carol J. Wikstrand and Darell D. Bigner

20 EGFR Mutations, Other Molecular Alterations Related to Sensitivity
    to EGFR Inhibitors, and Molecular Testing for EGFR-Targeted
    Therapies in Non-Small Cell Lung Cancer **293**
    David A. Eberhard

21 Crosstalk Between COX-2 and EGFR: A Potential Therapeutic
    Opportunity **337**
    Andrew J. Dannenberg and Kotha Subbaramaiah

22 Cellular Sensitivity to EGF Receptor Inhibitors **353**
    Stuart Thomson, John D. Haley and Robert Yauch

23 Utilizing Combinations of Molecular Targeted Agents to Sensitize
    Tumor Cells to EGFR Inhibitors **369**
    Elizabeth Buck, Alexandra Eyzaguirre, and Kenneth K. Iwata

CONTRIBUTORS

Marc A. Becker • Departments of Medicine and Pharmacology, University of Minnesota, Minneapolis, MN

Haley L. Bennett, PhD • Cancer Research Program, Garvan Institute of Medical Research, Sydney, NSW, Australia

Caterina Bianco • Cell Biology and Preclinical Models Unit, INT-Fondazione Pascale, Naples, IT

Darell D. Bigner, M.D PhD • Department of Pathology, Duke University Medical Center, Durham, NC

Blagoy Blagoev, PhD • Center for Experimental Bioinformatics (CEBI), Department of Biochemistry and Molecular Biology, University of Southern Denmark, Odense M, Denmark

Carol Box, PhD • Tumour Biology and Metastasis Team,CR-UK Centre For Cancer Therapeutics, McElwain Laboratories, Institute of Cancer Research, Belmont, Sutton, Surrey, UK

Tilman Brummer, PhD • Cancer Research Program, Garvan Institute of Medical Research, Sydney, NSW, Australia

Elizabeth Buck, PhD • Translational Research, OSI Pharmaceuticals Inc., Farmingdale, NY

Antony W. Burgess, PhD • Ludwig Institute for Cancer Research, Melbourne Branch, Royal Melbourne Hospital, Parkville Vic, Australia

Kermit L. Carraway, III, PhD • UC Davis Cancer Center, Sacramento, CA

Graham Carpenter PhD • Department of Biochemistry, Vanderbilt University School of Medicine, Nashville, TN

Roger J. Daly, PhD • Cancer Research Program, Garvan Institute of Medical Research, Sydney, NSW, Australia

Andrew J. Dannenberg, MD • Department of Medicine Weill Cornell Medical College, New York, NY

Jan Domin, PhD • Division of Medicine, Imperial College London, London UK

David A. Eberhard, MD PhD • Molecular Pathology and Diagnostics for Oncology, San Francisco, CA

Suzanne Eccles PhD • McElwain Laboratories, Institute of Cancer Research, Belmont, Sutton, Surrey, UK

Charles Eigenbrot, PhD • Department of Protein Engineering MS 27, Genentech, Inc., South San Francisco, CA

Alexandra Eyzaguirre, MS • Translational Research, OSI Pharmaceuticals Inc., Farmingdale, NY

Marianna Gallo • Cell Biology and Preclinical Models Unit, INT-Fondazione Pascale, Naples, IT

Thomas P.J. Garrett, PhD • The Walter and Eliza Hall of Medical Research, Parkville Vic, Australia

Julie Gavard, PhD • Oral and Pharyngeal Cancer Branch, National Institute of Dental and Craniofacial Research, National Institutes of Health, DHHS, Bethesda, MD

Jennifer Rubin Grandis, MD • University of Pittsburgh, Eye and Ear Institute, Pittsburgh, PA

William Gullick, PhD • Department of Biosciences, University of Kent, Canterbury, Kent, UK

J. Silvio Gutkind, PhD • Oral and Pharyngeal Cancer Branch, National Institute of Dental and Craniofacial Research, National Institutes of Health, Bethesda, MD

John D. Haley, PhD • Translational Research, OSI Pharmaceuticals Inc., Park Dr, Farmingdale, NY

Ellen IngallA • UC Davis Cancer Center, Sacramento, CA

Kenneth K. Iwata, PhD • Translational Research, OSI Pharmaceuticals Inc., Farmingdale, NY

Allison B. Jablonski, PhD • Biology Department, Lynchburg College, Lynchburg, VA

Colin G. Johnson, PhD • Computing Laboratory, University of Kent, Canterbury, Kent, UK

Priya Koppikar, PhD • Department of Otolaryngology, University of Pittsburgh, Pittsburgh, PA, USA.

Irina Kratchmarova, PhD • Center for Experimental Bioinformatics (CEBI), Department of Biochemistry and Molecular Biology, University of Southern Denmark, Odense M, Denmark

Jonathan M. Kurie, MD • Thoracic/Head and Neck Medical Oncology, UT M. D. Anderson Cancer Center, Houston, TX

Hong-Jun Liao, MD • Department of Biochemistry, Vanderbilt University School of Medicine, Nashville, TN

Antonella De Luca • Cell Biology and Preclinical Models Unit, INT-Fondazione Pascale, Naples, IT

Matthias Mann, PhD • Department of Proteomics and Signal Transduction, Max-Planck Institute for Biochemistry, Martinsried, Germany

Mario Mancino • Cell Biology and Preclinical Models Unit, INT-Fondazione Pascale, Naples, IT

Emmet McIntyre, PhD • Computing Laboratory, University of Kent, Canterbury, Kent, UK

Len Neckers, PhD • Urologic Oncology Branch, Center for Cancer Research, National Cancer Institute, NIH, Bethesda, MD

Nicola Normanno, MD • Cell Biology and Preclinical Models Unit, INT-Fondazione Pascale, Naples, IT

Jesper V. Olsen, PhD • Department of Proteomics and Signal Transduction, Max-Planck Institute for Biochemistry, Martinsried, Germany

Sarah J. Parsons, PhD • Department of Microbiology, University of Virginia Health System, Charlottesville, VA

Kate I. Patterson, PhD • Cancer Research Program, Garvan Institute of Medical Research, Sydney, NSW 2010, Australia

Joanna Peak, MSc • Tumour Biology and Metastasis Team, CR-UK Centre For Cancer Therapeutics, McElwain Laboratories, Institute of Cancer Research, Belmont, Sutton, Surrey, UK

Jessica E. Pritchard • Department of Microbiology and Cancer Center, University of Virginia Health System, Charlottesville, VA

Susanne Rogers, FRCR • Head and Neck Unit, Royal Marsden Hospital, London, UK

David S. Salomon, PhD • Tumor Growth Factor Section, Mammary Biology & Tumorigenesis Laboratory, NCI, NIH, Bethesda, MD

Alexander Sorkin, PhD • Department of Pharmacology, University of Colorado Health Sciences Center at Fitzsimmons, Aurora, CO

Howard M. Stern, MD, PhD • Department of Research Pathology, MS 72b, Genentech Inc., South San Francisco, CA

Luigi Strizzi • Cell Biology and Preclinical Models Unit, INT-Fondazione Pascale, Naples, IT

Kotha Subbaramaiah, PhD • Department of Medicine, Weill Cornell Medical College, New York, NY

Colleen Sweeney • UC Davis Cancer Center, Sacramento, CA

Stuart Thomson, PhD • Translational Research, OSI Pharmaceuticals Inc., Farmingdale, NY

Paul Timpson, PhD • Cancer Research Program, Garvan Institute of Medical Research, Sydney, NSW, Australia

Carol J. Wikstrand, PhD • Departments of Microbiology/Immunology, Saba University School of Medicine, Saba, Netherlands Antilles

Marie Wislez, MD, PhD • Department of Pulmonology, AP-HP Hôpital Tenon, Paris, France

Wanping Xu, PhD • Urologic Oncology Branch, Center for Cancer Research, National Cancer Institute, Bethesda, MD

Robert Yauch, PhD • Genentech Inc., South San Francisco, CA

Douglas Yee, MD • Departments of Medicine and Pharmacology, University of Minnesota, Minneapolis, MN

Lily Yen • UC Davis Cancer Center, Sacramento, CA

Section I:
EGFR Signaling Networks

1 EGF Receptor Family Extracellular Domain Structures and Functions

*Antony W. Burgess
and Thomas P.J. Garrett*

Contents

INTRODUCTION—EGFR STRUCTURE/FUNCTION
    STUDIES
EGFR
ERBB2
ERBB3 AND ERBB4
ANTIBODY BINDING TO THE EGFR FAMILY MEMBERS
REFERENCES

Abstract

From its discovery, the EGFR has been linked to the transformation events associated with oncogenic changes. Until recently, however, investigations on the 3-dimensional structures, cell surface configurations, and activation of the EGFR family members have yielded only limited insight into the biochemistry and biology of this receptor family. We now have the 3D-structures of the extracellular domains (ECDs) of all four family members. Surprisingly, when forming the activated, ligand-bound structures, the EGFR, ErbB3 and, ErbB4 undergo major conformational changes.

These family members appear to form tethered, low-affinity conformers and untethered, ligand-bound conformers that are capable of oligomerization. The 3D-structure of the ErbB2-ECD suggests that this family member only exists in the untethered form and is ready for oligomerization and consequential activation by ligand-associated untethered conformers of the other EGFR family members. The 3D-structures allow an understanding of the activation processes and the mechanisms by which several anti-EGFR and anti-ErbB2 antibodies inhibit the activation of these receptors.

Key Words: ErbB2, ErbB3, ErbB4, 3-dimensional structures, conformational transitions, antibody epitopes.

1. INTRODUCTION—EGFR STRUCTURE/FUNCTION STUDIES

Since the discovery of EGF by Stanley Cohen in the early 1950s, (*1*) cellular-signaling systems have intrigued both biochemists and cancer biologists. Once the EGF receptor was identified, it was quickly apparent that the biology of this receptor system was closely connected to transforming events associated with cancer (*2*). Pioneering work by biochemists, cell

From: *Cancer Drug Discovery and Development: EGFR Signaling Networks in Cancer Therapy*
Edited by: J. D. Haley and W. J. Gullick, DOI: 10.1007/978-1-59745-356-1_1
© 2008 Humana Press, a part of Springer Science+Business Media, LLC

biologists and biophysicists established a framework for the understanding of growth-factor signaling. In particular, the descriptions of high and low affinity EGFRs on the same cell (*3*), the discovery of ErbB2 (*4*), ErbB3 (*5*), and ErbB4 (*6*) (see also Chapter 2), as well as the down-regulation of the EGFR (*7*) and the induction of dimerization of sEGFR by ligand (*8*) allowed the development of sensible models for receptor activation and signal transduction (*9*). The validity of these models and progression of the molecular basis for regulation of the EGFR kinase (signaling) was hampered by the lack of reliable 3D-information relevant to either the extracellular domain (ECD) or the intracellular kinase.

In 2001/2002, the crystallographers finally broke through, solving a portion of the EGFR kinase domain (*10*), fragments of the EGFR-ECD bound to ligand (*11*), full-length erbB3-ECD (*12*), full-length EGFR-ECD in the presence of EGF (*13*, *14*), and the ErbB2-ECD (*15*, *16*). These structures revealed remarkable sub-domains and potential monomer-interaction sites, confirming a major conformational difference between unbound and ligand-bound ECDs (*17*, *18*). Most recently, the 3D-structures of ErbB4 (*19*) and the structures of the ECDs of the EGFR (*20*) and ErbB2 (*15*, *20*, *21*) with clinically relevant antibodies have been reported. In conjunction with analysis of the properties of site directed mutants and biophysical studies on the oligomerization state of the EGFR on the cell surface (*22*–*26*), it is possible to develop a much clearer model for the processes involved in the activation, regulation, and biology of signaling from the EGFR family in normal and transformed cells.

2. EGFR

Since the amino acid sequence of the EGFR was reported, there has been intensive investigation of its overall structure, the nature of the ligand-binding site(s), and the oligomerization state of the receptor in the presence and absence of the ligand. The recognition of the domain structure for the EGFR has been helpful in defining some the interactions that determined the functional roles for the receptor. The identification of two leucine-rich domains and two cystine-rich domains (Fig. 1.1) dominated our view of the EGFR family for a number of years. It was apparent that the leucine-rich domains were both involved in ligand binding, but the roles of the cystine-rich domains remained obscure. Despite many valiant attempts, the 3D-structures of the ECDs of EGFR family members were not available until a few years ago.

The breakthrough actually came when scientists at the CSIRO and the Biomolecular Research Institute in Melbourne, Australia determined the structure of a fragment of the insulin-like growth factor receptor ECD (IGF-IR) (*27*). Our understanding of the IGF-1R structure has improved substantially (as a result of the reporting of the 3D-structure for the insulin receptor (*28*)). When the structure of the IGF-1R was first published, however, it provided an example for the architecture of domains found in EGFR ECD. The juxtaposition of the "ligand-binding domains" suggested how a ligand could be bound by these domains but did not give us a detailed understanding of the mechanism by which dimerization occurred or signal transduction was activated.

At first sight, the dominating features of the extra-cellular domain of the IGF-1R are the two β-solenoid domains. These domains are structurally homologous, with each containing five turns of "rhomboidal" folds of the leucine-rich repeats and two capping turns. These domains are separated by a cystine-rich, rod-shaped β-solenoid consisting of seven disulfide-boned modules. A very similar arrangement occurs in all of the EGFR family members: β-solenoid(L1)-cystine-rich(CR1)-β-solenoid(L2)-cystine-rich(CR2).

In IGF1R, the ligand-binding faces of both β-solenoid domains are flat β-sheets with one protuberance in the middle turn. For EGFR β-solenoid domains, there more irregularities, and in many of these excursions from the β-solenoid fold, loops are formed, which, together

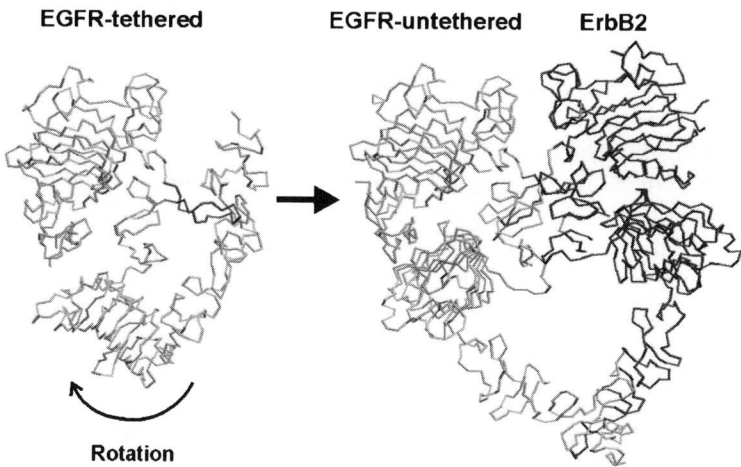

Fig. 1.1. The extracellular domains (ECDs) of the human EGFR and ErbB2. The left-hand model is the tethered form of the EGFR-ECD (*14*) with the CR1 loop highlighted in magenta and the C225 (cetuximab) epitope (lower part of the diagram) and the 806 epitope (*43*), (*56*) (below CR1 loop) are displayed in yellow. The EGF is colored green. On the right, the human, untethered EGFR-ECD conformer (blue) modeled from the conformation of the back-to-back ligand dimer (*11*), is docked in the back-to-back configuration with the human ErbB2-ECD (*15*) (red). The TGF-α is colored green and the CR1 loop is colored magenta. The antibody epitopes are colored yellow. For the EGFR-ECD, the C225 epitope is on the left, and the 806 epitope is on the right facing ErbB2. For ErbB2, the 2C4 epitope is close to the CR1 loop (magenta), and the herceptin epitope is at the C-terminus (at the bottom of the diagram) (*See Color Plate*).

with the flat β-sheets, constitute the ligand-binding surface. In the L1 domain, the first strand of the flat β-sheet extends in a V-shape, covering much of the face of the domain. In this position, it makes a crucial main chain to main chain contact with the different EGF-related ligands. This motif, in part, explains why EGFR can bind a number of ligands, even when they share relatively little sequence homology.

The cystine-rich domain (CR1), which joins the L1 and L2 domains, has a fascinating feature - a 17-amino acid loop that projects a substantial distance away from the body of the protein. In the insulin-receptor family, a similar-sized loop projects from CR1 into the ligand-binding site and may play a role in substrate specificity. The positioning of that loop would not be compatible with the EGFR structures. Instead, the EGFR loop projects in the opposite direction and makes no direct interaction with the ligand. The sequence of this CR1 loop, particularly the presence of some proline and asparagine residues, is essential for maintaining its structure and for the ability of the receptor to respond to ligands.

Amazingly, 18 years after the amino acid sequence of the EGFR was reported by Ullrich and his colleagues at Genentech (*29*), the HER3-ECD 3D-structure was published (*12*). One month later, two structures were reported simultaneously for the ligand-bound form of the EGFR-ECD (*11*, *13*). These three structures provided a major conundrum. While the domains were homologous, in the HER3 structure the second cystine-rich domain was folded back onto the first, occluding the CR1-loop and positioning the L domains in an orientation that could not be bridged by a ligand. In both the Garrett and Ogiso ligand-bound EGFR-ECD structures (*11*, *13*), the CR-1 loop did not interact with the same monomer but lay in a pocket of the juxtaposed receptor pair. It was not possible for the back-to-back EGFR dimer to form unless the CR2 domain folded out of the way. Although Ogiso's EGFR structure

(*13*) contained the CR2 domain, this part of the structure was not sufficiently ordered to trace the protein chain. The first two modules of the CR2 domain define the overall direction of the rod. Indeed, Jorissen was able to produce a model of the whole EGFR-ECD (residues 1-621) where the C-termini of the CR2 domains of both EGFR molecules would be closely juxtaposed in the membrane (*30*).

The reporting of the EGFR structures was followed closely by two independent reports of the 3D-structure of the full length ErbB2-ECD (i.e., L1-CR1-L2-CR2 (*15, 16, 30*)). ErbB2 formed a configuration almost identical to the expected structure for the full-length, untethered EGFR-ECD. The ErbB2 structure crystals packed as monomers, rather than the ligand-bound EGFR-dimer configuration that formed in the EGFR-TGF-α and EGFR-EGF crystals. Notably, the unbound CR1 loop in ErbB2 had a similar conformation to that of the EGFR.

These structures immediately generated models for the ligand binding, dimerization and consequent kinase activation on the cell surface (*31*). Even the configuration of the EGFR-ErbB2 heterodimer could be envisaged (see Fig. 1.1). The structures suggested, however, that there was more to learn about the EGFR both in solution and on the cell surface, in the presence and absence of ligand. In the same month, Ferguson and her colleagues published a low pH structure of the full length (residues 1-621) of the EGFR-ECD with EGF bound (*14*). Surprisingly, even in the presence of the EGF, the CR2 domain was tethered to the CR1 loop in the same way as HER3. The structure of the L1, and most of the CR1 domains were identical in the Garrett, Ogiso, and Ferguson EGFR-ECD structures, although the tethered structure was conformationally distinct in a small hinge region at the base of the CR1 domain. Clearly, when the EGFR-ECD forms the back-to-back dimeric configuration, the CR2 domain needs to untether from the CR1-loop. How is the transition from tethered to the untethered configuration induced? Is it through heterodimerization, ligand binding, thermodynamic fluctuation or even inside-out signaling? The Ferguson structure potentially provides a snapshot of one step in this transition. Here the ligand was bound only to the L1 domain, the second interaction apparently disrupted by crystallizing the protein at pH 5, which would protonate a number of receptor and ligand-histidine residues in the L2 ligand-binding interface. There is still much to be learned about EGFR dynamics, the activation of the cell surface structure, and about consequential activation of intracellular EGFR kinase signaling.

One the most surprising findings related to the EGFR-ligand complex was the distance between the two ligands in the back-to-back dimer – almost 80 Å. Clearly, the ligand was not directly involved in cross-linking the receptor dimer. As seen in the untethered form of the EGFR-ECD, however, the ligand links the L1 and L2 domains through close contacts to both surfaces. Indeed, there are backbone-to-backbone hydrogen bonds between the ligand and L1, which were maintained even at pH 5 as observed in the tethered, back-to-back configuration of the EGFR-ECD. The strong electrostatic and hydrophobic bonding between the ligand and the L2 domain, which includes the conserved amino acids in EGF (Arg 41 and Leu 47), appear to be equal contributors to ligand binding but could also provide a means of removing EGF during receptor recycling.

Apart from the beautiful β-solenoids, perhaps the most extraordinary feature of the EGFR is the CR1 loop. The CR1 loop (Pro241-Lys260) projects out from the CR1 axis. In the presence of ligand, apart from a sidechain-to-sidechain hydrogen bond between asn-86 and Thr-249, it interacts with the partner EGFR between residues 230 and 286. In particular, Tyr-251 interacts at van der Waals distance with Phe-263 of the partner EGFR, and the sidechain of Gln-252 forms a hydrogen bond with the partner backbone at residue 286. The docking and configuration of the CR1 loop are critical for both high-affinity ligand binding and activation of the intracellular EGFR kinase (*11, 13, 32*). It appears that the docking of the CR1 loop to the region 230-286 of its partner influences the juxtaposition of L1 and L2 (i.e., the conformation of the ligand-binding site), as well as the configuration of the intracellular domain (presumably through changes in the oligomerization state of either homo-oligomers or hetero-oligomers.

From the crystal structures it is obvious that the EGFR (1-621) can exist in two distinct conformations, namely, the tethered form, where the CR1 and CR2 loops interact, or the untethered form, where the hinge region at the C-terminus of the CR2 domain has rotated by 130 deg to bring the L1 and L2 close apposition *(14, 31, 32)*. When the C-terminal 120 residues of the EGFR-ECD are removed (EGFR-ECD$_{1-501}$), the EGFR-ECD$_{1-501}$ is not constrained to adopt a "tethered" conformation *(11)*. Indeed, this conformational transition is the most likely explanation for the dramatic increase in ligand affinity when the EGFR-ECD is truncated *(33)*. Truncation is not the only mechanism by which the EGFR-ECD can form the untethered conformation, however. When the EGFR-ECD$_{1-621}$ or EGFR-ECD$_{1-501}$ are produced as Fc fusion proteins, their affinity for ligand increases significantly, presumably by formation of the back-to-back EGFR-ECD untethered dimer. Although the EGFR-ECD-Fc fusion protein is a dimer, it appears possible to form the untethered conformation in the absence of further aggregation, as is the case for ErbB2.

In solution, the EGFR-ECD can adopt the tethered and untethered conformations seen in the crystal. It has been difficult, however, to measure transitions between these conformations or even confirm that it is the untethered form of the receptor that binds ligands with high affinity. At low concentrations in solution, the EGFR-ECD is monomeric; at high concentrations in the presence of ligand, the EGFR-ECD forms an [EGF:EGFR-ECD] dimer and perhaps higher-order oligomers *(8, 34)*. It has still not been determined whether the EGFR-ECD tethered or untethered conformations are in equilibrium, whether ligand binding shifts the equilibrium toward the untethered form, or whether ligand induces the untethering, allowing the back-to-back higher affinity conformation to form. It is important to emphasize, however, that EGFR-ECDs anchored to a cell membrane via the transmembrane and intracellular domain (ICD, including the transmembrane, juxtamembrane, kinase and C-terminal domains) are likely to be influenced differently than the EGFR-ECD in solution. In particular, in the unstimulated state, the EGFR appears to be present on the cell surface as a dimer (or even higher order oligomer). At low density and/or in the absence of ligands, the EGFR kinase is inactive *(35)*. Dimerization, therefore, does not require ligand, and dimerization does not appear to be sufficient to activate the EGFR kinase. Many cells, especially in tissue culture, either express the EGFR at high density and/or produce an endogenous EGFR ligand (e.g., TGF-α). These conditions can lead to EGFR kinase activation, stimulation of EGFR internalization, and intracellular docking to the phosphorylated forms of the EGFR, all of which confound the precise determination of the conformational events associated with ligand activation of the EGFR.

The EGFR was essentially the first growth factor receptor to be associated with cancer *(7)*. Stanley Cohen and his colleagues observed that the EGFR was down-regulated in animal cells transformed with acute oncogenic viruses. In fact, the EGFR in these cells was activated and internalized by autocrine secreted TGF-α, which increased the cell surface tyrosine kinase dependent signaling, but reduced the amount of receptor available for further ligand-induced stimulation. It was soon discovered that human cancer cells often secreted ligands for the EGFR and that the ligand initiated an autocrine loop that was part of the oncogenic process. Interfering with EGFR signaling can reduce the tumorigenic characteristics of both human cell lines *(7, 36, 37)* and cancers in patients. The first therapeutics to target the EGFR ECD have been antibodies directed against the ligand-binding region of the EGFR, e.g., cetuximab, this antibody was also called C225 *(7, 38)*. This antibody binds to the L2 domain, competes with ligand binding and inhibits the conformational changes necessary for activation of the ICD-EGFR kinase. Unfortunately, the expression of the EGFR on cells in normal organs such as the liver, lung, intestine, and skin means that the antibody is cleared from the circulation. When high concentrations of antibody are used, some side effects occur in both the skin and the intestines. In conjunction with other antitumor agents (e.g., 5-fluorouracil), the anti-EGFR antibodies such as cetuximab have been shown to be active anticancer agents. Ligand-induced activation is not the only mechanism by which the EGFR is activated in cancer. In glioma and head and neck tumors, the EGFR gene is often amplified. There is a common mutation that leads to truncation of the EGFR-ECD associated with this amplification (*7, 39–41*). This mutation, which is known as 2-7EGFR (also called EGFRvIII), leads to truncation of the EGFR-ECD such that the residues between 6 and 273 are missing, i.e., most of the L1 and CR1 domains, including the CR1 loop. The tyrosine kinase of this mutant form of the EGFR is constitutively active even in the absence of ligand. The specific activity of EGFRvIII is less than that of the ligand-activated receptor, but the activity appears to be sufficient to contribute to the malignancy of these cells. Antibodies that recognize the EGFRvIII have been developed: the exon 2-7 deletion mutation leads to a unique fusion-peptide sequence, which can be used to rise antibodies that bind to and kill cells expressing EGFRvIII (*40*). In another approach aimed at killing cells expressing EGFRvIII, cells expressing EGFRvIII and overexpressed wild-type receptor were used to raise monoclonal antibodies. One of these antibodies, mab806, recognized EGFRvIII and overexpressed EGFR, but not EGFR expressed at normal levels, i.e., below 100,000 copies per cell (*42*). These antibodies recognize an epitope at the C-terminus of the CR1 domain (residues 287-302) (*42, 43*). In both the tethered and untethered 3D-structures for the EGFR-ECD, it is difficult to see how the mab806 could bind to the epitope. Indeed, analysis of several EGFR-ECD mutants suggests that the mab806 epitope is only sterically available to the EGFRvIII or to the wild-type EGFR undergoing a conformational transition as a result of ligand (*32*) and/or interactions with other family members such as ErbB2. Interestingly, mab806 is capable of binding to cells that overexpress the EGFR and/or EGFRvIII and it can reduce the growth of human tumors xenografted into nude mice (*44*). When mab806 is administered in conjunction with an antibody that recognizes the ligand-binding site (i.e., cetuxumab/C225), tumor growth can be suppressed completely (*45*). Similar antitumor action is observed in animals when mab806 is administered with the EGFR kinase inhibitor AG1478 (*46*). The precise mechanism of this antitumor synergy is still being explored, but the principle should be considered when using anti-EGFR therapies for the treatment of human tumors.

3. ErbB2

ErbB2 was discovered as an oncogene (neu) associated with a rat brain tumor (*47*). While there are very few examples of ErbB2 mutation in human cancer, ErbB2 is often overexpressed in human breast tumors (*48*). Indeed, women diagnosed with breast cancers that overexpress the ErbB2 respond to treatments that include anti-ErbB2 antibodies (e.g., herceptin). The amino acid sequence of ErbB2 revealed that it was closely related to the EGFR. In particular, it appeared to be the receptor tyrosine kinase. Although the tyrosine kinase activity was confirmed, many years of searching for ligands that bind to the ErbB2-ECD and activate the intracellular kinase have proven unsuccessful. None of the EGFR ligands binds to ErbB2.

Through many elegant experiments it was determined that ErbB2 formed heteromers with the other EGFR family members (*48–50*). For example, ErbB2 heteromers with the EGFR have enhanced ligand binding and signals from the heteromer appear to be amplified in comparison to EGFR family homodimers. Similarly, when ErbB2 and ErbB3 form heteromers, strong intracellular signaling occurs in the presence of ligand. ErbB2 cannot bind the ligand, and the ErbB3 kinase is defective, but the combination of the two family members appears more potent than signaling when the receptors are expressed individually. It wasn't until the 3D-structure of ErbB2 was solved that the biochemistry and biology of ErbB2 became clearer (*15, 27, 31*).

of the ligand-binding site), as well as the configuration of the intracellular domain (presumably through changes in the oligomerization state of either homo-oligomers or hetero-oligomers.

From the crystal structures it is obvious that the EGFR (1-621) can exist in two distinct conformations, namely, the tethered form, where the CR1 and CR2 loops interact, or the untethered form, where the hinge region at the C-terminus of the CR2 domain has rotated by 130 deg to bring the L1 and L2 close apposition ($14, 31, 32$). When the C-terminal 120 residues of the EGFR-ECD are removed (EGFR-ECD$_{1-501}$), the EGFR-ECD$_{1-501}$ is not constrained to adopt a "tethered" conformation (11). Indeed, this conformational transition is the most likely explanation for the dramatic increase in ligand affinity when the EGFR-ECD is truncated (33). Truncation is not the only mechanism by which the EGFR-ECD can form the untethered conformation, however. When the EGFR-ECD$_{1-621}$ or EGFR-ECD$_{1-501}$ are produced as Fc fusion proteins, their affinity for ligand increases significantly, presumably by formation of the back-to-back EGFR-ECD untethered dimer. Although the EGFR-ECD-Fc fusion protein is a dimer, it appears possible to form the untethered conformation in the absence of further aggregation, as is the case for ErbB2.

In solution, the EGFR-ECD can adopt the tethered and untethered conformations seen in the crystal. It has been difficult, however, to measure transitions between these conformations or even confirm that it is the untethered form of the receptor that binds ligands with high affinity. At low concentrations in solution, the EGFR-ECD is monomeric; at high concentrations in the presence of ligand, the EGFR-ECD forms an [EGF:EGFR-ECD] dimer and perhaps higher-order oligomers ($8, 34$). It has still not been determined whether the EGFR-ECD tethered or untethered conformations are in equilibrium, whether ligand binding shifts the equilibrium toward the untethered form, or whether ligand induces the untethering, allowing the back-to-back higher affinity conformation to form. It is important to emphasize, however, that EGFR-ECDs anchored to a cell membrane via the transmembrane and intracellular domain (ICD, including the transmembrane, juxtamembrane, kinase and C-terminal domains) are likely to be influenced differently than the EGFR-ECD in solution. In particular, in the unstimulated state, the EGFR appears to be present on the cell surface as a dimer (or even higher order oligomer). At low density and/or in the absence of ligands, the EGFR kinase is inactive (35). Dimerization, therefore, does not require ligand, and dimerization does not appear to be sufficient to activate the EGFR kinase. Many cells, especially in tissue culture, either express the EGFR at high density and/or produce an endogenous EGFR ligand (e.g., TGF-α). These conditions can lead to EGFR kinase activation, stimulation of EGFR internalization, and intracellular docking to the phosphorylated forms of the EGFR, all of which confound the precise determination of the conformational events associated with ligand activation of the EGFR.

The EGFR was essentially the first growth factor receptor to be associated with cancer (7). Stanley Cohen and his colleagues observed that the EGFR was down-regulated in animal cells transformed with acute oncogenic viruses. In fact, the EGFR in these cells was activated and internalized by autocrine secreted TGF-α, which increased the cell surface tyrosine kinase dependent signaling, but reduced the amount of receptor available for further ligand-induced stimulation. It was soon discovered that human cancer cells often secreted ligands for the EGFR and that the ligand initiated an autocrine loop that was part of the oncogenic process. Interfering with EGFR signaling can reduce the tumorigenic characteristics of both human cell lines ($7, 36, 37$) and cancers in patients. The first therapeutics to target the EGFR ECD have been antibodies directed against the ligand-binding region of the EGFR, e.g., cetuximab, this antibody was also called C225 ($7, 38$). This antibody binds to the L2 domain, competes with ligand binding and inhibits the conformational changes necessary for activation of the ICD-EGFR kinase. Unfortunately, the expression of the EGFR on cells in normal organs such as the liver, lung, intestine, and skin means that the antibody is cleared from the circulation. When high concentrations of antibody are used, some side effects occur in both the skin and the intestines. In conjunction with other antitumor agents (e.g., 5-fluorouracil), the anti-EGFR antibodies such as cetuximab have been shown to be active anticancer agents. Ligand-induced activation is not the only mechanism by which the EGFR is activated in cancer. In glioma and head and neck tumors, the EGFR gene is often amplified. There is a common mutation that leads to truncation of the EGFR-ECD associated with this amplification (7, 39–41). This mutation, which is known as 2-7EGFR (also called EGFRvIII), leads to truncation of the EGFR-ECD such that the residues between 6 and 273 are missing, i.e., most of the L1 and CR1 domains, including the CR1 loop. The tyrosine kinase of this mutant form of the EGFR is constitutively active even in the absence of ligand. The specific activity of EGFRvIII is less than that of the ligand-activated receptor, but the activity appears to be sufficient to contribute to the malignancy of these cells. Antibodies that recognize the EGFRvIII have been developed: the exon 2-7 deletion mutation leads to a unique fusion-peptide sequence, which can be used to rise antibodies that bind to and kill cells expressing EGFRvIII (40). In another approach aimed at killing cells expressing EGFRvIII, cells expressing EGFRvIII and overexpressed wild-type receptor were used to raise monoclonal antibodies. One of these antibodies, mab806, recognized EGFRvIII and overexpressed EGFR, but not EGFR expressed at normal levels, i.e., below 100,000 copies per cell (42). These antibodies recognize an epitope at the C-terminus of the CR1 domain (residues 287-302) (42, 43). In both the tethered and untethered 3D-structures for the EGFR-ECD, it is difficult to see how the mab806 could bind to the epitope. Indeed, analysis of several EGFR-ECD mutants suggests that the mab806 epitope is only sterically available to the EGFRvIII or to the wild-type EGFR undergoing a conformational transition as a result of ligand (32) and/or interactions with other family members such as ErbB2. Interestingly, mab806 is capable of binding to cells that overexpress the EGFR and/or EGFRvIII and it can reduce the growth of human tumors xenografted into nude mice (44). When mab806 is administered in conjunction with an antibody that recognizes the ligand-binding site (i.e., cetuxumab/C225), tumor growth can be suppressed completely (45). Similar antitumor action is observed in animals when mab806 is administered with the EGFR kinase inhibitor AG1478 (46). The precise mechanism of this antitumor synergy is still being explored, but the principle should be considered when using anti-EGFR therapies for the treatment of human tumors.

3. ErbB2

ErbB2 was discovered as an oncogene (neu) associated with a rat brain tumor (47). While there are very few examples of ErbB2 mutation in human cancer, ErbB2 is often overexpressed in human breast tumors (48). Indeed, women diagnosed with breast cancers that overexpress the ErbB2 respond to treatments that include anti-ErbB2 antibodies (e.g., herceptin). The amino acid sequence of ErbB2 revealed that it was closely related to the EGFR. In particular, it appeared to be the receptor tyrosine kinase. Although the tyrosine kinase activity was confirmed, many years of searching for ligands that bind to the ErbB2-ECD and activate the intracellular kinase have proven unsuccessful. None of the EGFR ligands binds to ErbB2.

Through many elegant experiments it was determined that ErbB2 formed heteromers with the other EGFR family members (48–50). For example, ErbB2 heteromers with the EGFR have enhanced ligand binding and signals from the heteromer appear to be amplified in comparison to EGFR family homodimers. Similarly, when ErbB2 and ErbB3 form heteromers, strong intracellular signaling occurs in the presence of ligand. ErbB2 cannot bind the ligand, and the ErbB3 kinase is defective, but the combination of the two family members appears more potent than signaling when the receptors are expressed individually. It wasn't until the 3D-structure of ErbB2 was solved that the biochemistry and biology of ErbB2 became clearer (15, 27, 31).

The crystal structures of ErbB2-ECD fragments revealed an untethered conformation with many features similar to the ligand-bound, untethered conformer of the EGFR. The L1 and L2 domains are juxtaposed closely, with several L1 and L2 residues are in van der Waals contact, so there is no possibility of a ligand binding in the configuration observed in the EGFR-ECD:TGF-α of EGFR-ECD:EGF structures. The N-terminal residues of the L1 domain sit in contact with the bottom of the large β-sheet on L2. At the N-terminal end of the ErbB2 L2 surface, residues 16 and 17 of the ErbB2-ECD L1 approach his-449 so closely that a considerable conformational change would be needed to allow a ligand to align with the L2 surface. Furthermore, serine 15 of EGFR is replaced by arginine in ErbB2. In the EGFR, ErbB3, and ErbB4 sequences, a small residue such as serine or threonine is always present and the bulky arginine in this position for ErbB2 would disrupt ligand binding to L1. The hinge region between the CR1 module 7 and the L2 domain form similar angles for ErbB2 and the untethered conformation of the EGFR. The ErbB2 CR1-L2 hinge region is stabilized by a series of H-bonds, suggesting that there is unlikely to be a major conformational change in this region of ErbB2. Similarly, the CR2 loop, which interacts with the CR1 loop in the tethered conformations of EGFR, ErbB3, and ErbB4, is not conserved in ErbB2. The tethered conformation appears to be more stable for EGFR, ErbB3, and ErbB4 than for ErbB2. Interestingly, although the modules of the CR1 domain can vary considerably, the tips of the CR1 loop for the EGFR and ErbB2 are in similar juxtaposition with respect to the L2 domain. When the L2 domains of ErbB2 and the EGFR are superimposed, the tips of the CR1 loops are within 1 angstrom of each other (*15*, *16*).

Although the ErbB2 CR1 loop has a similar conformation to the EGFR CR1 loop, ErbB2 crystallizes as a monomer, not as a the back-to-back dimer found in the EGFR-ECD ligand complex (*15*). The binding pocket for the ErbB2 CR1 loop and the ErbB2 CR1 loop are negatively charged, so it is unlikely that ErbB2 will form a back-to-back dimer. Actually, it is difficult to form EGFR-ECD:ErbB2-ECD heterodimers in solution. Given that ErbB2 forms complexes with the other EGFR family members on the cell surface (*15*, *49*), it is likely that a considerable fraction of the binding energy between these family members must be associated with strong interactions between the transmembrane and/or intracellular domains of the receptors.

4. ErbB3 AND ErbB4

The 3D-structures of the ErbB3-ECD (*12*) and ErbB4-ECD (*19*) have also been determined. Although both receptor preparations are capable of binding ligands, these structures were solved in the absence of ligand and, not surprisingly, both were in the tethered conformation. The CR1 loops of EGFR-ECD and ErbB4-ECD have remarkably similar conformations (see Fig. 1.2). Although the EGFR structure was determined in the presence of ligand (i.e., untethered), the back-to-back dimer and the HER4 structure was determined in the tethered conformation. Both the backbone and sidechains of all of the residues at the nine residues at the tip of the CR1 loop are virtually superimposed (see Fig. 1.2).

In the tethered conformation, the CR1 loops of both ErbB3 and ErbB4 contact the same pocket near the C-terminus of the CR2 domain. The molecular contacts between the CR1 loop and the CR2 pocket are highly conserved between the EGFR, ErbB3, and ErbB4: specifically, a hydrogen-bonded network between the side-chain of a tyr at the end of the CR1 loop and an asp and lys in the LR2 pocket are conserved in all known vertebrate orthologs of EGFR, ErbB3, and ErbB4.

While ErbB3 binds neuregulins, ErbB4 binds both EGFR ligands and the neuregulins (*51*). The 3D-structure of the ErbB4 ligand-binding domain is considerably more basic than EGFR (*19*), but neither ErbB3 nor ErbB4 have a pH sensitive histidine in the ligand-binding

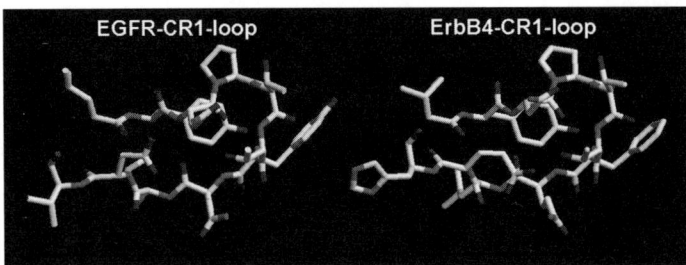

Fig. 1.2. The structural homology between the CR1 loop of the human EGFR (*11*) and ErbB4 (*19*) is remarkable. The amino acid sequences are similar, but not identical. Despite different quaternary contexts, both the backbone atoms and the sidechains adopt almost identical conformations. The EGFR-CR1 loop is involved in the crystal structure dimer interface in the ligand, untethered bound EGFR (*11*), whereas the ErbB4-CR1 loop is taken from the crystal structure of the tethered, monomeric form of ErbB4 (*19*) (*See Color Plate*).

surface of the L2 domain. The structural data suggests that ErbB3 and ErbB4 are less likely to release ligand at low pH, i.e., the ligand-bound structures are likely to be more stable in the endosomal compartment, thus altering the ability of these receptors to recycle.

5. ANTIBODY BINDING TO THE EGFR FAMILY MEMBERS

The EGFR family members are appropriate targets for cancer therapy. While small molecule kinase inhibitors are already being tested for their potential as cancer therapeutics (*38, 52–55*), it has not been possible to identify small molecules that will bind to and inhibit receptor activation by ligands. In part, the difficulties have been associated with significant conformational change between the unbound and ligand-associated states, but the complexity of the ligand-binding sites and the high affinity of the ligands make it difficult to design small molecules that can compete effectively. Antibodies directed toward the EGFR family members, however, have been developed (*48, 54*), and several of these antibodies have significant potential for development as anticancer therapeutics. Indeed, one of the most successful additions to the treatment of breast cancer is herceptin and antibody directed toward the CR2 domain of ErbB2 (*48*).

The Fab fragment of the herceptin/antibody (also known clinically as trastuzumab) binds to a site on the CR2 domain that includes the region of the pocket identified in EGFR, ErbB3, and ErbB4, which interacts with the CR1 loop (*15*). Binding close to the membrane appears to influence the biology of herceptin action. The complete herceptin antibody has an antiproliferative action, but the basis of this action is still being debated. The antibody appears to mediate cellular cytotoxicity (ADCC) as well as blocking receptor aggregation, stimulating cleavage of ErbB2 at the ECD-juxtamembrane and stimulating receptor endocytosis. The herceptin Fab fragments do not inhibit tumor growth, but it is not clear whether reduced affinity or a failure of its biological actions (e.g., stimulation of receptor endocytosis) is responsible for the loss of activity. The position of herceptin binding would be expected to modify the conformation of ErbB2-associated heteromers with the EGFR, ErbB3, and ErbB4. Another ErbB2 antibody, 2C4 (or pertuzumab), is being tested for its potential anticancer activity. The 3D-structure of the ErbB2-ECD and pertuzumab-Fab has been determined (*21*). The structure of the ErbB2-ECD is essentially identical to the structure in the absence of the 2C4-Fab; the antibody contacts the C-terminal end of the CR1 domain, including the CR1 loop. Binding of 2C4 to ErbB2 precludes binding of the CR1 loop to other EGFR

Color Plate

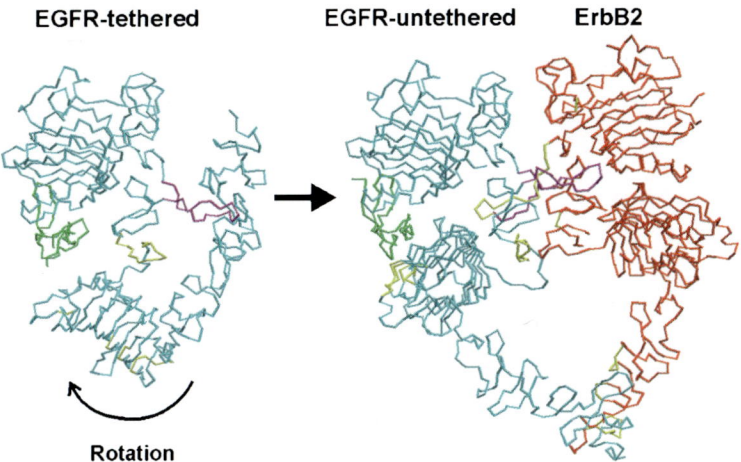

Fig. 1.1. The extracellular domains (ECDs) of the human EGFR and ErbB2. The left-hand model is the tethered form of the EGFR-ECD (*14*) with the CR1 loop highlighted in magenta and the C225 (cetuximab) epitope (lower part of the diagram) and the 806 epitope (*43*), (*56*) (below CR1 loop) are displayed in yellow. The EGF is colored green. On the right, the human, untethered EGFR-ECD conformer (blue) modeled from the conformation of the back-to-back ligand dimer (*11*), is docked in the back-to-back configuration with the human ErbB2-ECD (*15*) (red). The TGF-α is colored green and the CR1 loop is colored magenta. The antibody epitopes are colored yellow. For the EGFR-ECD, the C225 epitope is on the left, and the 806 epitope is on the right facing ErbB2. For ErbB2, the 2C4 epitope is close to the CR1 loop (magenta), and the herceptin epitope is at the C-terminus (at the bottom of the diagram).

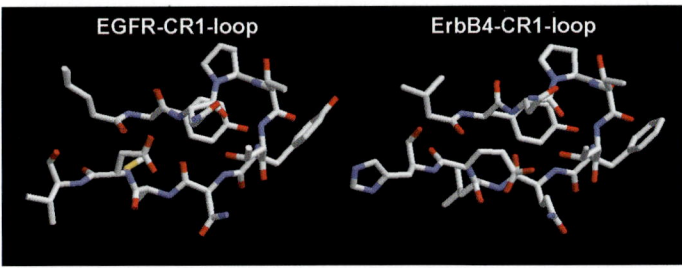

Fig. 1.2. The structural homology between the CR1 loop of the human EGFR (*11*) and ErbB4 (*19*) is remarkable. The amino acid sequences are similar, but not identical. Despite different quaternary contexts, both the backbone atoms and the sidechains adopt almost identical conformations. The EGFR-CR1 loop is involved in the crystal structure dimer interface in the ligand, untethered bound EGFR (*11*), whereas the ErbB4-CR1 loop is taken from the crystal structure of the tethered, monomeric form of ErbB4 (*19*).

family members and the binding also masks the pocket on ErbB2, which would be expected to dock the CR1 loop from other EGFR family members. From these studies it is now clear why both the full-length antibody and the Fab fragment of 2C4 interfere with back-to-back binding by ErbB2 to other EGFR family members.

EGFR antibodies have also been reported to have potential as anticancer therapeutics (*38*). The 3D-structure of an Fab fragment from the anti-EGFR antibody C225 complexed to the EGFR-ECD has been solved (*20*). As expected from epitope-mapping studies, this fragment binds to the L2 domain in a position that would prevent ligand binding. The antibody fragment is bound to the tethered configuration in this structure and Fab fragment it would prevent the formation of the ligand-binding site described in the back-to-back EGFR-ECD dimer that forms in the presence of ligand. While it is clear that the antibody can bind the tethered form of the EGFR, further experiments are required to explore the activity of C225 on EGFR-heterodimers on the cell surface. EGFR-ErbB2 heterodimers form higher affinity complexes, where the EGFR would be expected to be untethered. It is not clear whether the untethering would lead to a juxtaposition of the L1 and L2 domains, which would facilitate ligand binding and prevent antibody binding. Increased levels of ErbB2 (e.g., in a significant proportion of breast cancers) might lead to "priming" of the EGFR and a reduction in the effectiveness of C225. Similarly, tumors associated with elevated levels of ligand for EGFR may either compete for C225 binding or protect the receptor from C225 by inducing the untethered, back-to-back conformation.

Another anti-EGFR antibody, mab806, has a completely different mode of action (*42*). The epitope for this antibody is buried at the C-terminus of the CR1 domain (residues 287-302) (*43, 56*). Mab806 binds to the denatured EGFR, the D2-7-truncated-EGR found in many brain tumors, and EGFR-ECD1-501, but mab806 does not bind well to the tethered or untethered, back-to-back form of the EGFR. When the EGFR is expressed on cells at levels below 100,000 receptors per cell, mab806 binding is less than 5% of the binding by antibodies such as mab528, which bind to the native conformation of the L2 domain. On the other hand, when the receptor is overexpressed (e.g., head and neck tumors and brain tumors), mab806 binding increases. Furthermore, mutant forms of the EGFR, which are unable to form the back-to-back EGFR dimer, can be trapped by mab806 as the receptor is in transition to the (*32*) back-to-back conformation. This antibody has already been used in the clinic to detect overexpressed or truncated EGFR associated with tumors, and in animal studies mab806 synergizes effectively with other anti-EGFR antagonists/inhibitors and anticancer agents to prevent tumor growth (*44–46, 57*).

More than any other information over the last decade, the 3D-structures of the EGFR family ECDs has improved our understanding of the mechanisms involved in the activation of the EGFR. The 3D-structures have not only provided exciting explanations for the multiple-affinity states, the formation of heteromers between family members and the roles of the different family members in the absence of ligand binding (e.g., ErbB2), they have also provided the basis for biophysical determination of the conformation and aggregation state of the EGFR on both normal and cancer cells, in the presence and absence of different ligands, in the presence and absence of the different antibody probes, at different ratios of the various family members, and under different conditions of cell adhesion or metabolism. The distribution of tethered and untethered states on the cell surface is still a matter of conjecture, and the conformation of the untethered state in the presence and absence of ligand or heteromer association still needs to be determined. The availability of the 3D-structures of the ECDs for all four EGFR family members, the rich array of mutants based on these structures, the range of ligands, and the fluorescent derivatives of both the receptors and their ligands makes for an exciting time for scientists in the EGFR field.

REFERENCES

1. Cohen S. Isolation of a mouse submaxillary gland protein accelerating incisor eruption and eyelid opening in the newborn animal. J Biol Chem 1960;237:1555-1562.
2. Todaro GJ, Delarco JE, Cohen S. Transformation by Murine and Feline Sarcoma-Viruses Specifically Blocks Binding of Epidermal Growth-Factor to Cells. Nature 1976;264:26-31.
3. Holbrook MR, Slakey LL, Gross DJ. Thermodynamic mixing of molecular states of the epidermal growth factor receptor modulates macroscopic ligand binding affinity. Biochemical Journal 2000;352:99-108.
4. Schechter AL, Hung MC, Vaidyanathan L, Weinberg RA, Yang-Feng TL, Francke U et al. The neu gene: an erbB-homologous gene distinct from and unlinked to the gene encoding the EGF receptor. Science 1985;229:976-978.
5. Kraus MH, Issing W, Miki T, Popescu NC, Aaronson SA. Isolation and characterization of ERBB3, a third member of the ERBB/epidermal growth factor receptor family: evidence for overexpression in a subset of human mammary tumors. Proc Natl Acad Sci U S A 1989;86:9193-9197.
6. Plowman GD, Culouscou JM, Whitney GS, Green JM, Carlton GW, Foy L et al. Ligand-specific activation of HER4/p180erbB4, a fourth member of the epidermal growth factor receptor family. Proc Natl Acad Sci U S A 1993;90:1746-1750.
7. de Larco JE, Todaro GJ. Epithelioid and fibroblastic rat kidney cell clones: epidermal growth factor (EGF) receptors and the effect of mouse sarcoma virus transformation. J Cell Physiol 1978;94:335-342.
8. Yarden Y, Schlessinger J. Epidermal growth factor induces rapid, reversible aggregation of the purified epidermal growth factor receptor. Biochemistry 1987;26:1443-1451.
9. Schlessinger J. Ligand-induced, receptor-mediated dimerization and activation of EGF receptor. Cell 2002;%20;110:669-672.
10. Stamos J, Sliwkowski MX, Eigenbrot C. Structure of the epidermal growth factor receptor kinase domain alone and in complex with a 4-anilinoquinazoline inhibitor. J Biol Chem 2002;277:46265-46272.
11. Garrett TP, McKern NM, Lou M, Elleman TC, Adams TE, Lovrecz GO et al. Crystal structure of a truncated epidermal growth factor receptor extracellular domain bound to transforming growth factor alpha. Cell 2002;%20;110:763-773.
12. Cho HS, Leahy DJ. Structure of the extracellular region of HER3 reveals an interdomain tether. Science 2002;297:1330-1333.
13. Ogiso H, Ishitani R, Nureki O, Fukai S, Yamanaka M, Kim JH et al. Crystal structure of the complex of human epidermal growth factor and receptor extracellular domains. Cell 2002;%20;110:775-787.
14. Ferguson KM, Berger MB, Mendrola JM, Cho HS, Leahy DJ, Lemmon MA. EGF Activates Its Receptor by Removing Interactions that Autoinhibit Ectodomain Dimerization. Mol Cell 2003;11:507-517.
15. Cho HS, Mason K, Ramyar KX, Stanley AM, Gabelli SB, Denney DW, Jr. et al. Structure of the extracellular region of HER2 alone and in complex with the Herceptin Fab. Nature 2003;421:756-760.
16. Garrett TP, McKern NM, Lou M, Elleman TC, Adams TE, Lovrecz GO et al. The Crystal Structure of a Truncated ErbB2 Ectodomain Reveals an Active Conformation, Poised to Interact with Other ErbB Receptors. Mol Cell 2003;11:495-505.
17. De Crescenzo G, Grothe S, Lortie R, Debanne MT, O'Connor-McCourt M. Real-time kinetic studies on the interaction of transforming growth factor alpha with the epidermal growth factor receptor extracellular domain reveal a conformational change model. Biochemistry 2000;39:9466-9476.
18. Greenfield C, Hiles I, Waterfield MD, Federwisch M, Wollmer A, Blundell TL et al. Epidermal Growth-Factor Binding Induces A Conformational Change in the External Domain of Its Receptor. Embo Journal 1989;8:4115-4123.
19. Bouyain S, Longo PA, Li S, Ferguson KM, Leahy DJ. The extracellular region of ErbB4 adopts a tethered conformation in the absence of ligand. Proc Natl Acad Sci U S A 2005;102:15024-15029.
20. Li S, Schmitz KR, Jeffrey PD, Wiltzius JJ, Kussie P, Ferguson KM. Structural basis for inhibition of the epidermal growth factor receptor by cetuximab. Cancer Cell 2005;7:301-311.
21. Franklin MC, Carey KD, Vajdos FF, Leahy DJ, de Vos AM, Sliwkowski MX. Insights into ErbB signaling from the structure of the ErbB2-pertuzumab complex. Cancer Cell 2004;5:317-328.

22. Clayton AH, Walker F, Orchard SG, Henderson C, Fuchs D, Rothacker J et al. Ligand-induced dimer-tetramer transition during the activation of the cell surface epidermal growth factor receptor-A multi-dimensional microscopy analysis. J Biol Chem 2005;280:30392-30399.
23. Gadella TWJ, Jovin TM. Oligomerization of Epidermal Growth-Factor Receptors on A431 Cells Studied by Time-Resolved Fluorescence Imaging Microscopy - A Stereochemical Model for Tyrosine Kinase Receptor Activation. Journal of Cell Biology 1995;129:1543-1558.
24. Martin-Fernandez M, Clarke DT, Tobin MJ, Jones SV, Jones GR. Preformed oligomeric epidermal growth factor receptors undergo an ectodomain structure change during signaling. Biophysical Journal 2002;82:2415-2427.
25. Moriki T, Maruyama H, Maruyama IN. Activation of preformed EGF receptor dimers by ligand-induced rotation of the transmembrane domain. Journal of Molecular Biology 2001;311:1011-1026.
26. Yu XC, Sharma KD, Takahashi T, Iwamoto R, Mekada E. Ligand-independent dimer formation of epidermal growth factor receptor (EGFR) is a step separable from ligand-induced EGFR signaling. Molecular Biology of the Cell 2002;13:2547-2557.
27. Garrett TP, McKern NM, Lou M, Frenkel MJ, Bentley JD, Lovrecz GO et al. Crystal structure of the first three domains of the type-1 insulin-like growth factor receptor. Nature 1998;394:395-399.
28. McKern NM, Lawrence MC, Streltsov VA, Lou MZ, Adams TE, Lovrecz GO et al. Structure of the insulin receptor ectodomain reveals a folded-over conformation. Nature 2006;443: 218-221.
29. Ullrich A, Coussens L, Hayflick JS, Dull TJ, Gray A, Tam AW et al. Human epidermal growth factor receptor cDNA sequence and aberrant expression of the amplified gene in A431 epidermoid carcinoma cells. Nature 1984;309:418-425.
30. Jorissen RN, Walker FW, Pouliot N, Garrett TPJ, Ward CW, Burgess AW. Epidermal growth factor receptor: mechanisms of activation and signalling. Exp Cell Res 2003;284:31-53.
31. Burgess AW, Cho HS, Eigenbrot C, Ferguson KM, Garrett TP, Leahy DJ et al. An open-and-shut case? Recent insights into the activation of EGF/ErbB receptors. Mol Cell 2003;12:541-552.
32. Walker F, Orchard SG, Jorissen RN, Hall NE, Zhang HH, Hoyne PA et al. CR1/CR2 interactions modulate the functions of the cell surface epidermal growth factor receptor. J Biol Chem 2004;279:22387-22398.
33. Elleman TC, Domagala T, McKern NM, Nerrie M, Lonnqvist B, Adams TE et al. Identification of a determinant of epidermal growth factor receptor ligand-binding specificity using a truncated, high-affinity form of the ectodomain. Biochemistry 2001;40:8930-8939.
34. Domagala T, Konstantopoulos N, Smyth F, Jorissen RN, Fabri L, Geleick D et al. Stoichiometry, kinetic and binding analysis of the interaction between epidermal growth factor (EGF) and the extracellular domain of the EGF receptor. Growth Factors 2000;18:11-29.
35. Walker F, Hibbs ML, Zhang HH, Gonez LJ, Burgess AW. Biochemical characterization of mutant EGF receptors expressed in the hemopoietic cell line BaF/3. Growth Factors 1998;16:53-67.
36. Aboud-Pirak E, Hurwitz E, Pirak ME, Bellot F, Schlessinger J, Sela M. Efficacy of antibodies to epidermal growth factor receptor against KB carcinoma in vitro and in nude mice. J Natl Cancer Inst 1988;80:1605-1611.
37. Aboud-Pirak E, Hurwitz E, Bellot F, Schlessinger J, Sela M. Inhibition of human tumor growth in nude mice by a conjugate of doxorubicin with monoclonal antibodies to epidermal growth factor receptor. Proc Natl Acad Sci U S A 1989;86:3778-3781.
38. Arteaga CL. Overview of epidermal growth factor receptor biology and its role as a therapeutic target in human neoplasia. Semin Oncol 2002;29:3-9.
39. Ekstrand AJ, James CD, Cavenee WK, Seliger B, Pettersson RF, Collins VP. Genes for epidermal growth factor receptor, transforming growth factor alpha, and epidermal growth factor and their expression in human gliomas in vivo. Cancer Res 1991;51:2164-2172.
40. Humphrey PA, Wong AJ, Vogelstein B, Zalutsky MR, Fuller GN, Archer GE et al. Anti-synthetic peptide antibody reacting at the fusion junction of deletion-mutant epidermal growth factor receptors in human glioblastoma. Proc Natl Acad Sci U S A 1990;87:4207-4211.
41. Nishikawa R, Ji XD, Harmon RC, Lazar CS, Gill GN, Cavenee WK et al. A mutant epidermal growth factor receptor common in human glioma confers enhanced tumorigenicity. Proc Natl Acad Sci U S A 1994;91:7727-7731.

42. Jungbluth AA, Stockert E, Huang HJ, Collins VP, Coplan K, Iversen K et al. A monoclonal antibody recognizing human cancers with amplification/overexpression of the human epidermal growth factor receptor. Proc Natl Acad Sci U S A 2003;100:639-644.
43. Johns TG, Adams TE, Cochran JR, Hall NE, Hoyne PA, Olsen MJ et al. Identification of the epitope for the epidermal growth factor receptor-specific monoclonal antibody 806 reveals that it preferentially recognizes an untethered form of the receptor. J Biol Chem 2004;279:30375-30384.
44. Johns TG, Luwor RB, Murone C, Walker F, Weinstock J, Vitali AA et al. Antitumor efficacy of cytotoxic drugs and the monoclonal antibody 806 is enhanced by the EGF receptor inhibitor AG1478. Proc Natl Acad Sci U S A 2003;100:15871-15876.
45. Perera RM, Narita Y, Furnari FB, Gan HK, Murone C, Ahlkvist M et al. Treatment of human tumor xenografts with monoclonal antibody 806 in combination with a prototypical epidermal growth factor receptor-specific antibody generates enhanced antitumor activity. Clin Cancer Res 2005;11:6390-6399.
46. Gan HK, Walker F, Burgess AW, Rigopoulos A, Scott AM, Johns TG. The EGFR tyrosine kinase inhibitor AG1478 increases the formation of inactive untethered EGFR dimers: Implications for combination therapy with mab 806. J Biol Chem 2006.
47. Schechter AL, Stern DF, Vaidyanathan L, Decker SJ, Drebin JA, Greene MI et al. The neu oncogene: an erb-B-related gene encoding a 185,000-Mr tumour antigen. Nature 1984;312:513-516.
48. Slamon DJ, Leyland-Jones B, Shak S, Fuchs H, Paton V, Bajamonde A et al. Use of chemotherapy plus a monoclonal antibody against HER2 for metastatic breast cancer that overexpresses HER2. N Engl J Med 2001;344:783-792.
49. Holbro T, Hynes NE. ErbB receptors: directing key signaling networks throughout life. Annu Rev Pharmacol Toxicol 2004;44:195-217.:195-217.
50. Yen L, Benlimame N, Nie ZR, Xiao D, Wang T, Al Moustafa AE et al. Differential regulation of tumor angiogenesis by distinct ErbB homo- and heterodimers. Mol Biol Cell 2002;13:4029-4044.
51. Stein RA, Hustedt EJ, Staros JV, Beth AH. Rotational dynamics of the epidermal growth factor receptor. Biochemistry 2002;41:1957-1964.
52. Arteaga CL, Baselga J. Tyrosine kinase inhibitors: why does the current process of clinical development not apply to them? Cancer Cell 2004;5:525-531.
53. Baselga J. Targeting tyrosine kinases in cancer: the second wave. Science 2006;312:1175-1178.
54. Baselga J, Perez EA, Pienkowski T, Bell R. Adjuvant trastuzumab: a milestone in the treatment of HER-2-positive early breast cancer. Oncologist 2006;11 Suppl 1:4-12.:4-12.
55. Scaltriti M, Baselga J. The epidermal growth factor receptor pathway: a model for targeted therapy. Clin Cancer Res 2006;12:5268-5272.
56. Chao G, Cochran JR, Wittrup KD. Fine epitope mapping of anti-epidermal growth factor receptor antibodies through random mutagenesis and yeast surface display. J Mol Biol 2004;342:539-550.
57. Luwor RB, Johns TG, Murone C, Huang HJ, Cavenee WK, Ritter G et al. Monoclonal antibody 806 inhibits the growth of tumor xenografts expressing either the de2-7 or amplified epidermal growth factor receptor (EGFR) but not wild-type EGFR. Cancer Res 2001;61:5355-5361.Section I

2 EGFR Family Heterodimers in Cancer Pathogenesis and Treatment

Howard M. Stern

CONTENTS

> INTRODUCTION
> ERBB FAMILY DIMERIZATION AND ACTIVATION
> STRUCTURAL INSIGHTS ON ERBB FAMILY DIMERIZATION
> DIVERSITY OF ERBB DIMERS AND DOWNSTREAM EFFECTS
> ERBB HETERODIMERS IN DEVELOPMENT
> ERBB1/ERBB2 HETERODIMERS IN CANCER
> ERBB2/ERBB3 HETERODIMERS IN CANCER
> ATYPICAL HETERODIMERS—p95^{HER2}
> INHIBITION OF HETERODIMERS IN CANCER THERAPY
> CONCLUSIONS
> ACKNOWLEDGMENTS
> REFERENCES

Abstract

The ErbB family of receptor tyrosine kinases mediates oncogenic signaling in a variety of different cancer types. For example, ErbB1 (or EGFR) is thought to play an important role in the genesis of lung and colon cancer, and ErbB2 (or HER2) serves as a potent oncogene in a subset of breast cancer. Because of their role in cancer, ErbB1 and ErbB2 have long been a focus for drug development activities. Active signaling by the ErbB family of receptors requires formation of dimers including both homodimers and heterodimers. Mounting evidence in model systems suggests that ErbB heterodimers may be particularly oncogenic. Furthermore, recent structural analyses reveal how the receptors interact with ligands and with one another. These and other timely advances in ErbB heterodimer biology will be reviewed in detail in this chapter. Expanding knowledge of ErbB family signaling not only brings insight to the mechanism of action of existing therapies, but it also suggests that targeting specific heterodimers may have particular utility in treating cancer.

Key Words: EGFR, ErbB1, HER2, ErbB2, dimers, cancer, signaling.

1. INTRODUCTION

The human epidermal growth factor receptor (HER or ErbB) family plays a central role in driving neoplastic growth and has been a major focal point in cancer drug discovery (1–3). The formation of dimers among the ErbB family has long been known to be a critical event in receptor activation, but only recently has the mechanism of dimerization and activation been

From: *Cancer Drug Discovery and Development: EGFR Signaling Networks in Cancer Therapy*
Edited by: J. D. Haley and W. J. Gullick, DOI: 10.1007/978-1-59745-356-1_2
© 2008 Humana Press, a part of Springer Science+Business Media, LLC

elucidated (*4, 5*). The prototypical member of the family is known as HER1, EGFR, or ErbB1. A series of studies in the late 1970s and early 1980s revealed an association of ErbB1 with neoplastic transformation (*6–8*). These seminal findings culminated decades later in several targeted therapies for cancer patients, including the small-molecule inhibitors gefitinib and erlotinib and the monoclonal antibodies cetuximab and panitumumab. Subsequent to the discovery of ErbB1, closely related receptor tyrosine kinases were identified, including ErbB2, ErbB3, and ErbB4. The ErbB2 gene is amplified in approximately 20% of breast cancers and is another example of an ErbB family member that is known to drive tumorigenesis and is a target of the therapeutic monoclonal antibody trastuzumab and small-molecule tyrosine kinase inhibitor lapatinib (*2, 9–11*). The focus of this chapter is to review current knowledge of ErbB family dimerization and activation with an emphasis on the role of heterodimers in the pathogenesis of cancer and the impact of heterodimers on cancer treatment.

2. ErbB FAMILY DIMERIZATION AND ACTIVATION

As members of the receptor tyrosine kinase family, the ErbB family receptors are composed of an extracellular domain which in most cases binds growth-factor ligands, a single transmembrane domain, and an intracellular domain that is involved in activation of downstream signaling upon receptor dimerization. Although there is significant sequence-based and structural conservation among the ErbB family receptors, there are also significant functional differences. Both ErbB1 and ErbB4 are more typical members of the RTK family in that they both have the capability to bind ligand, and they both have intact intracellular kinase domains (*2, 3, 12*). ErbB2 is unusual because it lacks the capacity to bind ligand yet retains a functional kinase domain that can be activated via dimerization with other receptors (*13*). ErbB3 is unusual in a different way. It is known to bind ligand but lacks a functional intracellular kinase domain (*14*). Thus, ErbB3 is dependent on heterodimerization with kinase-intact family members to mediate signaling.

Several ligands are capable of inducing ErbB family dimerization and activation. These ligands fall into three major classes. One class specifically interacts with ErbB1 and includes EGF, TGF-α, and amphiregulin (*2, 15*). A second class consists of betacellulin, HB-EGF, and epiregulin, which interact with both ErbB1 and ErbB4 (*2, 15*). A third class, the heregulin or neuregulin (HRG or NRG) family, binds to ErbB3 and ErbB4, with NRG-1 and NRG-2 binding to both ErbB3 and ErbB4 and NRG-3 and NRG-4 binding to only ErbB4 (*16–20*). It was originally hypothesized that ligand-dependent ErbB receptor dimerization occurs via bivalent binding of a single ligand to cross-link two receptors (*21–23*). In that model, one high-affinity binding site on the ligand would interact with ErbB1 or ErbB3, and a second low-affinity binding site would interact more broadly with other HER family receptors, including ErbB2 (*22*). This proposed mechanism was analogous to the mechanism of activation for growth hormone receptors (*24, 25*). Subsequent studies examining the stoichiometry of EGF binding to ErbB1, however, indicated that receptor dimers contain not one, but two, ligands (*26–28*). This finding suggested that the process of ligand-induced ErbB receptor dimerization is more complicated than what was observed with growth hormone receptors. Data from X-ray crystal structures add further insight to this issue and will be described in more detail in the following section.

None of the three classes of ligand bind to ErbB2, but interestingly all ligands are capable of inducing phosphorylation of the ErbB2 intracellular domain (*29–32*), suggesting that ErbB2 participates in heterodimerization and trans-phosphorylation with other ligand-activated ErbB family receptors. In fact, evidence suggests that ErbB2 is the preferred dimerization partner for the other ErbB receptors. For example, in the T47D cell line that expresses all four ErbB receptors, neuregulin preferentially induces ErbB2/3 and ErbB2/4 heterodimers while EGF preferentially induces ErbB1/2 heterodimers (*33*). In the same model, neuregulin can induce ErbB1/3 and ErbB1/4 heterodimerization but only if ErbB2 is depleted via an endoplasmic reticulum targeted single-chain antibody (33, 34). For a long time, it was unclear how ErbB2 is able to act as the preferred dimerization partner in the absence of any ligand binding, but data from X-ray crystal structures of ErbB family members have helped to elucidate the mechanism.

3. STRUCTURAL INSIGHTS ON ErbB FAMILY DIMERIZATION

Recent data from a number of structural studies of ErbB family members provide significant insight into the mechanism by which receptor dimerization occurs and how this event is mediated by ligand binding. The extracellular portion of all four ErbB family members is organized into four domains – two large, leucine-rich repeat domains (also known as domains I and III) and two cysteine-rich domains (also known as domains II and IV) (35, 36). In the absence of ligand, ErbB1, ErbB3, and ErbB4 exist in a closed configuration in which there is a close interaction between domains II and IV (4, 37, 38) (Fig. 2.1). This interaction hides the dimerization arm

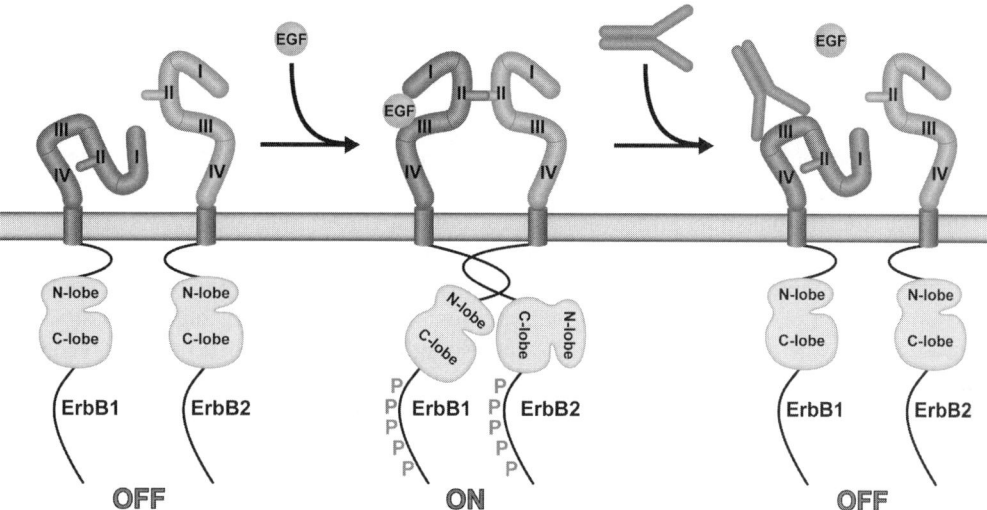

Fig. 2.1. The ErbB family of receptors consists of an extracellular portion that is divided into four domains – two leucine-rich repeat domains (I and III) and two cysteine-rich domains (II and IV). There is a single transmembrane domain, and an intracellular kinase domain consisting of an N-lobe and a C-lobe. An intracellular tail contains phosphorylation sites that enable recruitment and activation of downstream signaling molecules. ErbB1/ErbB2 heterodimers are depicted without ligand, with EGF, and with the ErbB1 monoclonal antibody cetuximab. ErbB2 is always locked in the open configuration even without ligand; whereas ErbB1 remains in the closed conformation with the domain II dimerization arm buried via an interaction with domain IV (4). Upon EGF binding a bridge is created between domains I and III, locking ErbB1 in the open configuration, allowing the domain II dimerization arm to interact with the analogous arm on ErbB2 (4). Upon receptor dimerization, there is an allosteric interaction that occurs between the N-lobe of one receptor and the C-lobe of the other receptor, resulting in kinase activation, much like the interaction that is observed with the CDK2/cyclin A cell cycle regulatory complex (44). Both ErbB1 and ErbB2 are capable of contributing either the N-lobe or the C-lobe to the interaction. The kinase domains phosphorylate the intracellular tails which then activate downstream signaling. In the presence of cetuximab, which binds to the ligand binding site in domain III of ErbB1, EGF is no longer able to interact with domain III. ErbB1 is thus locked in the closed conformation and both heterodimerization and downstream signaling are blocked, even in the presence of ligand.

located within domain II, thus preventing dimerization. The amino acid residues that mediate the domain II, IV interaction are conserved across ErbB1, ErbB3, and ErbB4, but interestingly are divergent in ErbB2 (*38*, *39*). Crystal structures in the setting of ligand-bound ErbB1 reveal a dramatic conformational change in which ligand interacts with both domains I and III within the same receptor, locking the receptor in an open configuration in which the domain II-IV interaction has been disrupted and the domain II dimerization arm is revealed (*4*, *39–41*) (Fig. 2.1). Of note, the crystal structure for ErbB2 is in the open configuration, providing a structural explanation for why ErbB2 does not require a ligand (*42*, *43*). Furthermore, being in the open configuration, ErbB2 would always be ready to dimerize, consistent with the observation that it is the preferred dimerization partner.

Once the ligand-induced receptors engage in heterodimerization or homodimerization, a trans-phosphorylation event occurs in the intracellular domain, leading to downstream pathway activation. Although initially assumed to be a symmetric cross-phosphorylation event, recent evidence, at least with EGFR, suggests that there is an asymmetric allosteric interaction similar to that seen with CDK2/cyclin A (*44*) (Fig. 2.1). In support of the allosteric model, amino acid residues that mediate the asymmetric intracellular domain interaction are conserved across the ErbB family. Interestingly, the one exception is ErbB3, where only one interaction face is conserved, which is perhaps consistent with the lack of an active kinase domain.

4. DIVERSITY OF ErbB DIMERS AND DOWNSTREAM EFFECTS

With four ErbB receptors, there are ten potential combinations of receptor pairs – four homodimers and six heterodimers. Although the numerous possibilities may seem redundant, there are a number of factors that differentiate the downstream effects of the receptor dimers. First, each of the receptors has a distinct affinity for specific downstream signaling effectors. Thus, various dimer combinations will result in differential activation of signaling pathways, which may in turn become integrated into distinct phenotypic consequences. Second, the predominant dimers in a particular cell at a given moment will depend upon the composition of ligands in the extracellular milieu. Finally, the level of expression of specific ErbB receptors in a cell can affect the predominant dimers that form.

The intracellular domains of ErbB1, ErbB2, and ErbB3 are well characterized in terms of the number of phospho-epitopes and the types of signaling modulators each phospho-epitope recruits (*15*). The ErbB1-intracellular domain can activate several downstream pathways, including PI3K, MAPK, PKC, and JNK. Although there are no binding sites for the p85 regulatory subunit of PI3K, ErbB1 can activate the PI3K pathway via GRB2, which recruits GAB1 and couples to the PI3K pathway (*2*). ErbB2 activates the MAPK pathway via GRB2, SHC, DOK-R, and CRK, and ErbB3 is a potent activator of the PI3K pathway with six binding sites for the p85 regulatory subunit of PI3K. With the diversity of homodimers and heterodimers, there is an open question regarding the mechanism by which the various pathway inputs are integrated to result in a specific cellular phenotype. Regardless of the mechanism, it is quite clear that there are dramatic differences in the phenotypic effect of receptor activation depending on the combination of dimers involved. This concept is well-illustrated by a study in which cells were transfected with various combinations of ErbB receptors and proliferation index was measured. The dimers most potent at stimulating proliferation are ErbB1/2, 2/3, and 1/3, the latter in the setting of heregulin stimulation (*1*, *45*).

Differential level of ErbB receptor expression is another feature that may impact the downstream sequelae of receptor activation. One dramatic example is the consequence of altered ErbB2 expression in breast cancer. Although ErbB2 is always in the open configuration with dimerization arms exposed, ErbB2 is not considered to be oncogenic unless activated by overexpression via gene amplification. The effect of ErbB receptor levels on cell signaling was recently illustrated in a study in which protein microarrays containing most SH2 and PTB domain proteins in the genome were used to survey the affinity of interaction with phophopeptides representing the phosphorylation sites in the intracellular domain of ErbB1, ErbB2, and ErbB3 (46). At any affinity threshold, ErbB3 consistently favored the PI3K pathway. For ErbB1 and ErbB2, however, the receptors engage an increasingly broad network of signaling components at increasing affinity thresholds. This observation may explain why overexpression of ErbB1 or ErbB2 can lead to active oncogenic signaling in some circumstances.

In a recent study, the importance of ErbB family heterodimerization was illustrated using a proximity-based assay to determine the level of interaction between specific ErbB dimer pairs. Chimeric receptors were engineered in which the intracellular domain consists of an inactive fragment of the β-gal enzyme. Enzymatic activity is restored when two inactive fragments are brought in proximity via receptor dimerization. With this technology, it was determined that association of ErbB2 with itself is relatively inefficient, whereas formation of ErbB1/2 and ErbB2/3 heterodimers is very efficient in the presence of ligand (47).

Despite the appearance of redundancy, there is considerable evidence suggesting a discrete biology attributable to specific dimer pairs, most frequently heterodimers. The following sections focus on the role of heterodimers in both development and cancer and will further highlight the distinct roles of specific ErbB heterodimers.

5. ErbB HETERODIMERS IN DEVELOPMENT

As with many genes involved in cancer pathogenesis, the ErbB family plays an important role in embryonic development. Some of the developmental biology discussed in this section serves as a nice illustration of discrete ErbB heterodimers being associated with specific phenotypes. In addition, some of the developmental phenotypes may be relevant to understanding specific adverse events observed with cancer therapies targeting ErbB family members.

Much of the information on ErbB receptors in embryonic development has come from studies in genetically engineered mice. Some homozygous ErbB1 knockout mice live until birth, but then all mice die shortly thereafter. Such mice exhibit a broad range of defects including abnormalities in the brain, lung, gastrointestinal tract, and skin (48–51). It is difficult from this information to glean the extent to which these phenotypes are due to loss of ErbB1 homodimers versus heterodimers. The phenotypes observed from knockouts of other ErbB family receptors do not overlap with that of the ErbB1 knockout, suggesting that the ErbB1 knockout phenotypes are attributable to ErbB1 homodimers. The ErbB2, ErbB3, and ErbB4 knockouts all are embryonic lethal, however, so one can't rule out the possibility that these receptors cooperate with ErbB1 in the perinatal phenotypes observed with ErbB1 knockout. One common adverse event observed with ErbB1 inhibition in humans is a skin rash. In that context, it is notable that the ErbB1 knockout mouse exhibits a skin phenotype.

Interestingly, the phenotype of ErbB2, ErbB4, and neuregulin knockout mice exhibits significant overlap. All such mice are embryonic lethal at E10.5 and exhibit a lack of trebeculation in the cardiac ventricle (52–55). Neuregulin is known to be expressed in the endocardium and ErbB2/ErbB4 is expressed in the myocardium. These observations have led to a model in which cardiac ventricular trebeculation is driven by paracrine activation of ErbB2/ErbB4 heterodimers in the myocardium via neuregulin produced in the endocardium (15). A role for ErbB2 in cardiac function of adult mice was revealed by an elegant experiment in which the cre-*loxP* system was utilized to produce a conditional knockout of ErbB2 in the cardiac ventricles. Although such mice were viable, they exhibited a physiological phenotype consistent with dilated cardiomyopathy (56). The observation of a cardiac phenotype in ErbB2 knockout mice is particularly notable given that administration of the ErbB2 inhibitor trastuzumab to HER2-positive breast cancer patients is associated with a risk of cardiac dysfunction (57–59).

In addition to the cardiac phenotype, there is also evidence for ErbB2/ErbB4 involvement in the mammary epithelium where expression of dominant negative ErbB2 or ErbB4 each results in a defect in lactation (60, 61). Similar observation of coincident developmental phenotypes suggests a role for ErbB2/ErbB3 heterodimers in peripheral nervous system development. Knockout of either of these genes leads to defects in Schwann cell development, hypoplasia of the sympathetic chain ganglia and cranial sensory ganglia (62–64). These peripheral nervous system phenotypes can all be attributed to cells of neural crest origin, and possibly a defect in neural crest migration (15).

6. ErbB1/ErbB2 HETERODIMERS IN CANCER

Numerous studies have been performed to examine the role of ErbB1 and ErbB2 in neoplastic progression. At least three mechanisms of activation have been proposed for ErbB1. First, several different types of ErbB1 mutations have been observed in non-small cell lung cancer patients. These mutations include exon 19 deletion and exon 21 L858R, both of which have been shown to activate in vitro signaling in the absence of ligand and are transforming (65–68). An extracellular domain deletion mutant called EGFRvIII has been observed most frequently in glioblastoma (69), and is also associated with constitutive activation. The significance of these and other mutations in EGFR are discussed in Chapters 19 and 20. In general, whether or not these mutations have any effect on the efficiency of homodimerization or heterodimerization has not been clearly established.

Another proposed mechanism of activation is increased ErbB1 mRNA and/or protein expression as observed in breast, ovarian, glioblastoma, non-small cell lung, colon, bladder, prostate, kidney, and head and neck tumors (3, 70). In many cases, however, it is not clear whether overexpression necessarily equates with activation. A third potential mechanism of activation is overexpression of ErbB1 ligands such as TGF-α. In vitro, the presence of ligand has clearly been shown to activate dimerization and downstream receptor signaling.

In the case of ErbB2, the main mechanism of activation is overexpression. Increased ErbB2 expression is well described in breast cancer and is a direct result of gene amplification. Although less common, ErbB2 overexpression with or without gene amplification has also been observed in lung, stomach, ovarian, colon, bladder and salivary gland carcinomas (3, 70). The detailed mechanism by which increased ErbB2 expression results in pathway activation is not entirely clear but is presumed to be due to a shift in equilibrium toward ErbB2 homodimerization or ligand-independent heterodimerization. Much less commonly observed are ErbB2 mutations (mostly insertion mutations), which have been described in non-small cell lung cancer and are predicted to activate the receptor (71).

Given the overlap of tumor types, there is the possibility that ErbB1 and ErbB2 could cooperate in tumorigenesis. In support of that concept, ErbB1 alone is not a very potent oncogene in some model systems. For example, ErbB1 expression in mouse mammary epithelial cells only rarely induces adenocarcinoma compared to ErbB2 expression (72, 73). Furthermore, in the MCF10A mammary epithelial cell line, introduction of chimeric ErbB1 receptors that can undergo homodimerization with a synthetic ligand do not show any evidence of transformation (74). In contrast, ErbB2 was potent at transformation in similar studies. Comparable observations have been made in fibroblast cell lines transfected with either ErbB1 or ErbB2 (75).

Despite the weak transforming activity of ErbB1 alone, there is considerable evidence suggesting potent cooperativity with ErbB2. First, experiments performed in the 1980s demonstrated that addition of the ErbB1 ligand EGF to various cell lines of rodent or human origin results in tyrosine phosphorylation of ErbB2, as well as an increase in the ErbB2 tyrosine kinase activity (*76–79*). Transforming activity was also examined in rodent fibroblast cell lines, such as NR6, in which it was found that neither ErbB1 nor ErbB2 alone had transforming capacity, but when co-transfected, the cells adopted a transformed phenotype (*80*). Mouse models also support the concept of cooperativity between ErbB1 and ErbB2. Mice in which both ErbB2 and TGF-α are overexpressed in mammary epithelial cells results in multiple mammary tumors with short latency compared to mice expressing either transgene alone (*81*).

There are several mechanisms that have been proposed to explain the cooperative interaction between ErbB1 and ErbB2. One key aspect of ErbB signaling regulation is the mode by which the signal is turned off. Ligand binding induces clustering of ErbB1 homodimers at clathrin-coated pits. Endocytic vesicles form, resulting in loss of ErbB1 from the plasma membrane and eventually degradation of the receptors, but the remaining ErbB family members do not follow the same fate (*3, 82*). Endocytosis of ErbB2, ErbB3, and ErbB4 occurs at a slower rate, and receptors are recycled to the cell surface rather than being degraded in endosomes. It has been observed that ErbB1 binding to ErbB2 reduces ErbB1 endocytosis and redirects ErbB1 to be recycled back to the cell membrane rather than being degraded in endosomes (*83, 84*).

A second mechanism of cooperative interaction is heterodimer-specific phosphorylation. NIH3T3 cells transfected with single ErbB receptors or combinations of ErbB receptors were treated with radiolabeled phosphate and stimulated with EGF. Phosphopeptide mapping was performed on immunoprecipitated ErbB receptors, and it was found that the spectrum of phosphopeptides in the context of ErbB1/ErbB2 co-expression was distinct from the spectrum observed in the setting of ErbB1 or ErbB2 expression alone (*85*). A third potential mechanism is increased affinity of ligand binding. In-depth studies of ligand-receptor interactions have demonstrated that ligands have higher affinity for ErbB2 containing heterodimers than for ErbB family homodimers, likely due to a slower off-rate (*86, 87*).

While the above observations and proposed mechanisms for cooperative interactions between ErbB1 and ErbB2 are interesting, a remaining question is whether ErbB1/ErbB2 heterodimers exhibit any evidence of unique downstream signaling properties compared to either receptor alone. This question was addressed in an MCF10A mammary epithelial cell line system. MCF-10A cells were transfected with chimeras of the intracellular domain of ErbB receptors fused to either wild-type or mutant FK506 binding protein (FKBP) derivatives. Using rapamycin-like small molecules that bind to FKBP, dimerization events can be initiated in the absence of ligand (*88*). In these experiments, it was found that both ErbB2 homodimers and ErbB1/ErbB2 heterodimers exhibit equal activation of the MAPK pathway, but that heterodimers are more effective at activating PI3K and phospholipase Cγ1 pathways. In three-dimensional cell culture, ErbB1/ErbB2 heterodimers were found to be more effective at inducing cell invasion into Matrigel than were ErbB2 homodimers (*88*).

Although ErbB1 and ErbB2 each independently play some role in neoplastic progression, the formation of ErbB1/ErbB2 heterodimers seems to be particularly oncogenic in some settings. Thus, therapies that target the ErbB1/ErbB2 heterodimer may have benefit in cancer therapy. In that regard, the small molecule lapatinib is a tyrosine kinase inhibitor that exhibits dual specificity for ErbB1 and ErbB2. Lapatinib was recently FDA-approved for use in HER2-positive metastatic breast cancer patients that have progressed on a trastuzumab-based regimen (*89*).

7. ErbB2/ErbB3 HETERODIMERS IN CANCER

Of all the ErbB receptor family dimer combinations, ErbB2/ErbB3 heterodimers are considered to be the most transforming. 32D cells, which are IL3 dependent and do not express endogenous ErbB receptors, were infected with recombinant retroviruses expressing ErbB receptors either singly or in pairs. Examination of all the permutations revealed that the most potent mitogenic signals eminate from the ErbB2/ErbB3 combination (*45*). Similarly, in NIH3T3 cells, it was found that co-expression of ErbB2 and ErbB3 exhibited an enhanced tumorigenic phenotype compared to expression of ErbB2 alone (*90*). The mitogenic effect of ErbB2/ErbB3 heterodimers may be due to very efficient activation of the PI3K pathway (*12, 91*). More specifically, the effects on cell proliferation have been linked to deregulation of the G1/S transition. This transition is regulated by the CDK2/cyclin E complex, which can be inhibited by the cyclin dependent kinase inhbitor p27^{Kip1}. PI3K pathway activation via ErbB2/ErbB3 heterodimers results in inhibition of p27^{Kip1} activity, resulting in derepression of the G1/S transition (*15, 92, 93*).

Some studies have explored the role of ErbB2/ErbB3 heterodimers in cell line models via downregulation of ErbB3. Expression of an artificial transcription factor E3 consisting of a polydactyl zinc finger domain that is designed to recognize an 18bp region of the ErbB3 5' untranslated region was used to decrease expression of ErbB3 in ErbB2 amplified cell lines (*94*). Cells with decreased expression of ErbB3 exhibited diminished cell proliferation. In another study, ErbB3 was examined via a short hairpin RNAi approach. Knockdown of ErbB3 in MDA-MB-435 cells was associated with a decrease in the incidence of metastasis when such cells were grown in vivo compared to separately selected control cell lines (*95*). Although often described as a breast cancer cell line, there have been some data suggesting that MDA-MB-435 may actually be a melanoma cell line (*96, 97*). Regardless of the cancer type, the data suggest that ErbB3 could play a role in driving tumorigenesis either by maintaining proliferation, promoting metastasis or perhaps both.

Involvement of ErbB3 in heterodimers is not only important for tumorigenesis, but it may also provide some insight into development of resistance to ErbB1 and ErbB2 targeted therapies. When ErbB2 amplified cell lines were treated with ErbB family tyrosine kinase inhibitors (TKIs), it was observed that phosphorylation of ErbB1 and ErbB2 was consistently reduced over the time period examined (up to 96 hours) (*98*). Phosphorylation of ErbB3, however, exhibited an initial decrease followed by a recovery to higher levels of phosphorylation between 12 and 24 hours of treatment. The recovery of ErbB3 phosphorylation was paralleled by a recovery in phosphorylation of AKT. These observations were accompanied by a shift in localization of ErbB3 from the cytoplasm to the membrane as determined by biochemical analysis of fractionated cells (*98*), raising the possibility that sub-cellular localization of ErbB3 participates in a regulatory feedback loop. Examination of ErbB3 status in human tumors will be needed to determine if these observations have relevance for development of resistance to TKIs in patients. Due to the difficulty in obtaining the on-therapy biopsies of tumor tissue needed to assay biomarkers in relation to therapeutic response and resistance, such questions are not trivial.

Many studies of ErbB3 have focused on breast cancer, but there is increasing evidence that ErbB3 may also play an important role in other cancer types. It is well documented that EGF can activate the androgen receptor in prostate cancer cell lines under conditions of androgen withdrawal (*99, 100*). This finding has led to a hypothesis that ErbB signaling could be associated with evolution of prostate cancer from androgen-dependent to androgen-independent growth. In a recent study of ErbB receptors in prostate cancer cells, a small molecule ErbB1/ErbB2 inhibitor, PKI-166, was used to study ErbB pathway signaling on androgen receptor activation. It was found that ErbB2/ErbB3 heterodimers were the main driver of androgen receptor activation even when ErbB1 was present (*101*). These findings suggest that the ErbB2/ErbB3 heterodimer could play a role in growth of androgen independent prostate cancer. Further examination of the status of ErbB3 in tissues from prostate cancer patients would be helpful in determining whether this apparent correlation translates to human tumors.

Less is known about the status of ErbB2/ErbB3 heterodimers in human cancer tissues. There have been some studies examining ErbB3 expression by immunohistochemistry and correlating to clinical outcome in cancer patients. These studies have suggested that ErbB3 expression is correlated with poor clinical outcome in breast cancer and ovarian cancer (*102, 103*). There is also some suggestion that high ErbB3 expression correlates with poor outcome in HER2-positive breast cancer after progression on the HER2 targeted antibody trastuzumab (*104*). Unfortunately, in some of these studies, it is not clear whether the immunohistochemical assay was validated to detect ErbB3 specifically in formalin-fixed, paraffin-embedded (FFPE) tissues.

8. ATYPICAL HETERODIMERS—p95^{HER2}

It is becoming increasingly evident that ErbB receptors are, at least in some cases, subject to cleavage of the extracellular domain. In the case of ErbB2, it is well-documented that a truncated form of the receptor known as p95^{HER2} is produced in breast cancer cell lines (*105–107*). In about 30% of HER2-positive breast cancer patients, p95HER2 is detected in tumor tissue by Western blot and is associated with poor clinical outcome (*108*). The truncated form of the receptor is structurally similar to the originally-described viral oncogene v-ErbB, and consistent with that observation, the receptor is constitutively active (*109, 110*). The therapeutic ErbB2 monoclonal antibody trastuzumab has been demonstrated to prevent the conversion of full length p185^{HER2} to truncated p95^{HER2} (*109*), suggesting that this may be one mechanism of trastuzumab activity.

The existence of a truncated form of ErbB2 raises the question of whether heterodimers with the truncated form of the receptor exist and whether they have any relevant biological role. One example of a heterodimer would be p185^{HER2} with p95^{HER2}, and in support of this model, there is evidence of an intracellular interacting domain that could mediate ligand-independent interaction of either full-length or truncated ErbB2 receptors (*111*). It is possible that this ErbB2 intracellular domain interaction could be mediated by the allosteric association of the kinase domain N and C-lobes. In addition, there is also the possibility that p95^{HER2} could associate with other ErbB family receptors. This concept is supported by a study in which p95^{HER2} heterodimers were examined in the HER2 amplified BT474 breast cancer cell line. In that setting, p95^{HER2} was found to heterodimerize specifically with ErbB3 but not with ErbB1 (*112*). Examination of p95^{HER2} containing heterodimers in a broader sampling of breast cancer cell lines and in human breast cancer tissues is warranted to determine the prevalence of such heterodimers. It would also be of interest to determine how the mitogenic potential of p95^{HER2}/ErbB3 heterodimers compare to that of full-length ErbB2/ErbB3 heterodimers, and if there are significant differences in the phosphopeptide profile of the activated p95^{HER2} containing heterodimers.

9. INHIBITION OF HETERODIMERS IN CANCER THERAPY

Given the substantial evidence for involvement of ErbB family members in oncogenesis, it is not surprising that this receptor family has been an area of significant activity with regard to drug development. Several approaches to inhibiting ErbB signaling have been exploited for therapeutic benefit. One approach is direct inhibition of tyrosine kinase activity by small molecule inhibitors of ErbB1 (e.g., erlotinib, gefitinib), as well as dual-specificity ErbB1/2 tyrosine kinase inhibitors such as lapatinib. Such inhibitors have exhibited efficacy in some patient populations such as erlotinib in non-small cell lung cancer (*113*) and lapatinib in HER2-positive metastatic breast cancer patients who have progressed on trastuzumab (*89*). Although these agents do not inhibit the ErbB dimerization process, they can effectively inhibit dimer-mediated signaling.

A second mechanism for inhibiting signaling from ErbB dimers includes blocking ligand-mediated activation via monoclonal antibody therapeutics (e.g., cetuximab, panitumumab). Although not direct, the inhibition of ligand binding to EGFR will leave the receptor extracellular domain in the closed configuration, thus inhibiting formation of ErbB1 homodimers and heterodimers. Cetuximab is known to bind to ErbB1 with high affinity and blocks ligand-mediated activation of the receptor *(114)*. A crystal structure reveals that cetuximab binds to the ligand-binding region within domain III of ErbB1, resulting in steric hindrance that prevents the receptor from adopting the open configuration and thus inhibiting heterodimerization *(115)* (Fig. 2.1). In cell lines, cetuximab has been shown to induce G1 arrest, potentiate apoptosis, as well as inhibit cancer cell invasion and metastasis *(114)*. Cetuximab has been found to have efficacy and is approved for use in metastatic colon cancer and head and heck cancer *(114)*.

Aside from cetuximab, other anti-ErbB1 monoclonal antibodies are in development. Preclinical data with panitumumab, a fully humanized monoclonal antibody directed against ErbB1, reveals efficacy in xenograft models with moderate to high levels of ErbB1 expression. Xenograft cell lines exhibiting efficacy are from a range of indications including colorectal, breast, prostate, renal, ovarian and pancreatic cancer *(116, 117)*. In general, efficacy was observed in xenograft lines in which cells express 17,000 receptors per cell or more, but was not observed in lines where there are fewer than 11,000 receptors per cell *(117)*. A phase III trial of best supportive care with or without panitumumab in metastatic colorectal cancer patients that had previously progressed on chemotherapy was presented at the 2006 Annual Meeting of the American Association for Cancer Research *(118)*. Panitumumab improved progression-free survival, and in September 2006, it was approved for this indication.

Direct inhibition of dimer formation is another strategy to inhibit ErbB family signaling. Pertuzumab is a monoclonal antibody that binds to the dimerization arm of ErbB2 and sterically interferes with formation of ErbB heterodimers *(119)* (Fig 2.2). In cell lines with

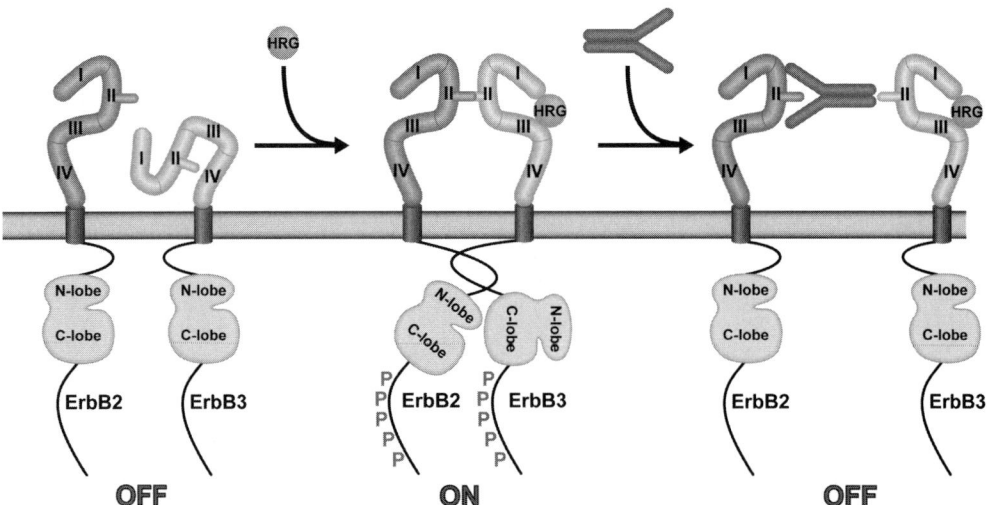

Fig. 2.2. ErbB2 / ErbB3 heterodimers are depicted without ligand, with heregulin (HRG), and with the monoclonal antibody pertuzumab. Induction of receptor signaling occurs by much the same mechanism as with ErbB1/2 heterodimers. HRG binding to domains I and III locks ErbB3 in the open configuration, thus allowing dimerization with ErbB2. One major difference is that ErbB3 lacks an active kinase, thus the phosphorylation of the intracellular tails must be mediated by the ErbB2 kinase. Perhaps consistent with this unique role for ErbB3, the N-lobe of ErbB3 is defective in its ability to interact with the C-lobe of other receptors *(44)*. Thus, ErbB3 can only present the C-lobe during allosteric activation, leaving ErbB2 to present the N-lobe. Pertuzumab binds to the dimerization arm in domain II of ErbB2. As such, it sterically hinders ErbB2 from participating in dimerization. This antibody-receptor interaction inhibits signaling even in the presence of ligand.

high HER2 expression (e.g., SKBR3) and those with low HER2 expression (e.g., MCF7), pertuzumab is capable of inhibiting formation of ErbB2/ErbB3 heterodimers upon heregulin treatment and also inhibits receptor tyrosine phosphorylation. These observations translate into inhibition of ligand-dependent growth in vitro and preclinical efficacy of pertuzumab in xenograft models of both HER2-positive and HER2-negative breast cancer (*119*). Pertuzumab was also capable of inhibiting ligand-dependent growth in both androgen-dependent and androgen-independent prostate cancer cell lines in vitro and in xenograft models (*120*). These data suggest that inhibition of ErbB family dimerization by targeting ErbB2, the preferred ErbB dimerization partner, may be clinically relevant in a wide range of tumor types, including tumors without HER2 amplification.

Pertuzumab was recently tested in a phase II monotherapy trial in heavily pretreated ovarian cancer. Of 117 patients over two dose cohorts that were evaluable for efficacy, there were five partial responses (4.3%), and eight patients exhibited stable disease (*121*). Five patients exhibited an asymptomatic decrease in left ventricular ejection fraction. In a fraction of patients where pretreatment biopsies were possible, phospho-HER2 (pHER2) was measured by ELISA. Interestingly, the median progression free survival in pHER2+ patients was 20.9 weeks compared to 5.8 weeks for pHER2- patients (*121*). These data suggest that pertuzumab is tolerable and that some heavily pre-treated ovarian cancer patients might benefit. An ongoing randomized phase II trial is evaluating pertuzumab in combination with chemotherapy in platinum refractory ovarian cancer. A qRT-PCR-based surrogate marker for pHER2 that can be assessed in archival FFPE tissues is being evaluated as a predictive diagnostic marker as part of this trial (*122*).

10. CONCLUSIONS

Over the past two decades, tremendous progress has been made in our understanding of the ErbB signaling pathway. This knowledge has led to the development of several clinically beneficial therapies, including both small molecule and monoclonal antibody inhibitors of ErbB1 and ErbB2. Evidence suggests that various ErbB family homodimers and heterodimers may have discrete biological function. In many cases, heterodimers exhibit stronger mitogenic signaling than do homodimers. ErbB1/ErbB2 and ErbB2/ErbB3 heterodimers in particular are the most oncogenic. Therapeutic strategies that prevent or disrupt heterodimer formation have the potential for clinical benefit. Cetuximab and panitumumab block ligand binding to ErbB1 and thus secondarily inhibit heterodimerization. Both have already shown significant efficacy in colorectal cancer. Pertuzumab is the first example of a distinct category of inhibitors that directly suppress ErbB dimerization via steric inhibition and is currently being evaluated in clinical trials. Undoubtedly, further insights into the biology of ErbB family signaling will help us understand in more detail how heterodimers impact cancer development and will allow more refined approaches to developing therapeutics that maximize clinical benefit for patients.

ACKNOWLEDGMENTS

I would like to thank Mark Sliwkowski for critical review of the manuscript and Jim Ligos for assistance with construction of figures.

REFERENCES

1. Arteaga CL. The epidermal growth factor receptor: from mutant oncogene in nonhuman cancers to therapeutic target in human neoplasia. J Clin Oncol 2001;19:32S-40S.
2. Hynes NE, Lane HA. ERBB receptors and cancer: the complexity of targeted inhibitors. Nat Rev Cancer 2005;5:341-54.

3. Yarden Y, Sliwkowski MX. Untangling the ErbB signalling network. Nat Rev Mol Cell Biol 2001;2:127-37.
4. Burgess AW, Cho HS, Eigenbrot C, et al. An open-and-shut case? Recent insights into the activation of EGF/ErbB receptors. Mol Cell 2003;12:541-52.
5. Schlessinger J. Ligand-induced, receptor-mediated dimerization and activation of EGF receptor. Cell 2002;110:669-72.
6. de Larco JE, Todaro GJ. Epithelioid and fibroblastic rat kidney cell clones: epidermal growth factor (EGF) receptors and the effect of mouse sarcoma virus transformation. J Cell Physiol 1978;94:335-42.
7. Downward J, Yarden Y, Mayes E, et al. Close similarity of epidermal growth factor receptor and v-erb-B oncogene protein sequences. Nature 1984;307:521-7.
8. Ushiro H, Cohen S. Identification of phosphotyrosine as a product of epidermal growth factor-activated protein kinase in A-431 cell membranes. J Biol Chem 1980;255:8363-5.
9. Braga S, dal Lago L, Bernard C, Cardoso F, Piccart M. Use of trastuzumab for the treatment of early stage breast cancer. Expert Rev Anticancer Ther 2006;6:1153-64.
10. Emens LA, Davidson NE. Trastuzumab in breast cancer. Oncology (Williston Park) 2004;18:1117-28; discussion 31-2, 37-8.
11. Moy B, Goss PE. Lapatinib: current status and future directions in breast cancer. Oncologist 2006;11:1047-57.
12. Citri A, Yarden Y. EGF-ERBB signalling: towards the systems level. Nat Rev Mol Cell Biol 2006;7:505-16.
13. Klapper LN, Glathe S, Vaisman N, et al. The ErbB-2/HER2 oncoprotein of human carcinomas may function solely as a shared coreceptor for multiple stroma-derived growth factors. Proc Natl Acad Sci U S A 1999;96:4995-5000.
14. Guy PM, Platko JV, Cantley LC, Cerione RA, Carraway KL, 3rd. Insect cell-expressed p180erbB3 possesses an impaired tyrosine kinase activity. Proc Natl Acad Sci U S A 1994;91:8132-6.
15. Olayioye MA, Neve RM, Lane HA, Hynes NE. The ErbB signaling network: receptor heterodimerization in development and cancer. Embo J 2000;19:3159-67.
16. Carraway KL, 3rd, Weber JL, Unger MJ, et al. Neuregulin-2, a new ligand of ErbB3/ErbB4-receptor tyrosine kinases. Nature 1997;387:512-6.
17. Chang H, Riese DJ, 2nd, Gilbert W, Stern DF, McMahan UJ. Ligands for ErbB-family receptors encoded by a neuregulin-like gene. Nature 1997;387:509-12.
18. Harari D, Tzahar E, Romano J, et al. Neuregulin-4: a novel growth factor that acts through the ErbB-4 receptor tyrosine kinase. Oncogene 1999;18:2681-9.
19. Riese DJ, 2nd, van Raaij TM, Plowman GD, Andrews GC, Stern DF. The cellular response to neuregulins is governed by complex interactions of the erbB receptor family. Mol Cell Biol 1995;15:5770-6.
20. Zhang D, Sliwkowski MX, Mark M, et al. Neuregulin-3 (NRG3): a novel neural tissue-enriched protein that binds and activates ErbB4. Proc Natl Acad Sci U S A 1997;94:9562-7.
21. Gullick WJ. A new model for the interaction of EGF-like ligands with their receptors: the new one-two. Eur J Cancer 1994;30A:2186.
22. Alroy I, Yarden Y. The ErbB signaling network in embryogenesis and oncogenesis: signal diversification through combinatorial ligand-receptor interactions. FEBS Lett 1997;410:83-6.
23. Pinkas-Kramarski R, Lenferink AE, Bacus SS, et al. The oncogenic ErbB-2/ErbB-3 heterodimer is a surrogate receptor of the epidermal growth factor and betacellulin. Oncogene 1998;16:1249-58.
24. Wells JA, Cunningham BC, Fuh G, et al. The molecular basis for growth hormone-receptor interactions. Recent Prog Horm Res 1993;48:253-75.
25. Wells JA, de Vos AM. Structure and function of human growth hormone: implications for the hematopoietins. Annu Rev Biophys Biomol Struct 1993;22:329-51.
26. Domagala T, Konstantopoulos N, Smyth F, et al. Stoichiometry, kinetic and binding analysis of the interaction between epidermal growth factor (EGF) and the extracellular domain of the EGF receptor. Growth Factors 2000;18:11-29.
27. Lemmon MA, Bu Z, Ladbury JE, et al. Two EGF molecules contribute additively to stabilization of the EGFR dimer. Embo J 1997;16:281-94.

28. Odaka M, Kohda D, Lax I, Schlessinger J, Inagaki F. Ligand-binding enhances the affinity of dimerization of the extracellular domain of the epidermal growth factor receptor. J Biochem (Tokyo) 1997;122:116-21.
29. Beerli RR, Hynes NE. Epidermal growth factor-related peptides activate distinct subsets of ErbB receptors and differ in their biological activities. J Biol Chem 1996;271:6071-6.
30. King CR, Borrello I, Bellot F, Comoglio P, Schlessinger J. Egf binding to its receptor triggers a rapid tyrosine phosphorylation of the erbB-2 protein in the mammary tumor cell line SK-BR-3. Embo J 1988;7:1647-51.
31. Plowman GD, Green JM, Culouscou JM, Carlton GW, Rothwell VM, Buckley S. Heregulin induces tyrosine phosphorylation of HER4/p180erbB4. Nature 1993;366:473-5.
32. Sliwkowski MX, Schaefer G, Akita RW, et al. Coexpression of erbB2 and erbB3 proteins reconstitutes a high affinity receptor for heregulin. J Biol Chem 1994;269:14661-5.
33. Graus-Porta D, Beerli RR, Daly JM, Hynes NE. ErbB-2, the preferred heterodimerization partner of all ErbB receptors, is a mediator of lateral signaling. Embo J 1997;16:1647-55.
34. Graus-Porta D, Beerli RR, Hynes NE. Single-chain antibody-mediated intracellular retention of ErbB-2 impairs Neu differentiation factor and epidermal growth factor signaling. Mol Cell Biol 1995;15:1182-91.
35. Lax I, Johnson A, Howk R, et al. Chicken epidermal growth factor (EGF) receptor: cDNA cloning, expression in mouse cells, and differential binding of EGF and transforming growth factor alpha. Mol Cell Biol 1988;8:1970-8.
36. Ward CW, Hoyne PA, Flegg RH. Insulin and epidermal growth factor receptors contain the cysteine repeat motif found in the tumor necrosis factor receptor. Proteins 1995;22:141-53.
37. Bouyain S, Longo PA, Li S, Ferguson KM, Leahy DJ. The extracellular region of ErbB4 adopts a tethered conformation in the absence of ligand. Proc Natl Acad Sci U S A 2005;102:15024-9.
38. Cho HS, Leahy DJ. Structure of the extracellular region of HER3 reveals an interdomain tether. Science 2002;297:1330-3.
39. Ferguson KM, Berger MB, Mendrola JM, Cho HS, Leahy DJ, Lemmon MA. EGF activates its receptor by removing interactions that autoinhibit ectodomain dimerization. Mol Cell 2003;11:507-17.
40. Garrett TP, McKern NM, Lou M, et al. Crystal structure of a truncated epidermal growth factor receptor extracellular domain bound to transforming growth factor alpha. Cell 2002;110:763-73.
41. Ogiso H, Ishitani R, Nureki O, et al. Crystal structure of the complex of human epidermal growth factor and receptor extracellular domains. Cell 2002;110:775-87.
42. Cho HS, Mason K, Ramyar KX, et al. Structure of the extracellular region of HER2 alone and in complex with the Herceptin Fab. Nature 2003;421:756-60.
43. Garrett TP, McKern NM, Lou M, et al. The crystal structure of a truncated ErbB2 ectodomain reveals an active conformation, poised to interact with other ErbB receptors. Mol Cell 2003;11:495-505.
44. Zhang X, Gureasko J, Shen K, Cole PA, Kuriyan J. An allosteric mechanism for activation of the kinase domain of epidermal growth factor receptor. Cell 2006;125:1137-49.
45. Pinkas-Kramarski R, Soussan L, Waterman H, et al. Diversification of Neu differentiation factor and epidermal growth factor signaling by combinatorial receptor interactions. Embo J 1996;15:2452-67.
46. Jones RB, Gordus A, Krall JA, MacBeath G. A quantitative protein interaction network for the ErbB receptors using protein microarrays. Nature 2006;439:168-74.
47. Wehrman TS, Raab WJ, Casipit CL, Doyonnas R, Pomerantz JH, Blau HM. A system for quantifying dynamic protein interactions defines a role for Herceptin in modulating ErbB2 interactions. Proc Natl Acad Sci U S A 2006;103:19063-8.
48. Miettinen PJ, Berger JE, Meneses J, et al. Epithelial immaturity and multiorgan failure in mice lacking epidermal growth factor receptor. Nature 1995;376:337-41.
49. Sibilia M, Steinbach JP, Stingl L, Aguzzi A, Wagner EF. A strain-independent postnatal neurodegeneration in mice lacking the EGF receptor. Embo J 1998;17:719-31.
50. Sibilia M, Wagner EF. Strain-dependent epithelial defects in mice lacking the EGF receptor. Science 1995;269:234-8.
51. Threadgill DW, Dlugosz AA, Hansen LA, et al. Targeted disruption of mouse EGF receptor: effect of genetic background on mutant phenotype. Science 1995;269:230-4.

52. Gassmann M, Casagranda F, Orioli D, et al. Aberrant neural and cardiac development in mice lacking the ErbB4 neuregulin receptor. Nature 1995;378:390-4.
53. Lee KF, Simon H, Chen H, Bates B, Hung MC, Hauser C. Requirement for neuregulin receptor erbB2 in neural and cardiac development. Nature 1995;378:394-8.
54. Meyer D, Birchmeier C. Multiple essential functions of neuregulin in development. Nature 1995;378:386-90.
55. Kramer R, Bucay N, Kane DJ, Martin LE, Tarpley JE, Theill LE. Neuregulins with an Ig-like domain are essential for mouse myocardial and neuronal development. Proc Natl Acad Sci U S A 1996;93:4833-8.
56. Crone SA, Zhao YY, Fan L, et al. ErbB2 is essential in the prevention of dilated cardiomyopathy. Nat Med 2002;8:459-65.
57. Chien KR. Herceptin and heart failure – a molecular modifier of cardiac failure. N Engl J Med 2006;354:789-90.
58. Piccart-Gebhart MJ, Procter M, Leyland-Jones B, et al. Trastuzumab after adjuvant chemotherapy in HER2-positive breast cancer. N Engl J Med 2005;353:1659-72.
59. Romond EH, Perez EA, Bryant J, et al. Trastuzumab plus adjuvant chemotherapy for operable HER2-positive breast cancer. N Engl J Med 2005;353:1673-84.
60. Jones FE, Stern DF. Expression of dominant-negative ErbB2 in the mammary gland of transgenic mice reveals a role in lobuloalveolar development and lactation. Oncogene 1999;18:3481-90.
61. Jones FE, Welte T, Fu XY, Stern DF. ErbB4 signaling in the mammary gland is required for lobuloalveolar development and Stat5 activation during lactation. J Cell Biol 1999;147:77-88.
62. Erickson SL, O'Shea KS, Ghaboosi N, et al. ErbB3 is required for normal cerebellar and cardiac development: a comparison with ErbB2-and heregulin-deficient mice. Development 1997;124:4999-5011.
63. Morris JK, Lin W, Hauser C, Marchuk Y, Getman D, Lee KF. Rescue of the cardiac defect in ErbB2 mutant mice reveals essential roles of ErbB2 in peripheral nervous system development. Neuron 1999;23:273-83.
64. Riethmacher D, Sonnenberg-Riethmacher E, Brinkmann V, Yamaai T, Lewin GR, Birchmeier C. Severe neuropathies in mice with targeted mutations in the ErbB3 receptor. Nature 1997;389:725-30.
65. Carey KD, Garton AJ, Romero MS, et al. Kinetic analysis of epidermal growth factor receptor somatic mutant proteins shows increased sensitivity to the epidermal growth factor receptor tyrosine kinase inhibitor, erlotinib. Cancer Res 2006;66:8163-71.
66. Greulich H, Chen TH, Feng W, et al. Oncogenic transformation by inhibitor-sensitive and -resistant EGFR mutants. PLoS Med 2005;2:e313.
67. Lynch TJ, Bell DW, Sordella R, et al. Activating mutations in the epidermal growth factor receptor underlying responsiveness of non-small-cell lung cancer to gefitinib. N Engl J Med 2004;350:2129-39.
68. Paez JG, Janne PA, Lee JC, et al. EGFR mutations in lung cancer: correlation with clinical response to gefitinib therapy. Science 2004;304:1497-500.
69. Moscatello DK, Holgado-Madruga M, Godwin AK, et al. Frequent expression of a mutant epidermal growth factor receptor in multiple human tumors. Cancer Res 1995;55:5536-9.
70. Holbro T, Hynes NE. ErbB receptors: directing key signaling networks throughout life. Annu Rev Pharmacol Toxicol 2004;44:195-217.
71. Stephens P, Hunter C, Bignell G, et al. Lung cancer: intragenic ERBB2 kinase mutations in tumours. Nature 2004;431:525-6.
72. Brandt R, Eisenbrandt R, Leenders F, et al. Mammary gland specific hEGF receptor transgene expression induces neoplasia and inhibits differentiation. Oncogene 2000;19:2129-37.
73. Guy CT, Webster MA, Schaller M, Parsons TJ, Cardiff RD, Muller WJ. Expression of the neu protooncogene in the mammary epithelium of transgenic mice induces metastatic disease. Proc Natl Acad Sci U S A 1992;89:10578-82.
74. Muthuswamy SK, Li D, Lelievre S, Bissell MJ, Brugge JS. ErbB2, but not ErbB1, reinitiates proliferation and induces luminal repopulation in epithelial acini. Nat Cell Biol 2001;3:785-92.
75. Di Fiore PP, Segatto O, Taylor WG, Aaronson SA, Pierce JH. EGF receptor and erbB-2 tyrosine kinase domains confer cell specificity for mitogenic signaling. Science 1990;248:79-83.

76. Akiyama T, Saito T, Ogawara H, Toyoshima K, Yamamoto T. Tumor promoter and epidermal growth factor stimulate phosphorylation of the c-erbB-2 gene product in MKN-7 human adenocarcinoma cells. Mol Cell Biol 1988;8:1019-26.
77. Kokai Y, Dobashi K, Weiner DB, Myers JN, Nowell PC, Greene MI. Phosphorylation process induced by epidermal growth factor alters the oncogenic and cellular neu (NGL) gene products. Proc Natl Acad Sci U S A 1988;85:5389-93.
78. Stern DF, Heffernan PA, Weinberg RA. p185, a product of the neu proto-oncogene, is a receptorlike protein associated with tyrosine kinase activity. Mol Cell Biol 1986;6:1729-40.
79. Stern DF, Kamps MP. EGF-stimulated tyrosine phosphorylation of p185neu: a potential model for receptor interactions. Embo J 1988;7:995-1001.
80. Kokai Y, Myers JN, Wada T, et al. Synergistic interaction of p185c-neu and the EGF receptor leads to transformation of rodent fibroblasts. Cell 1989;58:287-92.
81. Muller WJ, Arteaga CL, Muthuswamy SK, et al. Synergistic interaction of the Neu proto-oncogene product and transforming growth factor alpha in the mammary epithelium of transgenic mice. Mol Cell Biol 1996;16:5726-36.
82. Baulida J, Kraus MH, Alimandi M, Di Fiore PP, Carpenter G. All ErbB receptors other than the epidermal growth factor receptor are endocytosis impaired. J Biol Chem 1996;271:5251-7.
83. Lenferink AE, Pinkas-Kramarski R, van de Poll ML, et al. Differential endocytic routing of homo- and hetero-dimeric ErbB tyrosine kinases confers signaling superiority to receptor heterodimers. Embo J 1998;17:3385-97.
84. Worthylake R, Wiley HS. Structural aspects of the epidermal growth factor receptor required for transmodulation of erbB-2/neu. J Biol Chem 1997;272:8594-601.
85. Olayioye MA, Graus-Porta D, Beerli RR, Rohrer J, Gay B, Hynes NE. ErbB-1 and ErbB-2 acquire distinct signaling properties dependent upon their dimerization partner. Mol Cell Biol 1998;18:5042-51.
86. Karunagaran D, Tzahar E, Beerli RR, et al. ErbB-2 is a common auxiliary subunit of NDF and EGF receptors: implications for breast cancer. Embo J 1996;15:254-64.
87. Jones JT, Akita RW, Sliwkowski MX. Binding specificities and affinities of egf domains for ErbB receptors. FEBS Lett 1999;447:227-31.
88. Zhan L, Xiang B, Muthuswamy SK. Controlled activation of ErbB1/ErbB2 heterodimers promote invasion of three-dimensional organized epithelia in an ErbB1-dependent manner: implications for progression of ErbB2-overexpressing tumors. Cancer Res 2006;66:5201-8.
89. Geyer CE, Forster J, Lindquist D, et al. Lapatinib plus capecitabine for HER2-positive advanced breast cancer. N Engl J Med 2006;355:2733-43.
90. Alimandi M, Romano A, Curia MC, et al. Cooperative signaling of ErbB3 and ErbB2 in neoplastic transformation and human mammary carcinomas. Oncogene 1995;10:1813-21.
91. Wallasch C, Weiss FU, Niederfellner G, Jallal B, Issing W, Ullrich A. Heregulin-dependent regulation of HER2/neu oncogenic signaling by heterodimerization with HER3. Embo J 1995;14:4267-75.
92. Neve RM, Sutterluty H, Pullen N, et al. Effects of oncogenic ErbB2 on G1 cell cycle regulators in breast tumour cells. Oncogene 2000;19:1647-56.
93. Sherr CJ, Roberts JM. CDK inhibitors: positive and negative regulators of G1-phase progression. Genes Dev 1999;13:1501-12.
94. Holbro T, Beerli RR, Maurer F, Koziczak M, Barbas CF, 3rd, Hynes NE. The ErbB2/ErbB3 heterodimer functions as an oncogenic unit: ErbB2 requires ErbB3 to drive breast tumor cell proliferation. Proc Natl Acad Sci U S A 2003;100:8933-8.
95. Xue C, Liang F, Mahmood R, et al. ErbB3-dependent motility and intravasation in breast cancer metastasis. Cancer Res 2006;66:1418-26.
96. Rae JM, Ramus SJ, Waltham M, et al. Common origins of MDA-MB-435 cells from various sources with those shown to have melanoma properties. Clin Exp Metastasis 2004;21:543-52.
97. Ross DT, Scherf U, Eisen MB, et al. Systematic variation in gene expression patterns in human cancer cell lines. Nat Genet 2000;24:227-35.
98. Sergina NV, Rausch M, Wang D, et al. Escape from HER-family tyrosine kinase inhibitor therapy by the kinase-inactive HER3. Nature 2007;445:437-41.

99. Culig Z, Hobisch A, Cronauer MV, et al. Androgen receptor activation in prostatic tumor cell lines by insulin-like growth factor-I, keratinocyte growth factor, and epidermal growth factor. Cancer Res 1994;54:5474-8.
100. Freeman MR. HER2/HER3 heterodimers in prostate cancer: Whither HER1/EGFR? Cancer Cell 2004;6:427-8.
101. Mellinghoff IK, Vivanco I, Kwon A, Tran C, Wongvipat J, Sawyers CL. HER2/neu kinase-dependent modulation of androgen receptor function through effects on DNA binding and stability. Cancer Cell 2004;6:517-27.
102. Tanner B, Hasenclever D, Stern K, et al. ErbB-3 predicts survival in ovarian cancer. J Clin Oncol 2006;24:4317-23.
103. Witton CJ, Reeves JR, Going JJ, Cooke TG, Bartlett JM. Expression of the HER1-4 family of receptor tyrosine kinases in breast cancer. J Pathol 2003;200:290-7.
104. Robinson AG, Turbin D, Thomson T, et al. Molecular predictive factors in patients receiving trastuzumab-based chemotherapy for metastatic disease. Clin Breast Cancer 2006;7:254-61.
105. Lin YZ, Clinton GM. A soluble protein related to the HER-2 proto-oncogene product is released from human breast carcinoma cells. Oncogene 1991;6:639-43.
106. Pupa SM, Menard S, Morelli D, Pozzi B, De Palo G, Colnaghi MI. The extracellular domain of the c-erbB-2 oncoprotein is released from tumor cells by proteolytic cleavage. Oncogene 1993;8:2917-23.
107. Zabrecky JR, Lam T, McKenzie SJ, Carney W. The extracellular domain of p185/neu is released from the surface of human breast carcinoma cells, SK-BR-3. J Biol Chem 1991;266:1716-20.
108. Saez R, Molina MA, Ramsey EE, et al. p95HER-2 predicts worse outcome in patients with HER-2-positive breast cancer. Clin Cancer Res 2006;12:424-31.
109. Molina MA, Codony-Servat J, Albanell J, Rojo F, Arribas J, Baselga J. Trastuzumab (herceptin), a humanized anti-Her2 receptor monoclonal antibody, inhibits basal and activated Her2 ectodomain cleavage in breast cancer cells. Cancer Res 2001;61:4744-9.
110. Christianson TA, Doherty JK, Lin YJ, et al. NH2-terminally truncated HER-2/neu protein: relationship with shedding of the extracellular domain and with prognostic factors in breast cancer. Cancer Res 1998;58:5123-9.
111. Penuel E, Akita RW, Sliwkowski MX. Identification of a region within the ErbB2/HER2 intracellular domain that is necessary for ligand-independent association. J Biol Chem 2002;277:28468-73.
112. Xia W, Liu LH, Ho P, Spector NL. Truncated ErbB2 receptor (p95ErbB2) is regulated by heregulin through heterodimer formation with ErbB3 yet remains sensitive to the dual EGFR/ErbB2 kinase inhibitor GW572016. Oncogene 2004;23:646-53.
113. Shepherd FA, Rodrigues Pereira J, Ciuleanu T, et al. Erlotinib in previously treated non-small-cell lung cancer. N Engl J Med 2005;353:123-32.
114. Mendelsohn J, Baselga J. Epidermal growth factor receptor targeting in cancer. Semin Oncol 2006;33:369-85.
115. Li S, Schmitz KR, Jeffrey PD, Wiltzius JJ, Kussie P, Ferguson KM. Structural basis for inhibition of the epidermal growth factor receptor by cetuximab. Cancer Cell 2005;7:301-11.
116. Cohenuram M, Saif MW. Panitumumab the first fully human monoclonal antibody: from the bench to the clinic. Anticancer Drugs 2007;18:7-15.
117. Yang XD, Jia XC, Corvalan JR, Wang P, Davis CG. Development of ABX-EGF, a fully human anti-EGF receptor monoclonal antibody, for cancer therapy. Crit Rev Oncol Hematol 2001;38:17-23.
118. Van Cutsem E, Peeters M, Siena S, et al. Open-label phase III trial of panitumumab plus best supportive care compared with best supportive care alone in patients with chemotherapy-refractory metastatic colorectal cancer. J Clin Oncol 2007;25:1658-64.
119. Franklin MC, Carey KD, Vajdos FF, Leahy DJ, de Vos AM, Sliwkowski MX. Insights into ErbB signaling from the structure of the ErbB2-pertuzumab complex. Cancer Cell 2004;5:317-28.
120. Agus DB, Akita RW, Fox WD, et al. Targeting ligand-activated ErbB2 signaling inhibits breast and prostate tumor growth. Cancer Cell 2002;2:127-37.
121. Gordon MS, Matei D, Aghajanian C, et al. Clinical activity of pertuzumab (rhuMAb 2C4), a HER dimerization inhibitor, in advanced ovarian cancer: potential predictive relationship with tumor HER2 activation status. J Clin Oncol 2006;24:4324-32.
122. Amler L, Gordon MS, Strauss A, et al. Identification of predictive markers of cliinical activity from a phase II trial of single agent pertuzumab (rhuMab 2C4), a HER dimerization inhhibitor, in advanced ovarian cancer (OC). In: ASCO Annual Meeting; 2006; Atlanta, GA 2006.

3 Structure-Function of EGFR Kinase Domain and Its Inhibitors

Charles Eigenbrot

Contents

> INTRODUCTION
> GENERAL STRUCTURE OVERVIEW
> WILD-TYPE EGFR KINASE X-RAY STRUCTURES
> IMPLICATIONS FOR ESCAPE MUTANTS
> STRUCTURES OF ERLOTNIB & GEFITINIB SUSCEPTIBILITY
>   EGFR MUTANTS
> FUTURE DIRECTIONS IN EGFR SMI RESEARCH
> SUMMARY
> ACKNOWLEDGMENTS
> REFERENCES

Abstract

The EGF receptor is a key mediator of oncogenic transformation in a wide variety of solid tumors. Since 2002, there has been an explosion of X-ray crystallographic results that provide powerful insight into the activation and hyperactivation of this receptor and of its close homologues HER2, HER3, and HER4. The ability to catalyze phospho-transfer resides in the EGFR intracellular tyrosine kinase domain, which has proven a clinically useful target for therapeutic intervention. The rapidly expanding catalogue of EGFR kinase domain structures is surveyed with a focus on inhibitor activities and liabilities, as well as on control and dysregulation phenomena intrinsic to the protein.

Key Words: X-ray crystallography, small molecule inhibitor, escape mutation, kinase activation, allostery, L858R, T790M.

1. INTRODUCTION

There has been an explosion of structural insight into the molecular mechanics of activation of EGFR and closely related receptors since 2002. After decades of scrutiny as the most-studied family of cell-surface receptors, the new results have shown unprecedented arrangements (and rearrangements) of their extracellular domains (*1*) and the first structures of the EGFR kinase domain (both active (*2*) and inactive (*3*) forms). They have also given us powerful insight into the molecular connection between extracellular and intracellular compartments (*4*). Additionally, the structural origins of hyperactivity of some clinically important mutant kinase domains have been identified (*5*).

From: *Cancer Drug Discovery and Development: EGFR Signaling Networks in Cancer Therapy*
Edited by: J. D. Haley and W. J. Gullick, DOI: 10.1007/978-1-59745-356-1_3
© 2008 Humana Press, a part of Springer Science+Business Media, LLC

The topic before us in this work goes back about a decade, when information about small molecules targeting the EGFR kinase appeared from pharmaceutical companies' programs (6–8). Following successful clinical experiences derived from these efforts, we have now seen broader discussion of therapeutic strategies that include small molecule kinase inhibitors (9–11). This chapter will concentrate first on the structures of inhibitors in complex with the EGFR kinase domain, after which it will address hyperactivity of mutant kinases and the allosteric activation of the EGFR kinase arising from extracellular events.

The utility of small molecule inhibitors (SMI) of the catalytic domain of EGFR depends on their potency, specificity, and bioavailability. Potency is easily ascertained using an *in vitro* (or "biochemical") enzyme assay. High potency allows low doses to be effective. Specificity is also studied using biochemical assays with other kinases that are of interest, but the likely biological context in which an inhibitor is used can guide how important an off-target potency is perceived to be. A relatively low toxicity made possible by high specificity is the promise inherent in "targeted" therapies. Bioavailability, in the broadest sense, is a measure of how well an administered dose is delivered to the target kinase. All these properties arise from the chemical structure of the inhibitor and the resulting interactions with its target and with other components of the biological milieu.

Due to the wealth of X-ray crystal structures produced in drug discovery programs, potency and specificity are usually considered in light of structural information on the inhibitor bound to the target, as well as on available structures or models of off-target kinases of interest. Until 2002, there was no reported direct structural information for the EGFR kinase, which meant that extensive drug discovery efforts relied on the less robust structure-activity-relationship (SAR) paradigm. In a drug discovery program, SAR is the collected information about small molecules' properties and their activities. It arises from an iterative process where new molecules are designed and synthesized to test increasingly specific hypotheses about interactions between the small molecules and the target. In the absence of X-ray structures of the target kinase, the SAR data can arise in the light of computer models based on known structures of homologous proteins. This approach was successfully applied to the development of all three currently approved EGFR SMI drugs: erlotinib, gefitinib and lapatinib.

Nonetheless, achieving a deeper understanding of the activities of these medicines and others still in development has been aided significantly by X-ray structures of the EGFR kinase domain. In 2002, Stamos et al. reported the X-ray structure (2) of the kinase from EGFR in complex with the 4-anilinoquinazoline derivative discovered by OSI Pharmaceuticals, Inc. (OSI-774, erlotinib, Tarceva®). Based on the protein construct used by Stamos et al., subsequent X-ray structures have appeared, which include other inhibitors and ATP mimics (3–5). These structural results will serve as the basis for the following discussion of the features in the EGFR kinase domain and in the inhibitors that account for their potency. They will also serve as the basis of a limited discussion of inhibitor specificity, how clinically important mutations are related to inhibitor exposure, and future directions in developing additional useful or improved inhibitors.

2. GENERAL STRUCTURE OVERVIEW

There are approximately 500 protein kinases in the human genome (12, 13). The EGF receptor (EGFR) is one of about 60 transmembrane proteins that have a tyrosine kinase domain within their intracellular region and which in most cases act as receptors for soluble ligands presented to their extracellular region (receptor tyrosine kinases, RTK). Eukaryotic protein kinases act as catalysts for the transfer of the γ-phosphate group from the bound co-factor adenosine triphosphate (ATP) to a protein substrate, at a tyrosine (tyrosine kinase), serine, or threonine (serine/threonine kinase) amino acid side chain's hydroxyl group. Such reactions are integral to a myriad of cell-signaling processes. A great deal has been learned about protein kinases from X-ray structures (*14*) that started appearing in 1991, for instance the following prototypes: protein kinase A (*15*) (PKA or cyclic-AMP dependent kinase), the insulin receptor kinase domain (*16*), and Abelson tyrosine kinase (Abl) (*17*). Protein kinase catalytic domains share an overall structure incorporating about 300 amino acids, with an amino-terminal (N-terminal) lobe separated from a carboxy-terminal (C-terminal) lobe by the "ATP binding cleft" or inter-lobe cleft. The N-terminal lobe is mostly comprised of β-strands, but with an important α-helix (α_c), while the C-terminal lobe is mostly α-helical. The inter-lobe cleft is where ATP, the substrate segment of substrate proteins and most SMIs bind (Fig. 3.1).

The key role of protein phosphorylation in cell signaling is accompanied by mechanisms by which the enzyme activity of kinases is turned on and off. The most apparent "on switch" is the phosphorylation of the enzyme domain itself, in that one or more hydroxyl-containing side chains (tyrosine, serine, or threonine) within a long loop are often the first site(s) at which kinase domains are themselves phosphorylated and thereby turned on. This ~ 25 amino acid segment, called the Activation Loop (A-loop), is within the C-terminal lobe. It emerges from the back of the inter-lobe cleft and has at its beginning a highly-conserved tripeptide motif Aspartic Acid-Phenylalanine-Glycine ("DFG"– derived from the single-letter amino acid abbreviations for the amino acid residues). As they have been revealed in the large number of X-ray structures, the A-loop of protein kinases is highly variable conformationally, but since it supports substrate binding during phospho-transfer, we can presume a sharply restricted conformational space is relevant during the catalytic reaction. Phosphorylation within this

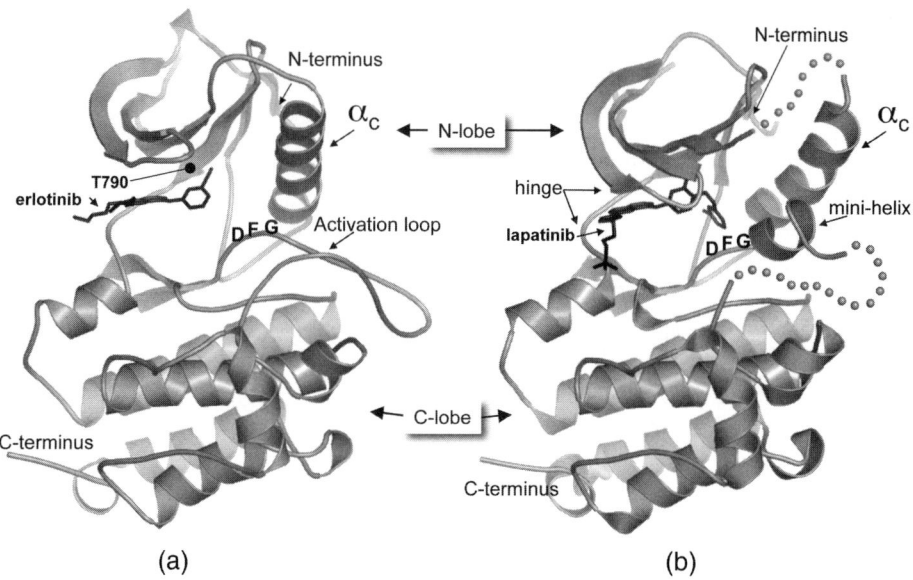

Fig. 3.1. Simplified representations of the kinase domain from EGFR. (a) The "active" conformation as seen in the complex with erlotinib (pdb accession code 1M17). (b) The "inactive" conformation as seen in the complex with lapatinib (pdb accession code 1XKK). The principal difference between the inhibitors is the greater extension (toward the right) of lapatinib, which is accommodated by a large shift of helix αc. Note also the additional short helix in front of αc. Dotted segments represent parts of the structure that were too highly flexible to be discerned in the X-ray experiment.

loop is associated with a large conformational change (20-30 Å) that either relieves an auto-inhibitory steric blockage of the substrate binding site, arranges key elements of the catalytic machinery for phospho-transfer, or both (*18*, *19*). Among the key elements are the α-helix in the N-terminal lobe ($α_c$), which can shift as a rigid body to provide important interactions with partners in the catalytic event and which can be associated with shifts of the entire N-terminal lobe, leading to a more "open" or more "closed" inter-lobe cleft. The simple picture of A-loop phosphorylation and rearrangement with $α_c$ and N-terminal lobe movement neglects control exerted via other domains in kinases where they exist, e.g., Src (*20*, *21*), but it serves well for discussion of the structure-function relationships of SMIs that bind in the ATP-binding cleft. EGFR and its close homologues HER2 and HER4 are themselves exceptional in this regard, as a phosphorylation event is not required for the catalytically competent conformation of the A-loop and $α_c$ (*2*, *22*). As for the other RTKs, EGFR enzyme activity is commonly turned off either due to de-phosphorylation by a phosphatase enzyme, or by internalization and degradation. Both these topics are covered elsewhere in this volume.

The structurally characterized EGFR kinase SMIs reported to date act by competing with ATP for binding in the inter-lobe cleft (Fig. 3.2). Almost all kinase SMIs use one or more hydrogen-bonds (H-bonds) to the polypeptide backbone in the segment connecting N- and C-terminal lobes (the "hinge") for part of their binding energy, a feature also used for binding by ATP. Beyond this, many kinase SMIs diverge from ATP and tend not to extend in the direction where ATP places its triphosphate chain. Instead, kinase SMIs usually extend more or less parallel to the hinge, which leads in one direction toward solvent, and in the opposite direction deeper into the inter-lobe cleft. These SMIs are discussed in terms of the core (H-bonds to hinge), the solubilizing group (extends toward solvent), and the "head group" (reaching into the cleft) (Fig. 3.3). The size of the head group can have important implications for the conformation of the protein to which a SMI will bind. The prototype example is the Abl kinase SMI imatinib (STI571, Gleevec® ,Glivec®, (Novartis)), which uses its relatively large head group to reach far into the cleft region

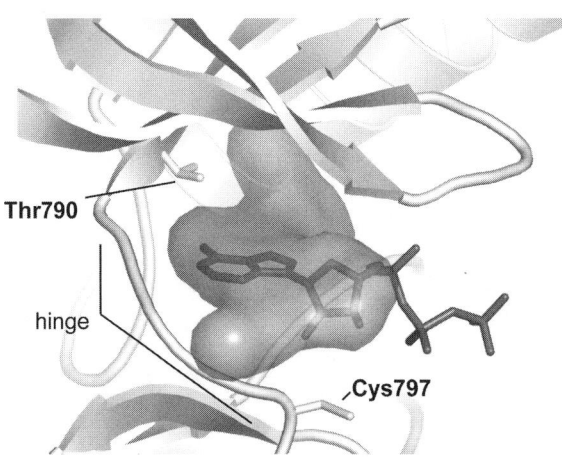

Fig. 3.2. The nature of inhibition in the ATP-binding cleft. An overlay of two EGFR kinase X-ray structures, one with erlotinib (pdb accession code 1M17) and the other with a close analogue of ATP (pdb accession code 2GS7). Erlotinib is depicted as a semi-transparent surface, and AMP-PNP as grey sticks. Both molecules establish H-bonds with the hinge region, and they cannot bind at the same time.

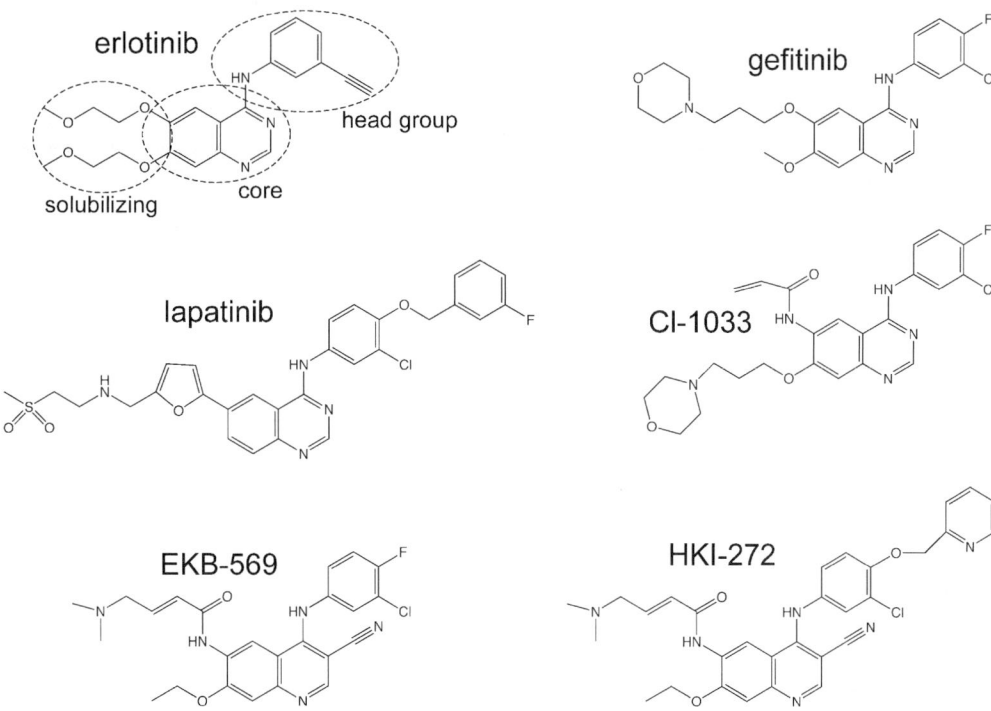

Fig. 3.3. The chemical structures of some potent inhibitors of the EGFR kinase. Erlotinib, gefitinib, lapatinib and Cl-1033 share a 4-anilino-quinazoline chemotype, while EKB-569 and HKI-272 share a 4-anilino-3-cyanoquinoline chemotype. Cl-1033, EKB-569 and HKI-272 all have a reactive moiety in their solubilizing sections designed to form a covalent bond with a cysteine amino acid near the ATP binding site that is characteristic of the erbB family kinase domains.

and bind to a protein conformation that requires the α_c helix and DFG to be in a catalytically incompetent arrangement (23). Other clinically effective kinase SMIs, like erlotinib and gefitinib (ZD-1829, Iressa®, (AstraZeneca)), have been captured in crystals binding tightly to the catalytically competent conformation, and so SMIs are sometimes described as binding to the "active" or "inactive" state.

The idea that every protein kinase target has an "inactive" conformation has given rise to the notion that targeting the "inactive" conformation may have an advantage regarding specificity. The reason is that as catalysts for ATP-dependent phospho-transfer, all kinase "active" forms must share certain features that make SMI specificity harder to obtain. Also, the many structures of inactive kinase conformations, which vary widely, have tended to support the logically opposite notion, namely, that inactive forms offered greater potential for specificity. Interestingly, recent developments in our understanding of the activation of the EGFR kinase rely, in part, on recognition of key similarities among the inactive forms of some kinase domains (Section 6).

One additional key feature of kinase/SMI interactions is the amino acid side chain presented by the protein at the "gatekeeper" position (Threonine 790 in EGFR, where the numbering system for reference to specific amino acid positions reflects inclusion of the 24 amino acids of signal peptide that are part of the EGFR gene but which are absent from the mature protein). In this numbering system, the Tyrosine residue referred to as Tyr845 (the "Src site", subject to phosphorylation by the cellular kinase Src and a target of commercial phospho-EGFR antibodies) is called Tyr869. The gatekeeper residue is in the beginning of the hinge, varies among protein kinases, and is commonly engaged in binding SMIs (Fig. 3.2). These attributes allow use of gatekeeper interactions to create specificity against some non-target kinases, but in the same way allow mutations of this residue to have very significant effects on SMI affinity (potency), as has been observed among patients treated with imatinib (24), and more recently, with gefitinib (25) and erlotinib (26).

3. WILD-TYPE EGFR KINASE X-RAY STRUCTURES

In spite of long-term and rather intense study of EGFR, it was not until 2002 that the first X-ray structures of the EGFR kinase (2) were reported, which used a protein construct of 327 amino acids extending between residue numbers 695 and 1022. The presence in this construct of approximately 40 amino acids C-terminal to the end on the canonical kinase domain seems to have been key to successful crystallization, as some of them are important mediators of crystal packing contacts. The structure with no inhibitor or ATP-like co-factor mimic ("apo") revealed the A-loop in a conformation closely similar to that observed for the insulin receptor kinase in its phosphorylated (active) form (18). The positions of other elements of the catalytic machinery, the DFG tripeptide and the α_c helix, were also consistent with catalytic competence. These details were in agreement with the finding that substitution of the hydroxyl-containing tyrosine residue within the A-loop (Tyr869) with phenylalanine (no hydroxyl) created an EGFR still competent for phospho-transfer activity (22). The same overall conformation was subsequently observed by Zhang et al. in a complex with an ATP analogue-peptide conjugate (4) that serves as a mimic of the phospho-transfer reaction.

Apo crystals were treated with erlotinib to provide the inhibitor complex structure in which the protein was found to be essentially unchanged from its apo parent. This mostly unchanged structure suggested, but did not prove, that erlotinib binds to the active protein conformation preferentially. Indeed, to this point there was no direct structural evidence that other conformations existed. Nonetheless, the interactions between erlotinib and the protein are entirely consistent with tight binding and there is no contrary evidence suggesting a different protein conformation is better suited to bind erlotinib.

The 4-anilinoquinazoline chemotype found in erlotinib had been structurally characterized earlier with the protein kinases CDK2 and p38 (27), and together with the erlotinib and gefitinib EGFR kinase structures, we can observe some common themes. These SMIs share the bicyclic quinazoline core substituted at one end with two ether-linkage containing groups (solubilizing groups) and at the other end with a substituted aniline moiety (head group) (Fig. 3.3). Structure/function analyses of kinase inhibitors generally discount contributions to binding affinity made by the "solubilizing" groups, although the significant differences in the solubilizing groups in erlotinib and gefitinib may be important in determining their bioavailability. Erlotinib and gefitinib both accept an H-bond from the main chain amide of residue Met793 to the N1 atom of their quinazoline cores. The other nitrogen atom within the core, N3, probably interacts with the Thr790 side chain indirectly via a water molecule (7, 27), although at the resolution of these structures (~2.6 – 2.7Å), such a water is not very reliably observed. Elsewhere, erlotinib and gefitinib differ only in the nature of the substituents on their respective anilino moieties. Erlotinib is meta-substituted with a 2-carbon acetylene group. Gefitinib is meta-substituted with a chlorine atom and para-substituted with a fluorine atom. As demonstrated with the CDK2 and p38 structures, the angle between the planes of the quinazoline core and the anilino head group is variable and is determined by details of the inter-lobe cleft it occupies. Erlotinib and gefitinib adopt very similar orientations in the EGFR kinase cleft, with an interplanar angle of about 40°. They both direct their meta-substituent into a hydrophobic pocket created by the relatively small side chain of Thr790. There are other potential weak interactions between the hinge and the quinazoline core that, based on comparisons with the CDK2 and p38 structures, seem to differ in detail according to the size of the side chain at the gatekeeper residue.

In stark contrast to the structures of erlotinib and gefitinib with (wild-type) EGFR kinase, the inhibitor lapatinib (GW-2016, Tykerb® (GlaxoSmithKline)) binds to an "inactive" form (*3*). Lapatinib is also a 4-substituted quinazoline, but it has a much larger head group than erlotinib or gefitinib (roughly twice as big) (Fig. 3.3). Wood et al. discount any influence of the poorly ordered solubilizing group on protein conformation, but the head group of lapatinib is not compatible with the "active" conformation (*3*) bound by the smaller inhibitors. The likelihood that the smaller erlotinib and gefitinib would also bind to the "inactive" conformation is less easily judged. A simple superposition of the relevant structures shows that the inactive conformation presents an altered environment to the head group of erlotinib and of gefitinib, but it seems possible that the resulting steric problem could be eliminated by relatively minor conformational changes.

As is true for erlotinib and gefitinib, the lapatinib quinazoline core H-bonds to the hinge via nitrogen atom N1. The water mediated H-bond from atom N3 in erlotinib (and perhaps gefitinib) is altered in the lapatinib structure, now associated with a different threonine residue, Thr854. The lapatinib head group is like that of gefitinib in having a meta-chlorine, but diverges at the para position, which is now a 3-fluorobenzyloxy moiety (nine atoms) rather than the lone fluorine atom of gefitinib. The much larger para-substitution of the anilino ring requires much more room, and the protein conformation is very different (Fig. 3.1). The α_c is shifted away from the catalytic machinery by about 9Å at the end distal to the hinge region, and the β-strands of the N-terminal lobe rotate by about 12° relative to the "active" conformation seen with erlotinib and gefitinib. This creates a hydrophobic pocket for the fluorobenzyloxy group while at the same time disrupting important elements of the catalytically competent conformation. As the distal end of α_c is shifted away from the site of catalysis, the vacancy created is partially filled by lapatinib but also by a changed conformation of the A-loop. The lapatinib-bound A-loop includes a short α-helical segment as it emerges from the inter-lobe cleft, reminiscent of the inactive form of the Src tyrosine kinase (*28, 29*).

4. IMPLICATIONS FOR ESCAPE MUTANTS

Clinical and research results involving the Abl kinase are defining a paradigm for the interplay between treatment using SMIs and biological effects, with direct relevance for the EGFR system. The use of imatinib in patients with chronic myeloid leukemia (CML) is associated with emergence of ~20 variant forms of the target Abl kinase (*30, 31*). These variant forms are less effectively inhibited by imatinib and thus are considered imatinib "escape" mutants (Fig. 3.4). This clinical experience is providing very important insights into the use of SMIs in the genetically labile environment characteristic of cancer. Imatinib binds to an inactive conformation of Abl (*23*). Among the origins of imatinib resistance are its relatively large size and its relatively low affinity. The large size is associated with contacts between imatinib and a relatively large number of Abl amino acid residues. The low affinity means that mutation at any contact residue has a relatively high likelihood of reducing the affinity to a point where clinical efficacy is lost. The effect of lower affinity may arise directly at a contact residue, but for some clinical Abl escape mutants it must arise allosterically, because the amino acid itself is not contacted by imatinib (Fig. 3.4). In response to the Abl escape mutants, drug designers have created a second generation imatinib (*32*) (AMN107, nilotinib (Novartis)), which benefits from a 20-fold increased affinity while remaining a close chemical relative of imatinib. As a result, nilotinib retains useful affinity for many of the escape mutants arising from imatinib treatment.

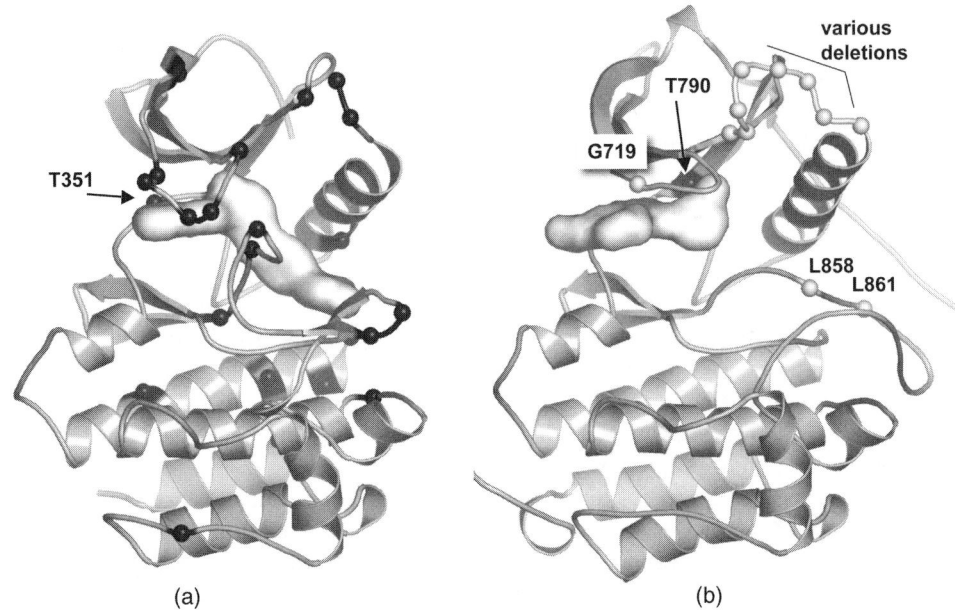

Fig. 3.4. Sites of mutations associated with the clinical experience following treatment with kinase inhibitors. (a) The Abl kinase complex with imatinib with black spheres at sites where mutations have arisen leading to imatinib escape (pdb accession code 2HYY). (b) The EGFR kinase complex with erlotinib with white spheres at sites where pre-treatment mutations confer heightened sensitivity to inhibitor treatment (pdb accession code 1M17). The single observed egfr kinase escape mutation is indicated with a black sphere at T790. The inhibitors are depicted as grey surfaces.

Another Abl SMI with good affinity for most clinical mutants of Abl is BMS-354825 (*33*) (dasatinib, Sprycel® (Bristol-Myers Squibb)). It is smaller than imatinib or nilotinib and is considered capable of binding with useful affinity to both active and inactive forms of the Abl kinase. The diminished conformational sensitivity is linked to dasatinib's smaller size. However, the smaller size is probably also a cause of reduced specificity, in that dasatinib is described as a dual Abl/Src SMI, indicative of diminished specificity toward Abl relative to the larger Abl SMIs. We might expect such a phenomenon to be general, because smaller SMIs will tend to have fewer contacts with a protein, and therefore will tend to probe fewer of its chemical and conformational idiosyncrasies. Such a concept would be useful during drug discovery and design efforts. Nonetheless, the EGFR SMIs erlotinib and gefitinib (smaller) and lapatinib (larger) argue against this notion. Erlotinib and gefitinib are relatively specific EGFR binders, while lapatinib is described as a dual EGFR/HER2 SMI (*3*).

Recently, a mutation in the EGFR kinase domain has been identified among patients treated with erlotinib or gefitinib, a change from threonine at position 790 to the larger methionine residue (T790M) (*26*, *34*, *35*). The affinity of erlotinib and gefitinib for T790M is drastically reduced (*35*, *36*), and this protein variant qualifies as an escape mutant. Interestingly, this mutation has also been identified in lung tumors at diagnosis (*37*) and in the germ line of a cancer-prone family (*38*). Nonetheless, T790M does not increase kinase activity in vitro (*34*) so its association with disease prior to treatment is not easy to understand. The position 790 in EGFR is homologous to position 315 in the Abl kinase, and among the ~20 imatinib escape mutants, the T315I mutation is the only one that second generation inhibitors nilotinib and dasatinib do not inhibit effectively (Fig. 3.4). These mutations occur at the respective gatekeeper residues. As a result, the affinities of many hinge-binding SMIs are likely to be easily and drastically reduced when a small side chain gatekeeper is mutated to a large one. Due to the close overall similarity between erlotinib, gefitinib and lapatinib and the way their cores are oriented with respect to the hinge, it is no surprise that lapatinib shares the reduced affinity for T790M seen for erlotinib and gefitinib (G. Schaefer, personal communication).

5. STRUCTURES OF ERLOTNIB & GEFITINIB SUSCEPTIBILITY EGFR MUTANTS

Quite different from the Abl and more recently EGFR escape mutants associated with SMI exposure, a series of EGFR mutations have been identified that confer special sensitivity to treatment with erlotinib and gefitinib (*39*, *40*) (Fig. 3.4). These mutations were identified among patients who experienced very dramatic positive responses to erlotinib or gefitinib treatment. Curiously, these mutations both increase the intrinsic activity of EGFR and increase sensitivity to erlotinib and gefitinib relative to the wild-type protein (*34*, *41*). In the context of the original apo and erlotinib complex structures of the "active" EGFR kinase, we lacked a molecular rationale for these characteristics, because the most interesting (hyperactive and but SMI sensitizing) mutations (L858R and deletions preceding α_c) are not very close to the bound inhibitor. The recent X-ray structure of the L858R mutant complexed with gefitinib (*5*) seems to have helped understanding of the hyperactivity of the mutant, but less about the special susceptibility this mutant has to erlotinib and gefitinib (*42*).

With the discovery of these sensitizing mutations, the lapatinib complex structure achieved greater relevance, because it characterized the inactive state of the protein (*3*). This inactive conformation, despite having been captured with bound lapatinib, is probably biologically relevant because of its kinship with other kinase structures that lack such a confounding influence. This inactive EGFR kinase structure revealed how mutations L858R or L861Q might augment kinase activity and thus be associated with hyperproliferation. In the lapatinib complex structure, these residues contribute to a mini-hydrophobic core, with other contributions from neighboring hydrophobic residues. The switch to polar or charged side chains will destabilize this assembly and as a result tend to favor the active state in which they would be solvent exposed.

Additionally, the structure of L858R with gefitnib (*5*) allows speculation regarding a higher inhibitory activity relative to wild-type. Yun et al. report an "active", erlotinib-complex-like protein conformation for gefitinib in complex with both wild-type and L858R proteins. The details of the gefitinib interactions with protein are essentially identical in both structures. With L858R, however, they also report an additional gefitinib structure in which the anilino ring of gefitinib rotates by about 180° relative to its orientation in the wild-type protein, thereby establishing an interaction between the meta-chlorine atom and the Asp855 side chain, which, via a water-mediated interaction, connects to the side chain of the mutated side chain (Arginine) at position 858. The net energetic difference of hydrophobic pocket/chlorine interactions versus hydrophilic Aspartyl/chlorine interactions is a subtle one, and the influence of the neighboring but indirectly-contacting L858R mutation is difficult to gauge. A similar rotation of the anilino-ring of erlotinib would allow the weakly acidic acetylenyl proton to partake in an H-bond with Asp855 of L858R. For both erlotinib and gefitinib, this kind of interaction could provide an incremental increase in potency relative to the wild-type protein.

The other most commonly seen erlotinib/gefitinib sensitivity mutations are G719S and deletions of several amino acids in the loop immediately preceding the important α_c helix. The structures of G719S reported by Yun et al. suggest a relatively subtle influence on catalytic activity and inhibitor sensitivity. So far, there is no reported structure of any of the deletion mutants and a clear rationale for their greater erlotinib/gefitinib sensitivity is not in hand. It seems likely, however, that the greater inherent catalytic activity of such mutants derives from a destabilization of the inactive conformation relative to the active one. For instance, Zhang et al. have reported an EGFR kinase structure in the inactive conformation in which residues subject to the deletion interact with the A-loop mini-helix characteristic of the inactive form (4). Without this contribution, the A-loop helix may be less favored. A different way of looking at it concerns the observed association between the mini-helix at the start of the inactive-form A-loop and the position of α_c. A deletion preceding α_c seems likely to alter, and probably reduce, its ability to shift as a rigid body. A shortened link to the preceding β-strand of the N-lobe will likely keep α_c closer to the "active" position, with an additional allosteric effect on the first part of the A-loop, probably destabilizing the mini-helical conformation and thereby the inactive state.

6. FUTURE DIRECTIONS IN EGFR SMI RESEARCH

The recent clinical history of erlotinib/gefitinib treatment and the subsequent escape mutation shows a clear parallel with imatinib/Abl. So far, only the T790M escape mutation has been seen in EGFR. Based on their tighter binding and smaller size relative to imatinib, one can argue that T790M may remain the only clinically important escape mutant that arises from treatment with erlotinib or gefitinib. Nonetheless, the issue facing patients with the hardest to address Abl mutation, T315I, is also faced by those with tumors expressing T790M EGFR. This mutation can only be addressed with SMIs significantly different from erlotinib, gefitinib or lapatinib. In this sense, it is useful to consider T790M a distinct target that will require a distinct SMI. It may be necessary to abandon a 4-anilinoquinazoline framework to discover hinge-binding SMIs that avoid contact with residue 790. Perhaps such an inhibitor would be effective regardless of the amino acid at position 790.

An interesting approach to EGFR inhibition with relevance to this problem was initiated before T790M was observed. Although we currently lack any structures of them in complex with EGFR kinase, a series of chemically reactive inhibitors have been described that show good activity against T790M (43–46). These SMIs take advantage of a cysteine residue near the ATP-binding site found in the erbB family kinase domains (Cys797 in EGFR, see Fig. 3.2), by forming a covalent link to the cysteine sulfur atom. Non-erbB-family protein kinase domains almost never have a cysteine in this position (47). These molecules are potent inhibitors of T790M (35, 36). Based on the high similarity of their chemical structures to those of erlotinib and gefitinib (Fig. 3.3), one can conclude that without a covalent attachment, they would probably not effectively inhibit T790M. It is interesting to ponder their exact relationship to the hinge when binding T790M, because the steric problem caused by a methionine at position 790 must be solved in some way. The answer to this question may be available in an X-ray structure in the near future.

It is also possible to conceive SMIs that are not hinge-binding. For instance, an X-ray structure shows the cellular kinase MEK1 is inhibited by an SMI that binds in the inter-lobe cleft, but that leaves the hinge region available for binding to ATP (48). Because this inhibitor is not ATP- or substrate-competitive, and it binds deep in the inter-lobe cleft more or less in the region between DFG and α_c, it is considered an allosteric inhibitor. Such a site in EGFR or other kinases offer potentially greater specificity as they avoid the more highly conserved ATP-binding residues.

There is strong evidence for an allosteric influence on EGFR kinase activity from a totally different site. Zhang et al. have reported a stunning insight into allosteric activation of EGFR kinase(*4*). They have shown that a site outside the inter-lobe cleft controls EGFR kinase domain activation. This insight explains how the formal activation, i.e., transition to the catalytically competent conformation, is effected for EGFR, HER2, and HER4 (HER3 has a catalytically incompetent amino acid sequence). The allosteric site lies between α_c and the rest of the N-terminal lobe, but on the outside of the inter-lobe cleft rather than within it. The shape of this site changes in accordance with the position of α_c, which, as discussed above, is associated with conformational change in the A-loop. A homologous site in the cellular kinase CDK2 is occupied by its endogenous activator CyclinA when they are in complex. The EGFR kinase story also involves an interacting protein, but this time it is provided by another copy of EGFR (Fig. 3.5). The other copy presents its C-terminal lobe, mostly the helix called α_H, to the interface. This interface appears in crystals that are isomorphous with those originally reported by Stamos et al. (the "active" conformation), but is incompatible with the position of α_c seen in the lapatinib structure ("inactive" conformation). Zhang et al. report that mutations of key residues on either side of this interface disrupt signal transduction in intact EGFR on cells. This finding also explains the influence of mutations in the tripeptide segment Leucine-Valine-Isoleucine ("LVI") reported by Penuel et al. (*49*), since LVI is part of the same interface. This new insight partitions EGFR-family kinase domains into two distinct functions, either as activator kinase or as activated kinase. Both functions are possible for EGFR, HER2, and HER4, but the dead catalytic site in HER3 restricts it to activator. Similarly, even with a SMI in their active site, EGFR, HER2, and HER4 can still act as activators because their C-terminal regions are not altered when erlotinib or similar

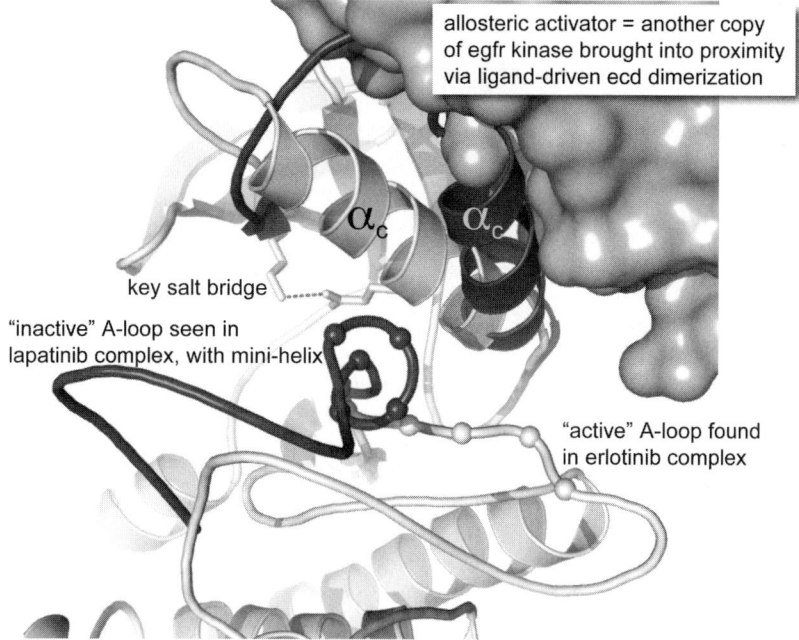

Fig. 3.5. Mechanism of activation of the EGFR kinase domain. Light gray ribbons depict the "active" conformation seen in the erlotinib complex. In dark gray ribbons are key parts from the "inactive" state seen in the lapatinib complex. The gray surface is a neighboring kinase domain seen in X-ray structures of the "active" state, in which it associates closely with α_c. The "inactive" α_c in dark gray is incompatible with this interaction. Extracellular dimerization brings another copy of the kinase domain into close proximity where it induces a shift into the "active" conformation, unwinding the A-loop mini-helix and allowing the key salt bridge to form.

SMIs bind in their inter-lobe cleft. Now that the allosteric influence exerted by sites outside the inter-lobe cleft are appreciated, attempts to exploit it for control of EGFR activity can be made.

7. SUMMARY

More than 20 years after the EGFR became the subject of intense research interest, we still are learning about the important control mechanisms required for its proper functioning. The unfortunate cause for this continuing interest is the dysregulation or hyperactivity of the EGFR and its close homologues found in many common cancers. There is reason for some optimism among medical researchers as treatments become available that are more tightly focused on these specific molecular mediators of oncogenesis and tumor progression. The success of antibody therapies (Herceptin® (Genentech), Erbitux® (ImClone), Vectibix® (Amgen) and others in development) directed against the extracellular parts of these receptors has been informed by X-ray crystallographic structures (50–55), and there is continuing effort along these lines. Additional and significant progress can be expected as structures of the catalytic kinase domain support continuing development of drugs directed at the intracellular compartment. With the already approved erlotinib, gefitinib and lapatinib, we have experienced a synergy between SMI treatment and clinical findings that promises to energize the discovery of next-generation medicines. Solutions to the T790M escape mutation will be found, and continuing developments regarding the success of T790M-inhibiting medicines will be informed by the rapidly unfolding Abl/imatinib experience. Highly specific allosteric inhibitors may be discovered. If it proves possible to determine structures of all or part of the other 200 amino acids of the intracellular domain, we may yet find completely new ways to control receptor signaling.

ACKNOWLEDGMENTS

Grateful acknowledgement is made to Professor M. J. Eck and to Dr. C-H Yun for access to their manuscript and coordinate files in advance of publication.

REFERENCES

1. Burgess AW, Cho HS, Eigenbrot C, Ferguson KM, Garrett TP, Leahy DJ, Lemmon MA, Sliwkowski MX, Ward CW, Yokoyama S. An open-and-shut case? Recent insights into the activation of EGF/ErbB receptors. Mol Cell 2003;12:541.
2. Stamos J, Sliwkowski MX, Eigenbrot C. Structure of the epidermal growth factor receptor kinase domain alone and in complex with a 4-anilinoquinazoline inhibitor. J Biol Chem 2002;277:46265-72.
3. Wood ER, Truesdale AT, McDonald OB, Yuan D, Hassell A, Dickerson SH, Ellis B, Pennisi C, Horne E, Lackey K, Alligood KJ, Rusnak DW, Gilmer TM, Shewchuk L. A unique structure for epidermal growth factor receptor bound to GW572016 (Lapatinib): relationships among protein conformation, inhibitor off-rate, and receptor activity in tumor cells. Cancer Res 2004;64:6652-9.
4. Zhang X, Gureasko J, Shen K, Cole PA, Kuriyan J. An allosteric mechanism for activation of the kinase domain of epidermal growth factor receptor. Cell 2006;125:1137-49.
5. Yun C-H, Boggon TJ, Li Y, Woo MS, Greulich H, Meyerson M, Eck MJ. Structures of lung cancer-derived EGFR mutants and inhibitor complexes: Mechanism of activation and insights into differential inhibitor sensitivity. Cancer Cell 2007;11:217-27.
6. Bridges AJ. Chemical inhibitors of protein kinases. Chem Rev 2001;101:2541-72.
7. Palmer BD, Trumpp-Kallmeyer S, Fry DW, Nelson JM, Showalter HD, Denny WA. Tyrosine kinase inhibitors. 11. Soluble analogues of pyrrolo- and pyrazoloquinazolines as epidermal growth factor receptor inhibitors: synthesis, biological evaluation, and modeling of the mode of binding. J Med Chem 1997;40:1519-29.
8. Wissner A, Berger DM, Boschelli DH, Floyd MB, Jr., Greenberger LM, Gruber BC, Johnson BD, Mamuya N, Nilakantan R, Reich MF, Shen R, Tsou HR, Upeslacis E, Wang YF, Wu B, Ye F, Zhang N.

4-Anilino-6,7-dialkoxyquinoline-3-carbonitrile inhibitors of epidermal growth factor receptor kinase and their bioisosteric relationship to the 4-anilino-6,7-dialkoxyquinazoline inhibitors. J Med Chem 2000;43:3244-56.
9. Ganti AK, Potti A. Epidermal growth factor inhibition in solid tumours. Expert Opin Biol Ther 2005;5:1165-74.
10. Heymach JV, Nilsson M, Blumenschein G, Papadimitrakopoulou V, Herbst R. Epidermal growth factor receptor inhibitors in development for the treatment of non-small cell lung cancer. Clin Cancer Res 2006;12:4441s-5s.
11. Mendelsohn J, Baselga J. Epidermal growth factor receptor targeting in cancer. Sem Oncol 2006;4:369-85.
12. Hanks SK. Genomic analysis of the eukaryotic protein kinase superfamily: a perspective. Genome Biol 2003;4:111.
13. Manning G, Whyte DB, Martinez R, Hunter T, Sudarsanam S. The protein kinase complement of the human genome. Science 2002;298:1912-34.
14. Cowan-Jacob SW. Structural biology of protein tyrosine kinases. Cell Mol Life Sci 2006;63:2608-25.
15. Knighton DR, Zheng JH, Ten Eyck LF, Ashford VA, Xuong NH, Taylor SS, Sowadski JM. Crystal structure of the catalytic subunit of cyclic adenosine monophosphate-dependent protein kinase. Science 1991;253:407-14.
16. Till JH, Ablooglu AJ, Frankel M, Bishop SM, Kohanski RA, Hubbard SR. Crystallographic and solution studies of an activation loop mutant of the insulin receptor tyrosine kinase: insights into kinase mechanism. J Biol Chem 2001;276:10049-55.
17. Levinson NM, Kuchment O, Shen K, Young MA, Koldobskiy M, Karplus M, Cole PA, Kuriyan J. A Src-like inactive conformation in the abl tyrosine kinase domain. PLoS Biol 2006;4:753-67.
18. Hubbard SR. Crystal structure of the activated insulin receptor tyrosine kinase in complex with peptide substrate and ATP analog. EMBO J 1997;16:5572-81.
19. Mohammadi M, McMahon G, Sun L, Tang C, Hirth P, Yeh BK, Hubbard SR, Schlessinger J. Structures of the tyrosine kinase domain of fibroblast growth factor receptor in complex with inhibitors. Science 1997;276:955-60.
20. Cowan-Jacob SW, Fendrich G, Manley PW, Jahnke W, Fabbro D, Liebetanz J, Meyer T. The crystal structure of a c-Src complex in an active conformation suggests possible steps in c-Src activation. Structure 2005;13:861-71.
21. Young MA, Gonfloni S, Superti-Furga G, Roux B, Kuriyan J. Dynamic coupling between the SH2 and SH3 domains of c-Src and Hck underlies their inactivation by C-terminal tyrosine phosphorylation. Cell 2001;105:115-26.
22. Gotoh N, Tojo A, Hino M, Yazaki Y, Shibuya M. A highly conserved tyrosine residue at codon 845 within the kinase domain is not required for the transforming activity of human epidermal growth factor receptor. Biochem Biophys Res Commun 1992;186:768-4.
23. Schindler T, Bornmann W, Pellicena P, Miller WT, Clarkson B, Kuriyan J. Structural mechanism for STI-571 inhibition of abelson tyrosine kinase. Science 2000;289:1938-42.
24. Branford S, Rudzki Z, Walsh S, Grigg A, Arthur C, Taylor K, Herrmann R, Lynch KP, Hughes TP. High frequency of point mutations clustered within the adenosine triphosphate-binding region of BCR/ABL in patients with chronic myeloid leukemia or Ph-positive acute lymphoblastic leukemia who develop imatinib (STI571) resistance. Blood 2002;99:3472-5.
25. Kosaka T, Yatabe Y, Endoh H, Yoshida K, Hida T, Tsuboi M, Tada H, Kuwano H, Mitsudomi T. Analysis of epidermal growth factor receptor gene mutation in patients with non-small cell lung cancer and acquired resistance to gefitinib. Cancer Ther Clin 2006;12:5764-9.
26. Pao W, Miller VA, Politi KA, Riely GJ, Somwar R, Zakowski MF, Kris MG, Varmus H. Acquired resistance of lung adenocarcinomas to gefitinib or erlotinib is associated with a second mutation in the EGFR kinase domain. PLoS Med 2005;2:e73.
27. Shewchuk L, Hassell A, Wisely B, Rocque W, Holmes W, Veal J, Kuyper LF. Binding mode of the 4-anilinoquinazoline class of protein kinase inhibitor: X-ray crystallographic studies of 4-anilinoquinazolines bound to cyclin-dependent kinase 2 and p38 kinase. J Med Chem 2000;43:133.
28. Schindler T, Sicheri F, Pico A, Gazit A, Levitzki A, Kuriyan J. Crystal structure of Hck in complex with a Src family-selective tyrosine kinase inhibitor. Mol Cell 1999;3:639-48.

29. Xu W, Harrison SC, Eck MJ. Three-dimensional structure of the tyrosine kinase c-Src. Nature 1997;385:595-602.
30. Burgess MR, Sawyers CL. Treating imatinib-resistant leukemia: the next generation targeted therapies. ScientificWorldJournal 2006;6:918-30.
31. Shah NP, Nicoll JM, Nagar B, Gorre ME, Paquette RL, Kuriyan J, Sawyers CL. Multiple BCR-ABL kinase domain mutations confer polyclonal resistance to the tyrosine kinase inhibitor imatinib (STI571) in chronic phase and blast crisis chronic myeloid leukemia. Cancer Cell 2002;2:117-25.
32. Weisberg E, Manley PW, Breitenstein W, Bruggen J, Cowan-Jacob SW, Ray A, Huntly B, Fabbro D, Fendrich G, Hall-Meyers E, Kung AL, Mestan J, Daley GQ, Callahan L, Catley L, Cavazza C, Azam M, Neuberg D, Wright RD, Gilliland DG, Griffin JD. Characterization of AMN107, a selective inhibitor of native and mutant Bcr-Abl. Cancer Cell 2005;7:129-41.
33. Shah NP, Tran C, Lee FY, Chen P, Norris D, Sawyers CL. Overriding imatinib resistance with a novel ABL kinase inhibitor. Science 2004;305:732-3.
34. Kobayashi S, Boggon TJ, Dayaram T, Janne PA, Kocher O, Meyerson M, Johnson BE, Eck MJ, Tenen DG, Halmos B. EGFR mutation and resistance of non-small-cell lung cancer to gefitinib. N Engl J Med 2005;352:786-92.
35. Kwak EL, Sordella R, Bell DW, Godin-Heymann N, Okimoto RA, Brannigan BW, Harris PL, Driscoll DR, Fidias P, Lynch TJ, Rabindran SK, McGinnis JP, Wissner A, Sharma SV, Isselbacher KJ, Settleman J, Haber DA. Irreversible inhibitors of the EGF receptor may circumvent acquired resistance to gefitinib. Proc Natl Acad Sci U S A 2005;102:7665-70.
36. Carter TA, Wodicka LM, Shah NP, Velasco AM, Fabian MA, Treiber DK, Milanov ZV, Atteridge CE, Biggs WH, 3rd, Edeen PT, Floyd M, Ford JM, Grotzfeld RM, Herrgard S, Insko DE, Mehta SA, Patel HK, Pao W, Sawyers CL, Varmus H, Zarrinkar PP, Lockhart DJ. Inhibition of drug-resistant mutants of ABL, KIT, and EGF receptor kinases. Proc Natl Acad Sci U S A 2005;102:11011-6.
37. Shih JY, Gow CH, Yang PC. EGFR mutation conferring primary resistance to gefitinib in non-small-cell lung cancer. N Engl J Med 2005;353:207-8.
38. Bell DW, Gore I, Okimoto RA, Godin-Heymann N, Sordella R, Mulloy R, Sharma SV, Brannigan BW, Mohapatra G, Settleman J, Haber DA. Inherited susceptibility to lung cancer may be associated with the T790M drug resistance mutation in EGFR. Nat Genet 2005;37:1315-6.
39. Lynch TJ, Bell DW, Sordella R, Gurubhagavatula S, Okimoto RA, Brannigan BW, Harris PL, Haserlat SM, Supko JG, Haluska FG, Louis DN, Christiani DC, Settleman J, Haber DA. Activating mutations in the epidermal growth factor receptor underlying responsiveness of non-small-cell lung cancer to gefitinib. N Engl J Med 2004;350:2129-39.
40. Paez JG, Janne PA, Lee JC, Tracy S, Greulich H, Gabriel S, Herman P, Kaye FJ, Lindeman N, Boggon TJ, Naoki K, Sasaki H, Fujii Y, Eck MJ, Sellers WR, Johnson BE, Meyerson M. EGFR mutations in lung cancer: correlation with clinical response to gefitinib therapy. Science 2004;304:1497-500.
41. Carey KD, Garton AJ, Romero MS, Kahler J, Thomson S, Ross S, Park F, Haley JD, Gibson N, Sliwkowski MX. Kinetic analysis of epidermal growth factor receptor somatic mutant proteins shows increased sensitivity to the epidermal growth factor receptor tyrosine kinase inhibitor, erlotinib. Cancer Res 2006;66:8163-71.
42. Greulich H, Chen TH, Feng W, Janne PA, Alvarez JV, Zappaterra M, Bulmer SE, Frank DA, Hahn WC, Sellers WR, Meyerson M. Oncogenic transformation by inhibitor-sensitive and -resistant EGFR mutants. PLoS Med 2005;2:e313.
43. Simon GR, Garrett CR, Olson SC, Langevin M, Eiseman IA, Mahany JJ, Williams CC, Lush R, Daud A, Munster P, Chiappori A, Fishman M, Bepler G, Lenehan PF, Sullivan DM. Increased bioavailability of intravenous versus oral CI-1033, a pan erbB tyrosine kinase inhibitor: results of a phase I pharmacokinetic study. Clin Cancer Res 2006;12:4645-51.
44. Smaill JB, Rewcastle GW, Loo JA, Greis KD, Chan OH, Reyner EL, Lipka E, Showalter HD, Vincent PW, Elliott WL, Denny WA. Tyrosine kinase inhibitors. 17. Irreversible inhibitors of the epidermal growth factor receptor: 4-(phenylamino)quinazoline- and 4-(phenylamino)pyrido[3,2-d]pyrimidine-6-acrylamides bearing additional solubilizing functions. J Med Chem 2000;43:1380-97.
45. Rabindran SK, Discafani CM, Rosfjord EC, Baxter M, Floyd MB, Golas J, Hallett WA, Johnson BD, Nilakantan R, Overbeek E, Reich MF, Shen R, Shi X, Tsou HR, Wang YF, Wissner A. Antitumor activity of HKI-272, an orally active, irreversible inhibitor of the HER-2 tyrosine kinase. Cancer Res 2004;64:3958-65.

46. Wissner A, Overbeek E, Reich MF, Floyd MB, Johnson BD, Mamuya N, Rosfjord EC, Discafani C, Davis R, Shi X, Rabindran SK, Gruber BC, Ye F, Hallett WA, Nilakantan R, Shen R, Wang YF, Greenberger LM, Tsou HR. Synthesis and structure-activity relationships of 6,7-disubstituted 4-anilinoquinoline-3-carbonitriles. The design of an orally active, irreversible inhibitor of the tyrosine kinase activity of the epidermal growth factor receptor (EGFR) and the human epidermal growth factor receptor-2 (HER-2). J Med Chem 2003;46:49-63.
47. Buzko O, Shokat KM. A kinase sequence database: sequence alignments and family assignment. Bioinformatics 2002;18:1274-5.
48. Ohren JF, Chen H, Pavlovsky A, Whitehead C, Zhang E, Kuffa P, Yan C, McConnell P, Spessard C, Banotai C, Mueller WT, Delaney A, Omer C, Sebolt-Leopold J, Dudley DT, Leung IK, Flamme C, Warmus J, Kaufman M, Barrett S, Tecle H, Hasemann CA. Structures of human MAP kinase kinase 1 (MEK1) and MEK2 describe novel noncompetitive kinase inhibition. Nat Struct Mol Biol 2004;11:1192-7.
49. Penuel E, Akita RW, Sliwkowski MX. Identification of a region within the ErbB2/HER2 intracellular domain that is necessary for ligand-independent association. J Biol Chem 2002;277:28468-73.
50. Bouyain S, Longo PA, Li S, Ferguson KM, Leahy DJ. The extracellular region of ErbB4 adopts a tethered conformation in the absence of ligand. Proc Natl Acad Sci U S A 2005;102:15024-9.
51. Cho H-S, Leahy DJ. Structure of the extracellular region of HER3 reveals an interdomain tether. Science 2002;297:1330-3.
52. Franklin MC, Carey KD, Vajdos FF, Leahy DJ, de Vos AM, Sliwkowski MX. Insights into ErbB signaling from the structure of the ErbB2-pertuzumab complex. Cancer Cell 2004;5:17-28.
53. Garrett TP, McKern NM, Lou M, Elleman TC, Adams TE, Lovrecz GO, Zhu HJ, Walker F, Frenkel MJ, Hoyne PA, Jorissen RN, Nice EC, Burgess AW, Ward CW. Crystal structure of a truncated epidermal growth factor receptor extracellular domain bound to transforming growth factor alpha. Cell 2002;110:763-73.
54. Li S, Schmitz KR, Jeffrey PD, Wiltzius JJ, Kussie P, Ferguson KM. Structural basis for inhibition of the epidermal growth factor receptor by cetuximab. Cancer Cell 2005;7:301-11.
55. Ogiso H, Ishitani R, Nureki O, Fukai S, Yamanaka M, Kim J-H, Saito K, Sakamoto A, Inoue M, Shirouzu M, Yokohama S. Crystal structure of the complex of human epidermal growth factor and receptor extracellular domains. Cell 2002;110:775-87.

4 Internalization and Degradation of the EGF Receptor

Alexander Sorkin

CONTENTS

INTRODUCTION
EGF-INDUCED ACCELERATION OF EGFR TURNOVER LEADING
  TO RECEPTOR DOWN-REGULATION
INITIAL STEP OF ENDOCYTOSIS: CLATHRIN-DEPENDENT
  AND -INDEPENDENT PATHWAYS OF INTERNALIZATION
CLATHRIN-DEPENDENT INTERNALIZATION: ROLE OF KINASE
  ACTIVITY AND PHOSPHORYLATION OF EGFR
PROTEINS MEDIATING EGFR INTERNALIZATION THROUGH
  CLATHRIN-COATED PITS
CLATHRIN-INDEPENDENT MECHANISMS OF EGFR INTERNALIZATION
PATHWAYS OF INTERNALIZED EGFR THROUGH THE ENDOSOMAL
  COMPARTMENT
MOLECULAR MECHANISMS OF EGFR SORTING IN MVB
PROTEINS MODULATING ENDOCYTOSIS AND SORTING OF EGFR
ACKNOWLEDGEMENTS
REFERENCES

Abstract

Activation of the EGF receptor (EGFR) at the cell surface results in acceleration of endocytosis of the receptor and rapid degradation of endocytosed receptors in lysosomes. The elevated internalization and lysosomal targeting result in down-regulation of the EGFR, which negatively regulates signaling by the receptor. This review describes the molecular mechanisms involved in EGFR trafficking, which lead to growth-factor-induced receptor down-regulation.

Key Words: EGF, receptor, endocytosis, clathrin, ubiquitination, degradation, endosome, lysosome.

1. INTRODUCTION

More than 30 years ago, the first comprehensive study of EGF endocytosis was published by Carpenter and Cohen (*1*). In this pivotal work, 125I-EGF was used to demonstrate saturative binding of EGF to cells, its uptake inside the cells and degradation by lysosomes. Subsequent studies in the late 1970s, mainly from Cohen's laboratory, have established key features of growth-factor induced endocytosis and the mechanisms underlying this process. For instance, a comparative analysis of EGF endocytosis in fibroblasts that express a low level of EGFR (2) and epidermoid carcinoma A-431 cells that express very high levels of EGFR suggested that EGF endocytosis occurs via clathrin-coated pits, as well as through the clathrin-independent pathway (3, 4). Early electron microscopy studies demonstrating the localization of EGF in the intralumenal vesicles of multivesicular bodies (MVB) created a basis for the current model of the endosomal sorting of EGFR (5). These studies remain the cornerstone of the current understanding of endocytosis of EGFR and other receptor tyrosine kinases (RTKs). Needless to say, EGFR remains one of the best characterized models for studying the kinetics and mechanisms of endocytosis, and it is still a prototypic receptor that is widely used to study general mechanisms of endocytosis, and in particular the endocytosis of the RTK family. Many key aspects of the molecular mechanisms of EGFR endocytic trafficking remain unclear, however. Our knowledge about the endocytosis of EGFR under physiological conditions in cell culture and in vivo is especially lapsing. This chapter will discuss the most recent discoveries in the field, which together with early classical studies, have shaped the current model of endocytic trafficking of EGFR.

2. EGF-INDUCED ACCELERATION OF EGFR TURNOVER LEADING TO RECEPTOR DOWN-REGULATION

In most types of cells studied, EGFR is constitutively internalized at a rate comparable to the rate of general membrane recycling (ke 0.02-0.05 min-1) (6–8), although there is one example of rapid constitutive internalization of EGFR (9). After internalization, receptors are mainly recycled back to cell surface. Because the recycling rate is several times higher than the internalization rate, the bulk of EGFR are present at the cell surface. Degradation of unoccupied receptors is very slow, which, together with slow internalization, results in a slow turnover of receptor protein. In cells expressing low levels of EGFR, receptors turn over with t1/2 in the range of 6-10 hrs whereas in cells overexpressing EGFR, such as A-431, t1/2 could be as long as 24 hs (10–12).

Binding of a growth factor to the receptor results in the dramatic acceleration of internalization (6). After internalization, EGF and EGFR are efficiently degraded, which results in the dramatic decrease of t1/2 of EGFR protein (11). Accelerated internalization and degradation of activated EGFR lead to the reduction of the amount of EGFR at the cell surface, a phenomenon referred to as EGF-induced down-regulation of EGFR. EGFR down-regulation is the major negative feedback regulatory mechanism that controls the intensity and duration of receptor signaling (13). In the following sections we describe the molecular mechanisms underlying ligand-induced down-regulation of the EGFR.

3. INITIAL STEP OF ENDOCYTOSIS: CLATHRIN-DEPENDENT AND -INDEPENDENT PATHWAYS OF INTERNALIZATION

Development of quantitative methods to measure the specific rates of EGF internalization has allowed detailed characterization of the kinetics of this process (14). These studies have led to two key findings. First, the specific internalization rates of labeled EGF were found to be within the range of these rates measured for nutrient receptors, such as transferrin receptor, which are internalized through clathrin-coated pits (ke ~0.2-0.5 min-1) (8). Second, the rapid internalization pathway was demonstrated to be saturable as revealed by the reduction of the internalization rates with the increase in the amount of EGFR occupied by EGF at the cell surface (15). The hypothesis was put forward that when the rapid internalization pathway is overwhelmed because of its low capacity and because of a large concentration of EGF:EGFR complexes at the cell surface, many of these complexes are internalized with a slow kinetics, and the contribution of the rapid pathway in the overall uptake of labeled EGF is minimal (14). This hypothesis received experimental support only recently. It was shown that the uptake of high concentrations of EGF (high receptor occupancy) was only minimally affected by overexpression of a dynamin mutant, known to inhibit clathrin vesicle formation, whereas the same mutant efficiently blocked internalization of low concentrations of EGF (16). Furthermore, knock-down of the clathrin-heavy chain by RNA interference (RNAi) significantly affected EGF internalization only when EGF was used at low concentrations (17). These data imply that under physiological conditions (low ligand concentrations and low/moderate expression levels of EGFR) EGFR is internalized mostly through the clathrin-dependent pathway, whereas under conditions of receptor overexpression and high ligand concentrations, clathrin-independent internalization is predominantly observed. It should be noted that in some cell types, the clathrin-dependent pathway appears to have sufficient capacity to internalize EGFR stimulated with high concentrations of EGF (18).

4. CLATHRIN-DEPENDENT INTERNALIZATION: ROLE OF KINASE ACTIVITY AND PHOSPHORYLATION OF EGFR

Endocytosis via clathrin-coated pits is the fastest and most highly regulated pathway of internalization by which plasma membrane proteins are taken up inside the cell. Numerous studies have detected an accumulation of EGF or EGFR in clathrin pits and vesicles (2, 19–22). These data, together with RNAi analysis, in which depletion of several proteins located in coated pits has been shown to inhibit EGFR endocytosis (23), strongly argue that clathrin-coated pits are the major physiological portal of EGFR internalization.

Binding of EGF to the receptor leads to activation of the tyrosine kinase in the cytoplasmic domain of the receptor (24). Inhibition of the kinase activity by mutations or specific chemical inhibitors demonstrated that EGFR kinase activity is required for rapid receptor endocytosis and, in particular, for recruitment of the receptors into coated pits (6, 25–28). Certainly, kinase-negative EGFR mutants and a wild-type EGFR inactivated by kinase inhibitors can be internalized and accumulate in endosomes; however, the specific rate of this internalization is significantly lower than that of the clathrin-dependent pathway and likely corresponds to a basal internalization of unoccupied EGFR (6). In the presence of a large amount of EGF, however, kinase-inactive, EGF-occupied receptors can accumulate in endosomes (29). Such accumulation is likely due to EGF-induced oligomerization of the receptors that slightly increases internalization and slows down recycling of endocytosed receptors back to the cell surface.

Kinase activity can be necessary for phosphorylation of cytoplasmic substrates and/or tyrosine phosphorylation of the receptor itself. Mutations of three or four major phosphorylation sites in the EGFR partially reduced internalization when expressed in mouse fibroblasts (7, 26). Surprisingly, mutation of Tyr1068 and Tyr1086, the major binding sites of Grb2 adaptor protein, was sufficient to strongly inhibit EGF internalization in porcine aortic endothelial (PAE) cells, thus implicating Grb2 in the internalization process (30). Furthermore, EGFR mutants, in which Grb2 binding sites are not present due to large carboxyl-terminal truncations, can be rapidly internalized in mouse fibroblasts (7) but are internalized very slowly in PAE cells (30). It is possible that truncations uncover cryptic internalization motifs leading to Tyr1068/86-independent endocytosis of truncated EGFR mutants. It is also possible that Grb2 can bind to truncated mutants by means other than pTyr1068/1086 in mouse fibroblastic but not PAE cells. Thus, a mutational analysis of EGFR endocytosis suggested that there might be multiple mechanisms of EGFR internalization through the clathrin-dependent pathway. Absence of such redundancy in PAE cells allowed revealing the importance of Grb2-dependent mechanisms. On the other hand, no clues to what the mechanisms of kinase-dependent but Grb2- and tyrosine phosphorylation-independent EGFR internalization could be are available.

Serine/threonine phosphorylation of EGFR has also been implicated in the regulation of receptor endocytosis. Protein kinase C-dependent phosphorylation of Thr654 results in decreased EGF endocytosis, presumably due to partial inhibition of the kinase activity of the receptor (*31*). Phosphorylation of Ser1046/1047 was proposed to be necessary for internalization (*32*). How exactly these and other phosphorylation sites contribute to the regulation of EGFR internalization is unknown, however. Recently, it was found that endocytosis of unoccupied EGFR can be induced by stress signals and chemical compounds that activate mitogen-activated protein kinase (MAPK)/p38 (*33–35*). It is possible that p38 participates in EGFR endocytosis by directly phosphorylating serines within the region between residues 1002-1020 of EGFR (*35*).

5. PROTEINS MEDIATING EGFR INTERNALIZATION THROUGH CLATHRIN-COATED PITS

In early studies, the interaction of EGFR with clathrin adaptor protein complex 2 (AP-2), a major cargo binding component of coated pits, was detected by co-immunoprecipitation and in vitro binding assays (*36, 37*). Functional studies, however, determined that neither the Y974RAL motif in the EGFR, which is responsible for binding to the µ2 subunit of AP2, nor the binding interface of this motif in the µ2 is essential for EGFR internalization (*38, 39*). Moreover, under certain experimental conditions, depletion of AP-2 by siRNA did not affect EGFR internalization, although there is disagreement among different reports regarding the effect of AP-2 depletion on EGFR endocytosis (*23, 40*). Nevertheless, while EGFR is capable of interaction with AP-2 and tyrosine phosphorylation of the β2 subunit of AP-2 (*41*), the role of EGFR:AP-2 interaction remains unknown. Interestingly, whereas EGF-receptor complexes are recruited into coated pits at 4oC, EGFR interaction with AP-2 requires 37°C, suggesting that this interaction occurs at the later stages of endocytosis.

The finding and characterization of proteins involved in the clathrin-dependent internalization of EGFR gained new life when RNAi methods were developed for the application in mammalian cells. The initial RNAi analysis revealed an essential and specific role of Grb2 in clathrin-dependent internalization of EGFR in PAE and human HeLa cells in agreement with the EGFR mutagenesis data obtained in PAE cells (*30*). siRNA experiments were also in agreement with the data obtained using dominant-negative mutants of Grb2 that have previously implicated this protein in regulation of EGFR trafficking in MDCK cells (*42*). Furthermore, Grb2-EGFR complexes were found in coated pits, and Grb2 was shown to be necessary for EGFR recruitment into coated pits (Fig. 4.1) (*21, 22, 30*). Depletion of Grb2 by siRNA caused a substantial (60–80%) decrease in the internalization rate in various cell lines (Sorkin A., unpublished observations), thus indicating that Grb2-dependent endocytosis is the major pathway of EGFR internalization.

Grb2 binds to EGFR via its SH2 domain and couples the receptor to proteins that are associated with the SH3 domains of Grb2. Several lines of evidence suggest that a Grb2-binding protein, Cbl, is critical for EGFR internalization. There are three members of the Cbl family in mammalian cells, c-Cbl, Cbl-b and Cbl-3; the first two species are capable of efficient binding to the SH3 domains of Grb2 (*43*). Cbl proteins function as E3 ubiquitin ligases for EGFR and other RTKs because Cbl contains a RING finger domain that can recruit E2 ubiquitin ligases (*44*). All three Cbls possess a tyrosine-kinase binding domain that can directly bind to phosphorylated Tyr1045 of EGFR (*44*). EGF-induced translocation of c-Cbl to clathrin-coated pits has been demonstrated (*45*), and overexpression of several c-Cbl mutants abrogated EGFR internalization (*16, 46*).

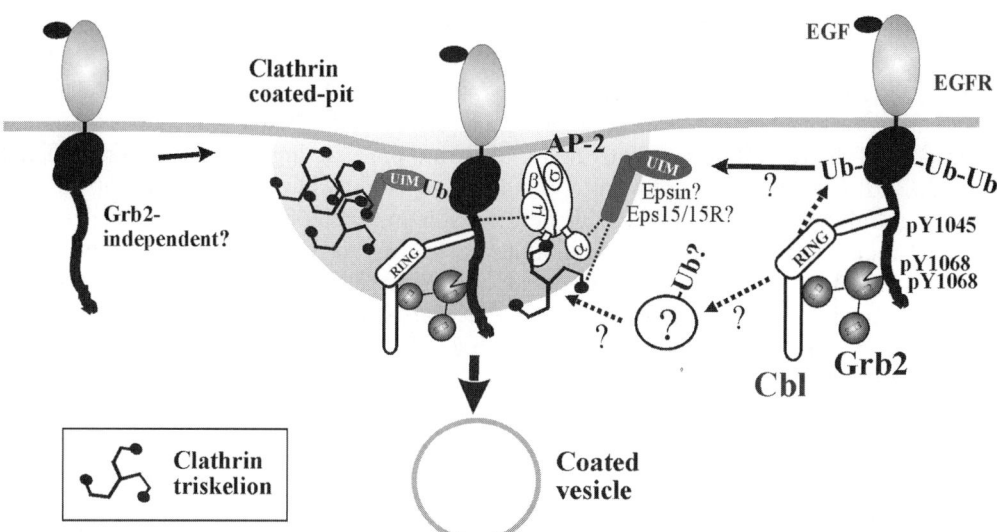

Fig. 4.1. **Putative mechanisms of EGFR internalization via clathrin-coated pits.** EGF binding leads to EGFR phosphorylation and recruitment of Grb2-Cbl complexes, which promotes EGFR ubiquitination. Ubiquitinated EGFR can be recognized by ubiquitin-inteacting motifs (UIMs) of epsin, Eps15 and Eps15R that are associated with AP-2 and clathrin heavy chain (component of *clathrin triskelion*) and located in coated pits. Alternatively, the EGFR-Grb2-Cbl complex can interact with an unknown protein ("?") that, in turn, interacts with clathrin or a clathrin-associated protein. This alternative adaptor may be ubiquitinated by Cbl. In the coated pit, EGFR can interact with the μ2 subunit of AP-2. EGFR-loaded pits that were either pre-existing or formed in response to EGFR activation, invaginate and constrict, leading to budding off a coated vesicle.

Importantly, chimeric proteins consisting of Grb2 SH2 domain and c-Cbl could rescue EGFR endocytosis in Grb2-depleted cells, confirming the function of Cbl downstream of Grb2 (*47*). Recently, the involvement of Cbl in the internalization step was directly demonstrated using siRNAs targeting both c-Cbl and Cbl-b (*48*). Interestingly, direct Cbl binding to EGFR pTyr1045 appears to play a minor role, if any, in clathrin-mediated internalization of EGR, whereas indirect interaction of Cbl with EGFR through Grb2 is critical (*16*). Studies in embryonic fibroblast cells derived from c-Cbl knockout mice revealed that c-Cbl is not necessary for EGF internalization (*49*). A significant amount of Cbl-b was present is these cells and could be sufficient for EGFR internalization. Altogether, the experimental data strongly suggest that Cbl is important for EGFR internalization and that both the Grb2 binding sites and an intact RING domain are essential for this Cbl function.

Because Cbl ubiquitinates EGFR, the logical hypothesis was that Cbl-mediated ubiquitination of EGFR is necessary for receptor internalization. An EGFR mutant, however, which lacks Tyr1045 and is weakly ubiquitinated, displayed a high rate of clathrin-dependent endocytosis (*16*). Recently, the ubiquitination sites in the EGFR kinase domain were mapped (*48*). Mutation of these sites did not affect EGFR internalization, confirming that EGFR ubiquitination is not essential for internalization. Because these EGFR mutants remained partially ubiquitinated (10–20% of wild-type EGFR ubiquitination), however, it is possible that this residual ubiquitination was sufficient to support internalization. Alternatively, a RING domain of Cbl is necessary for ubiquitination of another protein or an interaction with a protein other than an E2 ligase.

One of the fundamental questions in the field of clathrin-mediated endocytosis is whether ligand-induced internalization involves formation of new coated pits that are specialized for endocytosis of an activated receptor like EGFR. Early studies demonstrated co-localization of EGF and several other ligands in the same coated pit, thus arguing for the model of the recruitment of activated EGFR into pre-existing, non-specialized coated pits (20, 50). More recently, however, a number of studies have suggested that there is only a partial co-localization of EGFR and transferrin receptors in the same coated pits, and that there is a subset of coated pits that are formed in response to EGFR activation (22, 51, 52). These studies have proposed a model of an EGFR-specialized coated pit. The important conceptual aspect of this model is that recruitment of EGFR to these coated pits is coupled with the assembly of the coat, which would involve specific adaptor(s) that can bind both the receptor and clathrin coat. Epsin, Eps15 and Eps15R, proteins capable of binding to both the ubiquitin moieties and clathrin, are the candidates for being such adaptors. RNAi knock-down of these proteins, however, did not result in specific inhibition of clathrin-dependent EGFR internalization (17, 23). In light of the possibility that EGFR ubiquitination is not necessary for internalization, future research should focus on the search for a different class of proteins that can mediate internalization of the EGFR-Grb2-Cbl complex. An example of a potential candidate to be such an adaptor is intersectin, a protein that is present in clathrin-coated pits, capable of interaction with Cbl and shown to be necessary for internalization and/or degradation of EGFR (53). Another protein that can bind to Cbl and has been implicated in EGFR internalization is an SH3 domain adaptor CIN85 (54, 55). This protein is not detected in coated pits, however, and may be involved in post-endocytic trafficking of EGFR rather than internalization (56).

6. CLATHRIN-INDEPENDENT MECHANISMS OF EGFR INTERNALIZATION

Two types of clathrin-independent internalization of EGFR have been proposed: (i) pinocytosis-like endocytosis associated with actin cytoskeleton dynamics and (ii) lipid raft/caveolae dependent endocytosis. Electron microscopy studies demonstrated that EGF treatment causes actin rearrangement leading to dramatic plasma membrane ruffling and formation of micro- and macropinocytic vesicles containing EGF (3, 4). The formation of large vesicular structures containing EGFR in cells treated with high concentrations of EGF was also observed by fluorescence microscopy (57). Recently, dorsal ruffles were implicated in the formation of a heterogeneous vesicular-tubular endocytic compartment containing EGF and EGFR in several types of cells (58). The ruffle-associated pathway required the activity of the EGFR kinase, PI3 kinase and dynamin (58). Because measurements of the endocytic rates of ruffle-mediated endocytosis have not been performed, it is difficult to estimate the relative contribution of this pathway in the overall endocytosis of EGFR.

Endocytosis of EGFR involving cholesterol-rich lipid rafts and/or caveolae was demonstrated by Sigismund and co-workers (17). These authors observed cholesterol-dependent internalization under conditions of high EGFR occupancy in HeLa cells and proposed that EGFR ubiquitination is important for this internalization. In contrast, another study performed using HeLa cells demonstrated that cholesterol-rich rafts and caveolae play no role in EGFR endocytosis, and that the clathrin pathway has the major role under conditions of all occupancies of surface EGFR (18). One explanation of this discrepancy could be that the localization of EGFR in the caveolae and the contribution of lipid-raft/caveolae pathways is cell-specific and may even vary in different clones of HeLa cells. Such variability, together with the lack of specific inhibitors, makes it difficult to elucidate the mechanisms and evaluate the importance of clathrin-independent pathways of EGFR internalization.

7. PATHWAYS OF INTERNALIZED EGFR THROUGH THE ENDOSOMAL COMPARTMENT

After formation of a clathrin-coated vesicle, the clathrin coat rapidly dissociates from the vesicle in order for the vesicle to fuse with early endosomes. Early endosomes are morphologically heterogeneous compartments consisting of vesicular and tubular membranes and typically located at the periphery of the cell (*59–62*). EGF and EGFR accumulate in the early endosomal compartment after 2-5 minutes of continuous endocytosis. Early endosomes are a highly dynamic compartment and tend to fuse with each other, which leads to the formation of larger endosomes (reviewed in *63, 64*). These larger endosomes can be referred to as "intermediate" endosomes based on their size and time of delivery of cargo, or "sorting" endosomes according to their function. The pH in early and intermediate endosomes is mildly acidic (6.0-6.5). Importantly, this pH is not sufficient for significant dissociation of EGF-receptor complexes, and most of these complexes remain intact in endosomes (*65*). Consequently, receptors in endosomes remain dimerized, tyrosine phosphorylated, and associated with Grb2, Shc, and Cbl (*66–68*).

Fusion of early endosomes is a part of an endosome maturation process, which involves a gradual change of the composition and morphology of early endosomes to that of multivesicular bodies (MVBs) and late endosomes. Rab5 and EEA.1 protein complexes appear to play a key role in the early endosome fusion. Rab5 has been suggested to play a specific role in EGF receptor endocytosis (*69*). SiRNA knock-down of all three forms of Rab5, however, revealed that these proteins are also necessary for endocytosis of other receptors, such as the transferrin receptor (*23*). It is likely that the effects of Rab5 inhibition on internalization are due to the function of Rab5 during the fusion of primary endocytic vesicles with early endosomes.

In parallel with the endosome maturation process, receptors rapidly recycle back from early/intermediate endosomes to the cell surface. Since EGF does not significantly dissociate from the receptor, an intact EGF-receptor complex is recycled (*70*). When EGFR is occupied by another ligand, transforming growth factor (TGF), EGFR becomes rapidly inactivated in early endosomes because TGF-EGFR complexes are highly sensitive to an acidic pH and, therefore, readily dissociate in endosomes (*71*). This dissociation results in a substantially larger pool of recycled EGFR, which are mainly unoccupied, as opposed to this pool in the case of EGF-EGFR complexes.

No specific recycling signal has been identified in the EGFR, and therefore it is assumed that recycling is the default pathway of receptors from endosomes. In other words, receptors can be recycled unless they are retained from recycling by the specific interactions in sorting endosomes. Such interactions represent a part of a sorting process that has been recently analyzed in a large number of studies (reviewed in *72*).

In early studies, it was noticed that after 15–20 minutes of continuous EGF-induced endocytosis, EGF and EGFR accumulate in the intralumenal membranes of MVB that are mostly located in the perinuclear area of the cell (*5, 61, 62, 73*). A recent electron microscopy study, which used serial sectioning and tomography, demonstrated that these structures represent vesicles that are not connected to the limiting membrane of MVB (*74*). Therefore, EGFR incorporated into intralumenal membranes cannot recycle. MVBs have tubular extensions that are thought to be responsible for recycling of receptors that are not recruited into intralumenal vesicles (*59, 75*). Thus, recycling continues in MVB, albeit at lower rates than from early endosomes. This recycling is also highly temperature-dependent in comparison to rapid recycling from early endosomes (*70*).

8. MOLECULAR MECHANISMS OF EGFR SORTING IN MVB

Genetic analysis in yeast helped to identify sorting machineries (ESCRT complexes) in MVB that are responsible for the formation of internal vesicles and recruitment of cargo like EGFR into these vesicles. The following model of EGFR sorting in MVB is widely accepted

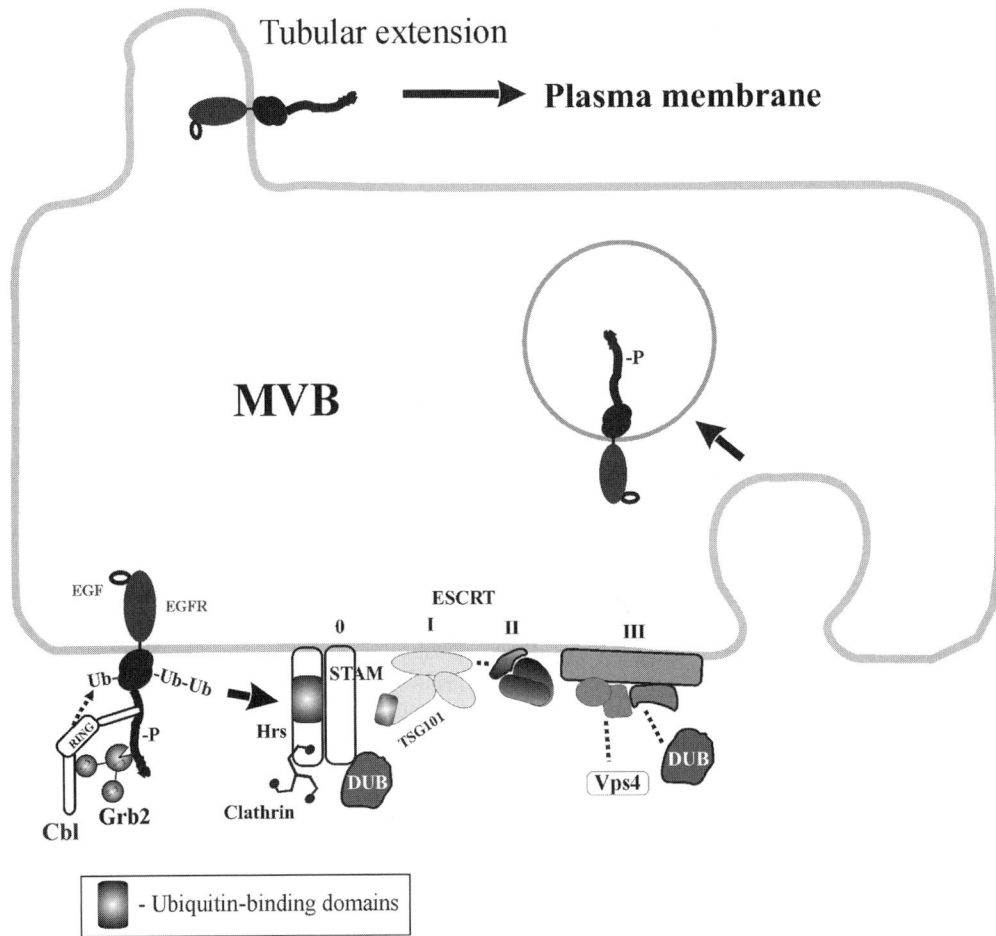

Fig. 4.2. Putative mechanisms of EGFR sorting in MVB. Ubiquitinated EGFR bind to the UIM domain of Hrs (ESCRT0 complex) and retained in the Hrs-STAM microdomains. Formation of these domains is facilitated by recruitment of clathrin to Hrs. ESCRTI, II and III complexes on the membrane of MVB participate in EGFR retention in the MVB and incorporation into inward forming vesicles. Receptors, that are not ubiquitinated, can be recycled back to the plasma membrane through the tubular extensions of the limiting membrane of MVB. *DUB*, deubiquitination enzyme.

(Fig. 4.2). Extensive EGFR ubiquitination was shown to be essential for lysosomal targeting of the receptor (*48*). Such ubiquitination requires direct binding of Cbl to pTyr1045 of the EGFR. Ubiquitinated EGFR is thought to interact with the ubiquitin-binding domain of Hrs that is associated with another protein, STAM1/2 (ESCRT0 complex). EGFR-Hrs interaction was shown using a co-immunoprecipitation assay (*17*). Hrs recruits clathrin that forms flat lattices, which presumably has a role in the formation of "Hrs microdomains". It is hypothesized that ubiquitinated EGFR can be sequentially "handed over" to ESCRTI, II and III complexes, although binding of EGFR to these complexes has not been demonstrated and the exact mechanism of this process is not understood (*72*). It is possible that the relative concentration of ESCRTI, II and III complexes increases whereas the concentration of ESCRT0 complex decreases during endosomes maturation, which may lead to a preferential association of EGFR with the former complexes as the MVB matures. Components of

ESCRTI and ESCRTIII complexes, TSG101 and hVps24, respectively, have been shown to be necessary for EGFR degradation (*76–80*). Although structural studies demonstrated the interaction of yeast ESCRTI and II complexes (*81*), the requirement of ESCRTII complex for EGFR sorting has not been confirmed using RNAi (*80*). ESCRTIII is thought to promote inward invagination of the limiting endosomal membrane, which is facilitated by oligomerization of CHMP (a component of ESCRTIII), leading to formation of a lattice-like structure (*81*). Membrane invagination results in the formation of internal vesicles containing trapped EGFR. It is proposed that ubiquitinated cargo is deubiquitinated prior to sorting into internal vesicles to prevent degradation of ubiquitin (*72*). EGFR deubiquitination during sorting in MVB, however, has not been directly demonstrated.

The last stage of EGFR sorting involves the fusion of MVBs with primary lysosomal vesicles that contain proteolytic enzymes, which leads to rapid proteolysis of intralumenal components of MVBs (*61*). Degradation of EGF and EGFR is blocked by lysosomal inhibitors (*1, 11*). Inhibitors of proteosome also have an effect on EGFR degradation (*82*). These inhibitors, however, may affect activity of lysosomal enzymes, turnover of ESCRT proteins and/or reduce the ubiquitin pool in the cell. Therefore, the effects of proteosomal inhibitors on EGFR degradation are likely indirect and do not imply that internalized EGFR is degraded by the proteosome.

Overall, whereas the model of EGFR sorting to lysosomes presented in Fig. 4.2 is widely accepted, a number of features of the model have been extrapolated from the model of the sorting process in yeast cells and have not been demonstrated experimentally in the case of EGFR sorting. RNAi analysis of ESCRT proteins should be interpreted with caution because depletion of these proteins has pleiotropic effects on the morphology of endosomes and many trafficking pathways through endosomes (*83, 84*). Furthermore, most of the studies of EGFR sorting and degradation were performed using non-physiological, high concentrations of EGF. Thus, it remains to be demonstrated that EGFR ubiquitination and ESCRT complexes are involved in the lysosomal targeting of the receptor in the presence of physiological concentrations of EGF. It is also unclear what the role is of several sequence motifs of EGFR that have been implicated in EGFR degradation, such as di-leicine motifs (*41, 85*). The components of the endocytic machinery interacting with these motifs remain unknown. Likewise, proteins other than ESCRT complexes, such sorting nexins and annexin 1, have been specifically implicated in EGFR sorting (*86, 87*). The exact role of these proteins in sorting process is unknown.

9. PROTEINS MODULATING ENDOCYTOSIS AND SORTING OF EGFR

In the previous sections, I described the mechanisms and the proteins that are thought to directly mediate internalization and degradation of activated EGFR. Recently, a number of proteins were identified that can modulate the rate of EGF-induced down-regulation of EGFR (Fig. 4.3). The central components of the down-regulation process are the Cbl proteins that ubiquitinate EGFR. Therefore, Cbls are an important node in the web of processes controlling EGFR trafficking, and modification of Cbl activity could yield a considerable change in EGFR down-regulation and signaling (*88*). For example, the Sprouty 2 protein is capable of binding to the RING and tyrosine kinase binding domains of Cbl, and it is proposed that such binding results in inhibition of Cbl activity, reduced EGFR ubiquitination and slow degradation (*89, 90*). Sprouty 2, however, also binds Grb2 and several other proteins downstream of EGFR, and it is possible that the mechanisms of Sprouty 2 effects are multifaceted (*91*). The effects of knock-out or knock-down of Sprouty 2 on EGFR degradation have not been examined in mammalian cells, and whether endogenous Sprouty2 is involved in the regulation of EGFR endocytosis is unknown.

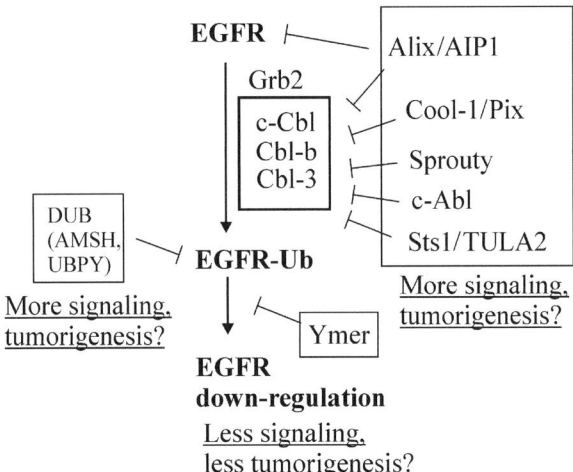

Fig. 4.3. **Putative modulators of EGFR down-regulation.** Grb2 and Cbl proteins are the key "positive" mediators of EGFR endocytosis and down-regulation. Putative modulators of EGFR down-regulation that inhibit Cbl or impose their effects at other steps of EGFR down-regulation are shown in boxes. Possible consequences of overexpression of these modulators for EGFR signal transduction are underlined.

An effector and a regulator of a small GTPase Cdc42, Cool-1, also binds to Cbl and inhibits its ubiquitination activity, thus inhibiting EGFR internalization and degradation (92). The EGFR-modulating function of Cool-1, however, was demonstrated only in the presence of v-Src (92). A number of other proteins that are capable of binding to Cbl and/or EGFR have been implicated in the regulation of EGFR internalization and degradation. Such proteins are Alix (93), c-Abl tyrosine kinase (94), Sts1/TULA2 (95), Lrig-1 (96), and supressors of cytokine signaling SOCS4/5 (97) (Fig. 4.3). The mechanisms of endocytosis-modulating effects of these proteins are not well understood. A novel tyrosine phosphorylation substrate of EGFR, Yme1, has recently been identified and shown to have an inhibitory effect on EGFR down-regulation (98). In general, most of the conclusions about the modulatory role of these proteins were obtained using their overexpression. There is a deficiency of experiments in cells, in which these proteins were knocked-out or depleted by siRNA.

An important family of proteins that regulates EGFR endocytosis and degradation are deubiquitination enzymes (DUBs) (99). Two DUBs have been implicated in the process of EGFR degradation, as well as regulation of ESCRT complexes. AMSH is the JAMM domain-containing DUB that is associated with STAM in endosomes and that can regulate EGFR degradation (Fig. 4.3) (100). UBPY is a DUB that was also found in endosomes and implicated in EGFR deubiquitination, though this enzyme appears to have wider substrate specificity (80, 101–103). Because the effects of siRNA knock-down of both AMSH and UBPY on EGFR degradation were either partial or absent, it is likely that there are other DUBs that can deubiquitinate EGFR.

ACKNOWLEDGMENTS

I thank Dr. Jason Duex and Ms. Melissa Adams for critical reading of the manuscript. This work was supported by NCI grant CA08915 and ACS grant RSG-00-247-04-CSM.

REFERENCES

1. Carpenter G, Cohen S. ^{125}I-Labeled human epidermal growth factor: binding internalization, and degradation in human fibroblasts. J. Cell Biol. 1976; 71:159-171.
2. Gorden P, Carpentier J-L, Cohen S, Orci L. Epidermal growth factor: Morphological demonstration of binding internalization and lydosomal association in human fibroblasts. Proc.Nat. Acad. Sci. USA 1978; 75:5025-5029.
3. Chinkers M, McKanna JA, Cohen S. Rapid induction of morphological changes in human carcinoma cells A-431 by epidermal growth factor. J. Cell Biol. 1979; 83:260-265.
4. Haigler HT, McKanna JA, Cohen S. Direct visualization of the binding and internalization of a ferritin conjugate of epidermal growth factor in human carcinoma cells A431. J. Cell Biol. 1979; 81:382-395.
5. McKanna JA, Haigler HT, Cohen S. Hormone receptor topology and dynamics: morphological analysis using ferritin-labeled epidermal growth factor. Proc Natl Acad Sci U S A 1979; 76:5689-93.
6. Wiley HS, Herbst JJ, Walsh BJ, Lauffenberger DA, Rosenfeld MG, Gill GN. The role of Tyrosine Kinase Activity in Endocytosis, Compartmentalization and Down-regulation of the Epidermal Growth Factor Receptor. J. Biol. Chem. 1991; 266:11083-11094.
7. Chang C-P, Lazar CS, Walsh BJ, et al. Ligand-induced internalization of the epidermal growth factor receptor is mediated by multiple endocytic codes analogous to the tyrosine motif found in constitutively internalized receptors. J. Biol. Chem. 1993; 268:19312-19320.
8. Resat H, Ewald JA, Dixon DA, Wiley HS. An integrated model of epidermal growth factor receptor trafficking and signal transduction. Biophys J 2003; 85:730-43.
9. Burke PM, Wiley HS. Human mammary epithelial cells rapidly exchange empty EGFR between surface and intracellular pools. J Cell Physiol 1999; 180:448-60.
10. Beguinot L, Lyall RM, Willingham MC, Pastan I. Down-regulation of the epidermal growth factor receptor in KB cells is due to receptor internalization and subsequent degradation in lysosomes. Proc. Natl. Acad. Sci. USA 1984; 81:2384-8.
11. Stoscheck CM, Carpenter G. "Down-regulation" of EGF receptors: Direct demonstration of receptor degradation in human fibroblasts. J. Cell Biol. 1984; 98:1048-1053.
12. Stoscheck CM, Carpenter G. Characterization of the metabolic turnover of epidermal growth factor receptor protein in A-431 cells. J. Cell Physiology 1984; 120:296-302.
13. Wells A, Welsh JB, Lazar CS, Wiley HS, Gill GN, Rosenfeld MG. Ligand-Induced Transformation By a Noninternalizing Epidermal Growth Factor Receptor. Science 1990; 247:962-964.
14. Lund KA, Opresko LK, Strarbuck C, Walsh BJ, Wiley HS. Quantitative analysis of the endocytic system involved in hormone-induced receptor internalization. J. Biol. Chem. 1990; 265:15713-13723.
15. Wiley HS. Anomalous Binding of Epidermal Growth Factor to A431 Cells Is Due to the Effect of High Receptor Densities and a Saturable Endocytic System. J. Cell Biol. 1988; 107:801-810.
16. Jiang X, Sorkin A. Epidermal growth factor receptor internalization through clathrin-coated pits requires Cbl RING finger and proline-rich domains but not receptor polyubiquitylation. Traffic 2003; 4:529-43.
17. Sigismund S, Woelk T, Puri C, et al. From the Cover: Clathrin-independent endocytosis of ubiquitinated cargos. Proc Natl Acad Sci U S A 2005; 102:2760-5.
18. Kazazic M, Roepstorff K, Johannessen LE, et al. EGF-induced activation of the EGF receptor does not trigger mobilization of caveolae. Traffic 2006; 7:1518-27.
19. Hanover JA, Willingham MC, Pastan I. Kinetics of transit of transferrin and epidermal growth factor through clathrin-coated membranes. Cell 1984; 39:283-293.
20. Carpentier J-L, Gorden P, Anderson RGW, Brown MS, Cohen S, Orci L. Co-localization of ^{125}I-epidermal growth factor and ferritin-low density lipoprotein in coated pits: A quantitative electron microscopic study in normal and mutant human fibroblasts. J. Cell Biol. 1982; 95:73-77.
21. Stang E, Blystad FD, Kazazic M, et al. Cbl-Dependent Ubiquitination is Required for Progression of EGF Receptors into Clathrin-coated Pits. Mol Biol Cell 2004.
22. Johannessen LE, Pedersen NM, Pedersen KW, Madshus IH, Stang E. Activation of the epidermal growth factor (EGF) receptor induces formation of EGF receptor- and grb2-containing clathrin-coated pits. Mol Cell Biol 2006; 26:389-401.
23. Huang F, Khvorova A, Marshall W, Sorkin A. Analysis of clathrin-mediated endocytosis of epidermal growth factor receptor by RNA interference. J Biol Chem 2004; 279:16657-61.

24. Schlessinger J. Cell signaling by receptor tyrosine kinases. Cell 2000; 103:211-25.
25. Chen WS, Lazar CS, Lund KA, et al. Functional Independence of the Epidermal Growth Factor Receptor From a Domain Required For Ligand-Induced Internalization and Calcium Regulation. Cell 1989; 59:33-43.
26. Sorkin A, Waters CM, Overholser KA, Carpenter G. Multiple autophosphorylation site mutations of the epidermal growth factor receptor. J. Biol. Chem. 1991; 266:8355-8362.
27. Lamaze C, Schmid SL. Recruitment of Epidermal Growth Factor Receptors into Coated Pits Requires Their Activated Tyrosine Kinase. J. Cell Biol. 1995; 129:47-54.
28. Sorkina T, Huang F, Beguinot L, Sorkin A. Effect of tyrosine kinase inhibitors on clathrin-coated pit recruitment and internalization of epidermal growth factor receptor. J Biol Chem 2002; 277:27433-41.
29. Honegger AM, Dull TJ, Felder S, et al. Point Mutation at the ATP Binding Site of EGF Receptor Abolishes Protein-Tyrosine Kinase Activity and Alters Cellular Routing. Cell 1987; 51:199-209.
30. Jiang X, Huang F, Marusyk A, Sorkin A. Grb2 Regulates Internalization of EGF Receptors through Clathrin-coated Pits. Mol Biol Cell 2003; 14:858-70.
31. Lund KA, Lazar CS, Chen WS, et al. Phosphorylation of the Epidermal Growth Factor Receptor at Threonine 654 Inhibits Ligand-induced Internalization and Down-regulation. J. Biol. Chem. 1990; 265:20517-20523.
32. Countaway JL, Nairn AC, Davis RJ. Mechanism of Desensitization of the Epidermal Growth Factor Receptor Protein-Tyrosine Kinase. J. Biol. Chem. 1992; 267:1129-1140.
33. Frey MR, Dise RS, Edelblum KL, Polk DB. p38 kinase regulates epidermal growth factor receptor downregulation and cellular migration. Embo J 2006; 25:5683-92.
34. Vergarajauregui S, San Miguel A, Puertollano R. Activation of p38 mitogen-activated protein kinase promotes epidermal growth factor receptor internalization. Traffic 2006; 7:686-98.
35. Zwang Y, Yarden Y. p38 MAP kinase mediates stress-induced internalization of EGFR: implications for cancer chemotherapy. Embo J 2006; 25:4195-206.
36. Sorkin A, Carpenter G. Interaction of activated EGF receptors with coated pit adaptins. Science 1993; 261:612-615.
37. Nesterov A, Kurten RC, Gill GN. Association of Epidermal Growth Factor Receptors with Coated Pit Adaptins via a Tyrosine Phosphorylation-regulated Mechanism. J. Biol. Chem. 1995; 270:6320-6327.
38. Nesterov A, Carter RE, Sorkina T, Gill GN, Sorkin A. Inhibition of the receptor-binding function of clathrin adaptor protein AP-2 by dominant-negative mutant mu2 subunit and its effects on endocytosis. Embo J 1999; 18:2489-99.
39. Sorkin A, Mazzotti M, Sorkina T, Scotto L, Beguinot L. Epidermal growth factor interaction with clathrin adaptors is mediated by the Tyr974-containing internalization motif. J. Biol. Chem. 1996; 271:13377-13384.
40. Motley A, Bright NA, Seaman MN, Robinson MS. Clathrin-mediated endocytosis in AP-2-depleted cells. J Cell Biol 2003; 162:909-918.
41. Huang F, Jiang X, Sorkin A. Tyrosine phosphorylation of the beta2 subunit of clathrin adaptor complex AP-2 reveals the role of a di-leucine motif in the epidermal growth factor receptor trafficking. J Biol Chem 2003; 278:43411-7.
42. Wang Z, Moran MF. Requirement for the adapter protein GRB2 in EGF receptor endocytosis. Science 1996; 272:1935-9.
43. Thien CB, Langdon WY. Cbl: many adaptations to regulate protein tyrosine kinases. Nat Rev Mol Cell Biol 2001; 2:294-307.
44. Levkowitz G, Waterman H, Ettenberg SA, et al. Ubiquitin ligase activity and tyrosine phosphorylation underlie suppression of growth factor signaling by c-Cbl/Sli-1 [In Process Citation]. Mol Cell 1999; 4:1029-40.
45. de Melker AA, van der Horst G, Calafat J, Jansen H, Borst J. c-Cbl ubiquitinates the EGF receptor at the plasma membrane and remains receptor associated throughout the endocytic route. J Cell Sci 2001; 114:2167-78.
46. Thien CB, Walker F, Langdon WY. RING finger mutations that abolish c-Cbl-directed polyubiquitination and downregulation of the EGF receptor are insufficient for cell transformation. Mol Cell 2001; 7:355-65.
47. Huang F, Sorkin A. Growth Factor Receptor Binding Protein 2-mediated Recruitment of the RING Domain of Cbl to the Epidermal Growth Factor Receptor Is Essential and Sufficient to Support Receptor Endocytosis. Mol Biol Cell 2005; 16:1268-81.

48. Huang F, Kirkpatrick D, Jiang X, Gygi S, Sorkin A. Differential regulation of EGF receptor internalization and degradation by multiubiquitination within the kinase domain. Mol Cell 2006; 21:737-48.
49. Duan L, Miura Y, Dimri M, et al. Cbl-mediated ubiquitinylation is required for lysosomal sorting of epidermal growth factor receptor but is dispensable for endocytosis. J Biol Chem 2003; 278: 28950-60.
50. Hanover JA, Beguinot L, Willingham MC, Pastan IH. Transit of receptors for epidermal growth factor and transferrin through clathrin-coated pits. Analysis of the kinetics of receptor entry. Journal of Biological Chemistry 1985; 260:15938-45.
51. Tsao PI, von Zastrow M. Type-specific sorting of G protein-coupled receptors after endocytosis. Journal of Biological Chemistry 2000; 275:11130-11140.
52. Confalonieri S, Salcini AE, Puri C, Tacchetti C, Di Fiore PP. Tyrosine phosphorylation of Eps15 is required for ligand-regulated, but not constitutive, endocytosis. J Cell Biol 2000; 150:905-12.
53. Martin NP, Mohney RP, Dunn S, Das M, Scappini E, O'Bryan JP. Intersectin regulates epidermal growth factor receptor endocytosis, ubiquitylation, and signaling. Mol Pharmacol 2006; 70:1643-53.
54. Soubeyran P, Kowanetz K, Szymkiewicz I, Langdon WY, Dikic I. Cbl-CIN85-endophilin complex mediates ligand-induced downregulation of EGF receptors. Nature 2002; 416:183-7.
55. Szymkiewicz I, Kowanetz K, Soubeyran P, Dinarina A, Lipkowitz S, Dikic I. CIN85 participates in Cbl-b-mediated downregulation of receptor tyrosine kinases. J Biol Chem 2002.
56. Haglund K, Shimokawa N, Szymkiewicz I, Dikic I. Cbl-directed monoubiquitination of CIN85 is involved in regulation of ligand-induced degradation of EGF receptors. Proc Natl Acad Sci U S A 2002; 99:12191-6.
57. Yamazaki T, Zaal K, Hailey D, Presley J, Lippincott-Schwartz J, Samelson LE. Role of Grb2 in EGF-stimulated EGFR internalization. J Cell Sci 2002; 115:1791-1802.
58. Orth JD, Krueger EW, Weller SG, McNiven MA. A novel endocytic mechanism of epidermal growth factor receptor sequestration and internalization. Cancer Res 2006; 66:3603-10.
59. Hopkins CR, Trowbridge IS. Internalization and processing of transferrin and the transferrin receptor in human carcinoma A-431 cells. J. Cell Biol. 1983; 97:508-521.
60. Hopkins CR, Miller K, Beardmore JM. Receptor-mediated endocytosis of transferrin and epidermal growth factor receptors: a comparison of constitutive and ligand-induced uptake. Journal of Cell Science - Supplement 1985; 3:173-86.
61. Miller K, Beardmore J, Kanety H, Schlessinger J, Hopkins CR. Localization of epidermal growth factor (EGF) receptor within the endosome of EGF-stimulated epidermoid carcinoma (A431) cells. J. Cell Biol. 1986; 102:500-509.
62. Dunn WA, Hubbard AC. Receptor-mediated endocytosis of epidermal growth factor by hepatocytes in the perfused rat liver: ligand and receptor dynamics. J. Cell Biol. 1984; 98:2148-2159.
63. Gruenberg J, Maxfield FR. Membrane transport in the endocytic pathway. Curr Opin Cell Biol 1995; 7:552-63.
64. Maxfield FR, McGraw TE. Endocytic recycling. Nat Rev Mol Cell Biol 2004; 5:121-32.
65. Sorkin A, Teslenko L, Nikolsky N. The endocytosis of epidermal growth factor in A431 cells: a pH of microenvironment and the dynamics of receptor complexes dissociation. Exp. Cell Res. 1988; 175:192-205.
66. Galperin E, Verkhusha VV, Sorkin A. Three-chromophore FRET micrsocopy to analyze multiprotein interactions in living cells. Nature Methods 2004; 1:209-217.
67. Di Gugliemo GM, Baass PC, Ou W-J, Posner B, Bergeron JJM. Compartmentalization of SHC, GRB2 and mSOS, and hyperphosphorylation of Raf-1 by EGF but not insulin in liver parenchyma. EMBO J. 1994; 13:4269-4277.
68. Sorkin A, Carpenter G. Dimerization of internalized growth factor receptors. J. Biol. Chem. 1991; 266:23453-23460.
69. Barbieri MA, Roberts RL, Gumusboga A, et al. Epidermal growth factor and membrane trafficking. EGF receptor activation of endocytosis requires Rab5a. J Cell Biol 2000; 151:539-50.
70. Sorkin A, Krolenko S, Kudrjavtceva N, et al. Recycling of epidermal growth factor-receptor complexes in A431 cells: identification of dual pathways. J. Cell Biology 1991; 112:55-63.
71. French AR, Tadaki DK, S.K. N, Lauffenberger DA. Intracellular trafficking of epidermal growth factor family ligands is directly influenced by the pH sensitivity of the receptor/ligand interaction. J. Biol. Chem. 1995; 270:4334-4340.
72. Slagsvold T, Pattni K, Malerod L, Stenmark H. Endosomal and non-endosomal functions of ESCRT proteins. Trends Cell Biol 2006; 16:317-26.

73. Carpentier JL, White MF, Orci L, Kahn CR. Direct visualization of the phosphorylated epidermal growth factor receptor during its internalization in A-431 cells. J. Cell Biol. 1987; 105:2751-2762.
74. Murk JL, Humbel BM, Ziese U, et al. Endosomal compartmentalization in three dimensions: implications for membrane fusion. Proc Natl Acad Sci U S A 2003; 100:13332-7.
75. Hopkins CR. Selective membrane protein trafficking: vectorial flow and filter [see comments]. Trends in Biochemical Sciences 1992; 17:27-32.
76. Babst M, Odorizzi G, Estepa EJ, Emr SD. Mammalian tumor susceptibility gene 101 (TSG101) and the yeast homologue, Vps23p, both function in late endosomal trafficking. Traffic 2000; 1:248-58.
77. Bishop N, Horman A, Woodman P. Mammalian class E vps proteins recognize ubiquitin and act in the removal of endosomal protein-ubiquitin conjugates. J Cell Biol 2002; 157:91-102.
78. Bache KG, Brech A, Mehlum A, Stenmark H. Hrs regulates multivesicular body formation via ESCRT recruitment to endosomes. J Cell Biol 2003; 162:435-42.
79. Bache KG, Stuffers S, Malerod L, et al. The ESCRT-III subunit hVps24 is required for degradation but not silencing of the epidermal growth factor receptor. Mol Biol Cell 2006; 17:2513-23.
80. Bowers K, Piper SC, Edeling MA, et al. Degradation of endocytosed epidermal growth factor and virally ubiquitinated major histocompatibility complex class I is independent of mammalian ESCRTII. J Biol Chem 2006; 281:5094-105.
81. Hurley JH, Emr SD. The ESCRT complexes: structure and mechanism of a membrane-trafficking network. Annu Rev Biophys Biomol Struct 2006; 35:277-98.
82. Longva KE, Blystad FD, Stang E, Larsen AM, Johannessen LE, Madshus IH. Ubiquitination and proteasomal activity is required for transport of the EGF receptor to inner membranes of multivesicular bodies. J Cell Biol 2002; 156:843-54.
83. Doyotte A, Russell MR, Hopkins CR, Woodman PG. Depletion of TSG101 forms a mammalian "Class E" compartment: a multicisternal early endosome with multiple sorting defects. J Cell Sci 2005; 118:3003-17.
84. Razi M, Futter CE. Distinct roles for Tsg101 and Hrs in multivesicular body formation and inward vesiculation. Mol Biol Cell 2006; 17:3469-83.
85. Tsacoumangos A, Kil SJ, Ma L, Sonnichsen FD, Carlin C. A novel dileucine lysosomal-sorting-signal mediates intracellular EGF-receptor retention independently of protein ubiquitylation. J Cell Sci 2005; 118:3959-71.
86. Kurten RC, Cadena DL, Gill GN. Enhanced degradation of EGF receptors by a sorting nexin, SNX-1. Science 1996; 272:1008-1010.
87. White IJ, Bailey LM, Aghakhani MR, Moss SE, Futter CE. EGF stimulates annexin 1-dependent inward vesiculation in a multivesicular endosome subpopulation. Embo J 2006; 25:1-12.
88. Rubin C, Gur G, Yarden Y. Negative regulation of receptor tyrosine kinases: unexpected links to c-Cbl and receptor ubiquitylation. Cell Res 2005; 15:66-71.
89. Wong ES, Fong CW, Lim J, et al. Sprouty2 attenuates epidermal growth factor receptor ubiquitylation and endocytosis, and consequently enhances Ras/ERK signalling. Embo J 2002; 21:4796-808.
90. Rubin C, Litvak V, Medvedovsky H, Zwang Y, Lev S, Yarden Y. Sprouty fine-tunes EGF signaling through interlinked positive and negative feedback loops. Curr Biol 2003; 13:297-307.
91. Hanafusa H, Torii S, Yasunaga T, Nishida E. Sprouty1 and Sprouty2 provide a control mechanism for the Ras/MAPK signalling pathway. Nat Cell Biol 2002; 4:850-8.
92. Feng Q, Baird D, Peng X, et al. Cool-1 functions as an essential regulatory node for EGF receptor- and Src-mediated cell growth. Nat Cell Biol 2006; 8:945-56.
93. Schmidt MH, Hoeller D, Yu J, et al. Alix/AIP1 antagonizes epidermal growth factor receptor downregulation by the Cbl-SETA/CIN85 complex. Mol Cell Biol 2004; 24:8981-93.
94. Tanos B, Pendergast AM. Abl tyrosine kinase regulates endocytosis of the epidermal growth factor receptor. J Biol Chem 2006; 281:32714-23.
95. Kowanetz K, Crosetto N, Haglund K, Schmidt MH, Heldin CH, Dikic I. Suppressors of T-cell receptor signaling Sts-1 and Sts-2 bind to Cbl and inhibit endocytosis of receptor tyrosine kinases. J Biol Chem 2004; 279:32786-95.
96. Gur G, Rubin C, Katz M, et al. LRIG1 restricts growth factor signaling by enhancing receptor ubiquitylation and degradation. Embo J 2004; 23:3270-81.
97. Kario E, Marmor MD, Adamsky K, et al. Suppressors of cytokine signaling 4 and 5 regulate epidermal growth factor receptor signaling. J Biol Chem 2005; 280:7038-48.

98. Tashiro K, Konishi H, Sano E, Nabeshi H, Yamauchi E, Taniguchi H. Suppression of the ligand-mediated down-regulation of epidermal growth factor receptor by Ymer, a novel tyrosine-phosphorylated and ubiquitinated protein. J Biol Chem 2006; 281:24612-22.
99. Urbe S, McCullough J, Row P, Prior IA, Welchman R, Clague MJ. Control of growth factor receptor dynamics by reversible ubiquitination. Biochem Soc Trans 2006; 34:754-6.
100. McCullough J, Clague MJ, Urbe S. AMSH is an endosome-associated ubiquitin isopeptidase. J Cell Biol 2004; 166:487-92.
101. Mizuno E, Iura T, Mukai A, Yoshimori T, Kitamura N, Komada M. Regulation of epidermal growth factor receptor down-regulation by UBPY-mediated deubiquitination at endosomes. Mol Biol Cell 2005; 16:5163-74.
102. Alwan HA, van Leeuwen JE. UBPY-mediated EGFR deubiquitination promotes EGFR degradation. J Biol Chem 2006.
103. Row PE, Prior IA, McCullough J, Clague MJ, Urbe S. The ubiquitin isopeptidase UBPY regulates endosomal ubiquitin dynamics and is essential for receptor down-regulation. J Biol Chem 2006; 281:12618-24.

5 Differential Dependence of EGFR and ErbB2 on the Molecular Chaperone Hsp90

Wanping Xu and Len Neckers

CONTENTS

THE MOLECULAR CHAPERONE HSP90
HSP90 IS SIMILARLY REQUIRED FOR MATURATION
    OF NASCENT EGFR AND ERBB2
HSP90 IS NECESSARY TO MAINTAIN STABILITY
    OF MATURE ERBB2 BUT NOT MATURE EGFR
WHAT DETERMINES THE RELIANCE OF MATURE ERBB2 ON HSP90?
SOMATIC MUTATIONS IN EGFR KINASE DOMAIN CONFER HSP90
    ASSOCIATION AND GA
CONCLUSION
REFERENCES

Abstract

EGFR and ErbB2 proteins are highly homologous in their amino acid sequence, yet they differ in their dependence on the molecular chaperone Hsp90. While both newly synthesized and mature ErbB2 proteins rely on Hsp90 for their stability, only the nascent form of the EGFR requires association with Hsp90 (*1–3*). Thus, blocking Hsp90 function with pharmacologic inhibitors, such as the benzoquinone ansamycin antibiotic geldanamycin (GA) and its derivatives, induces a rapid and dramatic decrease in the level of ErbB2 expression, but causes a much slower decline in the steady-state level of EGFR (Fig. 5.1).

Key Words: molecular chaperone, heat shock protein 90, benzoquinone ansamycins, geldanamycin, Hsp90 inhibitor, EGFR mutations, drug sensitivity.

1. THE MOLECULAR CHAPERONE HSP90

Hsp90 (90-kiloDalton Heat Shock Protein) is one of the most abundant proteins in the cell (*4*). As a molecular chaperone, Hsp90 guides the folding, assembly, intracellular disposition, and proteolytic turnover of many cellular proteins. To date, more than 100 proteins are known to be regulated by Hsp90. Most of these proteins, which are called "client proteins," serve as nodal points in multiple signal transduction pathways, and they include kinases (e.g., ErbB2, Akt, Raf-1), transcription factors (steriod receptors, HIF-1α, HSF1), and other signaling molecules (NO synthase, G$\beta\gamma$). Hsp90 modulates its client proteins by forming

From: *Cancer Drug Discovery and Development: EGFR Signaling Networks in Cancer Therapy*
Edited by: J. D. Haley and W. J. Gullick, DOI: 10.1007/978-1-59745-356-1_5
© 2008 Humana Press, a part of Springer Science+Business Media, LLC

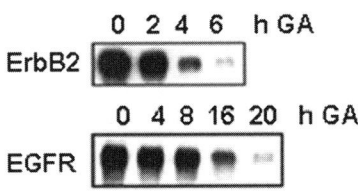

Fig. 5.1. **EGFR and ErbB2 proteins are differentially sensitive to GA-induced down-regulation.** A431 (lower panel) and SKBR3 (upper panel) cells were treated with 3 μM GA for increasing times. Cell lysates were separated by SDS-PAGE and Western-blotted for either EGFR (A431 lysates) or ErbB2 (SKBR3 lysates).

multi-component complexes with co-chaperones, which depends on its unique and flexible molecular structure. The ability to change conformation is likely important for the chaperoning function of Hsp90.

The mechanism of action of Hsp90 is best studied in the context of steroid receptors, including the glucocorticoid receptor, the androgen receptor and the progesterone receptor. In these cases, Hsp90 interacts with a pre-formed receptor·Hsp70·Hsp40 complex in an ATP-dependent process mediated by p60^{Hop} (5, 6). This Hsp90-containing complex promotes a conformational change of the receptor, producing an Hsp90·receptor heterocomplex, with Hsp90 in its ATP-bound conformation. The co-chaperone p23 and various immunophilins interact with Hsp90 to stabilize this complex. The receptor, probably together with the co-chaperone Aha1, stimulates the ATPase activity of Hsp90 (7, 8). Hydrolysis of ATP results in conformational change of Hsp90, allowing the release of the receptor protein. GA binds to the adenosine nucleotide-binding pocket in the N-terminal domain of Hsp90 and blocks the binding of ATP, thus interfering with conformational cycling of the chaperone complex and effectively inhibiting Hsp90 function (9–11).

For client protein kinases, immunophilins are replaced in the Hsp90 chaperone complex by the co-chaperone protein p50^{cdc37}. A ternary complex of Hsp90·p50^{cdc37}·kinase has been observed, in which three-way interactions exist. Hsp90 interacts with the kinase directly, most likely via its middle domain. Hsp90 also interacts with p50^{cdc37} via its N-terminal ATP-binding domain and the middle domain of p50^{cdc37} (12). Further, p50^{cdc37} interacts with the kinase through its N-terminal domain (13). It seems that p50^{cdc37} can sense conformational change in Hsp90 and is able to translate this change into enhanced affinity for the binding of kinases (14).

Hsp90 was first found to form a complex with the oncogenic v-Src protein together with p50^{cdc37} (15) and was shown to play a role in v-Src maturation. Immediately after translation, v-Src exists in a complex with Hsp90. In this complex, v-Src is unphosphorylated and is unable to phosphorylate itself and other substrates. After it is transported to and inserted into the plasma membrane, v-Src protein no longer requires association with Hsp90 and exhibits high kinase activity (16). Hsp90 also plays a role in the folding and maturation of the Src-related kinase Lck (17). A requirement of Hsp90 function for kinase maturation is well exemplified in the kinase GSK3β. In its mature form GSK3β is a serine/threonine kinase. Newly synthesized GSK3β however, instead displays tyrosine kinase activity. Autophosphorylation on tyrosine residue Tyr216 in the activation loop mediates the transition of GSK3β from a tyrosine kinase to a serine/threonine kinase. Importantly, this transition requires association with Hsp90 (18). In addition to assisting the folding and maturation of numerous nascent kinases, Hsp90 also associates with certain mature proteins and serves to regulate their activity. For example, Hsp90 binds to PKR and inhibits its phosphorylation of the substrate eIF-2alpha (19). Thus, Hsp90 function is differentially required by mature and newly synthesized kinase proteins.

2. Hsp90 IS SIMILARLY REQUIRED FOR MATURATION OF NASCENT EGFR AND ErbB2

The Hsp90 dependence of newly synthesized EGFR proteins was first suggested by the slow but steady decrease (similar to what was seen in the presence of the protein synthesis inhibitor cycloheximide) in EGFR level in the presence of GA, which could be explained by the cell's inability to replenish receptors naturally recycled from the cell surface (2). Direct evidence of the dependence of nascent EGFR on Hsp90 is supplied by the rapid decline of ^{35}S-labeled newly synthesized proteins, compared to total EGFR, in the presence of GA (20). Nascent ErbB2 proteins show a similar sensitivity to GA (3, 21). Evidence supporting a requirement for Hsp90 by nascent EGFR is supplied by their physical association, as recently shown by immunoprecipitation and mass spectrometry. Exploiting the unique observation that FLAG antibody lost interaction with FLAG-tagged EGFRvIII after glycosylation in the Golgi apparatus, Lavictoire et al. were able to immunopurify newly synthesized EGFRvIII proteins (22). Mass spectrometric analysis of the proteins co-immunoprecipitating with nascent EGFRvIII identified Hsp90 and $p50^{cdc37}$, providing support for the hypothesis that Hsp90 and its co-chaperone $p50^{cdc37}$ participate in the maturation of nascent EGFR proteins.

3. HSP90 IS NECESSARY TO MAINTAIN STABILITY OF MATURE ErbB2 BUT NOT MATURE EGFR

When EGFR matures, it becomes independent of Hsp90. This finding is supported by two observations. One is that mature EGFR proteins, in contrast to the nascent proteins, no longer associate with the Hsp90-$p50^{cdc37}$ complex, as shown by co-immunoprecipitation experiments. The other is that mature EGFR proteins are not sensitive to GA-induced degradation. In contrast to EGFR, mature ErbB2 proteins remain associated with the Hsp90-$p50^{cdc37}$ complex, and remain sensitive to rapid GA-induced degradation (2).

How does Hsp90 stabilize ErbB2? There are two competing models to explain this phenomenon. One is dynamic and the other is static, and each is supported by experimental data. In the dynamic model, mature ErbB2 proteins on the surface of the cell are constantly being endocytosed (23). Under normal conditions, these internalized ErbB2 proteins are recycled back to the cell surface. When Hsp90 function is inhibited by GA, however, this recycling is blocked, and the ErbB2 proteins are instead sorted to endosomes where they are degraded. In these experiments, inhibition of Hsp90 was not seen to affect the rate of ErbB2 internalization. In the static model, mature ErbB2 proteins are retained on the cell surface under normal conditions, without active recycling (24). ErbB2 proteins were shown to preferentially associate with membrane protrusions in untreated cells. Treatment with GA induces an increase in the amount of mobile ErbB2 and a redistribution of ErbB2 within the plasma membrane making the receptor accessible to endocytosis, as shown by FRAP (fluorescence recovery after photobleaching) analysis and electron microscopy. Interestingly, these authors also showed that internalization of ErbB2 proteins requires the normal function of the proteasome, consistent with previous observations that GA-induced ErbB2 degradation is blocked by specific proteasome inhibitors (1). Regardless of whether Hsp90 maintains the stability of mature ErbB2 proteins by promoting their recycling or by inhibiting their endocytosis, it seems that ubiquitination plays a key role in GA-induced ErbB2 degradation. GA treatment induces a rapid and dramatic increase in ErbB2 ubiquitination (1). Noticeably, ErbB2 ubiquitination occurs prior to decrease in ErbB2 protein level, and inhibition of proteasome activity prevents ErbB2 protein depletion while simultaneously increasing the fraction of ErbB2 that is ubiquitinated.

Ligand-induced EGFR ubiquitination has been shown to be mediated by the E3 ubiquitin ligase Cbl, which binds to EGFR via phosphorylated Tyr1045, an autophosphorylation site (*25*). Cbl also mediates ErbB2 ubiquitination by binding to ErbB2 via phosphorylated Tyr1112, the homologous site of EGFR Tyr1045 (*26*). GA treatment, however, decreases ErbB2 phosphorylation, including phosphorylation of Tyr1112, which suggests that Cbl is not likely to play a significant role in GA-induced degradation of mature ErbB2 (*27*). Indeed, overexpression of either wild-type or dominant-negative Cbl fails to affect GA-induced ErbB2 degradation (*28*). These data indicate that GA-induced ErbB2 ubiquitination is mediated by a mechanism unique from that induced by receptor ligands.

Several years ago, we along with others identified the unique E3 ubiquitin ligase CHIP (C-terminal Hsc70-interacting protein) as the mediator of GA-induced ErbB2 ubiquitination (*28, 29*). CHIP binds to the chaperones Hsp/Hsc70 and Hsp90 via an amino-terminal tetratricopeptide (TPR) domain, while its ubiquitin ligase activity is mediated by a carboxyl-terminal U box domain (*30*). We had previously shown that GA treatment disrupts ErbB2 binding to the Hsp90-p50^{cdc37} complex, while simultaneously favoring association of Hsp/Hsc70 (*2*). Concomitant with this process, we found ErbB2 to also associate with CHIP (*28*). Moreover, ectopic expression of CHIP was found to shorten the half-life of both nascent and mature ErbB2 protein, while in vitro ubiquitination assay revealed that purified CHIP protein serves as a ubiquitin ligase for ErbB2. Finally, both exogenously expressed and endogenous CHIP co-precipitate with the ErbB2 protein. ErbB2 association with CHIP is mediated by Hsp/Hsc70, as a point mutation in the TPR domain that disrupts CHIP interaction with Hsp/Hsc70 prevents complex formation. An inactivating point mutation in the U-box domain inhibits GA-induced ErbB2 ubiquitination without affecting association of the mutant CHIP protein with the kinase.

How did ErbB2 acquire its unique dependence on Hsp90? ErbB2 is likely to have arisen from EGFR through a gene duplication event since invertebrates contain only an EGFR-like ligand-activated protein (*31*). Analysis of the ErbB2 amino acid sequence reveals that it contains an insert not found in the other ErbB proteins, and this insert occurs near a residue in EGFR shown to be in close proximity to bound EGF (*32*). It has been speculated that this altered sequence in the ErbB2 extracellular domain may prevent it from binding ligand (*31*). The appearance of such a protein must surely have been considered a mutational event by the vertebrate organism in which it arose. Rutherford and Lindquist have proposed a model in which Hsp90 binding to mutated proteins may stabilize them while masking their phenotypic expression, thus allowing accumulation of multiple silent mutations during evolution and thus providing the organism with a greater diversity of responses when faced with unexpected environmental stress (*33*). If ErbB2 evolved by mutation from EGFR to become a ligandless heterodimerization partner, it may have simultaneously acquired dependence on Hsp90 for its stability. The growth and survival advantage conferred by ErbB2 would certainly favor its ultimate evolutionary selection.

4. WHAT DETERMINES THE RELIANCE OF MATURE ErbB2 ON Hsp90?

The differential dependence on Hsp90 for maintaining stability of mature EGFR and ErbB2 is determined by their amino acid sequences. Along with others, we first mapped the determinants of Hsp90 binding to the kinase domain of ErbB2 (*2, 34*). This was somewhat surprising since we expected the determinant to be contained within a region of significant sequence variation between EGFR and ErbB2, and the kinase domain is the most conserved region of both proteins. The Hsp90 binding motif was further localized to a short segment of eight amino acids that reside in a loop between the end of the C helix and the beginning of the 4 sheet in the N-lobe of the kinase domain, referred to as the M5 loop (*20, 35*). Conversion of five amino acid residues in the ErbB2 sequence to their counterparts in EGFR made ErbB2 refractory to GA, while preserving the normal functions of the kinase. Consistent with the loss of GA sensitivity, mutant ErbB2 lost association with the Hsp90 chaperone complex (20).

Computer modeling of the kinase domain of the two receptors revealed a surface-exposed hydrophobic strip and positively charged patch around the M5 loop of ErbB2. This hydrophobic strip, however, is interrupted by an aspartic acid residue in the M5 loop of EGFR, and the positively charged patch is simultaneously diminished (Fig. 5.2). Computer modeling indicated that mutation of Gly776 to aspartic acid would disrupt the hydrophobic strip in the ErbB2 kinase domain. Indeed, the ErbB2 mutant carrying a Gly776Asp mutation failed to associate with the Hsp90 chaperone complex and displayed significant resistance to GA-induced degradation (20). Conversely, mutation of the aspartic acid residue in EGFR to eliminate the positive charge disrupting the hydrophobic strip of the M5 loop conferred Hsp90 association on the mutant protein, as well as sensitivity to GA-induced degradation. These findings indicate that the electrostatic nature of the M5 loop determines dependence of mature ErbB2 on Hsp90.

It is interesting to note that the molecular features of the M5 loop seem to determine Hsp90 dependence of only the mature but not the nascent ErbB proteins. As transmembrane proteins, nascent EGFR and ErbB2 traverse the endoplasmic reticulum (ER) and Golgi apparatus after synthesis, before being transported to the cell surface. During maturation, the N-terminal extracellular domains, which are in the lumen of ER, are glycosylated with a 14-sugar precursor linked to asparagine residues (36). The sugar chains are further modified as

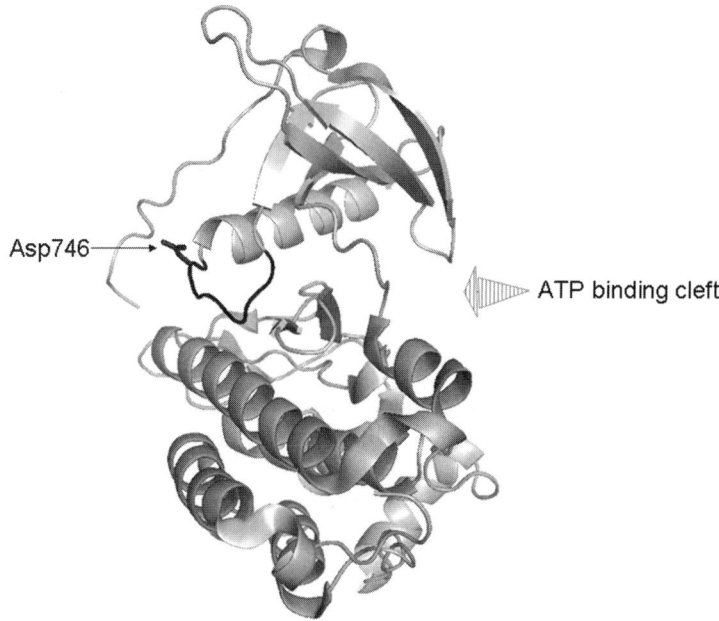

Fig. 5.2. A ribbon diagram of the ErbB kinase domain, oriented so that the Hsp90 binding loop (black) is facing out toward the reader. As drawn, the ATP binding is oriented away from the reader. The Hsp90 binding loop is primarily hydrophobic in nature in ErbB2, while in EGFR the presence of Asp746 disrupts the hydrophobic surface with a negative charge. Removal or insertion of this negative charge in the loop is sufficient to determine Hsp90 binding and GA sensitivity.

the receptor proteins are transported through the Golgi apparatus. The intracellular domains of both EGFR and ErbB2 are also modified post-translationally, mainly by phosphorylation (*37*). Together, these modifications may facilitate the attainment of the mature conformation. Upon maturation, EGFR is likely to adopt a conformation exposing the M5 loop, positioning Asp746 such that it hinders the association of the Hsp90-p50^{cdc37} complex. In contrast, when ErbB2 attains its mature conformation, it can associate with the chaperone complex due to lack of the hindering negative charge in the M5 loop region.

A recently published 3D structural model based on data from single-particle electron microscopy showed the interactions between Hsp90, p50^{cdc37} and the kinase CDK4 (*38*). This structure indicates that the kinase makes multiple interactions with Hsp90 and p50^{cdc37}, suggesting that other parts of the mature ErbB2 protein, in addition to the M5 loop, also participate in determining the interaction with the Hsp90-p50^{cdc37} complex. Given the high homology in amino acid sequences between the two kinase domains, Hsp90 association with ErbB2 but not EGFR raised the question whether the mature ErbB2 kinase domain assumes a different conformation compared to that of EGFR. Indeed, we recently showed that the activation loop of the ErbB2 kinase domain adopts a distinct configuration from that of EGFR (*39*). Crystallography data have demonstrated that the activation loop in the EGFR kinase domain assumes an activated, extended configuration in the absence of phosphorylation, similar to that of the phosphorylated insulin receptor (*40*). Consistent with these observations, EGFR phosphorylation in the activation loop mediated by Src kinase does not affect the intrinsic kinase activity of EGFR (*41*). In contrast, phosphorylation in the ErbB2 activation loop by Src kinases significantly elevates the intrinsic kinase activity of ErbB2 (*39*). A similar effect was also observed for the oncogenic rat ErbB2/*neu* protein (*42*). These data suggest that, unlike the EGFR, the ErbB2 activation loop adopts an inactive conformation in the absence of phosphorylation. Supporting this hypothesis, molecular modeling indicates that the EGFR kinase domain enjoys favorable intra-molecular interactions and interactions with solvent, which serve to maintain the activation loop in an activated conformation in the absence of phosphorylation (*39*). In contrast, the ErbB2 activation loop fails to do so due to lack of these favorable interactions. Instead, it adopts a configuration similar to that of inactive CDK6, with the loop flipping away from the ATP-binding cleft, making the kinase domain unable to align ATP with substrate. The inactive conformation of the mature ErbB2 protein, in addition to the electrostatic nature of the M5 loop, may contribute to complex formation with the Hsp90-p50^{cdc37} complex.

5. SOMATIC MUTATIONS IN EGFR KINASE DOMAIN CONFER Hsp90 ASSOCIATION AND GA

Since the surface features (hydrophobicity and positive charge) in the M5 loop region help determine ErbB association with the Hsp90 complex and sensitivity to GA-induced protein degradation, any mutations in this region that alter these surface features are likely to affect the chaperone dependence and drug sensitivity of the mutated receptor. Recently, somatic EGFR mutations were found in a subset of non-small cell lung cancers. These mutations often increase the kinase activity of the mutant EGFRs, and EGFR inhibition induces apoptosis in vitro and clinical responses in vivo (*43*). Interestingly, some of the reported mutations occur within or near the M5 loop region, such as the point mutations S768I (serine 768 mutated to isoleucine, amino acids numbered with the secretory leader peptide included) and R776C, and the insertion mutations M766ASV (alanine, serine and valine inserted after methionine 766), D770NPH, and D770NPG. As expected, EGFR proteins carrying these mutations were found to associate with Hsp90 and p50^{cdc37} and to be sensitive to degradation induced by Hsp90 inhibitors (Xu et al, unpublished data).

Somatic EGFR mutations have also been found in other regions of the kinase domain, the most common being the point mutation L858R in the activation loop and the deletion mutations in the loop between the 3 sheet and the C-helix. Surprisingly, all of these mutant EGFRs become sensitive to degradation induced by Hsp90 inhibition (*44*). It is likely that these mutations affect the conformation of the M5 loop and/or that of other parts of the kinase domain that determine Hsp90 association. Like the EGFRs carrying mutations in the M5 loop, these mutant EGFRs also readily associate with Hsp90 and p50^{cdc37}, supporting the notion that these mutations expose the kinase domain to structural stresses requiring chaperone stabilization.

Although most somatic mutations within the EGFR kinase domain result in increased sensitivity to EGFR inhibitors such as Iressa and Tarceva, resistance frequently develops. Furthermore, insertion mutations in the M5 loop render the EGFR resistant to these inhibitors (*45*). It is thus noteworthy to observe that, to date, all Iressa/Tarceva-resistant EGFR mutants remain dependent on Hsp90 and sensitive to degradation induced by Hsp90 inhibitors.

In the case of wild-type EGFR, ligand-induced receptor activation promotes autophosphorylation on tyrosine 1045, providing the docking site for the E3 ubiquitin ligase Cbl. Cbl mediates EGFR ubiquitination, which promotes EGFR internalization and targets the receptor to lysosomes for degradation (*46*). In addition, Cbl recruits CIN85 to activated EGFR. CIN85 is an adaptor protein, which constitutively interacts with endophilins, the regulatory component of clathrin-coated pits, and promotes internalization of EGFR (*47*). In the case of somatically mutated EGFRs, binding of CIN85 is inhibited (*48*). Furthermore, somatically mutated EGFRs induce phosphorylation of Cbl, which inhibits its ubiquitin ligase activity without affecting its binding to receptor tyrosine kinases. Thus, even though Cbl associates with somatically mutated EGFRs in the absence of ligand, it does not efficiently mediate the ubiquitination of these receptors, even when ligand is present. Inhibition of Hsp90 remedies these defects and restores ligand-induced degradation to somatically mutated EGFRs.

6. CONCLUSION

EGFR and ErbB2 are differentially dependent on the molecular chaperone Hsp90. While the nascent proteins of both receptors require the assistance of Hsp90 for their folding and maturation, only ErbB2 requires constitutive association with Hsp90 in order to maintain the stability of the mature protein. Even though mature wild-type EGFR does not require Hsp90, cancer cell-specific kinase domain mutations uniformly render the EGFR vulnerable to Hsp90 inhibition, even when those mutations confer resistance to more specific EGFR inhibitors.

REFERENCES

1. Mimnaugh EG, Chavany C, Neckers L. Polyubiquitination and proteasomal degradation of the p185c-erbB-2 receptor protein-tyrosine kinase induced by geldanamycin. J Biol Chem 1996; 271:22796-801.
2. Xu W, Mimnaugh E, Rosser MF, et al. Sensitivity of mature Erbb2 to geldanamycin is conferred by its kinase domain and is mediated by the chaperone protein Hsp90. J Biol Chem 2001; 276:3702-8.
3. Xu W, Mimnaugh EG, Kim JS, Trepel JB, Neckers LM. Hsp90, not Grp94, regulates the intracellular trafficking and stability of nascent ErbB2. Cell Stress Chaperones 2002; 7:91-6.
4. Neckers L. Chaperoning oncogenes: Hsp90 as a target of geldanamycin. Handb Exp Pharmacol 2006:259-77.
5. Hernandez MP, Sullivan WP, Toft DO. The assembly and intermolecular properties of the hsp70-Hop–hsp90 molecular chaperone complex. J Biol Chem 2002; 277:38294-304.

6. Murphy PJ, Morishima Y, Chen H, et al. Visualization and mechanism of assembly of a glucocorticoid receptor. Hsp70 complex that is primed for subsequent Hsp90-dependent opening of the steroid binding cleft. J Biol Chem 2003; 278:34764-73.
7. McLaughlin SH, Smith HW, Jackson SE. Stimulation of the weak ATPase activity of human hsp90 by a client protein. J Mol Biol 2002; 315:787-98.
8. Panaretou B, Siligardi G, Meyer P, et al. Activation of the ATPase activity of hsp90 by the stress-regulated cochaperone aha1. Mol Cell 2002; 10:1307-18.
9. Grenert JP, Sullivan WP, Fadden P, et al. The amino-terminal domain of heat shock protein 90 (hsp90) that binds geldanamycin is an ATP/ADP switch domain that regulates hsp90 conformation. J Biol Chem 1997; 272:23843-50.
10. Stebbins CE, Russo AA, Schneider C, Rosen N, Hartl FU, Pavletich NP. Crystal structure of an Hsp90-geldanamycin complex: targeting of a protein chaperone by an antitumor agent. Cell 1997; 89:239-50.
11. Zhang W, Hirshberg M, McLaughlin SH, et al. Biochemical and structural studies of the interaction of Cdc37 with Hsp90. J Mol Biol 2004; 340:891-907.
12. Roe SM, Ali MM, Meyer P, et al. The Mechanism of Hsp90 regulation by the protein kinase-specific cochaperone p50(cdc37). Cell 2004; 116:87-98.
13. Siligardi G, Panaretou B, Meyer P, et al. Regulation of Hsp90 ATPase activity by the co-chaperone Cdc37p/p50cdc37. J Biol Chem 2002; 277:20151-9.
14. Shao J, Irwin A, Hartson SD, Matts RL. Functional dissection of cdc37: characterization of domain structure and amino acid residues critical for protein kinase binding. Biochemistry 2003; 42:12577-88.
15. Brugge JS, Erikson E, Erikson RL. The specific interaction of the Rous sarcoma virus transforming protein, pp60src, with two cellular proteins. Cell 1981; 25:363-72.
16. Brugge J, Yonemoto W, Darrow D. Interaction between the Rous sarcoma virus transforming protein and two cellular phosphoproteins: analysis of the turnover and distribution of this complex. Mol Cell Biol 1983; 3:9-19.
17. Giannini A, Bijlmakers MJ. Regulation of the Src family kinase Lck by Hsp90 and ubiquitination. Mol Cell Biol 2004; 24:5667-76.
18. Lochhead PA, Kinstrie R, Sibbet G, Rawjee T, Morrice N, Cleghon V. A chaperone-dependent GSK-3beta transitional intermediate mediates activation-loop autophosphorylation. Mol Cell 2006; 24:627-33.
19. Donze O, Abbas-Terki T, Picard D. The Hsp90 chaperone complex is both a facilitator and a repressor of the dsRNA-dependent kinase PKR. Embo J 2001; 20:3771-80.
20. Xu W, Yuan X, Xiang Z, Mimnaugh E, Marcu M, Neckers L. Surface charge and hydrophobicity determine ErbB2 binding to the Hsp90 chaperone complex. Nat Struct Mol Biol 2005; 12:120-6.
21. Chavany C, Mimnaugh E, Miller P, et al. p185erbB2 binds to GRP94 in vivo. Dissociation of the p185erbB2/GRP94 heterocomplex by benzoquinone ansamycins precedes depletion of p185erbB2. J Biol Chem 1996; 271:4974-4977.
22. Lavictoire SJ, Parolin DA, Klimowicz AC, Kelly JF, Lorimer IA. Interaction of Hsp90 with the nascent form of the mutant epidermal growth factor receptor EGFRvIII. J Biol Chem 2003; 278:5292-9.
23. Austin CD, De Maziere AM, Pisacane PI, et al. Endocytosis and sorting of ErbB2 and the site of action of cancer therapeutics trastuzumab and geldanamycin. Mol Biol Cell 2004; 15:5268-82.
24. Lerdrup M, Hommelgaard AM, Grandal M, van Deurs B. Geldanamycin stimulates internalization of ErbB2 in a proteasome-dependent way. J Cell Sci 2006; 119:85-95.
25. Levkowitz G, Waterman H, Ettenberg SA, et al. Ubiquitin ligase activity and tyrosine phosphorylation underlie suppression of growth factor signaling by c-Cbl/Sli-1. Mol Cell 1999; 4:1029-40.
26. Klapper LN, Waterman H, Sela M, Yarden Y. Tumor-inhibitory antibodies to HER-2/ErbB-2 may act by recruiting c-Cbl and enhancing ubiquitination of HER-2. Cancer Res 2000; 60:3384-8.
27. Xu W, Yuan X, Jung YJ, et al. The heat shock protein 90 inhibitor geldanamycin and the ErbB inhibitor ZD1839 promote rapid PP1 phosphatase-dependent inactivation of AKT in ErbB2 overexpressing breast cancer cells. Cancer Res 2003; 63:7777-84.
28. Xu W, Marcu M, Yuan X, Mimnaugh E, Patterson C, Neckers L. Chaperone-dependent E3 ubiquitin ligase CHIP mediates a degradative pathway for c-ErbB2/Neu. Proc Natl Acad Sci U S A 2002; 99:12847-52.

29. Zhou P, Fernandes N, Dodge IL, et al. ErbB2 degradation mediated by the co-chaperone protein CHIP. J Biol Chem 2003; 278:13829-37.
30. Ballinger CA, Connell P, Wu Y, et al. Identification of CHIP, a novel tetratricopeptide repeat-containing protein that interacts with heat shock proteins and negatively regulates chaperone functions. Mol Cell Biol 1999; 19:4535-45.
31. Stein RA, Staros JV. Evolutionary analysis of the ErbB receptor and ligand families. J Mol Evol 2000; 50:397-412.
32. Woltjer RL, Lukas TJ, Staros JV. Direct identification of residues of the epidermal growth factor receptor in close proximity to the amino terminus of bound epidermal growth factor. Proc Natl Acad Sci U S A 1992; 89:7801-5.
33. Rutherford SL, Lindquist S. Hsp90 as a capacitor for morphological evolution. Nature 1998; 396:336-42.
34. Tikhomirov O, Carpenter G. Geldanamycin induces ErbB-2 degradation by proteolytic fragmentation. J Biol Chem 2000; 275:26625-31.
35. Tikhomirov O, Carpenter G. Identification of ErbB-2 kinase domain motifs required for geldanamycin-induced degradation. Cancer Res 2003; 63:39-43.
36. Medzihradszky KF. Characterization of protein N-glycosylation. Methods Enzymol 2005; 405:116-38.
37. Lee NY, Koland JG. Conformational changes accompany phosphorylation of the epidermal growth factor receptor C-terminal domain. Protein Sci 2005; 14:2793-803.
38. Vaughan CK, Gohlke U, Sobott F, et al. Structure of an Hsp90-Cdc37-Cdk4 complex. Mol Cell 2006; 23:697-707.
39. Xu W, Yuan X, Beebe K, Xiang Z, Neckers L. Loss of Hsp90 association up-regulates Src-dependent ErbB2 activity. Mol Cell Biol 2007; 27:220-8.
40. Stamos J, Sliwkowski MX, Eigenbrot C. Structure of the epidermal growth factor receptor kinase domain alone and in complex with a 4-anilinoquinazoline inhibitor. J Biol Chem 2002; 277:46265-72.
41. Tice DA, Biscardi JS, Nickles AL, Parsons SJ. Mechanism of biological synergy between cellular Src and epidermal growth factor receptor. Proc Natl Acad Sci U S A 1999; 96:1415-20.
42. Zhang HT, O'Rourke DM, Zhao H, et al. Absence of autophosphorylation site Y882 in the p185neu oncogene product correlates with a reduction of transforming potential. Oncogene 1998; 16:2835-42.
43. Riely GJ, Politi KA, Miller VA, Pao W. Update on epidermal growth factor receptor mutations in non-small cell lung cancer. Clin Cancer Res 2006; 12:7232-41.
44. Shimamura T, Lowell AM, Engelman JA, Shapiro GI. Epidermal growth factor receptors harboring kinase domain mutations associate with the heat shock protein 90 chaperone and are destabilized following exposure to geldanamycins. Cancer Res 2005; 65:6401-8.
45. Greulich H, Chen TH, Feng W, et al. Oncogenic transformation by inhibitor-sensitive and -resistant EGFR mutants. PLoS Med 2005; 2:e313.
46. Haglund K, Shimokawa N, Szymkiewicz I, Dikic I. Cbl-directed monoubiquitination of CIN85 is involved in regulation of ligand-induced degradation of EGF receptors. Proc Natl Acad Sci U S A 2002; 99:12191-6.
47. Soubeyran P, Kowanetz K, Szymkiewicz I, Langdon WY, Dikic I. Cbl-CIN85-endophilin complex mediates ligand-induced downregulation of EGF receptors. Nature 2002; 416:183-7.
48. Yang S, Qu S, Perez-Tores M, et al. Association with HSP90 inhibits Cbl-mediated down-regulation of mutant epidermal growth factor receptors. Cancer Res 2006; 66:6990-7.

6 Activation of STATs 3 and 5 Through the EGFR Signaling Axis

Priya Koppikar and Jennifer Rubin Grandis

CONTENTS

EPIDERMAL GROWTH FACTOR RECEPTOR (EGFR)
THE STAT SIGNALING PATHWAY
CONCLUSION
REFERENCES

Abstract

The living cell is a dynamic system, which is in a constant state of flux with the extracellular environment. Despite the intricacies of cellular interaction with its microenvironment, one striking feature of all biological systems remains their inherent unity in terms of signaling cascades. In the same cell, similar signaling pathways mediated through a common effector may give rise to a variety of cellular processes including differentiation, proliferation and apoptosis, depending upon the upstream regulator. Conversely, activation of the same downstream signaling pathway can occur via distinct upstream receptors. The various downstream effects mediated by interaction between the epidermal growth factor receptor (EGFR) and its numerous ligands are such an example.

Key Words: EGFR, STAT3, STAT5, STAT1, SCCHN, signal transduction

1. EPIDERMAL GROWTH FACTOR RECEPTOR (EGFR)

The epidermal growth factor receptor (EGFR), also known as HER1 or ErbB1, is a 170-kDa ubiquitous transmembrane glycoprotein that belongs to the type I receptor tyrosine kinases (RTKs) or the ErbB receptor family. Other family members include ErbB2 (HER2/neu), ErbB3 (HER3) and ErbB4 (HER4). These receptors are composed primarily of three domains: the extracellular domain, the hydrophobic transmembrane domain, and the cytoplasmic intracellular domain. EGFR was discovered approximately two decades ago as the proto-oncogenic counterpart of the oncogenic v-erbB tyrosine kinase, which causes avian erythroblastosis (*1*). In its proto-oncogenic form, EGFR requires binding of the growth factor molecule to enable its kinase activity. The oncogenic form of EGFR, however, produces a receptor that does not require binding of growth factor, but instead is constitutively active. Constitutive activation of EGFR can occur through various mutations. The most commonly studied mutation - EGFRvIII - occurs through an in-frame deletion mutation of exons 2 to 7

From: *Cancer Drug Discovery and Development: EGFR Signaling Networks in Cancer Therapy*
Edited by: J. D. Haley and W. J. Gullick, DOI: 10.1007/978-1-59745-356-1_6
© 2008 Humana Press, a part of Springer Science+Business Media, LLC

spanning the extracellular ligand-binding domain. This deletion produces a truncated 150-kDa protein that is weakly constitutively phosphorylated in a ligand-independent manner (*2, 3*). To date, EGFRvIII has only been detected in cancers, including gliomas, non-small cell lung carcinomas (NSCLC), breast cancer, ovarian cancer, and head and neck cancer, but not in normal tissue (*4, 5*).

Ligands that bind to EGFR include the epidermal growth factor (EGF), amphiregulin, transforming growth factor α (TGF-α), heparin-binding EGF-like growth factor (HB-EGF), amphiregulin, betacellulin, and epiregulin (*6*). EGFR is generally present on the cell membrane but has also been detected in the nucleus (*7*). The first step in EGFR activation is receptor dimerization. EGFR can both homodimerize and heterodimerize with other ErbB receptors (*8*) (also discussed in Chapters 1 and 2). Dimerized EGFR is internalized in the endosome and induces autophosphorylation of tyrosine residues in the carboxyl terminal of EGFR by its own kinase domain. The resulting phosphorylated tyrosine residues serve as binding sites for signaling molecules containing Src homology 2 (SH2) and phosphotyrosine binding domains (PTB), which further initiate intracellular signaling cascades linked to versatile cellular responses that include cellular proliferation, differentiation, migration, adhesion, anti-apoptotic survival mechanisms, and induction of angiogenesis.

Emerging evidence suggests that EGFR may also function as a nuclear transcription factor, where EGFR translocates to the nucleus and interacts with STAT3 leading to transcriptional activation of inducible nitric oxide synthase (iNOS) (*7, 9*). Other ErbB family members, including ErbB2 and ErbB4, have also been associated with nuclear transcription factor capabilities (*10, 11*). The precise role of membrane versus nuclear EGFR is not completely understood.

1.1. EGFR-Mediated Downstream Signaling Pathways

The most well-studied signaling routes affected by EGFR activation include the mitogen-activated protein kinase (MAPK), the phosphatidylinositol-3-OH kinase (PI3K)/Akt, the phospholipase Cγ (PLCγ) pathways, and the STAT mediated pathways (*12*). The precise pathway(s) activated downstream of EGFR depends upon the cellular context (Fig. 6.1).

1.1.1. THE MAPK PATHWAY

Binding of a cognate ligand to EGFR activates the tyrosine kinase activity of its cytoplasmic domain. Docking proteins such as GRB2 (growth factor receptor bound protein 2) contain SH2 domains that bind to the phosphotyrosines of the activated receptor. GRB2 binds to the guanine nucleotide exchange factor, SOS, through a SH3 domain in GRB2. When the GRB2-SOS complex docks to phosphorylated EGFR, SOS becomes activated (*13*). Activated SOS promotes the removal of GDP from Ras, which can then bind GTP and subsequently, become active.

Activated Ras induces the protein kinase activity of RAF kinase, a serine/threonine-selective protein kinase (*14*) (discussed also in Chapter 7). RAF kinase phosphorylates and activates MEK, another serine/threonine kinase. MEK, in turn, phosphorylates and activates mitogen activated protein kinase (MAPK- also known as Extracellular–signal regulated kinase or Erk).

Activation of the classical MAPK pathway leads to proliferation of many cell types. Two isoforms of MAPK- p44 MAPK (Erk-1) and p42 MAPK (Erk-2) - are generally expressed. The downstream targets of MAPK include various nuclear transcription factors like Ets and non-nuclear targets such as p90rsk (*15*) and cytosolic phospholipase A2 (*16*), which further activate various molecules associated with cell proliferation and differentiation.

Chapter 6 / EGFR-mediated Activation of STATs

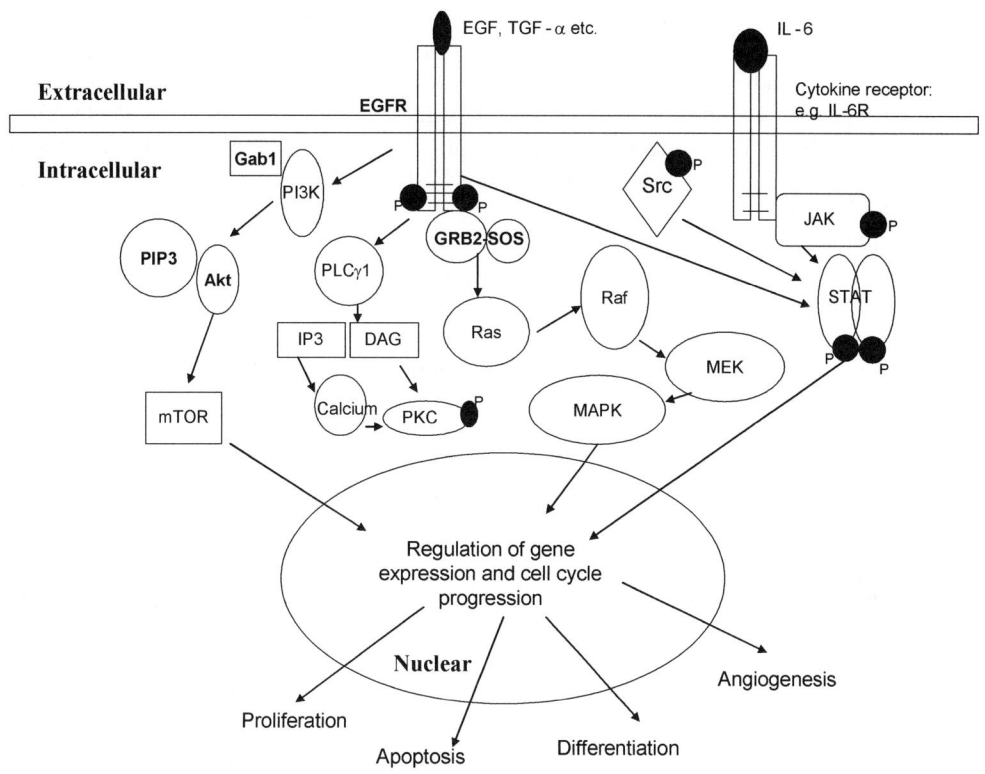

Fig. 6.1. Activation of EGFR through its ligand(s) triggers various signaling cascades depending upon the cellular context and the upstream regulating growth factor(s). Activation results in transactivation of any one of the four major pathways: the PI3K/Akt, MAPK, PLCγ, or the STAT signaling pathway. Each of these signaling molecules initiate further signaling cascades, resulting in regulation of gene transcription and cell cycle progression. STATs are also activated via EGFR independent mechanisms. The classical pathway for STAT activation is modulated by cytokine receptors and the JAK family of kinases. STATs could also be activated by cytoplasmic non-receptor tyrosine kinases like Src. The black ovals indicate phosphorylation/activation of various members in the signaling cascade.

1.1.2. THE PI3k/Akt PATHWAY

The other classical pathway activated by EGFR is the PI3 Kinase/Akt pathway. Upon activation by several growth factors, EGFR activates the phosphatidyl inositol-3 kinase, which in turn produces phosphatidyl inositol triphosphate (PIP3). PIP3 interacts with Akt (also known as Protein Kinase B: PKB) via the pleckstrin homology (PH) domain (*17*). Akt then, indirectly phosphorylates the mammalian target of rapamycin (mTOR) (*18*), which is a key regulator of eukaryotic cell growth and proliferation (see also Chapter 8). The activation of Akt provides cells with a survival signal that allows them to withstand apoptotic stimuli, through phosphorylation/inactivation of proapoptotic proteins, such as BAD and Caspase 9 (*19*).

1.1.3. THE PLCγ PATHWAY

Another prominent signaling protein activated by EGFR activation is the γ1 isoform of phospholipase C (PLC γ). Upon activation, PLC γ1 catalyses the hydrolysis of phosphatidyl inositol 4,5 biphosphate (PIP2) and generates the secondary messengers diacylglycerol (DAG) and inositol triphosphate (IP3) (*20*). IP3 is further recognized by the inositol triphosphate receptor (IP3R), a Ca2+ channel in the endoplasmic reticulum (ER) membrane. The binding of IP3 to IP3R releases the flow of calcium from the ER into the normally Ca2+-poor cytoplasm, which then triggers various events of calcium signaling (21). Calcium binds the protein calmodulin, which regulates a range of cellular targets, such as the Ca/calmodulin dependant protein kinases. Intracellular Ca2+ is also essential for activation of conventional Protein Kinase C (PKC) isoforms. DAG remains bound to the membrane, where it recruits and activates both conventional and novel members of the PKC family. PKC-α is a conventional PKC and requires both DAG and Ca2+ for activity. One of the targets activated by PKC-α is phospholipase D (PLD), which further hydrolyzes phosphatidylcholine (PC) to choline and phosphatidic acid.

EGFR thus activates PLCγ1 directly and Akt indirectly via PI3K. Recent evidence, however, indicates that there exists an interaction between PLCγ1 and Akt, which is mediated via the PLC γ1 SH3 domains through Akt proline-rich domains and is dependant on EGF stimulation (22).

1.2. EGFR Expression in Cancer

EGFR is overexpressed in a majority of epithelial tumors, including NSCLC, bladder, ovarian, kidney and pancreatic cancers and squamous cell carcinoma of the head and neck (SCCHN) (23). EGFR overexpression seems to be an early event in carcinogenesis since overexpression is detected in the histologically "normal" mucosa of SCCHN patients, as well as in premalignant dysplastic lesions (24, 25). Approximately 6% of breast carcinomas show EGFR amplification with EGFR protein overexpression (26). In breast cancer, EGFR overexpression is associated with reduced estrogen receptor content, advanced clinical stage and shortened relapse-free survival (27). In head and neck cancer, as well as in prostate cancer, EGFR overexpression correlates with poor prognosis and reduced survival (28, 29). Moreover, there is evidence for an association between resistance to ionizing radiation and EGFR overexpression in head and neck cancer (30). Protein overexpression is thought to result from enhanced transcription, and in some cases, from gene amplification (31), but not from enhanced mRNA stability (32, 33). EGFR can also be transactivated upon GPCR (G-protein-coupled receptor) stimulation via EGFR proligands including proHB-EGF and a metalloproteinase that is rapidly induced upon GPCR–ligand interaction (34, 35). This molecular cross talk provides evidence for cross-communication among different signalling systems (35) and represents new challenges for the design of therapeutic strategies (see also Chapters 17 and 18).

1.3. Downstream Effects of EGFR Overexpression

Increased expression of EGFR can lead to constitutive activation of several downstream signaling molecules. Downstream effectors often aberrantly activated include ERK1/-2, Akt, STAT3, and STAT5. Activated Erk has been correlated with EGFR overexpression and is associated with an advanced tumor stage in head and neck cancer (36). Phosphorylation of Akt, downstream of deregulated EGFR, has been observed in a majority of laryngeal cancers and is associated tumor development in the pharynx and larynx (37). The STAT family members, STAT3 and STAT5 are also upregulated, due, at least in part, to overexpression of EGFR. STAT3 is required for EGFR-mediated head and neck cancer cell growth in vitro (38), while STAT5b is constitutively activated through the EGFR axis and contributes to SCCHN tumorigenesis (39). STAT3 can also directly bind to tyrosine residues within the EGFR cytoplasmic domain and get activated directly (40). EGFR overexpression can also lead to increased invasion by way of a concomitant increase in phospholipase Cγ-1 (41). A recent report demonstrates evidence of Abl kinases being activated downstream of deregulated EGFR, as well as HER-2 and Src kinases in breast cancer cells (42). Abl kinases can further activate various signaling molecules resulting in increased migration and invasion (42).

2. THE STAT SIGNALING PATHWAY

STAT (signal transducers and activators of transcription) signaling pathways are key components of the EGFR-mediated signaling cascades. Overexpression or inactivation of various components of the pathway in a variety of human malignancies have provided valuable insights into the normal functioning of these molecules.

2.1. Structure and Function of the STAT Family Members

STATs are evolutionarily conserved dual-function proteins present in a latent state in the cytoplasm of all dividing cells. STATs serve as both signal transducers and as nuclear transcription factors. The cytokine activated Janus activated kinase-STAT (JAK-STAT) pathway is, in fact, considered a paradigm of signal transduction processes, as the signal is transduced directly to the nucleus from external stimuli, without the intervention of secondary messengers (*43*). STAT proteins were discovered about 16 years ago as mediators of interferon regulation, and their role has been best characterized in cytokine signaling. STATs can be activated by more than 20 different cytokines via their receptor association with the JAK family of kinases. Cumulative evidence supports a role for STATs in cancer progression (*44*).

2.2. STAT Family Members

There are seven members in the STAT family of proteins: STATs 1, 2, 3, 4, 5a, 5b, and 6. All STATs have a similar domain structure, with an amino terminal domain involved in tetramerization and phosphatase activity. Structure of STAT Family Members is linked to a coiled-coil domain, which is responsible for protein-protein interactions. The coiled-coil domain is followed by the DNA binding domain, a linker domain involved in DNA binding, a SH2 domain that mediates dimerization and receptor binding followed finally by the carboxy terminal transactivation domain (*45*). Though structurally similar, the STAT family proteins carry out different functions via their interactions with distinct cytokines and different downstream modulators. STAT5a and 5b are coded by two separate yet highly homologous genes localized to chromosome 17 of humans. Although STATs have been shown to interact with EGFR autophosphorylation sites (*46*), there is evidence that both wild-type (WT) and truncated EGF receptors that lack all autophosphorylation sites can activate STATs 1, 3, and 5 in response to either EGF or amphiregulin (*47*).

2.3. General Mechanism of STAT Activation in Signal Transduction

Signaling is initiated by binding of a specific ligand to its cognate receptor followed by aggregation of the receptor on the cell membrane. Cytokine receptors, like IL-6, which lack intrinsic tyrosine kinase activity, further recruit members of the JAK family of kinases (e.g., the members JAK1, JAK2, JAK3, and Tyk2), which act as intermediaries between the cytokine receptor and the STAT molecules (*48, 49*). The receptor activated JAK molecules further phosphorylate specific tyrosine residues within the cytoplasmic tails of receptors, which serve as docking sites for the recruitment of latent STAT molecules. Phosphorylation of the monomeric STAT molecules at critical tyrosine residues further induces STAT molecules to homo or heterodimerise via SH2 domains with other STAT molecules. This activated complex is then translocated to the nucleus, whereupon it binds to specific sequences in promoter regions of target genes.

Activation of STATs can also be mediated directly through the recruitment of STAT SH2 domains by activated growth factor receptor tyrosine kinases (e.g., EGFR and PDGFR). STAT1 activation by platelet derived growth factor receptor (PDGFR), however, seems to be biochemically distinct from that of STAT3, to which it is highly homologous. STAT1 activation seems to occur purely through PDGFR and does not require any cytosolic components, unlike STAT3, which requires the JAK family of kinases for maximal activation (50). STAT family members can also be directly activated via a third mechanism, i.e., through the cytoplasmic kinases, Src and Abl. v-Abl induced transformation of v-Src can bind to and phosphorylate STAT3 in vitro (51). Also, v-Abl mediated activation of STAT molecules via JAK1 suggests that the latter plays an important role in transformation of hematopoietic cells (52).

Though the conventional method of transcriptional activation by STAT molecules remains phosphorylation of key tyrosine residues, followed by dimerization and nuclear translocation, STATs can also induce target expression as unphosphorylated molecules (53). STAT1-null U3A cells did not undergo apoptosis on challenge until STAT1 expression was restored. The apoptotic response, however, was maintained even with the expression of STAT1 Y701F mutant (in which the critical tyrosine residue was mutated to a phenylalanine residue) (53).

2.3.1. PHOSPHORYLATION OF SERINE RESIDUES

Most STAT molecules (except probably STAT2 and STAT6) are also phosphorylated at specific serine residues in a stimulus-regulated manner (54). There seems to exist some interdependence of serine and tyrosine phosphorylation in some of these STAT molecules (54). The various steps involved in this complex interaction, however, still require complete elucidation.

2.4. Nuclear Translocation of Activated STATs and Downstream Effects

The mechanism of translocation of the activated STAT molecules to the nucleus is thought to be mediated via importins. The nuclear localization signal for STAT1 homodimers and STAT1–2 heterodimers has been identified (55). The phosphorylated dimer is actively transported in the nucleus via importin a/b and RanGDP complex. Once inside the nucleus, the active STAT dimer binds to cognate sequences contained within gene promoters such as TTN4-5AA (where N is any nucleotide base) sequence (56). Binding leads to transcription of specific target genes. Transcriptional targets of the STAT molecules are genes associated with cell proliferation, differentiation, motility, and apoptosis. Individual STATs differ in the physiological consequences of their activation. The precise spectrum of STAT activation is thought to be due to the regulating upstream cytokine, different growth factors, and the specific cellular context.

2.5. STAT1

STAT1 (Signal Transducer and Activator of Transcription 1) is activated by various cytokines and growth factors including interferon-alpha (IFN-α), interferon-gamma (IFN-γ), LIF (Leukemia Inhibitory Factor), growth hormone, EGF, PDGF, IL-10, and IL-6. The STAT1 gene, localized to human chromosome 2q32.2, gives rise to two differently processed RNA products that ultimately yield two proteins of sizes 91kDa and 84 kDa. Targeted disruption of the STAT1 gene delineates the important role that STAT1 plays in immunity and development. STAT1 deficient mice display no gross developmental defects; however, they fail to thrive and are susceptible to viral disease (57).

2.5.1. STAT1 IN CANCER

In contrast to STAT3 and STAT5, STAT1 negatively regulates cell proliferation and angiogenesis and thereby inhibits tumor formation. Consistent with its tumor suppressive properties, STAT1 and its downstream targets are reduced in a variety of human tumors. Moreover, STAT1 deficient mice are highly susceptible to tumor formation induced by chemical carcinogens (58). STAT1 restoration in RAD-105 tumor cells derived from a fibrosarcoma of STAT1 knockout mouse suppressed tumorigenecity and metastasis (59), indicating that

STAT1 is a negative regulator of tumor growth. STAT1 deficiency has been found in melanomas, gastric cancers and T cell lymphomas (*59*). On the other hand, constitutive activation of STAT1 has also been observed in tumors (*60*), indicating the complex role of STAT1 in tumorigenesis.

STAT1 homodimers are involved in type II interferon signalling and bind to the GAS (interferon-gamma activated sequence) promoter to induce expression of ISG (interferon stimulated genes). Previous studies indicate that IFN-γ mediated STAT1 activation leads to growth suppression via the induction of p21/waf1 (*61*). Our lab recently demonstrated that STAT 1 downregulation by promoter methylation via regulation of p21 contributes to tumor progression (*62*). Targeting of STAT1 using either antisense or dominant-negative strategies, however, had no effect on cell growth (*38*). Recently, the unphosphorylated form of STAT1 was crystallized (*63*), which should provide more insights into its structure and function.

2.6. STAT3

STAT3 can be activated by a number of cytokines, including IL-6, oncostatin M, LIF (*63*), and leptin (*64*). Receptor tyrosine kinases such as EGFR and c-met (*65*), as well as non-receptor tyrosine kinases like src (*66*) or JAK can phosphorylate STAT3, which leads to its activation. STAT3 is also the target of p210-BCR-ABL in a murine embryonic stem (ES) cell model and in primary CD34+ CML cells (*67*). Unlike the other STAT family members, STAT3 appears to be crucial for embryonic development, as STAT3 null mice fail to develop beyond embryonic day 7 (*68*). This finding has led to suggestions that STAT3 may be a primordial STAT protein (*69*). STAT3 target genes are implicated in all processes of tumorigenesis, including proliferation, apoptosis, angiogenesis, invasion, and migration (*70*). Intriguingly, recent evidence indicates a direct effect of non–tyrosine-phosphorylated, cytoplasmic STAT3 on cell motility (*71*), a small tubulin-binding protein that acts as a microtubule depolarization factor (*72*).

2.6.1. ACTIVATION OF STAT3

Like other STAT proteins, STAT3 is activated by tyrosine phosphorylation at a single tyrosine residue close to the carboxy-terminus (Y705), as well as by serine phosphorylation at a site within the transactivation domain (S727). Phosphorylation at Ser 727 augments the transcriptional activity of both STAT1 and STAT3 (*73*), presumably through interactions between STATs and co-activator proteins (*54*). Tyrosine phosphorylation in response to cytokine stimulation is mediated by JAK1 (*69*) and is required for STAT3 dimerization. After tyrosine phosphorylation, STAT3 forms a homodimer or a heterodimer with STAT1 and enters the nucleus, where it regulates the expression of a specific set of target genes such as Pim-1, c-Myc, Cyclin D2, Cyclin A etc., which associated with a diverse set of functions like proliferation, apoptosis and differentiation (*74*). Serine phosphorylation occurs within a mitogen-activated protein kinase consensus site (*69*) and has been shown to have an important role in oncogenesis. Dominant-negative STAT3 mutant with a Ser727 to Ala727 mutation was found to suppress STAT3 signaling and Src transformation (*75*). Moreover, activated STAT3 (Ser727) may also be involved in the pathogenesis of breast cancer in an estrogen receptor (ER)-dependent manner (*76*). In a study of 68 breast cancer tissues, a significant increase in phospho Ser 727 expression was observed in ER-negative breast cancer cells compared to corresponding non-cancer tissues, which correlated significantly with increased stage of cancer and tumor size. Recent evidence suggests that oncogenic STAT3 contributes to epigenetic silencing of a gene involved in negative regulation of T cell signaling (*77*), which may have important therapeutic implications.

2.6.2. STAT3 ACTIVATION IN CANCER

Elevated STAT3 levels have been detected in numerous malignancies including leukemias, lymphomas, multiple myeloma, breast cancer, prostate cancer, renal cell carcinoma, lung cancer, ovarian cancer, pancreatic adenocarcinoma, melanoma, and SCCHN (*49*). The constitutive active STAT3 molecule is sufficient to transform immortalized fibroblasts and induce tumors in nude mice (*78*), meaning that STAT3 possesses oncogenic potential.

In SCCHN, STAT3 activation has been found to be necessary for continued growth (*79*). Our lab previously demonstrated that activation of STAT1 and STAT3 was constitutive in transformed squamous epithelial cells, which produce elevated levels of TGF-α, and was enhanced by the addition of exogenous TGF-α (*38*). Targeting of STAT3 using antisense oligonucleotides directed against the translation initiation site resulted in significant growth inhibition (*38*).

High levels of activated STAT3 correlate with increased nodal metastases, clinical stage of tumor and poor patient prognosis in oral tongue carcinoma (*80*). High expression levels of STAT3 also seem to correlate with differentiation status of the tumor, with STAT3 expression levels the highest in poorly differentiated head and neck tumors and STAT1 levels highest in well-differentiated tumors (*81*). In fact, cells with a dominant-active STAT3 mutant proliferate independently of the upstream EGFR signaling axis (*82*). At the same time, transfection of SCCHN cells with dominant-negative STAT3 mutants or treatment with STAT3 antisense oligonucleotides resulted in growth inhibition, apoptosis, and decreased STAT3 target expression (*83*).

STAT3 can also interact with the Src family of kinases (e.g., lyn, fyn, yes and c-Src), which are activated via EGFR activation by TGF-α (*84*). Studies from our lab demonstrated that stable transfection of SCCHN cell lines with a dominant-negative c-Src mutant construct resulted in decreased levels of STAT3 activation. Furthermore, blocking activity of Src kinases using pyrrolopyrimidine Src kinase inhibitors inhibited SCCHN growth via abrogation of STAT3 activation (*84*). These data thus indicate activation of STAT molecules through the EGFR-Src signaling axis, and could be used to develop potential novel therapeutic targets. Residual ErbB2 activation by EGF has been reported to contribute to persistent downstream activation of STAT3. Also, combined exposure to an EGFR blocker and a JAK2 inhibitor (AG490) resulted in significantly greater tumor growth inhibition than either agent alone (*85*).

2.6.3. EGFR INDEPENDENT ACTIVATION OF STAT3

Constitutive activation of STAT3 can also occur through EGFR independent mechanisms (*43, 49*). Constitutive STAT3 activation is also capable of contributing to tumor growth in SCCHN independent of the EGFR autocrine axis (*86*).

STAT3 phosphorylation levels remain the same after treatment of several head and neck cancer cell lines with AG1478, a chemical inhibitor of EGFR activity (*87*). In fact, the same group determined that IL-6 is the major secretory ligand stimulating STAT3 activation by acting on the gp130 co-receptor in an autocrine/paracrine manner. Furthermore, interfering with this cytokine pathway resulted in abrogating cell growth and promoting apoptosis in head and neck cancer cell lines (*87*). Alternatively, this could also suggest that EGF continues to drive STAT3 phosphorylation through other receptors. Further investigations into the nature of molecular mechanisms involved in increased IL-6 production, however, resulted in identification of regulation of Il-6 by nuclear factor κB (NF-κB) (*88*). Blocking NF-κB reduced expression of phosphorylated STAT3 in SCCHN cells, indicating a convergence of two independent signaling pathways (*88*). These findings support the emerging view that a deregulated signaling network, rather than a single biochemical pathway, are involved in head and neck carcinogenesis and thus could be potential therapeutic targets (*88*).

2.7. STAT5

STAT5 was originally identified as a prolactin (PRL) activated mammary gland transcription factor (89). Shortly after this discovery, another highly homologous gene, STAT5b was identified and also found to be expressed in the mammary gland (90). STAT5a and STAT5b are encoded by two different highly homologous genes on the human chromosome 17q11.2 and mouse chromosome 11. STAT5 is activated by a variety of cytokines that include prolactin, IL-2, IL-3, IL-5, IL-7, granulocyte-macrophage colony stimulating factor (GM-CSF), G-CSF, M-CSF, erythropoietin (Epo), thrombopoietin, and growth hormone (GH) (91). Upon activation, the phosphorylated STAT molecules form either homo- or heterodimers through their SH2-domains and translocate into the nucleus to activate the transcription of various target genes including bcl-xL and cyclin D1. STAT5 recognizes the IFN-γ activated sequence TTCNNNGAA in the promoter region of the beta-casein gene.

STAT5a and 5b have been demonstrated to mediate PRL-induced mouse mammary gland development (92, 93). Studies on knockout mice have elucidated the diverse functional characteristics of STAT5. STAT5a and STAT5b knockout mice were generated in the laboratories of Dr. J. Ihle at St. Jude's Children's Hospital, Nashville, TN in 1998 (94). STAT5a knockout mice demonstrated impaired mammary gland development and lactogenesis (92). Their phenotype closely resembled the phenotype of PRL receptor deficient mice (95), which suggests that STAT5a is crucial for this aspect of prolactin function. (96).

The phenotype of STAT5b deficient mice, on the other hand, suggests an indispensable role in growth hormone (GH) action. The characteristics of STAT5b -/- mice were dwarfism, elevated plasma GH, low plasma insulin-like growth factor 1 and obesity. All these characteristics are similar to those of Laron-type dwarfism, a human disease associated with a defective GH receptor (96). Surprisingly, these double knockout mice showed almost intact hematopoeisis, given the crucial activation of STAT5 by various hematopoietic cytokines. In summary, knockout studies on STAT5 illustrate the essential, though redundant roles of both isoforms in a spectrum of physiological responses associated with GH and PRL signaling.

Activation of STAT5 is primarily involved in mediating either the growth promoting or transforming activities of a cytokine or oncogene or is involved in regulating apoptosis (97). Activation of STAT5 leads to downstream signal transduction events in a similar manner as those of the other STAT members. STAT5a and -b can form homodimers with itself or heterodimers with the adapter protein CrkL (98, 99).

2.7.1. STAT5 Activation in Cancer

STAT5 is constitutively activated in a wide range of human malignancies. STAT5 has been implicated as an oncogene, primarily in hematopoietic malignancies (100). In chronic myelogenous leukemia (CML), STAT5 activation has been shown to mediate the transforming activity of Bcr-Abl (101). Activation of STAT5a in myeloma and lymphoma associated with the TEL/JAK2 oncogenic gene fusion is independent of cell stimulus and has been shown to be essential for the tumorigenicity of the TEL/JAK2 oncogene (102). Indeed, activation of STAT5 is both necessary and sufficient for transformation by TEL/JAK2 and STAT5 activation, leading to induction of the single downstream target gene oncostatin M (OSM) and induction of a lethal myeloproliferative disease. STAT5 activation has been linked to transformation mediated by other fusion genes, including NPM/ALK and TEL/ABL (103, 104). The STAT5b/retinoic acid receptor alpha gene fusion has been detected in a small subset of acute promyelocytic-like leukemias (APLL) (105).

In solid tumors, there is emerging evidence for constitutive active STAT5 association with tumorigenesis (our observations and (106)). Constitutive activation of STAT5 has also been demonstrated in various solid tumors, including breast, prostate, nasopharyngeal cancer and head and neck cancers. In breast cancer, activation of STAT5 by prolactin caused increase in E-cadherin expression and reduced invasion through a Matrigel column (*107*). Constitutive activation of STAT5 has been associated with better prognosis in both breast cancer and nasopharyngeal cancer. In contrast, activated STAT5 correlated with high histological grade and early disease recurrence in prostate cancer (*106*). Activated STAT5 may also act as a survival factor in human melanoma via the EGFR signaling axis (*108*). In human melanomas, expression of activated STAT5 is driven by EGF, and is mediated through Src and JAK1 kinases (*108*). The seemingly different outcomes of STAT5 activation may be contributed to different tumor microenvironments, conflicting upstream regulating cytokines and other as yet unidentified factors.

STA5 activation appears to confer an advantage of growth proliferation to SCCHN cells (*39*). STAT5, in concert with Raf, has been shown to induce proliferation in IL-3 dependant cell lines, abrogating the need for the addition of exogenous cytokines. (*91*). Activated STAT5 has been demonstrated to play a role in cellular proliferation of a diverse phenotype of cells, including primary endothelial cells (*109*) and myeloid cells (*110*).

Targeting STAT5 using different approaches, including antisense oligonucleotides and dominant negative strategies, highlights the functional diversity between the STAT5 isoforms (*111*). Antisense oligos directed against STAT5 had no effect on growth rates of SCCHN cells, while targeting STAT5b inhibited SCCHN growth (*111*). In addition, SCCHN cells stably transfected with dominant-negative mutant STAT5b failed to proliferate in vitro, which further corroborated the generality of targteting approach.

2.7.2. EGFR Independent STAT5 Activation

STAT5, like STAT3, can be activated by various cytokines and growth factors apart from EGFR. STAT5 is essential for differentiation of erythroid cells through the erythropoietin (EPO) receptor cytoplasmic domain (*112*). STAT5 can also be activated by c-src, either directly or downstream of growth factor receptors. The src family of kinases was initially implicated in STAT activation by studies examining the molecular mechanisms associated with v-src mediated transformation of fibroblasts and hematopoietic cell lines (*51, 113*). Co-immunoprecipitation studies indicate an interaction between c-src and STAT5, as well as STAT3 and EGFR in SCCHN cell lines (*84*). c-src induced activation of STAT5 results in an as yet unidentified novel tyrosine phosphorylation site other than the well-characterized Y694 (for STAT5a) and Y699 for STAT5b) (*114*). Cumulative evidence suggests that STAT5a does not translocate to the nucleus after being phosphorylated in response to c-src, while STAT5b does (*66*). Despite being able to translocate to the nucleus, however, c-src activated STAT5b is unable to initiate transcription (*115, 116*). Thus, c-src activates STAT5 in a unique manner at novel tyrosine phosphorylation sites and exhibits different patterns of nuclear localization and transcriptional activation.

3. CONCLUSION

The highly conserved EGF receptor pathway comprises many levels of complex interactions mediated via its various downstream regulators, which is the norm rather than an exception in higher eukaryotic cellular signaling. These multiple layers, which ultimately execute distinct cellular fate in the form of cellular proliferation, differentiation, apoptosis, or cell migration, form a safeguard against aberrant kinase-phosphatase signaling cascades. The very versatile nature of these pathways, however, emphasizes the difficulties encountered in successful therapy of tumors. A complete understanding of the signaling networks in both normal physiological state and oncogenesis would lead to development of novel and more specific therapeutic targets.

REFERENCES

1. Ullrich A, Coussens L, Hayflick JS, et al. Human epidermal growth factor receptor cDNA sequence and aberrant expression of the amplified gene in A431 epidermoid carcinoma cells. Nature 1984;309(5967):418-25.
2. Wong AJ, Ruppert JM, Bigner SH, et al. Structural alterations of the epidermal growth factor receptor gene in human gliomas. Proc Natl Acad Sci U S A 1992;89(7):2965-9.
3. Moscatello DK, Montgomery RB, Sundareshan P, McDanel H, Wong MY, Wong AJ. Transformational and altered signal transduction by a naturally occurring mutant EGF receptor. Oncogene 1996;13(1):85-96.
4. Pedersen MW, Meltorn M, Damstrup L, Poulsen HS. The type III epidermal growth factor receptor mutation. Biological significance and potential target for anti-cancer therapy. Ann Oncol 2001;12(6):745-60.
5. Sok JC, Coppelli FM, Thomas SM, et al. Mutant epidermal growth factor receptor (EGFRvIII) contributes to head and neck cancer growth and resistance to EGFR targeting. Clin Cancer Res 2006;12(17):5064-73.
6. Yarden Y. The EGFR family and its ligands in human cancer. signalling mechanisms and therapeutic opportunities. Eur J Cancer 2001;37 Suppl 4:S3-8.
7. Lin SY, Makino K, Xia W, et al. Nuclear localization of EGF receptor and its potential new role as a transcription factor. Nat Cell Biol 2001;3(9):802-8.
8. Tzahar E, Yarden Y. The ErbB-2/HER2 oncogenic receptor of adenocarcinomas: from orphanhood to multiple stromal ligands. Biochim Biophys Acta 1998;1377(1):M25-37.
9. Lo HW, Hsu SC, Ali-Seyed M, et al. Nuclear interaction of EGFR and STAT3 in the activation of the iNOS/NO pathway. Cancer Cell 2005;7(6):575-89.
10. Carpenter G. Nuclear localization and possible functions of receptor tyrosine kinases. Curr Opin Cell Biol 2003;15(2):143-8.
11. Wang SC, Lien HC, Xia W, et al. Binding at and transactivation of the COX-2 promoter by nuclear tyrosine kinase receptor ErbB-2. Cancer Cell 2004;6(3):251-61.
12. Oliveira S, van Bergen en Henegouwen PM, Storm G, Schiffelers RM. Molecular biology of epidermal growth factor receptor inhibition for cancer therapy. Expert Opin Biol Ther 2006;6(6):605-17.
13. Pessin JE, Okada S. Insulin and EGF receptors integrate the Ras and Rap signaling pathways. Endocr J 1999;46 Suppl:S11-6.
14. Zhang XF, Settleman J, Kyriakis JM, et al. Normal and oncogenic p21ras proteins bind to the aminoterminal regulatory domain of c-Raf-1. Nature 1993;364(6435):308-13.
15. Avruch J, Khokhlatchev A, Kyriakis JM, et al. Ras activation of the Raf kinase: tyrosine kinase recruitment of the MAP kinase cascade. Recent Prog Horm Res 2001;56:127-55.
16. Ulisse S, Cinque B, Silvano G, et al. Erk-dependent cytosolic phospholipase A2 activity is induced by CD95 ligand cross-linking in the mouse derived Sertoli cell line TM4 and is required to trigger apoptosis in CD95 bearing cells. Cell Death Differ 2000;7(10):916-24.
17. Blume-Jensen P, Hunter T. Oncogenic kinase signalling. Nature 2001;411(6835):355-65.
18. Sekulic A, Hudson CC, Homme JL, et al. A direct linkage between the phosphoinositide 3-kinase-AKT signaling pathway and the mammalian target of rapamycin in mitogen-stimulated and transformed cells. Cancer Res 2000;60(13):3504-13.
19. Khwaja A. Akt is more than just a Bad kinase. Nature 1999;401(6748):33-4.
20. Majerus PW. Inositol phosphate biochemistry. Annu Rev Biochem 1992;61:225-50.
21. Berridge MJ. Inositol trisphosphate and calcium signalling. Nature 1993;361(6410):315-25.
22. Wang Y, Wu J, Wang Z. Akt binds to and phosphorylates phospholipase C-gamma1 in response to epidermal growth factor. Mol Biol Cell 2006;17(5):2267-77.
23. Zwick E, Bange J, Ullrich A. Receptor tyrosine kinase signalling as a target for cancer intervention strategies. Endocr Relat Cancer 2001;8(3):161-73.
24. Grandis JR, Tweardy DJ. Elevated levels of transforming growth factor alpha and epidermal growth factor receptor messenger RNA are early markers of carcinogenesis in head and neck cancer. Cancer Res 1993;53(15):3579-84.

25. Grandis JR, Tweardy DJ, Melhem MF. Asynchronous modulation of transforming growth factor alpha and epidermal growth factor receptor protein expression in progression of premalignant lesions to head and neck squamous cell carcinoma. Clin Cancer Res 1998;4(1):13-20.
26. Bhargava R, Gerald WL, Li AR, et al. EGFR gene amplification in breast cancer: correlation with epidermal growth factor receptor mRNA and protein expression and HER-2 status and absence of EGFR-activating mutations. Mod Pathol 2005;18(8):1027-33.
27. Nicholson RI, McClelland RA, Gee JM, et al. Epidermal growth factor receptor expression in breast cancer: association with response to endocrine therapy. Breast Cancer Res Treat 1994;29(1):117-25.
28. Grandis JR, Melhem MF, Gooding WE, et al. Levels of TGF-alpha and EGFR protein in head and neck squamous cell carcinoma and patient survival. J Natl Cancer Inst 1998;90(11):824-32.
29. Di Lorenzo G, Tortora G, D'Armiento FP, et al. Expression of epidermal growth factor receptor correlates with disease relapse and progression to androgen-independence in human prostate cancer. Clin Cancer Res 2002;8(11):3438-44.
30. Sheridan MT, O'Dwyer T, Seymour CB, Mothersill CE. Potential indicators of radiosensitivity in squamous cell carcinoma of the head and neck. Radiat Oncol Investig 1997;5(4):180-6.
31. Velu TJ. Structure, function and transforming potential of the epidermal growth factor receptor. Mol Cell Endocrinol 1990;70(3):205-16.
32. Zimmermann M, Zouhair A, Azria D, Ozsahin M. The epidermal growth factor receptor (EGFR) in head and neck cancer: its role and treatment implications. Radiat Oncol 2006;1:11.
33. Grandis JR, Tweardy DJ. TGF-alpha and EGFR in head and neck cancer. J Cell Biochem Suppl 1993:188-91.
34. Gschwind A, Zwick E, Prenzel N, Leserer M, Ullrich A. Cell communication networks: epidermal growth factor receptor transactivation as the paradigm for interreceptor signal transmission. Oncogene 2001;20(13):1594-600.
35. Prenzel N, Zwick E, Daub H, et al. EGF receptor transactivation by G-protein-coupled receptors requires metalloproteinase cleavage of proHB-EGF. Nature 1999;402(6764):884-8.
36. Albanell J, Codony-Servat J, Rojo F, et al. Activated extracellular signal-regulated kinases: association with epidermal growth factor receptor/transforming growth factor alpha expression in head and neck squamous carcinoma and inhibition by anti-epidermal growth factor receptor treatments. Cancer Res 2001;61(17):6500-10.
37. Ongkeko WM, Altuna X, Weisman RA, Wang-Rodriguez J. Expression of protein tyrosine kinases in head and neck squamous cell carcinomas. Am J Clin Pathol 2005;124(1):71-6.
38. Grandis JR, Drenning SD, Chakraborty A, et al. Requirement of Stat3 but not Stat1 activation for epidermal growth factor receptor- mediated cell growth in vitro. J Clin Invest 1998;102(7):1385-92.
39. Xi S, Zhang Q, Gooding WE, Smithgall TE, Grandis JR. Constitutive activation of Stat5b contributes to carcinogenesis in vivo. Cancer Res 2003;63(20):6763-71.
40. Xia L, Wang L, Chung AS, et al. Identification of both positive and negative domains within egf receptor cooh terminal region for stat activation. Journal of Biological Chemistry 2002: In Press.
41. Thomas SM, Coppelli FM, Wells A, et al. Epidermal growth factor receptor-stimulated activation of phospholipase Cgamma-1 promotes invasion of head and neck squamous cell carcinoma. Cancer Res 2003;63(17):5629-35.
42. Srinivasan D, Plattner R. Activation of Abl tyrosine kinases promotes invasion of aggressive breast cancer cells. Cancer Res 2006;66(11):5648-55.
43. Levy DE, Darnell JE, Jr. Stats: transcriptional control and biological impact. Nat Rev Mol Cell Biol 2002;3(9):651-62.
44. Yu H, Jove R. The STATs of cancer-new molecular targets come of age. Nat Rev Cancer 2004;4(2):97-105.
45. Meyer T, Vinkemeier U. Nucleocytoplasmic shuttling of STAT transcription factors. Eur J Biochem 2004;271(23-24):4606-12.
46. Shao H, Cheng HY, Cook RG, Tweardy DJ. Identification and characterization of signal transducer and activator of transcription 3 recruitment sites within the epidermal growth factor receptor. Cancer Res 2003;63(14):3923-30.
47. David M, Wong L, Flavell R, et al. STAT activation by epidermal growth factor (EGF) and amphiregulin. Requirement for the EGF receptor kinase but not for tyrosine phosphorylation sites or JAK1. J Biol Chem 1996;271(16):9185-8.

48. Ihle JN. Janus kinases in cytokine signalling. Philos Trans R Soc Lond B Biol Sci 1996;351(1336): 159-66.
49. Bowman T, Garcia R, Turkson J, Jove R. STATs in oncogenesis. Oncogene 2000;19(21):2474-88.
50. Vignais ML, Gilman M. Distinct mechanisms of activation of Stat1 and Stat3 by platelet-derived growth factor receptor in a cell-free system. Mol Cell Biol 1999;19(5):3727-35.
51. Cao X, Tay A, Guy GR, Tan YH. Activation and association of Stat3 with Src in v-Src-transformed cell lines. Mol Cell Biol 1996;16(4):1595-603.
52. Danial NN, Rothman P. JAK-STAT signaling activated by Abl oncogenes. Oncogene 2000;19(21): 2523-31.
53. Kumar A, Commane M, Flickinger TW, Horvath CM, Stark GR. Defective TNF-alpha-induced apoptosis in STAT1-null cells due to low constitutive levels of caspases. Science 1997;278(5343):1630-2.
54. Decker T, Kovarik P. Transcription factor activity of STAT proteins: structural requirements and regulation by phosphorylation and interacting proteins. Cell Mol Life Sci 1999;55(12):1535-46.
55. Melen K, Fagerlund R, Franke J, Kohler M, Kinnunen L, Julkunen I. Importin alpha nuclear localization signal binding sites for STAT1, STAT2, and influenza A virus nucleoprotein. J Biol Chem 2003;278(30):28193-200.
56. Bild AH, Turkson J, Jove R. Cytoplasmic transport of Stat3 by receptor-mediated endocytosis. Embo J 2002;21(13):3255-63.
57. Durbin JE, Hackenmiller R, Simon MC, Levy DE. Targeted disruption of the mouse Stat1 gene results in compromised innate immunity to viral disease. Cell 1996;84(3):443-50.
58. Kaplan DH, Shankaran V, Dighe AS, et al. Demonstration of an interferon gamma-dependent tumor surveillance system in immunocompetent mice. Proc Natl Acad Sci U S A 1998;95(13):7556-61.
59. Huang S, Bucana CD, Van Arsdall M, Fidler IJ. Stat1 negatively regulates angiogenesis, tumorigenicity and metastasis of tumor cells. Oncogene 2002;21(16):2504-12.
60. Widschwendter A, Tonko-Geymayer S, Welte T, Daxenbichler G, Marth C, Doppler W. Prognostic significance of signal transducer and activator of transcription 1 activation in breast cancer. Clin Cancer Res 2002;8(10):3065-74.
61. Chin YE, Kitagawa M, Su WC, You ZH, Iwamoto Y, Fu XY. Cell growth arrest and induction of cyclin-dependent kinase inhibitor p21 WAF1/CIP1 mediated by STAT1. Science 1996;272(5262): 719-22.
62. Xi S, Dyer KF, Kimak M, et al. Decreased STAT1 expression by promoter methylation in squamous cell carcinogenesis. J Natl Cancer Inst 2006;98(3):181-9.
63. Stahl N, Farruggella TJ, Boulton TG, Zhong Z, Darnell JE, Jr., Yancopoulos GD. Choice of STATs and other substrates specified by modular tyrosine- based motifs in cytokine receptors. Science 1995;267(5202):1349-53.
64. Ghilardi N, Skoda RC. The leptin receptor activates janus kinase 2 and signals for proliferation in a factor-dependent cell line. Mol Endocrinol 1997;11(4):393-9.
65. Yuan ZL, Guan YJ, Wang L, Wei W, Kane AB, Chin YE. Central role of the threonine residue within the p+1 loop of receptor tyrosine kinase in STAT3 constitutive phosphorylation in metastatic cancer cells. Mol Cell Biol 2004;24(21):9390-400.
66. Silva CM. Role of STATs as downstream signal transducers in Src family kinase-mediated tumorigenesis. Oncogene 2004;23(48):8017-23.
67. Coppo P, Flamant S, De Mas V, et al. BCR-ABL activates STAT3 via JAK and MEK pathways in human cells. Br J Haematol 2006;134(2):171-9.
68. Takeda K, Noguchi K, Shi W, et al. Targeted disruption of the mouse Stat3 gene leads to early embryonic lethality. Proc Natl Acad Sci U S A 1997;94(8):3801-4.
69. Levy DE, Lee CK. What does Stat3 do? J Clin Invest 2002;109(9):1143-8.
70. Gao SP, Bromberg JF. Touched and moved by STAT3. Sci STKE 2006;2006(343):pe30.
71. Ng DC, Lin BH, Lim CP, et al. Stat3 regulates microtubules by antagonizing the depolymerization activity of stathmin. J Cell Biol 2006;172(2):245-57.
72. Belmont LD, Mitchison TJ. Identification of a protein that interacts with tubulin dimers and increases the catastrophe rate of microtubules. Cell 1996;84(4):623-31.
73. Wen Z, Darnell JE, Jr. Mapping of Stat3 serine phosphorylation to a single residue (727) and evidence that serine phosphorylation has no influence on DNA binding of Stat1 and Stat3. Nucleic Acids Res 1997;25(11):2062-7.

74. Hirano T, Ishihara K, Hibi M. Roles of STAT3 in mediating the cell growth, differentiation and survival signals relayed through the IL-6 family of cytokine receptors. Oncogene 2000;19(21):2548-56.
75. Bromberg JF, Horvath CM, Besser D, Lathem WW, Darnell JE, Jr. Stat3 activation is required for cellular transformation by v-src. Mol Cell Biol 1998;18(5):2553-8.
76. Yeh YT, Ou-Yang F, Chen IF, et al. STAT3 ser727 phosphorylation and its association with negative estrogen receptor status in breast infiltrating ductal carcinoma. Int J Cancer 2006;118(12):2943-7.
77. Zhang Q, Wang HY, Marzec M, Raghunath PN, Nagasawa T, Wasik MA. STAT3- and DNA methyltransferase 1-mediated epigenetic silencing of SHP-1 tyrosine phosphatase tumor suppressor gene in malignant T lymphocytes. Proc Natl Acad Sci U S A 2005;102(19):6948-53.
78. Bromberg JF, Wrzeszczynska MH, Devgan G, et al. Stat3 as an oncogene. Cell 1999;98(3):295-303.
79. Leeman RJ, Lui VW, Grandis JR. STAT3 as a therapeutic target in head and neck cancer. Expert Opin Biol Ther 2006;6(3):231-41.
80. Masuda M, Suzui M, Yasumatu R, et al. Constitutive activation of signal transducers and activators of transcription 3 correlates with cyclin D1 overexpression and may provide a novel prognostic marker in head and neck squamous cell carcinoma. Cancer Res 2002;62(12):3351-5.
81. Arany I, Chen SH, Megyesi JK, et al. Differentiation-dependent expression of signal transducers and activators of transcription (STATs) might modify responses to growth factors in the cancers of the head and neck. Cancer Lett 2003;199(1):83-9.
82. Kijima T, Niwa H, Steinman RA, et al. STAT3 activation abrogates growth factor dependence and contributes to head and neck squamous cell carcinoma tumor growth in vivo. Cell Growth Differ 2002;13(8):355-62.
83. Rubin Grandis J, Zeng Q, Drenning SD. Epidermal growth factor receptor--mediated stat3 signaling blocks apoptosis in head and neck cancer. Laryngoscope 2000;110(5 Pt 1):868-74.
84. Xi S, Zhang Q, Dyer KF, et al. Src kinases mediate STAT growth pathways in squamous cell carcinoma of the head and neck. J Biol Chem 2003;278(34):31574-83.
85. Dowlati A, Nethery D, Kern JA. Combined inhibition of epidermal growth factor receptor and JAK/STAT pathways results in greater growth inhibition in vitro than single agent therapy. Mol Cancer Ther 2004;3(4):459-63.
86. Kijima T, Niwa H, Steinman RA, et al. Stat3-mediated EGFR-independent growth in SCCHN. Cell Growth Differ 2002;13:355-62.
87. Sriuranpong V, Park JI, Amornphimoltham P, Patel V, Nelkin BD, Gutkind JS. Epidermal growth factor receptor-independent constitutive activation of STAT3 in head and neck squamous cell carcinoma is mediated by the autocrine/paracrine stimulation of the interleukin 6/gp130 cytokine system. Cancer Res 2003;63(11):2948-56.
88. Squarize CH, Castilho RM, Sriuranpong V, Pinto DS, Jr., Gutkind JS. Molecular cross-talk between the NFkappaB and STAT3 signaling pathways in head and neck squamous cell carcinoma. Neoplasia 2006;8(9):733-46.
89. Wakao H, Gouilleux F, Groner B. Mammary gland factor (MGF) is a novel member of the cytokine regulated transcription factor gene family and confers the prolactin response. Embo J 1994;13(9):2182-91.
90. Liu X, Robinson GW, Gouilleux F, Groner B, Hennighausen L. Cloning and expression of Stat5 and an additional homologue (Stat5b) involved in prolactin signal transduction in mouse mammary tissue. Proc Natl Acad Sci U S A 1995;92(19):8831-5.
91. Onishi M, Nosaka T, Misawa K, et al. Identification and characterization of a constitutively active STAT5 mutant that promotes cell proliferation. Mol Cell Biol 1998;18(7):3871-9.
92. Liu X, Robinson GW, Wagner KU, Garrett L, Wynshaw-Boris A, Hennighausen L. Stat5a is mandatory for adult mammary gland development and lactogenesis. Genes Dev 1997;11(2):179-86.
93. Udy GB, Towers RP, Snell RG, et al. Requirement of STAT5b for sexual dimorphism of body growth rates and liver gene expression. Proc Natl Acad Sci U S A 1997;94(14):7239-44.
94. Teglund S, McKay C, Schuetz E, et al. Stat5a and Stat5b proteins have essential and nonessential, or redundant, roles in cytokine responses. Cell 1998;93(5):841-50.
95. Ormandy CJ, Camus A, Barra J, et al. Null mutation of the prolactin receptor gene produces multiple reproductive defects in the mouse. Genes Dev 1997;11(2):167-78.
96. Levy DE, Gilliland DG. Divergent roles of STAT1 and STAT5 in malignancy as revealed by gene disruptions in mice. Oncogene 2000;19(21):2505-10.

97. Bromberg JF. Activation of STAT proteins and growth control. Bioessays 2001;23(2):161-9.
98. Cella N, Groner B, Hynes NE. Characterization of Stat5a and Stat5b homodimers and heterodimers and their association with the glucocortiocoid receptor in mammary cells. Mol Cell Biol 1998;18(4):1783-92.
99. Schulze H, Ballmaier M, Welte K, Germeshausen M. Thrombopoietin induces the generation of distinct Stat1, Stat3, Stat5a and Stat5b homo- and heterodimeric complexes with different kinetics in human platelets. Exp Hematol 2000;28(3):294-304.
100. Moriggl R, Sexl V, Kenner L, et al. Stat5 tetramer formation is associated with leukemogenesis. Cancer Cell 2005;7(1):87-99.
101. Carlesso N, Frank DA, Griffin JD. Tyrosyl phosphorylation and DNA binding activity of signal transducers and activators of transcription (STAT) proteins in hematopoietic cell lines transformed by Bcr/Abl. J Exp Med 1996;183(3):811-20.
102. Schwaller J, Parganas E, Wang D, et al. Stat5 is essential for the myelo- and lymphoproliferative disease induced by TEL/JAK2. Mol Cell 2000;6(3):693-704.
103. Nieborowska-Skorska M, Slupianek A, Xue L, et al. Role of signal transducer and activator of transcription 5 in nucleophosmin/ anaplastic lymphoma kinase-mediated malignant transformation of lymphoid cells. Cancer Res 2001;61(17):6517-23.
104. Spiekermann K, Pau M, Schwab R, Schmieja K, Franzrahe S, Hiddemann W. Constitutive activation of STAT3 and STAT5 is induced by leukemic fusion proteins with protein tyrosine kinase activity and is sufficient for transformation of hematopoietic precursor cells. Exp Hematol 2002;30(3):262-71.
105. Arnould C, Philippe C, Bourdon V, Gr oire MJ, Berger R, Jonveaux P. The signal transducer and activator of transcription STAT5b gene is a new partner of retinoic acid receptor alpha in acute promyelocytic-like leukaemia. Hum Mol Genet 1999;8(9):1741-9.
106. Li H, Zhang Y, Glass A, et al. Activation of signal transducer and activator of transcription-5 in prostate cancer predicts early recurrence. Clin Cancer Res 2005;11(16):5863-8.
107. Sultan AS, Xie J, LeBaron MJ, Ealley EL, Nevalainen MT, Rui H. Stat5 promotes homotypic adhesion and inhibits invasive characteristics of human breast cancer cells. Oncogene 2005;24(5):746-60.
108. Mirmohammadsadegh A, Hassan M, Bardenheuer W, et al. STAT5 phosphorylation in malignant melanoma is important for survival and is mediated through SRC and JAK1 kinases. J Invest Dermatol 2006;126(10):2272-80.
109. Gomez D, Reich NC. Stimulation of primary human endothelial cell proliferation by IFN. J Immunol 2003;170(11):5373-81.
110. Ilaria RL, Jr., Hawley RG, Van Etten RA. Dominant negative mutants implicate STAT5 in myeloid cell proliferation and neutrophil differentiation. Blood 1999;93(12):4154-66.
111. Leong PL, Xi S, Drenning SD, et al. Differential function of STAT5 isoforms in head and neck cancer growth control. Oncogene 2002;21(18):2846-53.
112. Iwatsuki K, Endo T, Misawa H, et al. STAT5 activation correlates with erythropoietin receptor-mediated erythroid differentiation of an erythroleukemia cell line. J Biol Chem 1997;272(13):8149-52.
113. Yu CL, Prochownik EV, Jove R. Proximal promoter region of the junB gene mediates attenuation of serum inducibility in Src-transformed cells. Cell Growth Differ 1995;6(12):1513-21.
114. Olayioye MA, Beuvink I, Horsch K, Daly JM, Hynes NE. ErbB receptor-induced activation of stat transcription factors is mediated by Src tyrosine kinases. J Biol Chem 1999;274(24):17209-18.
115. Kazansky AV, Kabotyanski EB, Wyszomierski SL, Mancini MA, Rosen JM. Differential effects of prolactin and src/abl kinases on the nuclear translocation of STAT5B and STAT5A. J Biol Chem 1999;274(32):22484-92.
116. Kabotyanski EB, Rosen JM. Signal transduction pathways regulated by prolactin and Src result in different conformations of activated Stat5b. J Biol Chem 2003;278(19):17218-27.

7 The Intersection of EGFR and the Ras Signaling Pathway

Marie Wislez and Jonathan M. Kurie

CONTENTS

RAS CHARACTERISTICS AND FUNCTIONS
RAS ACTIVATION BY EGFR PATHWAY
RAS AND CANCER

Abstract

EGFR is a survival factor for a variety of cancer cell types. The mechanism by which EGFR is regulated and the downstream mediators of EGFR that regulate cell survival are the subjects of ongoing research. Here we highlight one important aspect of EGFR signaling, the bi-directional interaction between EGFR and Ras. We discuss the mechanistic basis for this interaction, its implications for cell biology, and its potential importance as a target for cancer therapy.

Key Words: lung cancer, Ras, EGFR, ligands.

1. RAS CHARACTERISTICS AND FUNCTIONS

Previous reviews provide a complete analysis of the Ras protein family (*1–5*). In brief, three human Ras genes encode the 21 kDa proteins H-ras, K-ras, and N-ras and have a high degree of homology in their sequences. Ras proteins are expressed in most adult and fetal tissues (*6*). Ras proteins are active when bound to guanosine triphosphate (GTP) and inactive when bound to guanosine diphosphate (GDP). When active, Ras hydrolyzes its bound GTP, which releases a phosphate and leaves itself inactive and bound to GDP. Two sets of proteins regulate Ras' activity: guanine-nucleotide exchange factors (GEFs) and GTPase-activating proteins (GAPs) (*7*). GEFs stimulate the release of Ras-bound GDP, resulting in the binding of GTP—naturally plentiful in the cell—to Ras. GAPs are negative regulators of Ras; they accelerate the hydrolysis of GTP into GDP. A balance between Ras-GDP and Ras-GTP regulates the function of Ras. In addition to its regulation by changes in the phosphorylation state of bound guanosine, Ras activity is regulated by changes in its cellular location. Ras can be fully active only when it is associated with the plasma membrane. The importance of this balance is shown by the fact that Ras dysregulation has been implicated in many cancers.

Once membrane-bound, Ras associates with downstream mediators (reviewed in (*2*)). For example, Ras associates with son of sevenless proteins (Sos1/2), which effect Ras signaling through, among others, the catalytic p110 subunit of type I phosphatidylinositol 3-kinase (PI3K). The PI3K then phosphorylates membrane phosphatidylinositides to recruit and activate one of the many factors containing a plekstrin homology domain, such as Akt (also known as protein kinase B), that transmit signals mediating cell survival, cell cycle progression, and glucose metabolism. Another key Ras effector is the Raf family of proteins, which activate mitogen-activated protein kinase (MAPK) via the phosphorylation of the MAPK kinase (MAPKK or MEK) (8). Activated MAPK then translocates to the nucleus and interacts with transcription factors, such as AP-1 (the jun/fos complex), to regulate the expression of genes that facilitate cell cycle progression and inhibit apoptosis (8, 9).

2. RAS ACTIVATION BY EGFR PATHWAY

2.1. ErbB Family Receptors and their Ligands

The ErbB family of receptor tyrosine kinases (RTKs) and their ligands are important regulators of tumor cell proliferation, angiogenesis, and metastasis. The four receptors in the ErbB family—EGFR (HER1 and ErbB1), HER2 (neu or ErbB2), HER3 (ErbB3), and HER4 (ErbB4)—are anchored in the cytoplasmic membrane and share a structure composed of an extracellular ligand-binding domain, a short hydrophobic transmembrane region, and an intracytoplasmic tyrosine kinase domain. The ErbB receptors form homodimers and heterodimers, and these dimeric complexes have distinct ligand-binding and signaling activities. Ligands that have been reported to bind to ErbB receptors include epidermal growth factor (EGF), transforming growth factor a (TGFa), heparin-binding EGF-like ligand (HB-EGF), amphiregulin (AR), betacellulin (BTC), epiregulin (EPR), epigen (EPG), heregulin (HRG), and neuregulin (NRG) (10). These ligands bind directly to EGFR, HER3, or HER4 (also see Chapter 2), which leads to the formation of homo- or heterodimers that trigger multiple downstream signaling cascades, including the RAS-ERK and PI3K-Akt pathways (11). Although HER2 lacks a functional ligand-binding domain, it is the preferred partner for heterodimerization upon ligand binding. HER3 is unique in that it lacks a functional kinase domain and can therefore send signals only when heterodimerized (12, 13). Furthermore, NRGs can bind only to HER4 (14).

2.2. Ras Activation by RTKs

EGF and other growth factors such as platelet-derived growth factor (PDGF) and cytokines all signal via Ras (15). In 1984, Kamata and Feramisco (16) showed that EGF stimulates the Ras oncoprotein to switch from its inactive GDP-bound form to its active GTP-bound form. Later, others showed Ras to be a downstream mediator of activated RTKs (17). In 1990, the missing links between Ras and RTKs were identified with the discovery of GEFs or Sos proteins (18, 19). Once activated via autophosphorylation, RTKs such as EGFR bind to the SH2 domain of growth-factor-receptor-bound protein 2 (GRB2) that is bound to SOS through its SH3 domain. The increased proximity of SOS and Ras in the plasma membrane increases the nucleotide exchange of Ras-bound GDP with GTP, completing the RTK-GRB2-SOS-Ras signal transduction cascade (20). In addition to its activation by RTKs through Ras, PI3K is able to couple directly with HER3 through docking sites for the p85 regulatory subunit (11). The redundancy of these signaling networks speaks to the importance of PI3K in RTK signaling.

2.3 ErbB Activation by Ras

Conditioned medium from ras-mutated cell lines has been shown to stimulate ErbB receptor activation. For example, transformation of NIH 3T3 fibroblasts by H-ras is dependent on soluble factors in the conditioned medium, which was inhibited by small molecule inhibitors of

EGFR and HER2 (21). In human colon cancer cells, mutant K-ras increased the expression of EPR and AR, thereby activating AKT, which led to the development of radioresistance in vitro (22). In Kras^{LA1} mice, a mouse model of lung adenocarcinoma that was developed through the somatic activation of a *Kras* allele carrying an activating mutation in codon 12 (G12D) (23), levels of EPR, RPG, and AR expression were 23.0-, 7.5-, and 5.0-fold higher, respectively, than in their wild-type littermates (24).

In addition to its effects on ErbB ligands, Ras activation can increase the expression and phosphorylation of ErbB family members. Constitutively active Ras induced HER4 phosphorylation, and this phosphorylation was ligand-independent (31). In an animal model carrying a conditionally activated mutant human Ha-ras (G12V) oncogene in the pancreatic ducts, many of the resulting pancreatic adenocarcinomas highly expressed EGF and EGFR (25). In Kras^{LA1} mice, the levels of HER3 expression were higher than in their wild-type littermates (24).

3. RAS AND CANCER

3.1. RAS Activation and Cancer

The most common ras mutations have been found in codons 12, 13, and 61, which permanently block Ras in its active, GTP-bound state. The Ras proteins with these mutations are resistant to GAPs, which consequently prevents the hydrolysis of their GTP into GDP (6). Apart from direct mutations in the ras genes, Ras is activated in cancer cells by the constitutive activation of GEF or loss of GAPs, which can result in the constitutive association of Ras with GTP (26).

Pancreatic cancer has the highest incidence of ras mutation in human tumors identified to date, with the frequencies of codon 12 mutations reported to range from 20% to 100%, depending on the technique used; the mutations also occurred early in the pancreatic tumor progression model (27). K-ras gene mutations have also been found in approximately 70% of colorectal cancers and 40% of colorectal adenomas (28). In lung adenocarcinomas, Kras mutations have been detected in 12-30% of specimens (29–31), more frequently in ever-smokers than never-smokers and in patients from western than east Asian countries (31), and predict shorter survival times (32).

3.2. RAS Activation by Mutant EGFR in Cancer

Somatic mutations in the EGFR kinase domain that constitutively activate the receptor have been found in the tumors of 10% to 40% of patients with NSCLC (33–36). While Ras activation has not been directly measured in these tumors, the phosphorylation of its downstream mediators Erk1/2 has been examined. Sordella et al. determined that Erk1/2 phosphorylation in stably transfected cells did not differ between cells that contained mutant receptors and cells that contained wild-type receptors (37). In contrast, Amann et al. (38) found that while no changes in the phosphorylation pattern of Erk1/2 were evident at 30 minutes, changes were evident at 2 hours, with lysates from cells transfected with mutant EGFRs having higher levels of phosphorylated Erk1/2 than those from cells transfected with wild-type receptors. Similarly, Erk1/2 phosphorylation was increased in tumors from transgenic mice that develop lung adenocarcinoma due to the expression of mutant EGFR (39). Lastly, Shc, a direct target of EGFR and an upstream activator of the Ras/MAPK pathway, also showed changes due to phosphorylation in cells transfected with mutant EGFR (38). Thus, while the results from in vitro data are mixed, Ras-dependent events appear to be activated as a consequence of EGFR mutations in cancer cells.

In cancer patients, however, the expression of phospho-ERK as a marker of EGFR activation seems more difficult to demonstrate. For example, the levels of EGFR expression in advanced gastric carcinoma cells significantly correlated with the levels of phospho-EGFR and Ki67 expression, but not with that of phospho-ERK expression. Also, the levels of phospho-EGFR in tumor cells were significantly reduced after gefitinib treatment, but this was not the case for phospho-ERK and phospho-Akt (*40*).

3.3. Clinical Significance

EGFR somatic mutations are associated with adenocarcinoma histology, female sex, and a non-smoking history. In keeping with this fact, patients who have lung cancer patients with EGFR mutations frequently experience rapid and sustained shrinkage of primary and metastatic disease in response to treatment with the EGFR tyrosine kinase inhibitors (TKIs) gefitinib or erlotinib (*33–36*). In addition, in a phase III trial, oral treatment with erlotinib conferred a survival benefit (*41*), whereas gefitinib did not confer a statistically significant effect on survival (*42*). The clinical benefits of treatment with oral TKIs do not appear limited to patients with EGFR-mutated disease, however. For example, a biological analysis of different phase III clinical trials and retrospective series of patients treated with oral TKI demonstrated clinical benefits in response to the treatment that could be associated with EGFR genomic gain (gene amplification or polysomy) or high protein expression (*43–45*).

K-ras mutations, on the other hand, have been shown to correlate with resistance to the anti-tumor effects of EGFR TKIs in NSCLC (*36*). In accordance with these results, K-ras mutations were also found to be associated with the resistance of the anti-EGFR antibody cetuximab in colorectal cancer (*46*). In NSCLC, a series of surgical patients with NSCLC showed that EGFR and Kras mutations occur in a mutually exclusive fashion (*31, 47*). This exclusivity is supported by epidemiologic data showing that Kras mutations occur most commonly in smokers, whereas EGFR mutations are more frequent in never smokers and distant quitters (*31, 48*). The exclusivity of these somatic mutations suggests that Ras-dependent pathways are crucial effectors of EGFR in the transformation of the bronchial epithelium.

Some speculate that, regardless of EGFR's activation level, cancer cells with somatic K-ras mutations will be resistant to anti-cancer drugs acting on targets upstream of the Ras protein, such as EGFR. This speculation was borne out by a recent study showing that the introduction of the K-ras12V mutant in cells with activating somatic EGFR mutations conferred gefitinib resistance on the cells (*49*). Several Ras-transformed cells, however, are sensitive to EGFR inhibitors. For example, Ras activation, as measured by the levels of phosphorylated Erk in head and neck cancer cell lines, correlated with high EGFR expression, and targeting EGFR in the cells with EGFR TKIs or with anti-EGFR antibodies was effective, as measured by inhibition of Erk phosphorylation and cell proliferation (*50*). In addition, some EGFR wild-type NSCLC cell lines with Kras somatic mutations are sensitive to erlotinib with a half maximal inhibitory concentration < 1 µM (*51*). Also, the treatment of Kras^{LA1} mice with gefitinib suppressed alveolar neoplasia expansion (*24*). Further, an immortalized human bronchial epithelial cell line that had been transfected with a retroviral vector expressing mutant K-ras did not become resistant to gefitinib (*24*). From this, we speculate that Ras mutations are not mechanistically associated with resistance to EGFR inhibitors but instead might occur coincidentally with other mutations that confer resistance to these inhibitors.

Potential molecular predictors of response to EGFR TKIs are markers of epithelial versus mesenchymal phenotypes, including E-cadherin expression (*51–53*). HER3 expression is associated with a tumor's epithelial phenotype, and high HER3 expression has been observed in gefitinib-sensitive NSCLC cell lines and in patients who achieved clinical benefits from gefitinib, even those with K-ras–mutated disease (*24, 51*).

From this, it appears that Ras is a major downstream protein effector of EGFR and its mutation is associated with a lack of sensitivity to EGFR inhibitors in NSCLCs. More studies need to be done, however, if we are to understand whether this lack of sensitivity is mechanistically associated or coincidental.

REFERENCES

1. Campbell SL, Khosravi-Far R, Rossman KL, Clark GJ, Der CJ. Increasing complexity of Ras signaling. Oncogene 1998;17:1395-413.
2. Downward J. Targeting RAS signalling pathways in cancer therapy. Nat Rev Cancer 2003;3:11-22.
3. Downward J. Signal transduction. Prelude to an anniversary for the RAS oncogene. Science 2006;314:433-434.
4. Reuther GW, Der CJ. The Ras branch of small GTPases: Ras family members don't fall far from the tree. Curr Opin Cell Biol 2000;12:157-165.
5. Weijzen S, Velders MP, Kast WM. Modulation of the immune response and tumor growth by activated Ras. Leukemia 1999;13:502-513.
6. Lowy DR, Willumsen BM. Function and regulation of ras. Annu Rev Biochem 1993;62:851-891.
7. Wittinghofer A, Scheffzek K, Ahmadian MR. The interaction of Ras with GTPase-activating proteins. FEBS Lett 1997;410:63-67.
8. Egan SE, Weinberg RA. The pathway to signal achievement. Nature 1993;365:781-3.
9. Edme N, Downward J, Thiery JP, Boyer B. Ras induces NBT-II epithelial cell scattering through the coordinate activities of Rac and MAPK pathways. J Cell Sci 2002;115:2591-2601.
10. Harris RC, Chung E, Coffey RJ. EGF receptor ligands. Exp Cell Res 2003;284:2-13.
11. Yarden Y, Sliwkowski MX. Untangling the ErbB signalling network. Nat Rev Mol Cell Biol 2001;2:127-137.
12. Schlessinger J. Ligand-induced, receptor-mediated dimerization and activation of EGF receptor. Cell 2002;110:669-672.
13. Citri A, Skaria KB, Yarden Y. The deaf and the dumb: the biology of ErbB-2 and ErbB-3. Exp Cell Res 2003;284:54-65.
14. Plowman GD, Culouscou JM, Whitney GS, et al. Ligand-specific activation of HER4/p180erbB4, a fourth member of the epidermal growth factor receptor family. Proc Natl Acad Sci U S A 1993;90:1746-1750.
15. Clark GJ, Der CJ. Aberrant function of the Ras signal transduction pathway in human breast cancer. Breast Cancer Res Treat 1995;35:133-144.
16. Kamata T, Feramisco JR. Epidermal growth factor stimulates guanine nucleotide binding activity and phosphorylation of ras oncogene proteins. Nature 1984;310:147-150.
17. Smith MR, DeGudicibus SJ, Stacey DW. Requirement for c-ras proteins during viral oncogene transformation. Nature 1986;320:540-3.
18. Downward J, Riehl R, Wu L, Weinberg RA. Identification of a nucleotide exchange-promoting activity for p21ras. Proc Natl Acad Sci U S A 1990;87:5998-6002.
19. Wolfman A, Macara IG. A cytosolic protein catalyzes the release of GDP from p21ras. Science 1990;248:67-69.
20. McCormick F. Signal transduction. How receptors turn Ras on. Nature 1993;363:15-16.
21. He H, Hirokawa Y, Manser E, Lim L, Levitzki A, Maruta H. Signal therapy for RAS-induced cancers in combination of AG 879 and PP1, specific inhibitors for ErbB2 and Src family kinases, that block PAK activation. Cancer J 2001;7:191-202.
22. Toulany M, Dittmann K, Kruger M, Baumann M, Rodemann HP. Radioresistance of K-Ras mutated human tumor cells is mediated through EGFR-dependent activation of PI3K-AKT pathway. Radiother Oncol 2005;76:143-150.
23. Johnson L, Mercer K, Greenbaum D, et al. Somatic activation of the K-ras oncogene causes early onset lung cancer in mice. Nature 2001;410:1111-1116.
24. Fujimoto N, Wislez M, Zhang J, et al. High Expression of ErbB Family Members and Their Ligands in Lung Adenocarcinomas That Are Sensitive to Inhibition of Epidermal Growth Factor Receptor. Cancer Res 2005;65:11478-11485.
25. Ueda S, Fukamachi K, Matsuoka Y, et al. Ductal origin of pancreatic adenocarcinomas induced by conditional activation of a human Ha-ras oncogene in rat pancreas. Carcinogenesis 2006;27:2497-2510. Epub 006 Jun 13.

26. Basu TN, Gutmann DH, Fletcher JA, Glover TW, Collins FS, Downward J. Aberrant regulation of ras proteins in malignant tumour cells from type 1 neurofibromatosis patients. Nature 1992; 356:713-715.
27. Schneider G, Schmid RM. Genetic alterations in pancreatic carcinoma. Mol Cancer 2003;2:15.
28. McDermott U, Longley DB, Johnston PG. Molecular and biochemical markers in colorectal cancer. Ann Oncol 2002;13:235-245.
29. Rodenhuis S, Slebos RJ, Boot AJ, et al. Incidence and possible clinical significance of K-ras oncogene activation in adenocarcinoma of the human lung. Cancer Res 1988;48:5738-41.
30. Suzuki Y, Orita M, Shiraishi M, Hayashi K, Sekiya T. Detection of ras gene mutations in human lung cancers by single-strand conformation polymorphism analysis of polymerase chain reaction products. Oncogene 1990;5:1037-1043.
31. Shigematsu H, Lin L, Takahashi T, et al. Clinical and biological features associated with epidermal growth factor receptor gene mutations in lung cancers. J Natl Cancer Inst 2005;97:339-346.
32. Mascaux C, Iannino N, Martin B, et al. The role of RAS oncogene in survival of patients with lung cancer: a systematic review of the literature with meta-analysis. Br J Cancer 2005;92:131-139.
33. Kosaka T, Yatabe Y, Endoh H, Kuwano H, Takahashi T, Mitsudomi T. Mutations of the epidermal growth factor receptor gene in lung cancer: biological and clinical implications. Cancer Res 2004;64:8919-8923.
34. Lynch TJ, Bell DW, Sordella R, et al. Activating mutations in the epidermal growth factor receptor underlying responsiveness of non-small-cell lung cancer to gefitinib. N Engl J Med 2004;350:2129-2139.
35. Paez JG, Janne PA, Lee JC, et al. EGFR mutations in lung cancer: correlation with clinical response to gefitinib therapy. Science 2004;304:1497-1500.
36. Pao W, Wang TY, Riely GJ, et al. KRAS Mutations and Primary Resistance of Lung Adenocarcinomas to Gefitinib or Erlotinib. PLoS Med 2005;2:e17.
37. Sordella R, Bell DW, Haber DA, Settleman J. Gefitinib-sensitizing EGFR mutations in lung cancer activate anti-apoptotic pathways. Science 2004;305:1163-1167.
38. Amann J, Kalyankrishna S, Massion PP, et al. Aberrant epidermal growth factor receptor signaling and enhanced sensitivity to EGFR inhibitors in lung cancer. Cancer Res 2005;65:226-235.
39. Ji H, Li D, Chen L, et al. The impact of human EGFR kinase domain mutations on lung tumorigenesis and in vivo sensitivity to EGFR-targeted therapies. Cancer Cell 2006;9:485-495.
40. Rojo F, Tabernero J, Albanell J, et al. Pharmacodynamic studies of gefitinib in tumor biopsy specimens from patients with advanced gastric carcinoma. J Clin Oncol 2006;24:4309-4316.
41. Shepherd FA, Rodrigues Pereira J, Ciuleanu T, et al. Erlotinib in previously treated non-small-cell lung cancer. N Engl J Med 2005;353:123-132.
42. Thatcher N, Chang A, Parikh P, et al. Gefitinib plus best supportive care in previously treated patients with refractory advanced non-small-cell lung cancer: results from a randomised, placebo-controlled, multicentre study (Iressa Survival Evaluation in Lung Cancer). Lancet 2005;366:1527-1537.
43. Eberhard DA, Johnson BE, Amler LC, et al. Mutations in the epidermal growth factor receptor and in KRAS are predictive and prognostic indicators in patients with non-small-cell lung cancer treated with chemotherapy alone and in combination with erlotinib. J Clin Oncol 2005;23:5900-5909.
44. Hirsch FR, Varella-Garcia M, Bunn PA, Jr., et al. Molecular predictors of outcome with gefitinib in a phase III placebo-controlled study in advanced non-small-cell lung cancer. J Clin Oncol 2006;24:5034-5042.
45. Tsao MS, Sakurada A, Cutz JC, et al. Erlotinib in lung cancer - molecular and clinical predictors of outcome. N Engl J Med 2005;353:133-144.
46. Lievre A, Bachet JB, Le Corre D, et al. KRAS mutation status is predictive of response to cetuximab therapy in colorectal cancer. Cancer Res 2006;66:3992-3995.
47. Marchetti A, Martella C, Felicioni L, et al. EGFR mutations in non-small-cell lung cancer: analysis of a large series of cases and development of a rapid and sensitive method for diagnostic screening with potential implications on pharmacologic treatment. J Clin Oncol 2005;23:857-865.
48. Tokumo M, Toyooka S, Kiura K, et al. The relationship between epidermal growth factor receptor mutations and clinicopathologic features in non-small cell lung cancers. Clin Cancer Res 2005;11:1167-1173.

49. Uchida A, Hirano S, Kitao H, et al. Activation of downstream epidermal growth factor receptor (EGFR) signaling provides gefitinib-resistance in cells carrying EGFR mutation. Cancer Sci 2007;98:357-363.
50. Albanell J, Codony-Servat J, Rojo F, et al. Activated extracellular signal-regulated kinases: association with epidermal growth factor receptor/transforming growth factor alpha expression in head and neck squamous carcinoma and inhibition by anti-epidermal growth factor receptor treatments. Cancer Res 2001;61:6500-6510.
51. Yauch RL, Januario T, Eberhard DA, et al. Epithelial versus mesenchymal phenotype determines in vitro sensitivity and predicts clinical activity of erlotinib in lung cancer patients. Clin Cancer Res 2005;11:8686-8698.
52. Witta SE, Gemmill RM, Hirsch FR, et al. Restoring E-cadherin expression increases sensitivity to epidermal growth factor receptor inhibitors in lung cancer cell lines. Cancer Res 2006;66:944-950.
53. Thomson S, Buck E, Petti F, et al. Epithelial to mesenchymal transition is a determinant of sensitivity of non-small-cell lung carcinoma cell lines and xenografts to epidermal growth factor receptor inhibition. Cancer Res 2005;65:9455-9462.

8 Phosphoinositide 3-Kinase Enzymes as Downstream Targets of the EGF Receptor

Jan Domin

CONTENTS

INTRODUCTION
CLASS I PI3K ENZYMES
CLASS II PI3K ENZYMES
CLASS III PI3K ENZYMES
SUBSTRATE SPECIFICITY OF PI3K ENZYMES
ERBB RECEPTOR-MEDIATED RECRUITMENT OF PI3K ENZYMES
DOWNSTREAM TARGETS OF PTDINS$(3, 4, 5)P_3$ AND PTDINS$(3, 4)P_2$
MAINTENANCE OF CELL VIABILTY
REGULATION OF TRANSCRIPTION
REGULATION OF METABOLISM
REGULATION OF CELL MIGRATION
REGULATION OF VESICLE TRANSPORT
CONCLUSION
REFERENCES

Abstract

Phosphoinositide 3-kinase (PI3K) activity plays a critical role downstream of the activated epidermal growth factor receptor (EGFR), regulating cell viability, proliferation, and migration. Here I will overview the components of the PI3K signaling pathway and its control. Emphasis is placed on the eight PI3K catalytic isoforms expressed in human tissue and grouped into three classes termed I, II, and III based on sequence similarity and substrate specificity. The nature and localization of the 3-phosphoinositide products of PI3K activity govern the translocation/activation of protein targets that include the serine/threonine kinases Akt and PDK-1. In this way the EGFR elicits its spectrum of intracellular effects that include altering cell migration, vesicle transport, cell cycle progression, metabolism, and transcription. Despite the intense focus, the mechanisms by which the activated EGFR stimulates PI3K activity are not completely understood. In addition, the possibility of EGF stimulated synthesis of phosphatidylinositol (3) phosphate could provide exciting new insights into the regulation of EGFR mediated vesicle transport.

From: *Cancer Drug Discovery and Development: EGFR Signaling Networks in Cancer Therapy*
Edited by: J. D. Haley and W. J. Gullick, DOI: 10.1007/978-1-59745-356-1_8
© 2008 Humana Press, a part of Springer Science+Business Media, LLC

Key Words: Epidermal growth factor, receptor, kinase, phosphoinositide, signal transduction, cell, cancer, Akt, mitogenesis, apoptosis, endocytosis.

1. INTRODUCTION

Phosphoinositide 3-kinase (PI3K) dependent signaling pathways downstream of the epidermal growth factor (EGF) receptor play a critical role in the maintenance of cell viability, control of vesicle transport, and cell migration. Although great advances have been made characterizing the enzymes responsible for 3-phosphoinositide production and their downstream targets, the full repertoire of mechanisms by which EGF receptor stimulates PI3K enzyme activity is not completely understood.

Some twenty years ago a novel kinase activity was identified that phosphorylated a minor eukaryotic cell membrane component termed phosphatidylinositol (PtdIns). Initially, this PtdIns kinase activity was found associated with oncogene products such as the polyoma middle T-antigen, v-src (1) and v-ros (2). Subsequent studies revealed co-immunoprecipitation of this lipid kinase activity with growth factor receptors for EGF and platelet-derived growth factor (PDGF) (3, 4). Interest in the PtdIns kinase enzyme was prompted by observations that its binding correlated with transforming potential (5–7). Fractionation of fibroblast extracts revealed two distinct PtdIns kinases termed type I and type II (8), but only the type I PtdIns kinase associated with activated tyrosine kinases and specifically phosphorylated the 3' –OH group on the inositol ring to generate PtdIns(3)P in vitro (9). Detailed analysis of intracellular PtdIns derivatives revealed that synthesis of PtdIns(3,4)P_2 and PtdIns(3,4,5)P_3 but not PtdIns(3)P increased markedly following growth factor stimulation (10–12). Large scale purification of the phosphoinositide 3-kinase (PI3K) enzyme from bovine brain identified a heterodimer consisting of 85 kDa (p85) and 110 kDa (p110) subunits (13). Two isoforms of the p85 protein termed p85α and p85β were described (14–16) and the sequence of the catalytic subunit p110 was published shortly thereafter (17). Stimulation with EGF allowed immunoprecipitation of PI3K activity with anti-phosphotyrosine antibody and stimulated tyrosine phosphorylation of p85 and p110 subunits to varying degrees depending upon cell type (18).

Analysis of yeast *Saccharomyces cerevisiae* defective in membrane traffic revealed that the product of one mutant gene termed Vps34 also had PI3K activity (19,20). Alignment of the p110 and vps34p sequences allowed development of cloning strategies to identify novel cDNAs by RT-PCR that encoded PI3K enzymes. Degenerate oligonucleotides amplified sequences that were then used to screen mammalian cDNA libraries. This approach identified p110β and p110δ (21,22). Probing *Drosophila* cDNA identified Drosophila 68_D a PI3K enzyme distinct from any of the p110 isozymes or vps34p (23). This led to the identification of human PI3K-C2α, HsC2-PI3K and PI3K-C2γ(24–27), mouse PI3K-C2α termed p170 (28) and cpk (29) and rat PI3K-C2γ (30). A nomenclature developed to stratify the eight mammalian PI3K isoforms into three classes termed I, II and III based on sequence similarity and in vitro substrate specificity was proposed that remains in use today (31–33) (Fig. 8.1).

2. CLASS I PI3K ENZYMES

These enzymes are all 110 kDa apparent molecular mass and bind an adaptor subunit. Class I PI3K enzymes are subdivided into two types termed class IA, which bind a p85-like adaptor, and class IB enzymes, which do not.

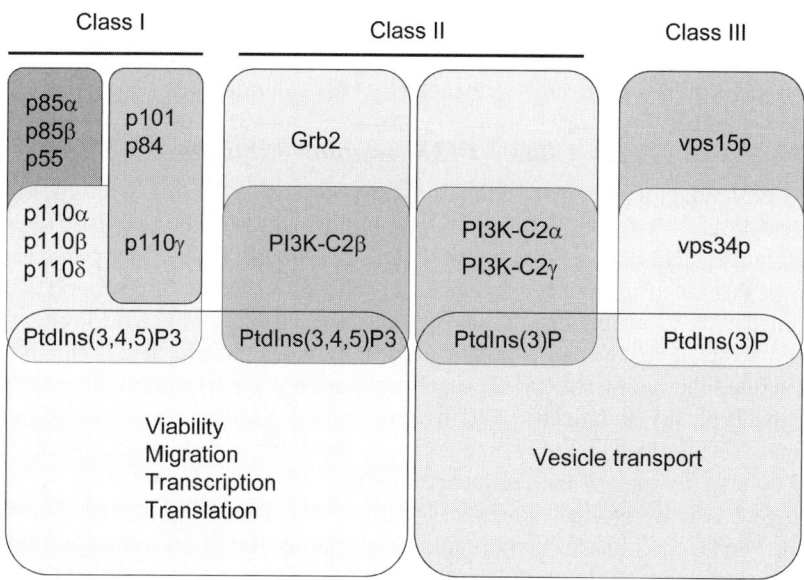

Fig. 8.1. **Schematic Relationship between PI3K Enzymes, Their Adaptor Proteins and in vivo 3-Phosphoinositide Products.** Although the 3-phosphoinositide produced by the class II PI3K enzymes in vivo remain unclear one possibility is shown.

2.1. Class I PI3K Catalytic Subunits

Class IA PI3K comprises p110α (17), p110 β (21), and p110 δ (22) isozymes, each of which is encoded by a separate gene. All class IA enzymes contain an N-terminal binding site (residues 20-108) for the helical inter- SH2 domain region of p85 (34). Adjacent to this region lies a binding site for the small GTPase ras (35). PI3K enzymes all contain an internal C2 (CalB) domain (36, 37). C2 domains are found within proteins involved in phospholipid mediated signal transduction such as phospholipase C (PLC), cytosolic phospholipase A2 (cPLA2), and protein kinase C (PKC) (38). C2 domains are divided into two types - those present in enzymes such as cPLA2 and PLCδ1 whose binding to phospholipids is dependent on Ca^{2+} (type I) and those such as the C2 domain in PKCδ whose interaction with phospholipids occurs independent of Ca^{2+} (type II). The phosphoinositide kinase (PIK) and catalytic domains form the C-terminus. Both p110α and β isoforms have a wide tissue distribution, whereas expression of the δ isoform is largely restricted to cells of haematopoietic origin (22). The ras binding site in PI3K enzymes has the same conformation as the ras binding site in raf (39) and ralGDS (40). Upon binding, ras either stabilizes the p110 catalytic subunit at the plasma membrane or induces a conformational change to alter substrate or co-factor binding.

p110γ is the only class IB PI3K isoform in mammalian cells. In contrast to class IA enzymes, p110γ does not bind a p85 like adaptor but instead a 101 kDa protein termed p101 (41). Resolution of p110γ crystal structure has allowed important insight into regulatory mechanisms of its lipid kinase activity (37). Residues 1-143 of p110γ contain the binding site for the adaptor protein p101 (42), a ras binding domain, a C2 domain, a helical domain similar to HEAT repeats involved in protein-protein interactions (43) and the catalytic domain. The C2 domain present in the class IB PI3K p110γ is similar to the Ca^{2+} insensitive type II C2 domain of phospholipase Cδ1 (44). As in the case of the class IA PI3K enzymes, stimulation of p110γ activates both phosphoinositide and protein kinase activity, which leads to autophosphorylation of p110γ on serine 1101 (45). In contrast to the class IA PI3K isoforms, however, autophosphorylation of p110γ does not attenuate lipid kinase activity and autophosphorylation is significantly enhanced by Gβγ subunits (46).

2.2. Class I PI3K Adaptor Subunits

Class IA PI3K adaptor proteins contain two phosphotyrosine binding Src homology 2 (SH2) domains, two proline-rich motifs, a region of homology to the breakpoint cluster region (BCR), and an N-terminal SH3 domain that binds proline-rich motifs (14). Biophysical analysis has demonstrated that the affinity of this interaction is also governed by three amino acid residues that lie immediately C-terminal to the phosphotyrosine itself. For the SH2 domains of p85 a methionine residue at position +4 is preferred (47). Between the two SH2 domains lies a helical region termed the inter-SH2 (iSH2) sequence that binds p110α (34) and contains residue serine 608 that is phosphorylated by p110 thereby regulating kinase activity (48). The N-terminus contains a SH3 domain that may bind components of the actin cytoskeleton (49). Adjacent to the SH3 domain lies a motif with sequence similarity to the breakpoint cluster region (BCR) flanked on each side by proline-rich motifs (P1 and P2). This BCR domain binds the small GTPases Rac and Cdc42 (50, 51) and regulates reorganization of the actin cytoskeleton (52). Each proline-rich region could provide an intramolecular binding site for the N-terminal SH3 domain to either alter conformation or serve as a binding site for regulatory proteins.

A total of eight class IA adaptors have been described that are derived from three distinct genes termed p85α, p85β and p55γ. In addition to p85α and p85β, AS53 (also known as p55α) (53, 54), and p50α (55, 56) are splice variants derived from the gene encoding p85 (Pik3r1). These contain both p85α SH2 domains but lack the SH3 domain, amino-terminal proline-rich domain, and BCR domain. Instead, they have unique amino-terminal sequences consisting of 34 and six amino acids, respectively. Another isoform p55[PIK] is homologous to AS53/p55α but is encoded by a different gene (57). p85α shows the widest tissue distribution and is expressed at the highest levels (14). In contrast, AS53 and p50α, appear to play specific roles in selected tissues and are of particular relevance to signaling downstream of the insulin receptor and may play a significant role in diabetes (58). Although each class IA adaptor can bind all class IA catalytic subunits in vitro, some receptors and their adaptors appear to display a preference for specific adaptor subunits (59).

The class IB adaptor p101 has no sequence similarity to other class I PI3K adaptors. In contrast to phosphotyrosine binding, p101 confers sensitivity upon the p101/p110γ complex to G-protein stimulation (41, 60). An additional p110γ adaptor termed p84 was recently identified (61). Like p101, binding of p84 to p110γ increases the ability of Gβγ to stimulate lipid kinase activity both in vitro and in vivo. The p84/p110γ heterodimer, however, is approximately four times less sensitive to Gβγ. Consequently, p110γ appears to have two regulatory subunits and their significance is unclear.

3. CLASS II PI3K ENZYMES

Mammalian cells contain three class II PI3K enzymes termed PI3K-C2α, PI3K-C2β and PI3K-C2γ (24–27). Each is encoded by a separate gene and the enzymes are characterized by their high molecular mass >170kDa and two phospholipid-binding motifs termed a Phox (PX) domain and C2 domain that form their C-terminal region. Class II PI3K enzymes also contain the internal C2 domain, a PIK domain, and the catalytic domain described above for the class I PI3K enzymes. The catalytic region provides the greatest sequence similarity with the class I and class III PI3K enzymes.

The first phospholipid-binding domain identified in the class II PI3K enzymes was the type II C2 domain at the C-terminus (23) that binds phosphoinositides including PtdIns(4,5)P_2

in a Ca²+ independent manner. A PI3K-C2β mutant lacking the C-terminal C2 domain displayed increased specific activity using PtdIns as substrate (*26*). Despite its ability to bind phospholipids, deletion of the C2 domain did not alter the subcellular localization of PI3K-C2α (*62*). The C-terminus of class II PI3K enzymes also contains a PX domain that in mouse and human PI3K-C2α preferentially binds PtdIns(*4,5*)P$_2$ (*63, 64*).

Class II PI3K enzymes show no sequence similarity to other proteins at their N-terminus however, this region contains several proline-rich motifs, through which PI3K-C2β binds the SH3 domain containing adaptor protein Grb-2, a putative ras-binding motif and a region that binds clathin. (*65*).

4. CLASS III PI3K ENZYMES

Only a single class III PI3K enzyme exists in each species and both the yeast and human vps34p enzymes produce PtdIns(*3*)P (*19, 20*). Since the steady state levels of PtdIns(*3*)P alter little following receptor stimulation, many investigators concluded that activation of this PI3K isoform is constitutive (*10*).

Mammalian vps34p is of a similar molecular mass to the class I PI3K enzymes. Like the class II enzymes, however, its sequence similarity with the class I PI3K isoforms decreases sharply outside the internal C2 and PIK/kinase domains. Its C-terminus binds a protein kinase termed vps15p, and this association is dependent on vps15p catalytic activity (*66, 67*). Both yeast and human vps34p are post-translationally modified by the addition of a myristoyl moiety at their N-terminus that targets the class III PI3K enzyme to the membrane. The N-terminus of vps15p contains its protein kinase domain and the vps34p binding site. Toward the C-terminus vps15 contains HEAT repeats that mediate its interaction with vps34p (*66*) and WD40 domains that bind the small GTPase Rab5 (*68*).

5. SUBSTRATE SPECIFICITY OF PI3K ENZYMES

The assignment of the mammalian PI3K enzymes into their respective classes was based in part on their lipid substrate specificity in vitro. Class I PI3K enzymes can phopshorylate either PtdIns, PtdIns(*4*)P, or PtdIns(*4,5*)P$_2$, the class II PI3K enzymes predominantly PtdIns and PtdIns(*4*)P and the class III PI3K PtdIns only. Both class I and class III PI3K enzymes require Mg²+ as a divalent cation for this reaction, but class II PI3K enzymes can also use Ca²+ (*69*). Uniquely, the class II PI3K isoform PI3K-C2α is refractory to the inhibitory effects of wortmannin and LY294002, which are two commonly used PI3K inhibitors that are approximately 10 times less sensitive than the other PI3K enzymes (*24*).

In vivo, class I PI3K enzymes produce PtdIns(*3,4,5*)P$_3$ (*10*) and the class III PI3K vps34p PtdIns(*3*)P. In contrast, the 3-phosphoinositide generated by class II PI3K enzymes remains controversial. Unlike class I PI3K enzymes, expression of recombinant class II PI3K enzymes does not increase the production of either PtdIns(*3,4*)P$_2$ or PtdIns(*3,4,5*)P$_3$. Activation of integrin alphaIIb beta3 on platelets or their incubation with Ca²+ stimulates both the production of PtdIns(*3,4*)P$_2$ and PI3K-C2β kinase activity (*70*). An increasing volume of data supports the hypothesis that class II PI3K enzymes produce PtdIns(*3*)P. When cell nuclei purified from liver were harvested 20 hours after hepatectomy and depleted of their envelope to remove class I PI3K enzymes, increased production of PtdIns(*3*)P and PI3K-C2 activity was observed (*71*). Furthermore, increased PtdIns(*3*)P synthesis and stimulation of PI3K-C2 enzyme activity correlated during cell cycle progression (*72*). Stimulation of renal cortical slices with hepatocyte growth factor transiently elevates PtdIns(*3*)P production in brush-border plasma membranes and this hypothesis also increased PI3K-C2β activity in this fraction (73). Most recently, PI3K-C2β stimulated cell migration was observed via a PtdIns(3)P dependent pathway (74, 75). Since expression of a kinase-inactive form of PI3K-C2β inhibited PtdIns(3,4,5)P$_3$ dependent phosphorylation of Akt and cell growth in a small cell cancer cell line, this suggests that PI3K-C2β may also contribute to PtdIns(3,4,5)P$_3$ production in vivo (76).

6. ERBB RECEPTOR-MEDIATED RECRUITMENT OF PI3K ENZYMES

Phosphoinositide kinase activity was originally co-purified with the EGF receptor in A431 cells and its activity was stimulated upon ligand binding (77, 78). Characterization of PI3K activity allowed this to be distinguished from PI4K and PI4-5K also present in anti-phosphotyrosine (79–81) and anti-EGF receptor immunoprecipitates (82, 83). One of the original approaches used to clone the p85 adaptor was based on an assay that used the tyrosine-phosphorylated carboxyl terminus of the EGF receptor as bait (15). Furthermore, EGF receptor was affinity purified using either SH2 domain of p85 expressed as a GST fusion protein (83). Co-immunoprecipitation of recombinant p85 and EGF receptor in insect cells that had not been stimulated with EGF, however, raised concerns about the physiological relevance of this interaction (84). For many groups co-immunoprecipitation of PI3K activity with anti-EGF receptor antisera was problematic. Furthermore, binding of p85 to the EGF receptor, ErbB2, or ErbB4 was difficult to explain (85) given that each receptor contains only a single YxxM motif, the preferred consensus for p85 SH2 domain binding, in their kinase domain that is not thought to be phosphorylated (86, 87). In contrast, ErbB3 contains six YxxM motifs, and immunoprecipitation of ErbB3 from EGF stimulated A431 cells efficiently co-precipitated phosphoinositide 3-kinase activity (88). Expression of a chimeric receptor, consisting of the extracellular domain of EGF receptor and the transmembrane and intracellular region of ErbB3, confirmed p85 binding sites to pYxxM motifs following EGF stimulation (89). Use of p85 tagged with green fluorescent protein (GFP) demonstrated that stimulation of the EGF receptor/ErbB3 chimera resulted in clustering of p85 at the cell membrane in a concentration dependent manner (90). Translocation of p85 to ErbB3, however, did not explain the isolation of PI3K activity in anti-phosphotyrosine immunoprecipitates from lysates of many other EGF stimulated cultures indicating the existence of alternative mechanisms (Fig. 8.2).

One alternative involves the adaptor protein p120^{Cbl} (91). Originally isolated as a tyrosyl phosphoprotein that complexed with Fyn, Grb2, and p85 in T cells c-Cbl encodes a 120kDa protein that is phosphorylated on tyrosine residues following EGF stimulation and binds directly to the phosphorylated EGF receptor (92–94). Another is the Grb2-associated binder-1 (Gab-1). Gab-1 is a multi-substrate docking protein that was identified from a cDNA library of glioblastoma tumors and plays a role in cellular growth, transformation, and apoptosis (95). Gab-1 binds phosphorylated tyrosine 1068 and 1086 residues in the carboxyl tail of the EGF receptor to allow binding of p85. Overexpression of Gab1 potentiates EGF-induced activation of the mitogen-activated protein kinase and Jun kinase signaling pathways. A mutant of Gab1 unable to bind p85 was defective in potentiating EGF receptor signaling and this effect involves PtdIns(3,4,5)P$_3$ binding to the PH domain of Gab1 (96). Furthermore, the PH domain mediates Gab1 translocation to the plasma membrane in response to EGF. In certain cell types, stimulation of cells including rat hepatocytes with EGF also causes tyrosine phosphorylation of insulin receptor substrate (IRS)-1 and IRS-2 and their binding to p85 (97). IRS-1 contains 9 p85 consensus-binding motifs.

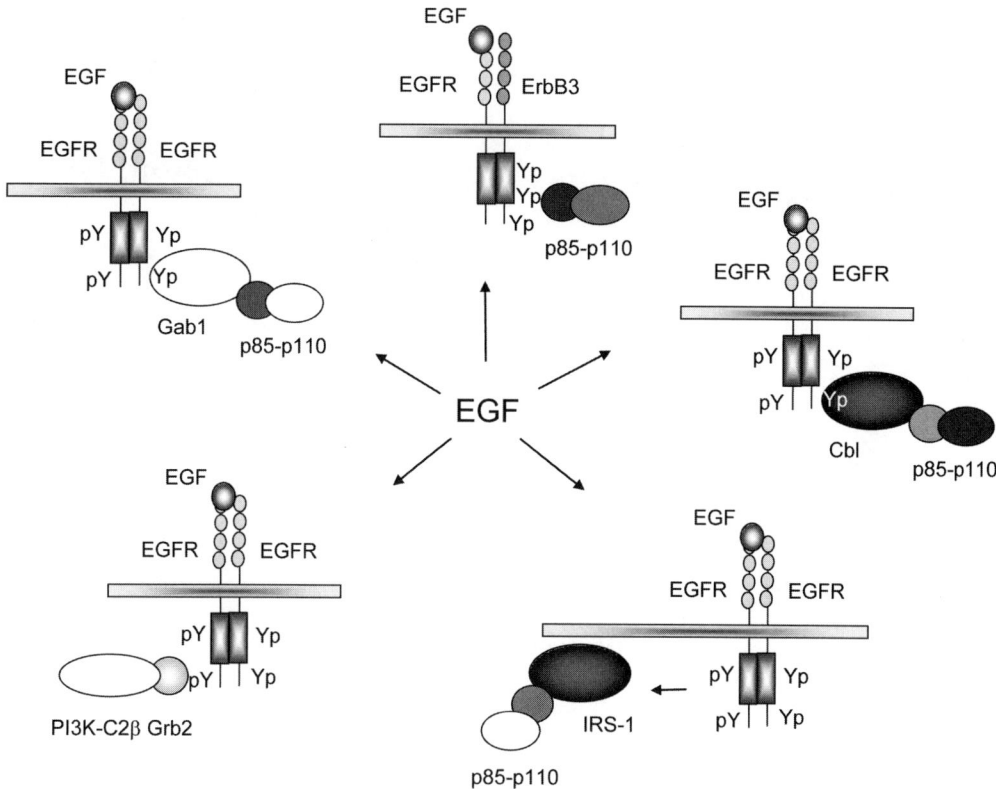

Fig. 8.2. Options for Recruitment of PI3K Enzymes to the Activated EGF Receptor. ErbB receptors are shown localized in the plasma membrane with phosphotyrosine residues (pY) shown.

Isolation of activated EGF receptor has also demonstrated co-immunoprecipitation of class II PI3K enzymes in a manner analogous to class IA PI3K enzymes (*69*). Association of the PI3K-C2β isoform with EGFR is mediated by the adaptor Grb-2 (*65*), co-immunoprecipitates Shc and requires phosphorylation of EGF receptor on residues tyrosine992, tyrosine1068, and tyrosine1173 (*69*). More recently, it was proposed that PI3K-C2β is recruited to the EGF receptor as part of a multiprotein signaling complex that includes Eps8, Abi1, Sos1, and Shc and Grb2 (*98*).

7. DOWNSTREAM TARGETS OF PTDINS(*3, 4, 5*)P$_3$ AND PTDINS(*3, 4*)P$_2$

A limited number of distinct protein domains that bind PtdIns(*3,4,5*)P$_3$ and PtdIns(*3,4*)P$_2$ have been identified in serine/threonine protein kinases, tyrosine kinases, phospholipases, and molecules that regulate the exchange of guanine nucleotides to GTPases (Fig. 8.3).

The plekstrin homology (PH) domain was originally identified as binding small GTPases (*99, 100*), but inositol phosphate headgroups are their major target (*101*). Approximately 100 amino acid residues long PH domains are found in a large number of proteins and their binding to PtdIns(*3,4*)P$_2$ and PtdIns(*3,4,5*)P$_3$ allows translocation to membranes. PH domains bind PtdIns(*3*)P with low affinity and in vivo appear to preferentially bind PtdIns(*3,4,5*)P$_3$.

The epsin N-terminal homology (ENTH) domain is conserved in eukaryotes and found in several proteins involved in vesicle transport and reorganization of the actin cytoskeleton

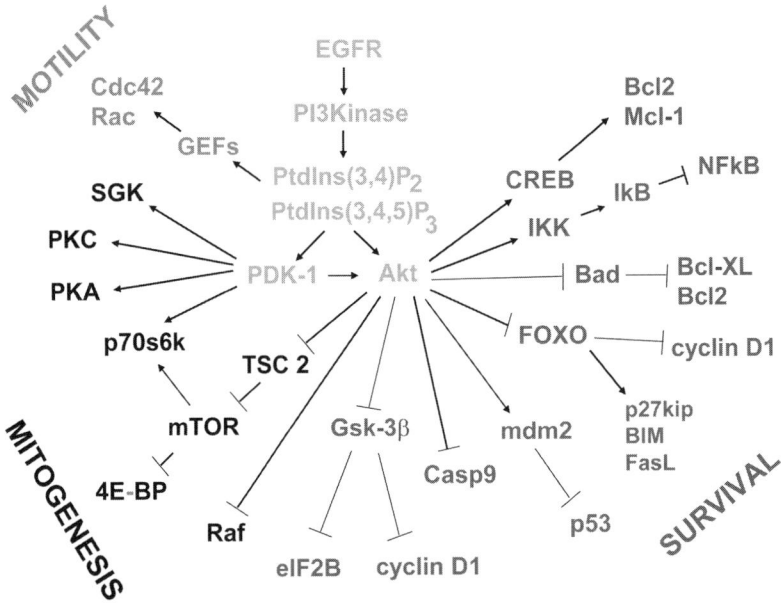

Fig. 8.3. **Downstream Targets of PDK-1 and Akt** Substrates of the PDK-1 and Akt kinases are shown. Arrows indicate where phosphorylation has a positive effect on substrate, bars indicate inhibitory effect.

(*102, 103*). These proteins include Epsin and its homologues, adaptor protein 180 (AP180), Huntingtin-interacting protein 1 (HIP1), and the clathrin assembly lymphoid myeloid leukemia protein (CALM) (*104*). Whilst ENTH domains bind PtdIns(*4,5*)P$_2$ (*105, 106*), the ENTH domain of HIP1 and HIP1 related proteins binds PtdIns(*3,5*)P$_2$ and PtdIns(*3,4*)P$_2$ (*107, 108*).

7.1. Akt (PKB)

Akt (also known as protein kinase B – PKB and RAC related to protein kinase A and C) was identified independently as both the cellular homologue of the viral oncoprotein v-Akt (*109*) and as a protein kinase with sequence similarity to protein kinase A and protein kinase C (*110, 111*). This 57kDa serine/threonine kinase exists in three isoforms termed Akt1, Akt2, and Akt3 each encoded by separate genes on chromosomes 14q32, 19q13, and 1q44 (*109–113*). The sequence similarity of Akt2 and Akt3 to Akt1 is 81% and 83%, respectively. Growth factor and cytokine stimulated production of PtdIns(*3,4,5*)P$_3$ and PtdIns(*3,4*)P$_2$ results in the translocation of Akt to the plasma membrane and the binding of these 3-phosphoinositides via its PH domain (*114*). Wortmannin and LY294002 both attenuate EGF stimulated Akt kinase activity. Mutations within the Akt PH domain block activation of catalytic activity in vivo (*115*). Akt is constitutively phosphorylated on residues serine 124 and threonine 450, but ligand induced phosphorylation on threonine308 within the kinase domain and serine 473 at the C-terminus confers maximal specific activity (*116*). In oesophageal cancer cells where EGF receptor is frequently overexpressed, EGF stimulated phosphorylation of Akt1 and Akt2 but did not alter the phosphorylation of Akt3 (*117*). Akt immunoprecipitated from serum starved cells is inactive, but its specific activity is rapidly increased following EGF stimulation (*115, 118*). The Akt PH domain binds both PtdIns(*3,4,5*)P$_3$ and PtdIns(*3,4*)P$_2$ (*119*). Once activated, Akt translocates to the nucleus (*120*).

7.2. Phosphoinositide-dependent Kinase – PDK-1

PDK-1 was isolated from bovine brain and rabbit skeletal muscle as a 63kDa kinase that phosphorylates Akt on residue threonine 308 (*119, 121*). This serine/threonine kinase contains an N-terminal catalytic domain and a PH domain at the C-terminus that binds PtdIns(3,4,5)P$_3$ with high affinity (*122*). The catalytic activity of PDK1 appears constitutive since cell stimulation does not appear to alter catalytic activity (*123*). Phosphorylation of Akt by PDK1 occurs at the plasma membrane and is dependent on 3-phosphoinositide production. Membrane localized Akt is constitutively phosphorylated and activated (*124*). Translocation of PDK1 to the nucleus has also been shown to occur in a PI3K dependent manner (*125*).

7.3. Additional Downstream Targets of PDK-1

Residues threonine 308 and serine 473 of Akt lie within consensus sequences shared by the AGC family of protein kinases. These include protein kinase A, protein kinase G and protein kinase C (*126*), p70S6-kinases (p70S6K), p90 ribosomal S6-kinases (p90RSK) and serum and glucocorticoid induced protein kinase (SGK) (*127*). Following receptor stimulation, several of these kinases are also phosphorylated by PDK-1 on a residue equivalent to threonine 308 (*128–132*) in a 3-phosphoinositide dependent manner. p70S6K is encoded by 2 genes termed p70S6K α and p70S6K β. There are 2 isoforms of p70S6K, p70S6K α is mainly found in the cytoplasm, whilst p85S6K is primarily nuclear. The activity of p70S6K in situ is inhibited by rapamycin and wortmannin (*133, 134*). p70S6K regulates G1 to S phase cell cycle progression and the translocation of mRNA messages that contain a polypyrimidine tract at their translational start site (*135*). These genes include transcripts for ribosomal proteins and elongation factors of protein synthesis. The principal p70S6K substrate is the S6 ribosomal protein that comprises the 40S ribosomal subunit.

The family of PKC enzymes regulate protein synthesis, transcription, cell growth, differentiation, and apoptosis (*136*). The kinase activity of several PKC isoforms is activated directly by 3-phosphoinositides in vitro and inhibited in vivo by PI3K inhibitors (*129, 137, 138*). Phosphorylation of PKC α and PKC β II by PDK1 is stimulated by PtdIns(3,4,5)P$_3$ in vitro (*139*).

cAMP dependent protein kinase (PKA) is a complex kinase family consisting of at least three catalytic and two regulatory subunits (*140*). PKA is activated by cAMP produced downstream of G-protein coupled receptors. Once activated, PKA phosphorylates a number of downstream targets that regulate cell growth, differentiation and metabolism (*141*). PDK-1 mediated phosphorylation of PKA on residue threonine 197 increases kinase activity (*128*). PDK1 also phosphorylates the serum and glucocorticoid inducible kinase (SGK) (*123*)

7.4. Other Kinases that Phosphorylate Akt

Identification of the kinase responsible for phosphorylating Akt on serine 473 has proved problematic. Several candidates have been proposed as the PDK-2, including MAPKAP kinase-2, several PKC isoforms, integrin-linked kinase (ILK), DNA-dependent protein kinase, Ataxia-telangiectasia mutant (ATM), and PDK-1 (*142*). Others suggest that phosphorylation of serine 473 is the result of Akt autophosphorylation (*143*). RNA interference (siRNA) and conditional knockouts of ILK shows that loss of ILK abolishes phosphorylation of serine 473, suppresses phosphorylation of GSK-3 β and expression of cyclin D1 and simulated apoptosis (*144*). A complex of proteins raptor, Gβ L, and the mammalian target of rapamycin (mTOR) phosphorylates several proteins in a hydrophobic motif equivalent to the serine 473 consensus (*145, 146*). Although phosphorylation of this residue is not sensitive to rapamycin treatment, a rapamycin-insensitive form of the mTOR was characterized in a complex with Rictor and GβL and found to phosphorylate Akt/PKB at serine 473 (*147*). Knockdown of mTOR or Rictor expression by siRNA ablate serine 473 phosphorylation.

7.5. Akt Targets

Mice null for Akt1 are small due to placental abnormalities (*148*) and have a shorter life expectancy than wild-type littermates (*149*). These animals also have increased apoptotic cell death in thymus and testis and impaired platelet responses to thrombin and collagen (*150*). Conversely, knockout of Akt2 produces insulin resistance and a condition equivalent to diabetes mellitus (*151*). A wide spectrum of proteins in both the cytoplasm and nucleus act as Akt substrates.

8. MAINTENANCE OF CELL VIABILTY

Expression of recombinant Akt delays cell death (*152*) and it is frequently over-expressed in tumors (*112*). In its non-phosphorylated form, the Bcl-2/Bcl-XL antagonist causing cell death (BAD) protein is localized in mitochondria where it forms a complex with two anti-apoptotic proteins termed Bcl-2 and Bcl-XL and inhibits their activity (*153*). Phosphorylation of BAD on either serine 112 or serine 136 prevents its association with Bcl-2 and Bcl-XL leading to its release into the cytoplasm where it binds 14-3-3 proteins (*154*). Akt phosphorylates BAD on serine 136 (*155, 156*).

Caspase 9, a pro-apoptotic protease is phosphorylated and inhibited by Akt (*157*). Akt phosphorylates p21(Waf1/Cip1) and p27 (Kip2) and inhibits their anti-proliferative effects by retaining them in the cytoplasm (*158–160*). In this way, activation of cyclin/Cdk complexes that include cyclin D1/Cdk4 is inhibited. Akt also phosphorylates the murine double minute-2 (mdm-2) protein leading to its translocation into the nucleus and destabilizing the tumor suppressor protein p53 (*161, 162*). Degradation of p53 inhibits the stress response to increase cell survival. Phosphorylation of Raf by Akt inhibited activation of the Raf-MEK-ERK signaling pathway and in a human breast cancer cell line shifted the cellular response from cell cycle arrest to proliferation (*163*).

9. REGULATION OF TRANSCRIPTION

The forkhead box O (FOXO) family of transcription factors are targets of Akt (*164, 165*). FOXO1 (FKHR), FOXO3 (FKHRL1), FOXO4 (AFX), and FOXO6 are localized in the nucleus of quiescent cells (*166*) but upon stimulation they translocate to the cytosol and bind 14-3-3 that sequesters them away from the nucleus (*167*). Phosphorylation of FOXO proteins by Akt occurs on three highly conserved consensus motifs (RxRxxS/T) (*164, 165, 168*). FOXO proteins increase expression of the pro-apoptotic factors Fas ligand and Bim. Since FOXOs inhibit transcription of cyclin D1 and cyclin D2 their phosphorylation by Akt increases rates of transcription (*169*). FOXO3a increases the transcription of the p27kip¹ gene (*170*) and Akt phosphorylates p27kip¹ inhibiting its anti-proliferative activity (*171*). FOXO proteins are also phosphorylated by serum and glucocorticoid–regulated kinase (SGK) (*172*), that is activated by 3-phosphoinisitides and PDK-1.

Nuclear Factor kB (NFkB) is a transcription factor for several anti-apoptotic genes (*173*). When bound to its inhibitor IkB, NFkB is inactive and retained in the cytoplasm. Akt phosphorylates and activates an IkB kinase (IKK) (*174*). Phosphorylation of IkB results in its dissociation from NFkB targeting IkB for degradation in the proteosome allowing movement of NFkB to the nucleus where it activates NFkB dependent pro-survival genes that include Bcl-XL, caspase inhibitors and c-Myb (*175*).

Akt directly phosphorylates the cyclic nucleotide response element binding (CREB) protein on serine 133 (*176*). Phosphorylated CREB binds the co-activator CREB binding protein (CBP) to promote expression of genes that suppress apoptosis, including Bcl-2, Mcl-1 and Akt itself (*176–179*). In tumor cell lines lacking the 3-phosphoinositide phosphatase PTEN, FOXO proteins are constitutively activated (*180*). Akt regulates the activity of the c-fos promoter downstream of Rho and Rac dependent signals through the serum response element (SRE) (*181, 182*).

10. REGULATION OF METABOLISM

Following stimulation of the insulin receptor Akt directly phosphorylates and inactivates glycogen synthase kinase 3 (GSK3) on serine 9 (*183, 184*). Inhibition of GSK3 prevents phosphorylation of β-catenin inhibiting its degradation allowing it translocation to the nucleus. There β-catenin binds transcription factors that include TCF/LEF-1 to induce expression of genes such as cyclin D1. GSK-3 phosphorylates and inactivates the translational initiation factor eIF2B (*185*). Since GSK3 is inactivated following growth factor stimulation, this mechansism could explain their effects on translation initiation (*186*). Akt also phosphorylates and activates 6-phosphofructo-2-kinase (PFK-2), an enzyme responsible for synthesis of fructose 2,6-biphosphate (*187*). Fructose 2,6-biphosphate in turn stimulates 6-phosphofructo-1-kinase, a potent activator of glycolysis (*188*).

The growth of eukaryotic cells is regulated not only by intercellular growth factors but also by the availability of nutrients (*189–191*). The Akt substrate tuberous sclerosis complex-2 (TSC2), which forms part of the TSC1/TSC2 protein complex, constitutes a nutrient sensitive signaling pathway that alters cell size and growth (*192, 193*). Phosphorylated TSC2 fails to bind TSC1, thereby inhibiting p70S6K and activating 4E-BP1. Germline mutations in either tumor suppressor genes TSC1 or TSC2 result in tuberous sclerosis, an autosomal dominant human genetic disorder characterized by hamartoma development (*194*). The TSC1/TSC2 complex has GAP activity for the Rheb GTPase (a member of the ras family), and activated Rheb-GTP activates the mammalian target of rapamycin (mTOR) (*195, 196*). mTOR promotes translation of cyclin D mRNA and p70 S6K and inhibits the eukaryotic initiation factor 4E-binding protein 1 (4E-BP1).

11. REGULATION OF CELL MIGRATION

The binding of GTP to GTPases is regulated by GTP/GDP exchange factors (GEFs) and GTPase activating proteins (GAPs) (*197*). GEFs catalyze the exchange of GDP for GTP while GAPs accelerate the intrinsic GTPase activity. GEFs of the Rho GTPase family and Arf contain a PH domain (*198*). There are over 60 Rho GEFs characterized by a Dbl homology (DH) domain, followed almost invariably by a PH domain. Treatment of cells with PI3K inhibitors inhibits receptor-mediated induced reorganization of the actin cytoskeleton and Rac GTP binding (*199*). Since expression of constitutively activated Rac reverses the effect of PI3K inhibitors on F-actin polymerization it suggests that Rac lies downstream of 3-phosphoinositide production. Vav and Tiam1 are two Rac GEFs that may be regulated in a PI3K dependent manner (*200, 201*). Although ARF GTPases are involved in intracellular vesicle transport three ARF GEFs termed General Receptor for Phosphoinositides (GRP1), ARF nucleotide binding site opener (ARNO) and cytohesin-1 contain PH domains that preferentially bind PtdIns$(3,4,5)P_3$ thereby allowing receptor stimulated translocation of these GEFs from the cytoplasm to the plasma membrane (*202*). GAP1^m and GAP1IP4BP are GAPs for Ras and their binding to the plasma membrane is regulated by PtdIns$(3,4,5)P_3$ (*203*). Centaurins also bind PtdIns$(3,4,5)P_3$ in vivo (*204*) and have homology to the ARF GAP in yeast.

12. REGULATION OF VESICLE TRANSPORT

Following their stimulation, EGF receptors are internalized and delivered to multivesicular bodies where they are sorted prior to delivery to lysosomes and degraded. Since PI3K inhibitors lead to enlarged endosomes containing EGF receptors, PI3K enzymes were thought to regulate EGF receptor endocytosis. Although expression of kinase inactive p110 δ did not inhibit targeting of EGF receptor to lysosomes (205), microinjection of anti-vps34p antibody inhibited internal vesicle formation (206). Silencing of human vps34 gene expression using siRNA reveals no effect on receptor internalization but slows initial receptor degradation and potentiates signaling (207).

PI3K-C2 α and PI3K-C2β are both recruited to complexes containing activated EGF receptor (69). Immunofluorescence staining of PI3K-C2α revealed a punctate distribution with a perinuclear localization (62) and this enzyme is enriched upon purification of clathrin-coated vesicles (62, 208). Interestingly both PI3K-C2α and PI3K-C2β bind clathrin directly via clathrin-binding motif at their N-termini (208, 209). In this way, clathrin functions as an adaptor for class II PIK enzymes and stimulating their catalytic activity. Since expression of PI3K-C2α affects clathrin-mediated endocytosis and sorting in the trans-Golgi network (208), these data indicate that class II PI3K enzymes provide a mechanism for growth factor receptor-mediated vesicle transport.

13. CONCLUSION

Binding of EGF to its receptor stimulates both class IA and class II PI3K enzymes to initiate a number of intracellular signaling events mediated through the generation of 3-phopsphoinositides. As a consequence, an intricate balance between cell viability, proliferation, migration, and vesicle transport is maintained. Although greatest emphasis has been placed on understanding the role of class IA PI3K enzymes, attention is now shifting to the class II isozymes where significant opportunities remain to gain exciting insight into regulation of EGF receptor function. In addition to the success of EGF receptor antagonists, significant potential exists to fine tune future therapeutic approaches with PI3K isoform specific antagonists (210).

REFERENCES

1. Sugimoto Y, Whitman M, Cantley LC, Erikson RL. Evidence that the Rous sarcoma virus transforming gene product phosphorylates phosphatidylinositol and diacylglycerol. Proc Natl Acad Sci U S A 1984; 81:2117-2121.
2. Macara IG, Marinetti GV, Balduzzi PC. Transforming protein of avian sarcoma virus UR2 is associated with phosphatidylinositol kinase activity: possible role in tumorigenesis. Proc Natl Acad Sci USA 1984; 84:2728-2732.
3. Auger KR, Serunian LA, Soltoff SP, Libby P, Cantley LC. PDGF-dependent tyrosine phosphorylation stimulates production of novel polyphosphoinositides in intact cells. Cell 1989; 57:167-175.
4. Varticovski L, Druker B, Morrison D, Cantley L, Roberts T. The colony stimulating factor-1 receptor associates with and activates phosphatidylinositol-3 kinase. Nature 1989; 342:699-702.
5. Whitman M, Kaplan DR, Schaffhausen B, Cantley L, Roberts TM. Association of phosphatidylinositol kinase activity with polyoma middle-T competent for transformation. Nature 1985; 315:239-42.
6. Courtneidge SA, Heber A. An 81 kd protein complexed with middle T antigen and pp60c-src: a possible phosphatidylinositol kinase. Cell 1987; 50:1031-1037.
7. Talmage DA, Freund R, Young AT, Dahl J, Dawe CJ, Benjamin TL. Phosphorylation of middle T by pp60c-src: a switch for binding of phosphatidylinositol 3-kinase and optimal tumorigenesis. Cell 1989; 59:55-65.
8. Endemann G, Dunn SN, Cantley LC. Bovine brain contains two types of phosphatidylinositol kinase. Biochemistry 1987; 26:6845-6852.
9. Whitman M, Downes CP, Keeler M, Keller T, Cantley L. Type I phosphatidylinositol kinase makes a novel inositol phospholipid, phosphatidylinositol-3-phosphate. Nature 1988; 332:644-646.
10. Stephens LR, Hughes KT, Irvine RF. Pathways of phosphatidylinositol (3,4,5)-trisphosphate synthesis in activated neutrophils. Nature 1991; 351:33-39.

11. Hawkins PT, Jackson TR, Stephens LR. Platelet-derived growth factor stimulates synthesis of PtdIns(3,4,5)P3 by activating a PtdIns(4,5)P2 3-OH kinase. Nature 1992; 358:157-9.
12. Jackson TR, Stephens LR, Hawkins PT. Receptor specificity of growth factor-stimulated synthesis of 3-phosphorylated inositol lipids in Swiss 3T3 cells. J Biol Chem 1992; 267:16627-36.
13. Morgan SJ, Smith AD, Parker PJ. Purification and characterization of bovine brain type I phosphatidylinositol kinase. Eur J Biochem 1990; 191:761-767.
14. Otsu M, Hiles ID, Gout I, Fry MJ, Ruiz-Larrea F, Panayotou G et al. Chracterization of two 85 kd proteins that associate with receptor tyrosine kinases, middle-T/pp60c-src complexes, and PI3-kinase. Cell 1991; 65:91-104.
15. Skolnik EY, Margolis B, Mohammadi M, Lowenstein E, Fisher R, Drepps A et al. Cloning of PI3-kinase-associated p85 utilizing a novel method for expression/cloning of target proteins for receptor tyrosine kinases. Cell 1991; 65:83-90.
16. Escobedo J, Navankasattusas S, Kavanaugh WM, Milfay D, Fried VA, Williams LT. cDNA cloning of a novel 85 kd protein that has SH2 domains and regulates binding of PI3-kinase to the PDGF beta-receptor. Cell 1991; 65:75-82.
17. Hiles ID, Otsu M, Volinia S, Fry MJ, Gout I, Dhand R et al. Phosphatidylinositol 3-kinase : structure and expression of the 110 kd catalytic subunit. Cell 1992; 70:419-429.
18. Downing JR, Reynolds AB. PDGF, CSF-1, and EGF induce tyrosine phosphorylation of p120, a pp60src transformation-associated substrate. Oncogene 1991; 6:607-613.
19. Herman PK, Emr SD. Characterization of VPS34, a gene required for vacuolar protein sorting and vacuole segregation in Saccharomyces cerevisiae. Mol Cell Biol 1990; 10:6742-6754.
20. Schu PV, Takegawa K, Fry MJ, Stack JH, Waterfield MD, Emr SD. Phosphatidylinositol 3-kinase encoded by the yeast VPS34 gene essential for protein sorting. Science 1993; 260:88-92.
21. Hu P, Mondino A, Skolnik EY, Schlessinger J. Cloning of a novel, ubiquitously expressed human phosphatidylinositol 3-kinase and identification of its binding site on p85. Mol Cell Biol 1993; 13:7677-88.
22. Vanhaesebroeck B, Welham MJ, Kotani K, Stein R, Warne PH, Zvelebil MJ et al. p110d, a novel phosphoinositide 3-kinase in leukocytes. Proc Natl Acad Sci 1997; 94:4330-5.
23. MacDougall LK, Domin J, Waterfield MD. A family of phosphoinositide 3-kinases in Drosophila identifies a new mediator of signal transduction. Curr Biol 1995; 5:1404-1415.
24. Domin J, Pages F, Volinia S, Rittenhouse SE, Zvelebil MJ, Stein RC et al. Cloning of a human phosphatidylinositol 3-kinase with a C2 domain which displays reduced sensitivity to the inhibitor wortmannin. Biochem J 1997; 326:139-47.
25. Brown RA, Ho LK, Weber-Hall SJ, Shipley JM, Fry MJ. Identification and cDNA cloning of a novel mammalian C2 domain-containing phosphoinositide 3-kinase, HsC2-PI3K. Biochem Biophys Res Commun 1997; 233:537-544.
26. Arcaro A, Volinia S, Zvelebil MJ, Stein R, Watton SJ, Layton MJ et al. Human PI3-kinase C2β - The role of calcium and the C2 domain in enzyme activity. J Biol Chem 1998; 273:33082-33091.
27. Rozycka M, Lu YJ, Brown RA, Lau MR, Shipley JM, Fry MJ. cDNA cloning of a third human C2-domain-containing class II phosphoinositide 3-kinase, PI3K-C2gamma, and chromosomal assignment of this gene (PIK3C2G) to 12p12. Genomics 1998; 54:569-574.
28. Virbasius JV, Guilherme A, Czech MP. Mouse p170 is a novel phosphatidylinositol 3-kinase containing a C2 domain. J Biol Chem 1996; 271:13304-13307.
29. Molz L, Chen YW, Hirano M, Williams LT. Cpk is a novel class of drosophila PtdIns 3-kinase containing a C2 domain. J Biol Chem 1996; 271:13892-99.
30. Ono F, Nakagawa T, Saito S, Owada Y, Sakagami H, Goto K et al. A novel class II phosphoinositide 3-kinase predominantly expressed in the liver and its enhanced expression during liver regeneration. J Biol Chem 1998; 273:7731-7736.
31. Domin J, Waterfield MD. Using structure to define the function of phosphoinositide 3-kinase family members. FEBS Lett 1997; 410:91-95.
32. Vanhaesebroeck B, Leevers SJ, Ahmadi K, Timms J, Katso R, Driscoll PC et al. Synthesis and function of 3-phosphorylated inositol lipids. Annu Rev Biochem 2001; 70:535-602.
33. Fruman DA, Meyers RE, Cantley LC. Phosphoinositide kinases. Annu Rev Biochem 1998; 67:481-507.
34. Dhand R, Hara K, Hiles I, Bax B, Gout I, Panayotou G et al. PI 3-kinase: structural and functional analysis of intersubunit interactions. EMBO J 1994; 13:511-521.

35. Rodriguez-Viciana P, Warne PH, Dhand R, Vanhaesebroeck B, Gout I, Fry MJ et al. Phosphatidylinositol-3-OH kinase as a direct target of Ras. Nature 1994; 370:527-532.
36. Ponting CP. Novel domains in NADPH oxidase subunits, sorting nexins and PtdIns 3-kinases: Binding partners of SH3 domains? Protein Sci 1996; 5:2353-7.
37. Walker E, Perisic O, Ried C, Stephens L, Williams R. Structural insights into phosphoinositide 3-kinase catalysis and signalling. Nature 1999; 402:313-20.
38. Katan M, Allen VL. Modular PH and C2 domains in membrane attachment and other functions. FEBS Lett 1999; 452:36-40.
39. Rojas E, Nassar-Gentina V, Luxoro M, Pollard ME, Carrasco MA. Inositol 1,4,5-trisphosphate-induced Ca2+ release from the sarcoplasmic reticulum and contraction in crustacean muscle. Can J Physiol Pharmacol 1987; 65:672-680.
40. Huang L, Hofer F, Martin GS, Kim SH. Structural basis for the interaction of Ras with RalGDS. Nat Struct Biol 1998; 5:422-426.
41. Stephens LR, Eguinoa A, Erdjument-Bromage H, Lui M, Cooke F, Coadwell J et al. The Gβγ sensitivity of a PI3K is dependent upon a tightly associated adaptor, p101. Cell 1997; 89:105-114.
42. Krugmann S, Hawkins PT, Pryer N, Braselmann S. Characterizing the interactions between the two subunits of the p101/p110gamma phosphoinositide 3-kinase and their role in the activation of this enzyme by G beta gamma subunits. J Biol Chem 1999; 274:17152-17158.
43. Andrade MA, Petosa C, O'Donoghue SI, Muller CW, Bork P. Comparison of ARM and HEAT protein repeats. J Mol Biol 2001; 309:1-18.
44. Essen LO, Perisic O, Lynch DE, Katan M, Williams RL. A ternary metal binding site in the C2 domain of phosphoinositide-specific phospholipase C-delta1. Biochemistry 1997; 36:2753-2762.
45. Czupalla C, Culo M, Muller EC, Brock C, Reusch HP, Spicher K et al. Identification and characterization of the autophosphorylation sites of phosphoinositide 3-kinase isoforms beta and gamma. J Biol Chem 2003; 278:11536-11545.
46. Brock C, Schaefer M, Reusch HP, Czupalla C, Michalke M, Spicher K et al. Roles of G beta gamma in membrane recruitment and activation of p110 gamma/p101 phosphoinositide 3-kinase gamma. J Cell Biol 2003; 160:89-99.
47. Marengere LE, Songyang Z, Gish GD, Schaller MD, Parsons JT, Stern MJ et al. SH2 domain specificity and activity modified by a single residue. Nature 1994; 369:502-505.
48. Dhand R, Hiles I, Panayotou G, Roche S, Fry MJ, Gout I et al. PI 3-kinase is a dual specificity enzyme: autoregulation by an intrinsic protein-serine kinase activity. EMBO J 1994; 13:522-533.
49. Bunday L. Membrane-targeting of signalling molecules by SH2/SH3 domain-containing adaptor proteins. Biochim Biophys Acta 1999; 1422:187-204.
50. Zheng Y, Bagrodia S, Cerione RA. Activation of phosphoinositide 3-kinase activity by Cdc42Hs binding to p85. J Biol Chem 1994; 269:18727-18730.
51. Tolias KF, Cantley LC, Carpenter CL. Rho family GTPases bind to phosphoinositide kinases. J Biol Chem 1995; 270:17656-17659.
52. Hill KM, Huang Y, Yip SC, Yu J, Segall JE, Backer JM. N-terminal domains of the class ia phosphoinositide 3-kinase regulatory subunit play a role in cytoskeletal but not mitogenic signaling. J Biol Chem 2001; 276:16374-16378.
53. Antonetti DA, Algenstaedt P, Kahn CR. Insulin receptor substrate 1 binds two novel splice variants of the regulatory subunit of phosphatidylinositol 3-kinase in muscle and brain. Mol Cell Biol 1996; 16:2195-2203.
54. Inukai K, Anai M, Van Breda E, Hosaka T, Katagiri H, Funaki M et al. A novel 55-kDa regulatory subunit for phosphatidylinositol 3-kinase structurally similar to p55PIK Is generated by alternative splicing of the p85alpha gene. J-Biol-Chem 1996; 271:5317-20.
55. Fruman DA, Cantley LC, Carpenter CL. Structural organization and alternative splicing of the murine phosphoinositide 3-kinase p85 alpha gene. Genomics 1996; 37:113-121.
56. Inukai K, Funaki M, Ogihara T, Katagiri H, Kanda A, Anai M et al. p85alpha gene generates three isoforms of regulatory subunit for phosphatidylinositol 3-kinase (PI 3-Kinase), p50alpha, p55alpha, and p85alpha, with different PI 3-kinase activity elevating responses to insulin. J Biol Chem 1997; 272:7873-7882.
57. Pons S, Asano T, Glasheen E, Miralpeix M, Zhang Y, Fisher TL et al. The structure and function of p55PIK reveal a new regulatory subunit for phosphatidylinositol 3-kinase. Mol Cell Biol 1995; 15:4453-4465.

58. Kerouz NJ, Horsch D, Pons S, Kahn CR. Differential regulation of insulin receptor substrates-1 and -2 (IRS-1 and IRS-2) and phosphatidylinositol 3-kinase isoforms in liver and muscle of the obese diabetic (ob/ob. mouse. J Clin Invest 1997; 100:3164-3172.
59. Xia X, Serrero G. Multiple forms of p55PIK, a regulatory subunit of phosphoinositide 3-kinase, are generated by alternative initiation of translation. Biochem J 1999; 341 (Pt 3):831-837.
60. Stoyanov B, Volinia S, Hanck T, Rubio I, Loubtchenkov M, Malek D et al. Cloning and characterisation of a G protein-activated human phosphatidlinositol 3-kinase. Science 1995; 269:690-693.
61. Suire S, Coadwell J, Ferguson GJ, Davidson K, Hawkins P, Stephens L. p84, a new Gbetagamma-activated regulatory subunit of the type IB phosphoinositide 3-kinase p110gamma. Curr Biol 2005; 15:566-570.
62. Domin J, Gaidarov I, Smith M, Keen J, Waterfield M. The class II phosphoinositide 3-kinase PI3K-C2alpha is concentrated in the trans-Golgi network and present in clathrin-coated vesicles. J Biol Chem 2000; 275:11943-50.
63. Song X, Xu W, Zhang A, Huang G, Liang X, Virbasius JV et al. Phox homology domains specifically bind phosphatidylinositol phosphates. Biochemistry 2001; 40:8940-8944.
64. Bravo J, Karathanassis D, Pacold CM, Pacold ME, Ellson CD, Anderson KE et al. The crystal structure of the PX domain from p40(phox) bound to phosphatidylinositol 3-phosphate. Mol Cell 2001; 8:829-839.
65. Wheeler M, Domin J. Recruitment of the class II phosphoinositide 3-kinase C2beta to the epidermal growth factor receptor: role of Grb2. Mol Cell Biol 2001; 21:6660-6667.
66. Budovskaya YV, Hama H, DeWald DB, Herman PK. The C terminus of the Vps34p phosphoinositide 3-kinase is necessary and sufficient for the interaction with the Vps15p protein kinase. J Biol Chem 2002; 277:287-294.
67. Panaretou C, Domin J, Cockcroft S, Waterfield MD. Characterization of p150, an adaptor protein for the human phosphatidylinositol (PtdIns) 3-kinase. Substrate presentation by phosphatidylinositol transfer protein to the p150.Ptdins 3-kinase complex. J Biol Chem 1997; 272:2477-2485.
68. Murray JT, Panaretou C, Stenmark H, Miaczynska M, Backer JM. Role of Rab5 in the recruitment of hVps34/p150 to the early endosome. Traffic 2002; 3:416-427.
69. Arcaro A, Zvelebil MJ, Wallasch C, Ullrich A, Waterfield MD, Domin J. Class II phosphoinositide 3-kinase are downstream targets of activated polypeptide growth factor receptors. Mol Cell Biol 2000; 20:3817-30.
70. Zhang J, Banfic H, Straforini F, Tosi L, Volinia S, Rittenhouse S. A type II phosphoinositide 3-kinase is stimulated via activated integrin in platelets. A source of phosphatidylinositol 3-phosphate. J Biol Chem 1998; 273:14081-14084.
71. Sindic A, Aleksandrova A, Fields AP, Volinia S, Banfic H. Presence and activation of nuclear phosphoinositide 3-kinase C2beta during compensatory liver growth. J Biol Chem 2001; 276:17754-17761.
72. Visnjic D, Curic J, Crljen V, Batinic D, Volinia S, Banfic H. Nuclear phosphoinositide 3-kinase C2beta activation during G2/M phase of the cell cycle in HL-60 cells. Biochim Biophys Acta 2003; 1631:61-71.
73. Crljen V, Volinia S, Banfic H. Hepatocyte growth factor activates phosphoinositide 3-kinase C2beta in renal brush-border plasma membranes. Biochem J 2002; 365:791-799.
74. Domin J, Harper L, Aubyn D, Wheeler M, Florey O, Haskard D et al. The class II phosphoinositide 3-kinase PI3K-C2beta regulates cell migration by a PtdIns(3)P dependent mechanism. J Cell Physiol 2005.
75. Maffucci T, Cooke FT, Foster FM, Traer CJ, Fry MJ, Falasca M. Class II phosphoinositide 3-kinase defines a novel signaling pathway in cell migration. J Cell Biol 2005; 169:789-799.
76. Arcaro A, Khanzada UK, Vanhaesebroeck B, Tetley TD, Waterfield MD, Seckl MJ. Two distinct phosphoinositide 3-kinases mediate polypeptide growth factor-stimulated PKB activation. EMBO J 2002; 21:5097-5108.
77. Thompson DM, Cochet C, Chambaz EM, Gill GN. Separation and characterization of a phosphatidylinositol kinase activity that co-purifies with the epidermal growth factor receptor. J Biol Chem 1985; 260:8824-8830.
78. Pike LJ, Eakes AT. Epidermal growth factor stimulates the production of phosphatidylinositol monophosphate and the breakdown of polyphosphoinositides in A431 cells. J Biol Chem 1987; 262:1644-1651.
79. Carter AN, Downes CP. Phosphatidylinositol 3-kinase is activated by nerve growth factor and epidermal growth factor in PC12 cells. J Biol Chem 1992; 267:14563-14567.

80. Miller ES, Ascoli M. Anti-phosphotyrosine immunoprecipitation of phosphoinositol 3'kinase activity in different cell types after exposure to epidermal growth factor. Biochem Biophys Res Commun 1990; 173:289-295.
81. Raffioni S, Bradshaw RA. Activation of phosphatidylinositol 3 kinase by epidermal growth factor, basic fibroblast growth factor and nerve growth factor in PC12 phaeochromocytoma cells. Proc Natl Acad Sci 1992; 89:9121-9125.
82. Bjorge JD, Chan TO, Antczak M, Kung HJ, Fujita DJ. Activated type I phosphatidylinositol kinase is associated with the epidermal growth factor (EGF) receptor following EGF stimulation. Proc Natl Acad Sci U S A 1990; 87:3816-3820.
83. Hu P, Margolis B, Skolnik EY, Lammers R, Ullrich A, Schlessinger J. Interaction of phosphatidylinositol 3-kinase-associated p85 with epidermal growth factor and platelet-derived growth factor receptors. Mol Cell Biol 1992; 12:981-990.
84. Gout I, Dhand R, Panayotou G, Fry MJ, Hiles I, Otsu M et al. Expression and characterization of the p85 subunit of the phosphatidylinositol 3-kinase complex and a related p85 beta protein by using the baculovirus expression system. Biochem J 1992; 288:395-405.
85. King CR, Borrello I, Bellot F, Comoglio P, Schlessinger J. Egf binding to its receptor triggers a rapid tyrosine phosphorylation of the erbB-2 protein in the mammary tumor cell line SK-BR-3. EMBO J 1988; 7:1647-1651.
86. Songyang Z, Shoelson SE, Chaudhuri M, Gish G, Pawson T, Haser WG et al. SH2 domains recognize specific phosphopeptide sequences. Cell 1993; 72:767-778.
87. Panayotou G, Bax B, Gout I, Federwisch M, Wroblowski B, Dhand R et al. Interaction of the p85 subunit of PI 3-kinase and its N-terminal SH2 domain with a PDGF receptor phosphorylation site: structural features and analysis of conformational changes. EMBO J 1992; 11:4261-4272.
88. Soltoff SP, Carraway SA, Prigent SA, Gullick WG, Cantley LC. ErbB3 is involved in activation of phosphatidylinositol 3-kinase by epidermal growth factor. Mol Cell Biol 1994; 14:3550-3558.
89. Prigent SA, Gullick WJ. Identification of c-erbB-3 binding sites for phosphatidylinositol 3'-kinase and SHC using an EGF receptor/c-erbB-3 chimera. Embo J 1994; 13:2831-2841.
90. Gillham H, Golding MCHM, Pepperkok R, Gullick WJ. Intracellular movement of green flourescent protein-tagged phosphatidylinositol 3-kinase in response to growth factor receptor signaling. J Cell Biol 1999; 146:869-880.
91. Soltoff SP, Cantley LC. p120cbl is a cytosolic adaptor protein that associates with phosphoinositide 3-kinase in response to epidermal growth factor in PC12 and other cells. J Biol Chem 1996; 271:563-567.
92. Fukazawa T, Reedquist KA, Trub T, Soltoff S, Panchamoorthy G, Druker B et al. The SH3 domain-binding T cell tyrosyl phosphoprotein p120. Demonstration of its identity with the c-cbl protooncogene product and in vivo complexes with Fyn, Grb2, and phosphatidylinositol 3-kinase. J Biol Chem 1995; 270:19141-19150.
93. Galisteo ML, Dikic I, Batzer AG, Langdon WY, Schlessinger J. Tyrosine phosphorylation of the c-cbl proto-oncogene protein product and association with epidermal growth factor (EGF) receptor upon EGF stimulation. J Biol Chem 1995; 270:20242-20245.
94. Bowtell DD, Langdon WY. The protein product of the c-cbl oncogene rapidly complexes with the EGF receptor and is tyrosine phosphorylated following EGF stimulation. Oncogene 1995; 11:1561-1567.
95. Lehr S, Kotzka J, Herkner A, Klein E, Siethoff C, Knebel B et al. Identification of tyrosine phosphorylation sites in human Gab-1 protein by EGF receptor kinase in vitro. Biochemistry 1999; 38:151-159.
96. Rodrigues GA, Falasca M, Zhang Z, Ong SH, Schlessinger J. A novel positive feedback loop mediated by the docking protein Gab1 and phosphatidylinositol 3-kinase in epidermal growth factor receptor signaling. Mol Cell Biol 2000; 20:1448-1459.
97. Fujioka T, Ui M. Involvement of insulin receptor substrates in epidermal growth factor induced activation of phosphatidylinositol 3-kinase in rat hepatocyte primary culture. Eur J Biochem 2001; 268:25-34.
98. Katso RM, Pardo OE, Palamidessi A, Franz CM, Marinov M, De Laurentiis A et al. Phosphoinositide 3-Kinase C2beta regulates cytoskeletal organization and cell migration via Rac-dependent mechanisms. Mol Biol Cell 2006; 17:3729-3744.

99. Mayer BJ, Ren R, Clark KL, Baltimore D. A putative modular domain present in diverse signaling proteins. Cell 1993; 73:629-630.
100. Haslam RJ, Koide HB, Hemmings BA. Pleckstrin domain homology. Nature 1993; 363:309-310.
101. Harlan JE, Hajduk PJ, Yoon HS, Fesik SW. Pleckstrin homology domains bind to phosphatidylinositol-4,5-bisphosphate. Nature 1994; 371:168-170.
102. Kay BK, Yamabhai M, Wendland B, Emr SD. Identification of a novel domain shared by putative components of the endocytic and cytoskeletal machinery. Protein Sci 1999; 8:435-438.
103. Legendre-Guillemin V, Wasiak S, Hussain NK, Angers A, McPherson PS. ENTH/ANTH proteins and clathrin-mediated membrane budding. J Cell Sci 2004; 117:9-18.
104. Rosenthal JA, Chen H, Slepnev VI, Pellegrini L, Salcini AE, Di Fiore PP et al. The epsins define a family of proteins that interact with components of the clathrin coat and contain a new protein module. J Biol Chem 1999; 274:33959-33965.
105. Itoh T, Koshiba S, Kigawa T, Kikuchi A, Yokoyama S, Takenawa T. Role of the ENTH domain in phosphatidylinositol-4,5-bisphosphate binding and endocytosis. Science 2001; 291:1047-1051.
106. Ford MG, Pearse BM, Higgins MK, Vallis Y, Owen DJ, Gibson A et al. Simultaneous binding of PtdIns(4,5)P2 and clathrin by AP180 in the nucleation of clathrin lattices on membranes. Science 2001; 291:1051-1055.
107. Hyun TS, Rao DS, Saint-Dic D, Michael LE, Kumar PD, Bradley SV et al. HIP1 and HIP1r stabilize receptor tyrosine kinases and bind 3-phosphoinositides via epsin N-terminal homology domains. J Biol Chem 2004; 279:14294-14306.
108. Friant S, Pecheur EI, Eugster A, Michel F, Lefkir Y, Nourrisson D et al. Ent3p Is a PtdIns(3,5.P2 effector required for protein sorting to the multivesicular body. Dev Cell 2003; 5:499-511.
109. Bellacosa A, Testa JR, Staal SP, Tsichlis PN. A retroviral oncogene, akt, encoding a serine-threonine kinase containing an SH2-like region. Science 1991; 254:274-277.
110. Coffer PJ, Woodgett JR. Molecular cloning and characterisation of a novel putative protein-serine kinase related to the cAMP-dependent and protein kinase C families. Eur J Biochem 1991; 201:475-481.
111. Jones PF, Jakubowicz T, Pitossi FJ, Maurer F, Hemmings BA. Molecular cloning and identification of a serine/threonine protein kinase of the second-messenger subfamily. Proc Natl Acad Sci U S A 1991; 88:4171-4175.
112. Cheng JQ, Godwin AK, Bellacosa A, Taguchi T, Franke TF, Hamilton TC et al. AKT2, a putative oncogene encoding a member of a subfamily of protein-serine/threonine kinases, is amplified in human ovarian carcinomas. Proc Natl Acad Sci U S A 1992; 89:9267-9271.
113. Konishi H, Kuroda S, Tanaka M, Matsuzaki H, Ono Y, Kameyama K et al. Molecular cloning and characterization of a new member of the RAC protein kinase family: association of the pleckstrin homology domain of three types of RAC protein kinase with protein kinase C subspecies and beta gamma subunits of G proteins. Biochem Biophys Res Commun 1995; 216:526-534.
114. Franke TF, Kaplan DR, Cantley LC, Toker A. Direct regulation of the Akt proto-oncogene product by phosphatidylinositol-3,4-bisphosphate. Science 1997; 275:665-668.
115. Franke TF, Yang S-I, Chan TO, Datta K, Kazlauskas A, Morrison DK et al. The protein kinase encoded by the Akt proto-oncogene is a target of the PDGF-ativated phosphatidylinositol 3-kinase. Cell 1995; 81:727-736.
116. Alessi DR, Andjelkovic M, Caudwell B, Cron P, Morrice N, Cohen P et al. Mechanism of activation of protein kinase B by insulin and IGF-1. EMBO J 1996; 15:6541-6551.
117. Okano J, Gaslightwala I, Birnbaum MJ, Rustgi AK, Nakagawa H. Akt/protein kinase B isoforms are differentially regulated by epidermal growth factor stimulation. J Biol Chem 2000; 275:30934-30942.
118. Burgering BM, Coffer PJ. Protein kinase B (c-Akt) in phosphatidylinositol-3-OH kinase signal transduction. Nature 1995; 376:599-602.
119. Alessi DR, James SR, Downes CP, Holmes AB, Gaffney PRJ, Reese CB et al. Characterization of a 3-phosphoinositide-dependent protein kinase which phosphorylates and activates protein kinase Bα. Current Biology 1997; 7:261-269.
120. Meier R, Alessi DR, Cron P, Andjelkovic M, Hemmings BA. Mitogenic activation, phosphorylation, and nuclear translocation of protein kinase Bbeta. J Biol Chem 1997; 272:30491-30497.
121. Stokoe D, Stephens LR, Copeland T, Gaffney PR, Reese CB, Painter GF et al. Dual role of phosphatidylinositol-3,4,5-trisphosphate in the activation of protein kinase B. Science 1997; 277:567-570.

122. Stephens L, Anderson K, Stokoe D, Erdjument-Bromage H, Painter GF, Holmes AB et al. Protein kinase B kinases that mediate phosphatidylinositol 3,4,5-trisphosphate-dependent activation of protein kinase B. Science 1998; 279:710-714.
123. Mora A, Komander D, van Aalten DM, Alessi DR. PDK1, the master regulator of AGC kinase signal transduction. Semin Cell Dev Biol 2004; 15:161-170.
124. Kohn AD, Summers SA, Birnbaum MJ, Roth RA. Expression of a constitutively active Akt Ser/Thr kinase in 3T3-L1 adipocytes stimulates glucose uptake and glucose transporter 4 translocation. J Biol Chem 1996; 271:31372-31378.
125. Lim MA, Kikani CK, Wick MJ, Dong LQ. Nuclear translocation of 3'-phosphoinositide-dependent protein kinase 1 (PDK-1): a potential regulatory mechanism for PDK-1 function. Proc Natl Acad Sci U S A 2003; 100:14006-14011.
126. Komander D, Fairservice A, Deak M, Kular GS, Prescott AR, Peter DC et al. Structural insights into the regulation of PDK1 by phosphoinositides and inositol phosphates. EMBO J 2004; 23:3918-3928.
127. Frodin M, Antal TL, Dummler BA, Jensen CJ, Deak M, Gammeltoft S et al. A phosphoserine/threonine-binding pocket in AGC kinases and PDK1 mediates activation by hydrophobic motif phosphorylation. EMBO J 2002; 21:5396-5407.
128. Cheng X, Ma Y, Moore M, Hemmings BA, Taylor SS. Phosphorylation and activation of cAMP-dependent protein kinase by phosphoinositide-dependent protein kinase. Proc Natl Acad Sci U S A 1998; 95:9849-9854.
129. Le Good JA, Ziegler WH, Parekh DB, Alessi DR, Cohen P, Parker PJ. Protein kinase C isotypes controlled by phosphoinositide 3-kinase through the protein kinase PDK1. Science 1998; 281:2042-2045.
130. Pullen N, Dennis PB, Andjelkovic M, Dufner A, Kozma SC, Hemmings BA et al. Phosphorylation and activation of p70s6k by PDK1. Science 1998; 279:707-710.
131. Jensen CJ, Buch MB, Krag TO, Hemmings BA, Gammeltoft S, Frodin M. 90-kDa ribosomal S6 kinase is phosphorylated and activated by 3-phosphoinositide-dependent protein kinase-1. J Biol Chem 1999; 274:27168-27176.
132. Park J, Leong ML, Buse P, Maiyar AC, Firestone GL, Hemmings BA. Serum and glucocorticoid-inducible kinase (SGK. is a target of the PI 3-kinase-stimulated signaling pathway. EMBO J 1999; 18:3024-3033.
133. Terada N, Lucas JJ, Szepesi A, Franklin RA, Takase K, Gelfand EW. Rapamycin inhibits the phosphorylation of p70 S6 kinase in IL-2 and mitogen-activated human T cells. Biochem Biophys Res Commun 1992; 186:1315-1321.
134. Wilson M, Burt AR, Milligan G, Anderson NG. Wortmannin-sensitive activation of p70s6k by endogenous and heterologously expressed Gi-coupled receptors. J Biol Chem 1996; 271:8537-8540.
135. Jefferies HB, Reinhard C, Kozma SC, Thomas G. Rapamycin selectively represses translation of the "polypyrimidine tract" mRNA family. Proc Natl Acad Sci U S A 1994; 91:4441-4445.
136. Parker PJ, Murray-Rust J. PKC at a glance. J Cell Sci 2004; 117:131-132.
137. Akimoto K, Takahashi R, Moriya S, Nishioka N, Takayanagi J, Kimura K et al. EGF or PDGF receptors activate atypical PKClambda through phosphatidylinositol 3-kinase. EMBO J 1996; 15:788-798.
138. Kotani K, Ogawa W, Matsumoto M, Kitamura T, Sakaue H, Hino Y et al. Requirement of atypical protein kinase clambda for insulin stimulation of glucose uptake but not for Akt activation in 3T3-L1 adipocytes. Mol Cell Biol 1998; 18:6971-6982.
139. Dutil EM, Toker A, Newton AC. Regulation of conventional protein kinase C isozymes by phosphoinositide-dependent kinase 1 (PDK-1). Curr Biol 1998; 8:1366-1375.
140. Taylor SS, Yang J, Wu J, Haste NM, Radzio-Andzelm E, Anand G. PKA: a portrait of protein kinase dynamics. Biochim Biophys Acta 2004; 1697:259-269.
141. Michel JJ, Scott JD. AKAP mediated signal transduction. Annu Rev Pharmacol Toxicol 2002; 42:235-257.
142. Bayascas JR, Alessi DR. Regulation of Akt/PKB Ser473 phosphorylation. Mol Cell 2005; 18:143-145.
143. Toker A, Newton AC. Cellular signaling: pivoting around PDK-1. Cell 2000; 103:185-188.
144. Troussard AA, Mawji NM, Ong C, Mui A, Arnaud R, Dedhar S. Conditional knock-out of integrin-linked kinase demonstrates an essential role in protein kinase B/Akt activation. J Biol Chem 2003; 278:22374-22378.
145. Hara K, Maruki Y, Long X, Yoshino K, Oshiro N, Hidayat S et al. Raptor, a binding partner of target of rapamycin (TOR), mediates TOR action. Cell 2002; 110:177-189.

146. Kim DH, Sarbassov DD, Ali SM, King JE, Latek RR, Erdjument-Bromage H et al. mTOR interacts with raptor to form a nutrient-sensitive complex that signals to the cell growth machinery. Cell 2002; 110:163-175.
147. Sarbassov DD, Guertin DA, Ali SM, Sabatini DM. Phosphorylation and regulation of Akt/PKB by the rictor-mTOR complex. Science 2005; 307:1098-1101.
148. Yang ZZ, Tschopp O, Hemmings-Mieszczak M, Feng J, Brodbeck D, Perentes E et al. Protein kinase B alpha/Akt1 regulates placental development and fetal growth. J Biol Chem 2003; 278:32124-32131.
149. Chen WS, Xu PZ, Gottlob K, Chen ML, Sokol K, Shiyanova T et al. Growth retardation and increased apoptosis in mice with homozygous disruption of the Akt1 gene. Genes Dev 2001; 15:2203-2208.
150. Chen J, De S, Damron DS, Chen WS, Hay N, Byzova TV. Impaired platelet responses to thrombin and collagen in AKT-1-deficient mice. Blood 2004; 104:1703-1710.
151. Cho H, Mu J, Kim JK, Thorvaldsen JL, Chu Q, Crenshaw EB, III et al. Insulin resistance and a diabetes mellitus-like syndrome in mice lacking the protein kinase Akt2 (PKB beta). Science 2001; 292:1728-1731.
152. Franke TF, Kaplan DR, Cantley LC. PI3K: downstream AKTion blocks apoptosis. Cell 1997; 88:435-437.
153. Chao DT, Korsmeyer SJ. BCL-2 family: regulators of cell death. Annu Rev Immunol 1998; 16:395-419.
154. Fang X, Yu S, Eder A, Mao M, Bast RC, Jr., Boyd D et al. Regulation of BAD phosphorylation at serine 112 by the Ras-mitogen-activated protein kinase pathway. Oncogene 1999; 18:6635-6640.
155. del PL, Gonzalez-Garcia M, Page C, Herrera R, Nunez G. Interleukin-3-induced phosphorylation of BAD through the protein kinase Akt. Science 1997; 278:687-689.
156. Datta SR, Dudek H, Tao X, Masters S, Fu H, Gotoh Y et al. Akt phosphorylation of BAD couples survival signals to the cell-intrinsic death machinery. Cell 1997; 91:231-241.
157. Cardone MH, Roy N, Stennicke HR, Salvesen GS, Franke TF, Stanbridge E et al. Regulation of cell death protease caspase-9 by phosphorylation. Science 1998; 282:1318-1321.
158. Shin I, Yakes FM, Rojo F, Shin NY, Bakin AV, Baselga J et al. PKB/Akt mediates cell-cycle progression by phosphorylation of p27(Kip1) at threonine 157 and modulation of its cellular localization. Nat Med 2002; 8:1145-1152.
159. Viglietto G, Motti ML, Bruni P, Melillo RM, D'Alessio A, Califano D et al. Cytoplasmic relocalization and inhibition of the cyclin-dependent kinase inhibitor p27(Kip1) by PKB/Akt-mediated phosphorylation in breast cancer. Nat Med 2002; 8:1136-1144.
160. Zhou BP, Liao Y, Xia W, Spohn B, Lee MH, Hung MC. Cytoplasmic localization of p21Cip1/WAF1 by Akt-induced phosphorylation in HER-2/neu-overexpressing cells. Nat Cell Biol 2001; 3:245-252.
161. Mayo LD, Donner DB. A phosphatidylinositol 3-kinase/Akt pathway promotes translocation of Mdm2 from the cytoplasm to the nucleus. Proc Natl Acad Sci U S A 2001; 98:11598-11603.
162. Zhou BP, Liao Y, Xia W, Zou Y, Spohn B, Hung MC. HER-2/neu induces p53 ubiquitination via Akt-mediated MDM2 phosphorylation. Nat Cell Biol 2001; 3:973-982.
163. Zimmermann S, Moelling K. Phosphorylation and regulation of Raf by Akt (protein kinase B). Science 1999; 286:1741-1744.
164. Brunet A, Bonni A, Zigmond MJ, Lin MZ, Juo P, Hu LS et al. Akt promotes cell survival by phosphorylating and inhibiting a Forkhead transcription factor. Cell 1999; 96:857-868.
165. Kops GJ, de Ruiter ND, Vries-Smits AM, Powell DR, Bos JL, Burgering BM. Direct control of the Forkhead transcription factor AFX by protein kinase B. Nature 1999; 398:630-634.
166. Van Der Heide LP, Hoekman MF, Smidt MP. The ins and outs of FoxO shuttling: mechanisms of FoxO translocation and transcriptional regulation. Biochem J 2004; 380:297-309.
167. Biggs WH, III, Meisenhelder J, Hunter T, Cavenee WK, Arden KC. Protein kinase B/Akt-mediated phosphorylation promotes nuclear exclusion of the winged helix transcription factor FKHR1. Proc Natl Acad Sci U S A 1999; 96:7421-7426.
168. Takaishi H, Konishi H, Matsuzaki H, Ono Y, Shirai Y, Saito N et al. Regulation of nuclear translocation of forkhead transcription factor AFX by protein kinase B. Proc Natl Acad Sci U S A 1999; 96:11836-11841.
169. Schmidt M, Fernandez de MS, van der HA, Klompmaker R, Kops GJ, Lam EW et al. Cell cycle inhibition by FoxO forkhead transcription factors involves downregulation of cyclin D. Mol Cell Biol 2002; 22:7842-7852.

170. Dijkers PF, Medema RH, Pals C, Banerji L, Thomas NS, Lam EW et al. Forkhead transcription factor FKHR-L1 modulates cytokine-dependent transcriptional regulation of p27(KIP1). Mol Cell Biol 2000; 20:9138-9148.
171. Liang J, Zubovitz J, Petrocelli T, Kotchetkov R, Connor MK, Han K et al. PKB/Akt phosphorylates p27, impairs nuclear import of p27 and opposes p27-mediated G1 arrest. Nat Med 2002; 8:1153-1160.
172. Brunet A, Park J, Tran H, Hu LS, Hemmings BA, Greenberg ME. Protein kinase SGK mediates survival signals by phosphorylating the forkhead transcription factor FKHRL1 (FOXO3a). Mol Cell Biol 2001; 21:952-965.
173. Aggarwal BB. Nuclear factor-kappaB: the enemy within. Cancer Cell 2004; 6:203-208.
174. Khwaja A. Akt is more than just a Bad kinase. Nature 1999; 401:33-34.
175. Lauder A, Castellanos A, Weston K. c-Myb transcription is activated by protein kinase B (PKB) following interleukin 2 stimulation of Tcells and is required for PKB-mediated protection from apoptosis. Mol Cell Biol 2001; 21:5797-5805.
176. Du K, Montminy M. CREB is a regulatory target for the protein kinase Akt/PKB. J Biol Chem 1998; 273:32377-32379.
177. Pugazhenthi S, Nesterova A, Sable C, Heidenreich KA, Boxer LM, Heasley LE et al. Akt/protein kinase B up-regulates Bcl-2 expression through cAMP-response element-binding protein. J Biol Chem 2000; 275:10761-10766.
178. Wang JM, Chao JR, Chen W, Kuo ML, Yen JJ, Yang-Yen HF. The antiapoptotic gene mcl-1 is up-regulated by the phosphatidylinositol 3-kinase/Akt signaling pathway through a transcription factor complex containing CREB. Mol Cell Biol 1999; 19:6195-6206.
179. Mayr B, Montminy M. Transcriptional regulation by the phosphorylation-dependent factor CREB. Nat Rev Mol Cell Biol 2001; 2:599-609.
180. Nakamura N, Ramaswamy S, Vazquez F, Signoretti S, Loda M, Sellers WR. Forkhead transcription factors are critical effectors of cell death and cell cycle arrest downstream of PTEN. Mol Cell Biol 2000; 20:8969-8982.
181. Kim BC, Lee MN, Kim JY, Lee SS, Chang JD, Kim SS et al. Roles of phosphatidylinositol 3-kinase and Rac in the nuclear signaling by tumor necrosis factor-alpha in rat-2 fibroblasts. J Biol Chem 1999; 274:24372-24377.
182. Wang Y, Falasca M, Schlessinger J, Malstrom S, Tsichlis P, Settleman J et al. Activation of the c-fos serum response element by phosphatidyl inositol 3-kinase and rho pathways in HeLa cells. Cell Growth Differ 1998; 9:513-522.
183. Coffer PJ, Jin J, Woodgett JR. Protein kinase B (c-Akt): a multifunctional mediator of phosphatidylinositol 3-kinase activation. Biochem J 1998; 335 (Pt 1):1-13.
184. Delcommenne M, Tan C, Gray V, Rue L, Woodgett J, Dedhar S. Phosphoinositide-3-OH kinase-dependent regulation of glycogen synthase kinase 3 and protein kinase B/AKT by the integrin-linked kinase. Proc Natl Acad Sci U S A 1998; 95:11211-11216.
185. Welsh GI, Miller CM, Loughlin AJ, Price NT, Proud CG. Regulation of eukaryotic initiation factor eIF2B: glycogen synthase kinase-3 phosphorylates a conserved serine which undergoes dephosphorylation in response to insulin. FEBS Lett 1998; 421:125-130.
186. Proud CG. eIF2 and the control of cell physiology. Semin Cell Dev Biol 2005; 16:3-12.
187. Deprez J, Vertommen D, Alessi DR, Hue L, Rider MH. Phosphorylation and activation of heart 6-phosphofructo-2-kinase by protein kinase B and other protein kinases of the insulin signaling cascades. J Biol Chem 1997; 272:17269-17275.
188. Rider MH, Bertrand L, Vertommen D, Michels PA, Rousseau GG, Hue L. 6-phosphofructo-2-kinase/fructose-2,6-bisphosphatase: head-to-head with a bifunctional enzyme that controls glycolysis. Biochem J 2004; 381:561-579.
189. Gingras AC, Raught B, Sonenberg N. Regulation of translation initiation by FRAP/mTOR. Genes Dev 2001; 15:807-826.
190. Shamji AF, Nghiem P, Schreiber SL. Integration of growth factor and nutrient signaling: implications for cancer biology. Mol Cell 2003; 12:271-280.
191. Fingar DC, Blenis J. Target of rapamycin (TOR): an integrator of nutrient and growth factor signals and coordinator of cell growth and cell cycle progression. Oncogene 2004; 23:3151-3171.
192. Inoki K, Li Y, Zhu T, Wu J, Guan KL. TSC2 is phosphorylated and inhibited by Akt and suppresses mTOR signalling. Nat Cell Biol 2002; 4:648-657.

193. Potter CJ, Pedraza LG, Xu T. Akt regulates growth by directly phosphorylating Tsc2. Nat Cell Biol 2002; 4:658-665.
194. Gao X, Pan D. TSC1 and TSC2 tumor suppressors antagonize insulin signaling in cell growth. Genes Dev 2001; 15:1383-1392.
195. Harris TE, Lawrence JC, Jr. TOR signaling. Sci STKE 2003; 2003:re15.
196. Kwiatkowski DJ. Rhebbing up mTOR: new insights on TSC1 and TSC2, and the pathogenesis of tuberous sclerosis. Cancer Biol Ther 2003; 2:471-476.
197. Wittinghofer A. Signal transduction via Ras. Biol Chem 1998; 379:933-937.
198. Worthylake DK, Rossman KL, Sondek J. Crystal structure of the DH/PH fragment of Dbs without bound GTPase. Structure (Camb) 2004; 12:1078-1086.
199. Welch HC, Coadwell WJ, Stephens LR, Hawkins PT. Phosphoinositide 3-kinase-dependent activation of Rac. FEBS Lett 2003; 546:93-97.
200. Rameh LE, Cantley LC. The role of phosphoinositide 3-kinase lipid products in cell function. J Biol Chem 1999; 274:8347-50.
201. Han J, Luby-Phelps K, Das B, Shu X, Xia Y, Mosteller RD et al. Role of substrates and products of PI 3-kinase in regulating activation of Rac-related guanosine triphosphatases by Vav. Science 1998; 279:558-560.
202. Venkateswarlu K, Oatey PB, Tavare JM, Cullen PJ. Insulin-dependent translocation of ARNO to the plasma membrane of adipocytes requires phosphatidylinositol 3-kinase. Curr Biol 1998; 8:463-466.
203. Lockyer PJ, Wennstrom S, Kupzig S, Venkateswarlu K, Downward J, Cullen PJ. Identification of the ras GTPase-activating protein GAP1(m) as a phosphatidylinositol-3,4,5-trisphosphate-binding protein in vivo. Curr Biol 1999; 9:265-268.
204. Venkateswarlu K, Oatey PB, Tavare JM, Jackson TR, Cullen PJ. Identification of centaurin-alpha1 as a potential in vivo phosphatidylinositol 3,4,5-trisphosphate-binding protein that is functionally homologous to the yeast ADP-ribosylation factor (ARF) GTPase-activating protein, Gcs1. Biochem J 1999; 340 Pt 2):359-363.
205. Chen X, Wang Z. Regulation of intracellular trafficking of the EGF receptor by Rab5 in the absence of phosphatidylinositol 3-kinase activity. EMBO Rep 2001; 2:68-74.
206. Futter CE, Collinson LM, Backer JM, Hopkins CR. Human VPS34 is required for internal vesicle formation within multivesicular endosomes. J Cell Biol 2001; 155:1251-1264.
207. Johnson EE, Overmeyer JH, Gunning WT, Maltese WA. Gene silencing reveals a specific function of hVps34 phosphatidylinositol 3-kinase in late versus early endosomes. J Cell Sci 2006; 119:1219-1232.
208. Gaidarov I, Smith ME, Domin J, Keen JH. The class II phosphoinositide 3-kinase C2alpha is activated by clathrin and regulates clathrin-mediated membrane trafficking. Mol Cell 2001; 7:443-449.
209. Wheeler M, Domin J. The N-terminus of phosphoinositide 3-kinase-C2beta regulates lipid kinase activity and binding to clathrin. J Cell Physiol 2006; 206:586-593.
210. Knight ZA, Gonzalez B, Feldman ME, Zunder ER, Goldenberg DD, Williams O et al. A pharmacological map of the PI3-K family defines a role for p110alpha in insulin signaling. Cell 2006; 125:733-747.

9 Convergence of EGF Receptor and Src Family Signaling Networks in Cancer

Jessica E. Pritchard, Allison B. Jablonski, and Sarah J. Parsons

CONTENTS

AN INTRODUCTION TO C-SRC
C-SRC INTERACTIONS WITH THE EGFR
EFFECTS OF THE CONVERGENCE OF EGFR AND C-SRC SIGNALING ON ONCOGENESIS
MECHANISMS OF C-SRC SIGNALING UPSTREAM OF THE EGFR: TRANSACTIVATION OF THE EGFR
MECHANISMS OF C-SRC SIGNALING DOWNSTREAM OF THE EGFR
INHIBITION OF SRC SIGNALING THAT CONVERGES WITH THE EGFR
REFERENCES

Abstract

EGF receptor (EGFR) and c-Src are tyrosine kinases of the receptor and non-receptor classes, respectively, which are frequently co-overexpressed or co-activated in multiple human cancers, including those of breast, prostate, lung, and colon. Most of these cancers express non-mutated forms of each kinase, and overexpression of either is weakly or non-oncogenic. However, when co-overexpressed, they exhibit profound synergism that up-regulates many neoplastic processes, including cell proliferation, survival, and metastasis. This synergism is dependent upon or greatly enhanced by physical association between c-Src and ligand-stimulated EGFR, which leads to activation of both kinases, phosphorylation of the EGFR by c-Src, and enhanced phosphorylation of EGFR and c-Src substrates. Non-EGFR ligands, such as agonists for G-protein coupled-, steriod hormone-, and cytokine receptors, also induce association between EGFR and c-Src and subsequent oncogenic consequences of this interaction. Because of their important roles in the etiology and progression of a broad spectrum of cancers, EGFR and c-Src represent signaling molecules that are ripe for combinatorial therapeutic targeting.

Key Words: EGF Receptor (EGFR), c-Src, Cancer, Synergism, Signaling, Phosphorylation, Transactivation, Inhibitors.

1. AN INTRODUCTION TO C-SRC

Cellular-Src, or c-Src, is the proto-oncogenic homolog to oncogenic viral-Src (v-Src), originally isolated from the avian Rous Sarcoma Virus (*1, 2*). C-Src is a membrane-associated non-receptor tyrosine kinase that has been shown to have numerous protein substrates.

These substrates regulate many cellular processes, including adhesion, migration, proliferation, apoptosis, and differentiation (3).

C-Src is the founding member of a family that includes Fyn, Yes, Fgr, Hck, Lck, Blk, Yrk, Lyn, and the Frk subfamily, composed of Frk/Rak and Lyk/Bsk. Src, Fyn, Yes, and Yrk are ubiquitously expressed in the body, while Fgr, Hck, Lck, Blk, and Lyn are predominately expressed in hematopoietic cells. Primary epithelial cells are the favored sites of Frk subfamily expression. In many cases, Src family members have demonstrated aberrant expression patterns and levels in cancer (3).

C-Src is a 60 kD protein composed of six functional regions (Fig. 9.1A). At its N-terminus is the Src-homology 4 (SH4) domain, which contains myristoylation and palmitoylation sites for membrane anchoring. Adjacent to this domain is the poorly-conserved "unique"

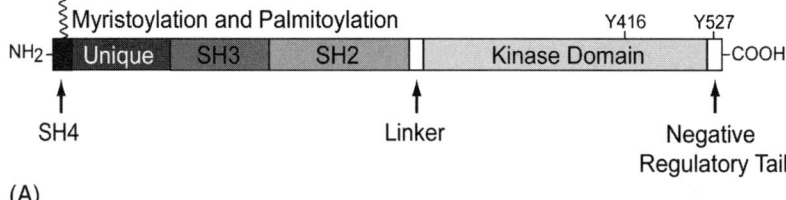

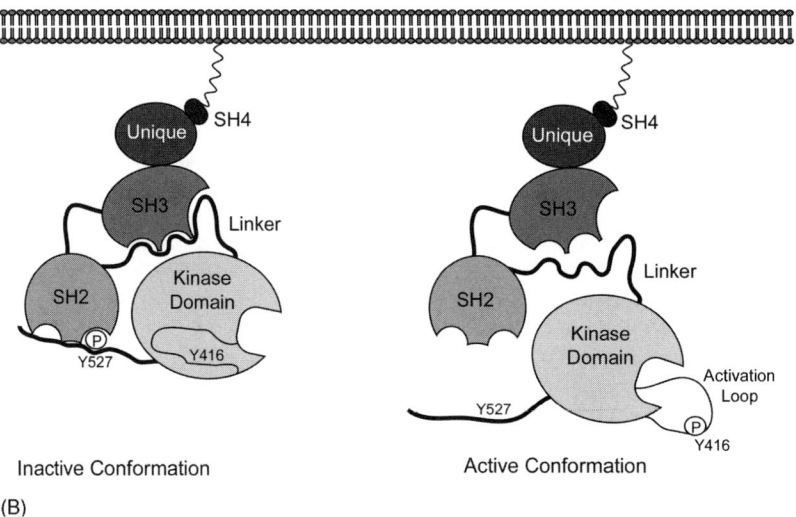

Fig. 9.1. **C-Src Structure and Autoregulation.** A) The functional domains of c-Src. Myristoylation and palmitoylation are post-translational modifications of the Src homology 4 (SH4) domain that aid in membrane anchoring. The unique region is the most variable domain among Src family members and contains regulatory sites of phosphorylation. The SH2 and SH3 domains mediate protein-protein interactions as detailed in the text. The SH1 or kinase domain catalyzes the transfer of the gamma phosphate of ATP to tyrosine residues on substrate proteins. The C-terminal tail contains Y527, which plays an important role in autoinhibition of the molecule. B) Autoregulation of c-Src. C-Src assumes an inactive conformation when phosphorylated Y527 engages the SH2 domain in an intramolecular fashion, the SH3 domain binds the pseudo-proline-rich region in the linker, and Y416 is unphosphorylated. Dephosphorylation of Y527 or competitive binding of other signaling molecules to the SH2 and/or SH3 domains releases the autoinhibition and promotes ATP binding, autophosphorylation of Y416, and transphosphorylation of substrate proteins.

region, followed by the SH3 domain that binds proline-rich regions of interacting proteins and the SH2 domain that binds phospho-tyrosine residues. At the C-terminus is a short tail containing a conserved tyrosine (Y527 in chicken c-Src; Y530 in human c-Src) that contributes to the autoregulation of the molecule. Protein interactions with the various domains of c-Src affect its activation state and cellular localization, as well as those of its binding partners (*1, 3*).

C-Src is autoinhibited by the interactions of the phosphorylated Y527 with its own SH2 domain and by SH3 domain binding to both the linker region (which connects the SH2 and catalytic domains) and the backbone of the catalytic domain (Fig. 9.1B). It must be noted, however, that the phosphorylation of Y527 is not always required for inactivation. Activity is restored upon engagement of its SH2 and/or SH3 domains by interacting proteins, dephosphorylation of Y527, autophosphorylation of Y416 (Y419 in human c-Src) in the activation loop of the catalytic domain, or any combination of these three events (*3*).

2. C-SRC INTERACTIONS WITH THE EGFR

One of the most extensively studied binding partners of c-Src is the EGFR. This association has been demonstrated with endogenous proteins in EGF-stimulated breast and colorectal cancer cell lines, as well as in breast tumor tissue (*5, 6*). In C3H10T1/2 murine fibroblasts that stably co-overexpress the EGFR and c-Src, these proteins form a complex upon EGF stimulation that occurs independently of c-Src kinase activity (*4*). Phosphorylation of the EGFR facilitates c-Src association with the EGFR (*6*). This interaction is thought to be mediated by the SH2 domain of c-Src binding to an EGFR phosphotyrosine, although an indirect association remains a possibility. Phosphopeptide competition studies suggest that Y992 is a preferred site of binding the c-Src SH2 domain (*6–8*), but Y891, Y920 (*6*) and Y1101 (*9*) have also been implicated.

Though no reports indicate that c-Src can be phosphorylated directly by the EGFR or ErbB2, c-Src-specific phosphorylation of the EGFR has been reported multiple times. Utilizing tryptic phosphopeptide mapping and mass spectrophotometric analysis of the phosphorylated EGFR from MCF-7 breast cancer cells, Stover et al. (*6*) identified the non-autophosphorylation sites, Y891 and Y920, as well as the autophosphorylation sites, Y992 and Y1086, of the EGFR as EGF-induced c-Src phosphorylation sites. Additionally, phosphospecific antibodies were employed to detect weak Src family-dependent phosphorylation of the autophosphorylation site Y1148 in the EGFR of normal human keratinocytes treated with EGF (*10*). All these sites are located in the C-terminal tail of the EGFR.

Two additional c-Src-specific sites, Y845 and Y1101, were revealed by tryptic phosphopeptide mapping and mass spectrophotometry of the EGFR from C3H10T½ murine fibroblasts stably overexpressing c-Src and EGFR and stimulated with EGF (reviewed in *11, 12*). Tyrosine 1101 resides in the C-terminal tail, and its function is as yet undetermined. Tyrosine 845 is located in the activation loop of the catalytic domain and is a conserved residue among all tyrosine kinases. Homologues of Y845 are autophosphorylated by their respective kinases and required for the kinases' full catalytic and biological activities. In contrast, mutation of Y845 in the EGFR has little to no effect on the catalytic activity of the receptor but inhibits EGF-induced mitogenesis and cell survival (*4, 11*). It is of interest to note that the context of Y845 EGFR is not conducive to SH2 domain binding. In addition to the aforementioned study, Y845 EGFR has been shown to be a c-Src-specific phosphorylation site in A431, MDA-MB-231, normal human keratinocytes, and tamoxifen-resistant MCF-7 cells (*5, 7, 10, 13*). By utilizing catalytically inactive mutants of the EGFR and c-Src, as well as pharmacological inhibitors and purified components of each kinase multiple groups have demonstrated that the catalytic activity of the EGFR is required for phosphorylation of Y845, despite the fact that the EGFR has weak or undetectable activity toward this residue (*14–17*). These findings are consistent with a model in which autophosphorylation of the EGFR is necessary for c-Src binding of the receptor and subsequent phosphorylation of Y845 by c-Src, although under certain circumstances, activated c-Src can phosphorylate Y845 independently of the EGFR kinase activity (*18*). In either situation, EGFR and c-Src appear to cooperate with one another to mediate the biochemical events that regulate EGF-induced biological processes.

3. EFFECTS OF THE CONVERGENCE OF EGFR AND C-SRC SIGNALING ON ONCOGENISIS

The first in-depth test of the hypothesis that the biochemical co-operativity between the EGFR and c-Src had biological consequences was carried out in the context of cancer. From a historical perspective, the EGFR was known to be frequently overexpressed in a variety of human malignancies (*11, 12*). These findings suggested that it may play an etiological role in the genesis of these diseases. This idea was examined by Velu and colleagues (*19*), who demonstrated that overexpression of the EGFR in immortalized but non-transformed murine fibroblasts conferred a transformed phenotype to the cells when they were grown in the presence of EGF. Further studies in cell culture and animal models revealed, however, that the EGFR is a relatively weak oncogene. That the activated EGFR was found to physically associate with c-Src in fibroblasts and in a variety of human tumor cell lines (*5, 7, 20, 21*) suggested that c-Src may contribute to EGFR signaling, particularly if it too were overexpressed.

Indeed, a survey of a large number of human breast tumor tissues by Ottenhalf-Kalff and colleagues (*22*) showed that all tumors tested exhibited elevated tyrosine kinase activity compared to normal controls and that greater than 70% of the elevated activity was due to overexpressed c-Src. Elevations in c-Src tyrosine kinase activity were also documented by other groups of investigators and in other human cancers, most notably those of the colon (*23–25*), lung (*26*), and breast (*25, 27, 28*). Overexpression of c-Src alone, however, was known to be insufficient to transform fibroblasts in culture (*29*).

One hypothesis derived from these findings was that overexpressed EGFR required overexpressed c-Src (and vice versa) to confer a strong malignant phenotype. Subsequent studies demonstrated that c-Src and the EGFR are concomitantly overexpressed in a substantial subset of multiple human tumor types, including breast, squamous cell carcinoma, ovary, colon, prostate, head and neck (HNSCC), lung (non-small cell and adenocarcinoma), pancreas, nervous system, gall bladder, melanoma, and kidney (*30–33*), lending support to the hypothesis. A direct test of the hypothesis was conducted first in a murine fibroblast model where the oncogenic growth characteristics of a panel of matched cell lines were assessed. Cells that overexpressed both c-Src and the EGFR exhibited striking synergism in EGF-induced DNA synthesis, growth in soft agar, and tumor formation in nude mice when compared to cells overexpressing c-Src or EGFR alone or not overexpressing either kinase (*21*). These findings were extended by Biscardi and colleagues (*5*) who determined that co-overexpression of EGFR and c-Src in human breast tumors and breast cancer cell lines correlated with higher grade in the former and enhanced xenograft tumor growth in the latter, as compared to tumors or cell lines that overexpressed only one of the pair. Phosphorylation of Y845 and Y1101 of the EGFR, hyper-activation of the MAPK pathway, and enhanced phosphorylation of EGFR substrates occurred concomitantly with co-overexpression of c-Src and the EGFR. These data indicated that the interplay between these two kinases can contribute in significant ways to tumorigenesis. Further tests of the c-Src/EGFR synergism in oncogenesis require testing of recently derived small molecule inhibitors specific for each kinase in animal models and human patients.

4. MECHANISMS OF C-SRC SIGNALING UPSTREAM OF THE EGFR: TRANSACTIVATION OF THE EGFR

In addition to stimulation by EGF and structurally related ligands, the EGFR can also be activated by agonists specific to several other receptors (*34*). In multiple instances this process, known as transactivation, is mediated by the kinase activity of a Src family member. A common mechanism entails activation by c-Src of a member or members of the metalloproteinase (MMP) family, which leads to ectodomain shedding of an EGFR ligand from a membrane-bound precursor form and subsequent binding of the released ligand to the EGFR (Fig. 9.2). The MMP-mediated mechanism of EGFR transactivation does not always require the Src family, however, and there are several examples of EGFR transactivation that occur independently of the MMP family.

4.1. GPCR-mediated EGFR Transactivation

By far, the largest and best characterized group of receptors that transactivate the EGFR is the G-protein coupled receptor (GPCR) family. Ligand-activated GPCRs function as guanine nucleotide exchange factors for associated heterotrimeric complexes of guanine nucleotide-binding (G) proteins. GPCRs regulate a plethora of processes contributing to oncogenesis, including cell proliferation, survival, metastasis, and differentiation. Src family kinases can directly and indirectly associate with GPCRs (in some instances through β-arrestin) and are activated following ligand binding to several GPCRs. Upon activation, Src family kinases mediate signaling downstream of GPCRs, including the phosphorylation and regulation of specific GPCRs, their associated G proteins, and activation of MMP family members (Reviewed in (*34*)).

Bioactive lipids constitute one class of GPCR agonists, and some of these molecules are implicated in Src family-dependent transactivation of the EGFR. Lysophosphatidic acid (LPA), for example, is the major mitogenic component of serum that signals in a plethora of cancer types (*35, 36*). Through its receptor, LPA promotes the phosphorylation of the EGFR on Y845, Y992, Y1068, and Y1173 (*37, 38*). The requirement for Src family kinases in this process has been described in several models, but the involvement of MMPs is uncertain

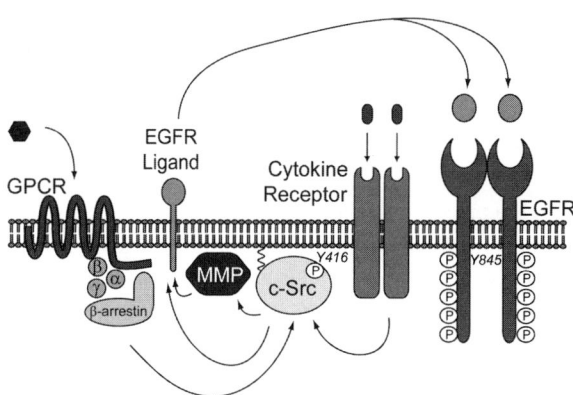

Fig. 9.2. C-Src Signaling Upstream of the EGFR. G-protein coupled receptor (GPCR) ligands can signal through the GPCR complex to activate c-Src, as indicated by phosphorylation of Y416. The GPCR complex contains a serpentine GPCR, the α, β, γ subunits of a heterotrimeric G protein, and β-arrestin (see text). Activated c-Src promotes either metalloproteinase (MMP)-dependent or –independent cleavage of a membrane-localized EGFR ligand, which in turn binds to and transactivates the EGFR. Ligand activated cytokine receptors and specific growth factor receptors transactivate the EGFR in a similar fashion.

(37–39). In human breast cancer cells, pY845 is required for LPA-induced DNA synthesis, indicating a critical role for EGFR in LPA-induced mitogenesis *(37, 38)*. Eicosanoids, such as prostaglandin E2 (PGE2), are derivatives of arachadonic acid. Signaling from EP4, the PGE2 receptor, requires c-Src action upstream of the EGFR *(40)*, but involvement of the MMP family in this pathway is unclear. Studies by Pia and colleagues *(41)* demonstrated that MMPs are involved upstream of the EGFR in normal and transformed colon cell lines, while in a different colorectal cancer cell line, MMP activity is downstream of the Src family and EGFR and mediates PGE2-stimulated invasion but not migration *(40)*.

Peptides are another class of GPCR agonists that are capable of transactivating the EGFR. In head and neck cancer cells, gastrin-releasing peptide (GRP) activates c-Src, which in turn promotes MMP-mediated amphiregulin and transforming growth factor-α (TGF-α) release (both ligands of the EGFR); c-Src also signals downstream of the GRP-activated EGFR and is required for GRP-induced cell proliferation *(42)*. Similarly, gonadotropin-releasing hormone (GnRH) binds its receptor, which stimulates c-Src, MMP2, and MMP9 activities and facilitates phosphorylation of Y845 on the EGFR*(16)*. Although Y845 phosphorylation is typically associated with mitogenesis, GnRH is growth inhibitory for prostate and ovarian cancer cells *(43, 44)*. Stromal cell-derived factor-1α (SDF-1α), a chemokine, signals through CXCR4 in ovarian adenocarcinoma cells and promotes Src family-dependent EGFR activation and DNA synthesis *(45)*.

Endothelin and angiotensin II regulate vascular constriction and dilation but are also mitogenic for multiple types of cancer cells and capable of transactivating the EGFR *(46–48)*. Work in ovarian carcinoma cells by Spinella and colleagues *(49)* suggests that endothelin requires c-Src, MMP, and EGFR activities to promote PGE2 release, which in turn activates c-Src, MMP, and EGFR and increases Y845 phosphorylation on the EGFR. Both c-Src and EGFR kinase activities are required for endothelin or PGE2-induced migration of these cells. In addition, Boerner and colleagues *(37, 49)* have demonstrated that Y845 phosphorylation is required for endothelin-induced DNA synthesis of breast cancer cells. Angiotensin II acts via the AT11 receptor and causes HB-EGF to stimulate phosphorylation of Y1173 on the EGFR in C9 rat liver epithelial cells. In this model system c-Src acts upstream of HB-EGF release and subsequent EGFR transactivation *(50)*.

While estrogen is best known for its actions through the canonical estrogen receptor, it can also bind and activate the GPCR, GPR30. Estrogen-induced GPR30 transactivation of the EGFR involves $G\beta_\gamma$ stimulation of c-Src, which in turn activates the MMP family, releasing HB-EGF to activate EGFR *(51)*. In Ishikawa endometrial cells, GPR30-mediated transcription in response to estrogen requires the Src family and EGFR kinase activity but is independent of steroid hormone receptors *(52)*. Similarly, estrogen signaling through GPR30 and/or the canonical estrogen receptor(s) in MCF-7 breast cancer cells releases sphingosine-1-phosphate, which binds to its receptor, a GPCR, Edg-3. Signaling through this pathway requires sphingosine kinase-1, MMPs, and the Src family for EGFR phosphorylation. EGFR kinase activity and Edg-3 are required for estrogen-induced cell proliferation in this breast cancer model *(53)*.

4.2. Nuclear Steroid Hormone Receptor-mediated EGFR Transactivation

Although nuclear hormone receptors were so named based on their ligand-dependent transcriptional activity, these receptors are found in both the nucleus and cytoplasm and participate in ligand-dependent and ligand-independent protein-protein interactions. This family of proteins includes the estrogen receptors, ER-α and ER-β, and the androgen receptor. Hormones binding these receptors are key regulators of cancer cell growth, metastasis, and survival, particularly in the hormone-responsive tissues, such as breast, uterus, cervix and prostate *(54)*. While there is ample evidence of crosstalk between the EGFR and steroid hormone receptors (reviewed in (54, 55)), there is little direct evidence of transactivation of the EGFR by liganded hormone receptors. Steroid hormone receptors, however, have been shown to interact with both EGFR and Src family members. For example, it is known that c-Src and Lck phosphorylate Y537 in the ligand-binding domain of ER-α, *in vitro* and *in vivo* (56). The c-Src SH2 domain binds phosphorylated Y537 of ER-α, while the SH3 domain of c-Src basally associates with modulator of nongenomic activity of the ER (MNAR), a scaffolding protein, forming a multimeric complex (57). In MCF-7 cells, EGF stimulates the formation of a complex comprised of ER-α or ER-β, androgen receptor, c-Src, MNAR, and EGFR, which facilitates EGFR phosphorylation, increases proliferation, and induces cytoskeletal changes (58). These findings suggest a biological significance for this complex that has not yet been fully investigated.

4.3. Transactivation of the EGFR by other Receptors and Molecules

In addition to the receptors discussed above, several other types of receptors and chemical moieties lead to Src-mediated EGFR activation and phosphorylation. These include cytokine and growth factor receptors, intracellular kinases, as well as charged molecules, such as Zn^+ and hydrogen peroxide.

Cytokines, growth hormone and interferon-γ (IFN-γ), are highly expressed in specific cancers, and their ligand-bound receptors are capable of transactivating the EGFR (59–61). Growth hormone stimulates c-Src and Y845 phosphorylation of the EGFR, as well as c-Src-dependent association of c-Src with the EGFR (37). Phosphorylation of Y845 is required for growth hormone-induced DNA synthesis in breast cancer cells (37). A 24- hour IFN-γ treatment of colonic epithelial cells results in activation of the Src family and TGF-α release from the basolateral surface, both of which promote EGFR phosphorylation (62).

Crosstalk between the EGFR and insulin-like growth factor receptor (IGFR) is extensively characterized and is discussed in greater detail in Chapter 11. Ligand-activated IGFR promotes the growth of tamoxifen-resistant breast cancer cells (63, 64) and concomitantly induces tyrosine phosphorylation of c-Src, c-Src-dependent phosphorylation of Y845 and Y1068 on the EGFR, and association of the EGFR with the IGFR and c-Src (13). C-Src and EGFR kinase activities are required for IGF-induced growth of these cells.

Protein kinase C is a family of eleven phospholipid-dependent serine / threonine kinases that bind the carcinogenic phorbol esters. In glioblastoma cell lines phorbol 12-myristate 13-acetate (PMA) activates the Ca^{2+}-independent isoform of PKC, PKCδ which results in phosphorylation of c-Src on serines 12 and 48, c-Src activation, and c-Src-dependent phosphorylation of Y845 and Y1068 on the EGFR. Involvement of both the EGFR and c-Src are required for PMA-induced DNA synthesis in these tumor cells (65). In contrast, in primary mouse keratinocytes, activation of PKCη by the Src family kinase, Fyn, has the opposite effect, decreasing EGFR tyrosine phosphorylation and DNA synthesis (66).

Small, charged molecules, such as Zn^{2+} and hydrogen peroxide (H_2O_2), also have the capability of transactivating the EGFR. Zn^{2+} has repeatedly been shown to induce a c-Src-dependent phosphorylation of Y845 on the EGFR and activation of the MAP kinase pathway, but there is some disagreement over whether the autophosphorylation sites of the EGFR are phosphorylated (14, 15). Further work suggests the involvement of the MMP family in EGFR transactivation, but the mechanism by which c-Src becomes activated by Zn^{2+} has not been elucidated (14). Similar to Zn^{2+} treatment, H_2O_2 activates c-Src upstream of the EGFR, resulting in phosphorylation of Y845 and Y1068 via an MMP-independent mechanism (67). Some evidence supports the notion that H_2O_2 activates c-Src through inhibition of protein tyrosine phosphatases, which would enhance retention of the phosphate on Y416/419 of c-Src, favoring the activated conformation (68, 69). The full relevance of Zn^{2+} and H_2O_2 activation of c-Src and the EGFR to cancer initiation or progression are not understood at the present time.

In summary, a wide variety of ligands for cell surface receptors are capable of transactivating the EGFR in a Src family-dependent manner. Where examined, biological responses to these extracellular cues invariably require c-Src, the activated EGFR and frequently phosphorylation of Y845, a c-Src-specific site. These findings have potentially far-reaching implications not only for normal physiological responses but also for pathological conditions, many of which are the result of aberrant receptor signaling.

5. MECHANISMS OF C-SRC SIGNALING DOWNSTREAM OF THE EGFR

5.1. Signaling from the c-Src-mediated Phosphorylation Site on the EGFR, Tyrosine 845

Substitution of Y845 with phenylalanine creates a mutant EGFR that inhibits EGF-induced DNA synthesis, growth in soft agar, and survival following induction of apoptotic stress (4, 11, 37, 70). Interestingly, neither the catalytic activity of the receptor nor signaling to Shc, ERK2, and a number of other EGFR effectors is affected by this mutation (4), suggesting that the canonical EGFR signaling pathways are not sufficient for EGF-induced proliferation/survival and that other effectors downstream of pY845 are required. Indeed, several downstream mediators of pY845 have been identified, including STAT5b, a transcription factor involved in mitogenesis (71), and cytochrome c oxidase subunit II (Cox II) (70), a mitochondrially encoded protein involved in oxidative phosphorylation and postulated to regulate cytochrome c release during apoptosis (72, 73).

5.1.1. STATs

Signal transducers and activators of transcription (STATs) are transcription factors that reside in the cytoplasm, where they can be activated by growth factors or cytokines. Activation entails phosphorylation on critical tyrosine residues, dimerization, and translocation to the nucleus, where the proteins modulate transcriptional programs and regulate a range of biological processes, including proliferation, differentiation, and survival (74). Of the seven STAT proteins, three (STATs 3, 5a, and 5b) are repeatedly implicated in playing critical roles in hematologic cancers, as well as solid tumors of the prostate, pancreas, breast, and head and neck (75, 76).

In breast cancer cells pY845 of the EGFR activates STAT5b (71). Overexpression of the liganded EGFR, c-Src kinase activity, and phosphorylation of Y845 on the EGFR are required for this activation. Dominant-negative STAT5b inhibits EGF-induced proliferation in these cells, demonstrating that STAT5b is required for EGF-stimulated mitogenesis in breast cancer cells and that both c-Src and the EGFR play critical roles in its activation.

In contrast to STAT5b, constitutive activation of STAT3 is dependent upon c-Src and JAK tyrosine kinases but not upon the EGFR (77). However, EGF stimulation, further increases STAT3 DNA binding activity in murine fibroblasts modeled to overexpress the EGFR and/or c-Src, suggesting that STAT3 may also play a role in EGF-inducible events in breast cancers. Importantly, expression of a dominant negative STAT3 leads to growth inhibition and apoptosis of breast cancer cells, as does inhibition of c-Src or JAK tyrosine kinases (77).

Similar relationships between the EGFR, c-Src, and STATs 3 and 5 are seen in squamous cell carcinoma of the head and neck (SCCHN) (78). Constitutive activation of STATs 3 and 5 is linked to constitutive phosphorylation of the EGFR in these cancers, and c-Src, EGFR, and STATs3/5 form a stable, co-immunoprecipitatable complex. In nine SCCHN cell lines examined, c-Src phosphotyrosine levels were found to correlate with activation levels of STATs 3 and 5, and growth rates of these cell lines were reduced by inhibitors of c-Src. Together, these studies demonstrate a role for c-Src in mediating activation of STATs 3 and 5 in concert with the EGFR.

5.1.2. Cytochrome c oxidase II (Cox II)

Phosphorylated Y845 of the EGFR also mediates EGFR binding to the mitochondrial protein, cytochrome c oxidase subunit II (Cox II) (70). Cox II is encoded by mitochondrial DNA and located in the inner mitochondrial membrane. It is a critical component of the fourth complex of the electron transport chain and through its affinity for cytochrome c is speculated to play a role in regulating apoptosis (72, 73). Following EGF stimulation of murine fibroblasts or breast cancer cells, the EGFR translocates to the mitochondria, where it associates with Cox II in a pY845-dependent manner. A mitochondrial function for the EGFR is implicated by its ability to protect breast cancer cells from chemotherapy-induced apoptosis. Specifically, transient, ectopic expression of the Y845F mutant EGFR renders the cells more sensitive to adriamycin-induced death, suggesting that the ability of the EGFR to bind Cox II through pY845 plays a key role in EGFR-mediated resistance to the drug. Mutant or dominant negative STAT5b fails to reverse the inhibition by Y845F EGFR, indicating that signaling to STAT5b from Y845F is insufficient for this event (70).

The presence of c-Src in mitochondria of osteoclasts has been described previously (79, 80), and in EGF-stimulated murine fibroblasts, ongoing studies show that c-Src translocates to the mitochondria with the same time course as the EGFR (Demory et al., in preparation). Translocation of the EGFR requires the catalytic activity of both c-Src and the EGFR, a putative mitochondrial targeting sequence, and endocytosis of the receptor (Demory et al., in preparation). Furthermore, in osteoclasts, c-Src can tyrosine phosphorylate Cox II, a modification that appears to regulate its activity and association with cytochrome c. This finding suggests that tyrosine kinases can regulate Cox II and possibly mitochondrial function. Additional studies are needed to verify and extend these findings, as the outcomes have potentially important applications to our understanding of drug-induced cell death and therapeutic resistance.

5.2. Signaling from Other c-Src-phosphorylated Sites on the EGFR

C-Src has been demonstrated to phosphorylate *in vitro* all five EGFR autophosphorylation sites, as well as five novel sites, four of which have been shown to occur in intact cells (Y845, Y891, Y920, and Y1101) (6, 10, 11, Biscardi, J.S., M.E. Cox, S. Parsons, unpublished). Site mapping, combined with *in vitro* affinity precipitation and Far Western analyses (8, 9, 11) demonstrate that the c-Src SH2 domain can bind activated EGFR specifically and directly. Furthermore, full-length c-Src can co-immunoprecipitate with activated EGFR (21, 81). These findings place c-Src in a position to phosphorylate other signaling molecules that bind the EGFR, such as the adapter molecules Shc, Gab1 and 2, as well as PLCγ, the p85 subunit of PI-3 kinase, Cbl, and others. In several instances, direct phosphorylation of these molecules by c-Src is implicated (particularly with PI-3 kinase), but not verified by *in vitro* and/or *in situ* studies.

5.2.1. PI-3 Kinase

Early studies by Stover and colleagues (6) demonstrated that the SH2 domain of the regulatory subunit of PI-3 kinase (p85) exhibited preferred binding to one of the *in vivo* c-Src phosphorylation sites on the EGFR, namely Y920. Subsequent attempts to co-immunoprecipitate p85 with EGFR, however, met with variable success, suggesting that the interaction may not be direct. More recent studies have revealed the propensity of p85 to interact on a constitutive basis with cytosolic adaptor proteins (such as Gab1, Gab2, and Shc), which in turn localize to the membrane following EGF stimulation and bind the EGFR indirectly (or also directly in the case of Shc) through Grb2 (82–84). Gab1, Gab2, and Shc are all tyrosine phosphorylated, and at least one kinase capable of mediating this phosphorylation is c-Src (85–87). Multiple reports link c-Src to tyrosine phosphorylation of p85 and activation of PI-3 kinase signaling pathways (including activation of Akt), but evidence for direct phosphorylation of p85 by c-Src is lacking. Rather, cumulative data in several different signaling systems (including the EGFR), suggest that the link is indirect, being as it is upstream of p85 and likely at the level of the adaptor protein associated with the receptor (*88–90*).

5.2.2. MAP KINASE and PLCγ

Similarly, c-Src is implicated as an activator of MAP kinase. Again, there is no evidence that c-Src phosphorylates this molecule directly. Rather, it is likely that c-Src, along with the EGFR, phosphorylates Shc, which in turn binds Grb2 and activates the SOS, Ras, Raf, MEK, MAPK cascade. Likewise, a few references describe c-Src as regulating PLCγ activity, but the mechanism again appears to be indirect. The preferred means of phosphorylating and activating PLCγ is by the EGFR itself, following binding of PLCγ to the C-terminal tail of the receptor (*91*).

5.3. Other EGFR Effectors Phosphorylated and Regulated by c-Src

To date, a variety of proteins have been identified and characterized as substrates for c-Src. Among the numerous c-Src targets, examples of those that are known to participate in signaling conveyed from the EGFR/c-Src interaction are featured here (Fig. 9.3).

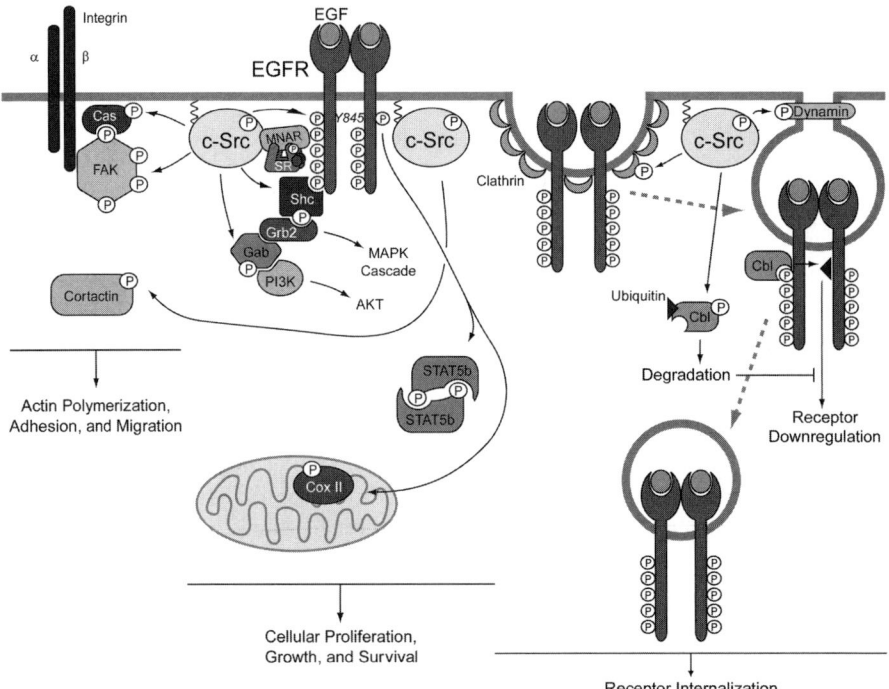

Fig. 9.3. C-Src Signaling Downstream of the EGFR. C-Src regulates many EGF-initiated events, such as (1) cell adhesion and migration, (2) cell proliferation, growth, and survival, and (3) EGFR endocytosis by phosphorylating critical sites on the EGFR (including Y845) and cellular substrates involved in each of the processes. See text for a detailed description of the substrates and how phosphorylation by c-Src affects each of them. Definitions: Integrin – receptor for extracellular matrix; FAK – Focal Adhesion Kinase; P130 Cas – 130 kDa scaffolding protein in focal adhesions; Cortactin – an actin binding protein; MNAR – Modulator of Nongenomic Activity of the Estrogen Receptor; SR – Steroid hormone Receptor; Shc, Gab1,2, Grb2 – adaptor proteins; STAT5b – Signal Transducer and Activator of Transcription 5b; Cox II – cytochrome c oxidase subunit II; Clathrin – a protein involved in coated pit formation; Dynamin – a GTPase involved in cleavage of endocytic vesicles from the plasma membrane; Cbl – an E3 ligase that binds the EGFR and mediates its ubiquitination and targeting for lysosomal degradation.

5.3.1. c-Src Substrates that Regulate EGFR Internalization and Degradation

Cbl, clathrin, dynamin, and caveolin are *bona fide* substrates of c-Src that regulate EGFR internalization and degradation.

5.3.1.1. Cbl

Cbl is an E3-ligase that binds to and ubiquitinates ligand-activated EGFR. Ubiquitination promotes both receptor endocytosis and degradation (*92*). Phosphorylation of Cbl by c-Src facilitates the ubiquitination and proteasomal degradation of Cbl, thereby reducing levels of Cbl, promoting receptor recycling back to the plasma membrane, and extending EGFR signaling (*93*).

5.3.1.2. Clathrin

Clathrins assemble in a protein lattice to form coated pits into which ligand-bound receptors are sorted and internalized. C-Src phosphorylates Y1477 on the clathrin heavy chain; this site is located in a domain critical for clathrin self-assembly. Some evidence suggests that phosphorylation of clathrin by c-Src enhances the endosomal pool of activated receptors that continue to signal until degraded (*94*). This is supported by the findings of Ware and colleagues (*95*) that cells overexpressing c-Src show an increased rate of EGFR endocytosis and a larger pool of internalized receptors than controls.

5.3.1.3. Dynamin

Dynamin is a GTPase that governs separation of the endocytic vesicles from the plasma membrane (*96*). C-Src phosphorylation of dynamin at Y597 increases both dynamin self-assembly and GTPase activity and is required for EGF-mediated EGFR internalization.

5.3.1.4. Caveolin

Caveolin, a small integral membrane protein, is a principal component of caveolae membrane invaginations and is suggested to have a scaffolding function. EGFR and c-Src are components of caveolae, with caveolin having the capacity to bind EGFR directly and inhibit its kinase activity (*97*). EGF binding to its receptor induces migration from caveolae, a movement that occurs independently of internalization by clathrin-coated pits and is dependent on c-Src phosphorylation of caveolin on Y14 (*98, 99*). Phosphorylation of Y14 is postulated to release EGFR from the inhibitory effects of caveolin and confer binding to Grb7, both of which functionally augment anchorage-independent growth and EGF-stimulated cell migration.

5.3.2. C-Src Substrates that Link Actin Cytoskeletal Dynamics to the EGFR

Multiple c-Src substrates mediate changes in the actin cytoskeleton that are set into motion by stimulation with EGF. These include cortactin, focal adhesion kinase (FAK), p130Cas, paxillin, p190RhoGAP, PIPKIγ661, tensin, and others. Below is an abbreviated discussion of representatives of this group. More in-depth descriptions can be found in Playford and Schaller (*100*) and Schlaepfer and Mitra (*101*).

5.3.2.1. Cortactin

Cortactin is an F-actin binding protein that plays a role in enhancing nucleation of actin filaments by Arp2/3 and in cross-linking F-actin (*102, 103*). As such, it is postulated to contribute to filopodia or lamellipodia formation. Tyrosines 421 and 466 of cortactin have been identified as *in vivo* and *in vitro* c-Src phosphorylation sites (*104, 105*), but the exact role these sites play in cellular movement is somewhat unclear. Overall, tyrosyl phosphorylation of cortactin can reduce its F-actin cross-linking activity, but the impact on cell spreading, migration or invasion is not well understood. Cortactin becomes highly tyrosine phosphorylated following EGF stimulation (*106*), an event that is regulated by levels and activity of c-Src (*106, 107*).

5.3.2.2. Focal Adhesion Kinase

Focal adhesion kinase (FAK) is a tyrosine kinase that interacts with multiple cellular proteins to translate integrin engagement by the extracellular matrix (ECM) into intracellular actin cytoskeletal alterations that promote key components of cancer metastasis: cell spreading, motility, and invasion (*108*). FAK and c-Src form a transient, active complex following integrin activation by ECM proteins or ligand stimulation of the EGF or PDGF receptors, which results in phosphorylation of FAK by c-Src on tyrosines 576, 577, 861, and 925. These sites in turn enhance FAK kinase activity and generate docking sites for multiple proteins, including paxillin and p130Cas, which regulate cell motility and invasion (*101*). Integrin activation also results in phosphorylation of EGFR at multiple tyrosines, including Y845 (*109*), which in turn can activate proliferation and survival signals.

5.3.2.3. p130 Cas

Cas is an adapter protein involved in multiple cell functions, including cell migration and invasion, as well as proliferation and resistance to chemotherapeutic agents (*18, 100*). C-Src is activated by binding to Cas, which results in phosphorylation of Cas by c-Src on multiple tyrosine residues. C-Src can bind Cas in the context of the focal adhesion or in other membrane sites. Phosphorylation of Cas by c-Src generates multiple unidentified docking sites on Cas for SH2-containing signaling proteins, and it is this interplay that is thought to play a role in the ability of p130Cas to confer tamoxifen resistance to breast cancer cells. Interestingly, phosphorylation of Y845 on the EGFR by Cas-activated c-Src is required for Cas to mediate tamoxifen resistance (*18*).

5.3.3. STEROID HORMONE RECEPTORS AS C-SRC SUBSTRATES DOWNSTREAM OF EGFR

5.3.3.1. Estrogen Receptor

In specific reproductive tissues, such as the uterus, EGF-induced proliferation is dependent upon the canonical ER and estrogen-induced proliferation is dependent upon the EGFR (*110, 111*). As discussed above, mechanistic studies have revealed that estrogen transactivates the EGFR via a c-Src-dependent mechanism (*112*) and c-Src also functions downstream of the EGFR to mediate its activation of MAP kinase and phosphorylation of ER-α in its activation function 1 (AF1) domain, a phosphorylation important for ER-dependent transcriptional activity (*113, 114*). Furthermore, c-Src can phosphorylate ER-α directly on Y537 (*56, 115*), but as yet this phosphorylation has no consensus effect on ER-α function.

5.3.3.2. Androgen Receptor

Similarly, activated c-Src can phosphorylate the androgen receptor on Y534, a phosphorylation that is required for androgen-independent progression in prostate cancer cells. One mechanism of activation of c-Src in this system is by growth factors, such as EGF (*116, 117*).

6. INHIBITION OF C-SRC SIGNALING THAT CONVERGES WITH THE EGFR

Given the overwhelming evidence that Src and EGFR signaling networks converge at multiple levels from direct interaction between the two molecules to collaborative activation of shared downstream effectors, one strategy for interdicting this interplay in cancer cells is to target both kinases with inhibitors. Indeed, small molecule inhibitors have been developed for both the EGFR and Src family kinases (SFKs). The predominant type of inhibitor is one that inserts into the catalytic cleft of the enzymes and competitively inhibits ATP binding and substrate phosphorylation. Several ATP competitors for the EGFR, such as Gefitinib, Erlotinib, and Lapatinib, have undergone fairly extensive testing in the clinic and are the subject of Chapter 3 within this volume. The data emerging from these studies indicate the need for combinatorial therapies, perhaps some involving drugs that target the SFKs along with the EGFR inhibitors. Below is a short description of representative SFK inhibitors of the ATP competitor class and their uses both in experimental cell culture systems and in some instances in human clinical trials. To date, few studies have been conducted that utilize both EGFR and SFK inhibitors simultaneously, although this strategy appears to be imminent.

6.1. Molecules that Function as ATP Competitive Inhibitors for SFK

6.1.1. PP1 and PP2

PP1 and PP2 were identified in 1995 as novel chemical ATP competitors of SFKs (*118*). PP2 is the more selective for SFKs since PP1 also inhibits the PDGF-β receptor kinase with a nearly equal IC_{50} as that of SFKs (*119*). Both PP1 and PP2 have limited membrane permeability and thus are rarely used in animal studies and not at all in clinical trials. Nevertheless, the relatively high specificity of the agents has prompted their extensive application in cell culture studies, studies which have provided much of the proof of principle needed for development of agents with equal or greater specificity and bioavailability. For example, in studies of MDA-MB-468 breast carcinoma cells which overexpress EGFR, Li and colleagues (*120*) demonstrated that ionizing radiation causes ERK1/2 activation and EGFR tyrosine phosphorylation, but not auto-phosphorylation or phosphorylation at Y845, the c-Src-specific site. Both PP2 and AG1478 (EGFR inhibitor) but not wortmannin (PI-3 kinase inhibitor) suppressed activation of ERK, in this system, suggesting involvement of both c-Src and EGFR in a novel pathway activated by ionizing radiation.

In squamous carcinoma and A431 cells, Y14 of caveolin is phosphorylated upon EGF treatment. This effect can be blocked by PP1 or PP2, but not MEK inhibitors, PI3K inhibition or cytoskeleton-disruption agents (*121*).

6.1.2. AZD0530

AZD0530 is a highly selective, dual-specificity inhibitor of c-Src and BCR-ABL. Hiscox and colleagues (*122*) have shown that acquisition of tamoxifen-resistance by MCF-7 breast carcinoma cells results in elevated EGFR signaling, as well as increased c-Src kinase activity, independently of c-Src protein levels or gene expression. In this cell system, treatment with AZD0530 reduces c-Src activity, FAK activity, and levels of phosphorylated paxillin and suppresses motility and invasion. The EGFR inhibitor gefitinib is additive for these effects.

6.1.3. Dasatanib

Dasatanib (BMS-354825) is a potent, orally-active inhibitor of SFKs and a less potent inhibitor of other tyrosine kinases, including c-Kit, PDGFR and BCR-ABL. Song and colleagues (*123*) reported that in non-small cell lung carcinoma (NSCLC) cells with activating EGFR mutations, Dasatinib induced apoptosis, but not in NSCLC that express wild-type EGFR. In the apoptotic cells, Akt and STAT3 activation were also down-regulated, which suggests that Dasatinib is inhibiting Src family- and EGFR-regulated PI-3 K/PTEN/Akt and STAT pathways. In cells expressing wild-type EGFR, Dasatinib causes a G1/S cell cycle arrest. A Phase I dose-escalation study of Dasatinib in treatment-resistant gastrointestinal stromal tumors (GIST) was recently published as an abstract at American Society of Clinical Oncology (ASCO). Evans and colleagues (*124*) report that Dasatinib can be safely administered at doses of up to 70mg BID on a 5-days on, 2-days off, weekly schedule. No objective tumor responses were seen by CT analysis, although the abstract suggests that the clinical benefits in a subset of patients were encouraging. Shah (*125*) reports that clinical trials of Dasatinib in chronic myelogenous leukemia (CML) patients who are resistant to Imatinib (a front-line therapy) show remarkable promise.

6.2. Alternate Means of Inhibiting SFKs

6.2.1. EXPRESSION of DOMINANT NEGATIVE c-Src

Head and neck cancer cell lines (HNSCC), which overexpress the EGFR and demonstrate enhanced GRP signaling, can induce phosphorylation of the EGFR and MAPK, likely via release of membrane-bound TGF-α. Inhibiting c-Src activity by means of an ATP competitive inhibitor or by expression of dominant negative c-Src decreases GRP-induced MAPK activation, as well as cell invasion, growth, and secretion of TGF-α and amphiregulin (42).

Inhibition by ATP competitors or expression of a dominant negative c-Src prevents invasion of U251 glioma cells. The authors suggest that inhibition of invasion is likely due to c-Src-dependent changes in actin dynamics (126).

In glioma cell lines PMA transactivates the EGFR and induces serine/threonine phosphorylation of c-Src, as well as phosphorylation of Y845 and Y1068 on the EGFR, resulting in enhanced cell proliferation. Competitive ATP inhibitors of c-Src or expression of dominant negative c-Src prevents this enhancement, indicating a role for a PKC/c-Src/EGFR pathway in glioma cell growth (65).

Substance P is a neurotransmitter expressed in glioblastomas that leads to activation of MAPK and cell proliferation. PP2 or expression of dominant negative c-Src prevents this activation, whereas AG1478 (an EGFR inhibitor) only partially decreases it. Data suggest that the Substance P receptor works through the PKCδ pathway (127).

6.2.2. Src HOMOZYGOUS NULL MICE

Glioblastoma are brain cancers that do not overexpress c-Src but require c-Src activity for EGFR signaling. In c-Src -/- knock-out mice, glioma growth is blocked by a mechanism involving vascular endothelial growth factor (VEGF). C-Src -/- mice also exhibit reduced glioma cell invasion and infiltration in mouse brain tumor xenografts (128).

Overall, the results of preclinical tissue culture and animal studies employing SFK inhibitors point to critical roles played by c-Src and its related family members in the genesis and progression of human cancers. These findings, derived from a variety of different tumor types, provide in many ways the "proof of principle" that movement of the SFK inhibitors into the clinic, particularly in combination with EGFR inhibitors, is warranted.

REFERENCES

1. Brown MT, Cooper JA. Regulation, substrates and functions of src. Biochim Biophys Acta 1996; 1287:121-49.
2. Martin GS. The road to Src. Oncogene 2004; 23:7910-7.
3. Thomas SM, Brugge JS. Cellular functions regulated by Src family kinases. Annu Rev Cell Dev Biol 1997; 13:513-609.
4. Tice DA, Biscardi JS, Nickles AL, Parsons SJ. Mechanism of biological synergy between cellular Src and epidermal growth factor receptor. Proc Natl Acad Sci U S A 1999; 96:1415-20.
5. Biscardi JS, Belsches AP, Parsons SJ. Characterization of human epidermal growth factor receptor and c-Src interactions in human breast tumor cells. Mol Carcinog 1998; 21:261-72.
6. Stover DR, Becker M, Liebetanz J, Lydon NB. Src phosphorylation of the epidermal growth factor receptor at novel sites mediates receptor interaction with Src and P85 alpha. J Biol Chem 1995; 270:15591-7.
7. Sato K, Sato A, Aoto M, Fukami Y. c-Src phosphorylates epidermal growth factor receptor on tyrosine 845. Biochem Biophys Res Commun 1995; 215:1078-87.
8. Sierke SL, Longo GM, Koland JG. Structural basis of interactions between epidermal growth factor receptor and SH2 domain proteins. Biochem Biophys Res Commun 1993; 191:45-54.
9. Lombardo CR, Consler TG, Kassel DB. In vitro phosphorylation of the epidermal growth factor receptor autophosphorylation domain by c-src: identification of phosphorylation sites and c-src SH2 domain binding sites. Biochemistry 1995; 34:16456-66.
10. Kansra S, Stoll SW, Johnson JL, Elder JT. Src family kinase inhibitors block amphiregulin-mediated autocrine ErbB signaling in normal human keratinocytes. Mol Pharmacol 2005; 67:1145-57.

11. Biscardi JS, Tice DA, Parsons SJ. c-Src, receptor tyrosine kinases, and human cancer. Adv Cancer Res 1999; 76:61-119.
12. Biscardi JS, Ishizawar RC, Silva CM, Parsons SJ. Tyrosine kinase signalling in breast cancer: epidermal growth factor receptor and c-Src interactions in breast cancer. Breast Cancer Res 2000; 2:203-10.
13. Knowlden JM, Hutcheson IR, Barrow D, Gee JM, Nicholson RI. Insulin-like growth factor-I receptor signaling in tamoxifen-resistant breast cancer: a supporting role to the epidermal growth factor receptor. Endocrinology 2005; 146:4609-18.
14. Wu W, Graves LM, Gill GN, Parsons SJ, Samet JM. Src-dependent phosphorylation of the epidermal growth factor receptor on tyrosine 845 is required for zinc-induced Ras activation. J Biol Chem 2002; 277:24252-7.
15. Samet JM, Dewar BJ, Wu W, Graves LM. Mechanisms of $Zn(2^+)$-induced signal initiation through the epidermal growth factor receptor. Toxicol Appl Pharmacol 2003; 191:86-93.
16. Roelle S, Grosse R, Aigner A, Krell HW, Czubayko F, Gudermann T. Matrix metalloproteinases 2 and 9 mediate epidermal growth factor receptor transactivation by gonadotropin-releasing hormone. J Biol Chem 2003; 278:47307-18.
17. Reich H, Tritchler D, Herzenberg AM, et al. Albumin activates ERK via EGF receptor in human renal epithelial cells. J Am Soc Nephrol 2005; 16:1266-78.
18. Riggins RB, Thomas KS, Ta HQ, et al. Physical and functional interactions between Cas and c-Src induce tamoxifen resistance of breast cancer cells through pathways involving epidermal growth factor receptor and signal transducer and activator of transcription 5b. Cancer Res 2006; 66:7007-15.
19. Velu TJ, Beguinot L, Vass WC, et al. Epidermal-growth-factor-dependent transformation by a human EGF receptor proto-oncogene. Science 1987; 238:1408-10.
20. Luttrell DK, Lee A, Lansing TJ, et al. Involvement of pp60c-src with two major signaling pathways in human breast cancer. Proc Natl Acad Sci U S A 1994; 91:83-7.
21. Maa MC, Leu TH, McCarley DJ, Schatzman RC, Parsons SJ. Potentiation of epidermal growth factor receptor-mediated oncogenesis by c-Src: implications for the etiology of multiple human cancers. Proc Natl Acad Sci U S A 1995; 92:6981-5.
22. Ottenhoff-Kalff AE, Rijksen G, van Beurden EA, Hennipman A, Michels AA, Staal GE. Characterization of protein tyrosine kinases from human breast cancer: involvement of the c-src oncogene product. Cancer Res 1992; 52:4773-8.
23. Cartwright CA, Kamps MP, Meisler AI, Pipas JM, Eckhart W. pp60c-src activation in human colon carcinoma. J Clin Invest 1989; 83:2025-33.
24. Bolen JB, Veillette A, Schwartz AM, Deseau V, Rosen N. Analysis of pp60c-src in human colon carcinoma and normal human colon mucosal cells. Oncogene Res 1987; 1:149-68.
25. Rosen N, Bolen JB, Schwartz AM, Cohen P, DeSeau V, Israel MA. Analysis of pp60c-src protein kinase activity in human tumor cell lines and tissues. J Biol Chem 1986; 261:13754-9.
26. Mazurenko NN, Kogan EA, Sukhova NM, Zborovskaia IB. [Synthesis and distribution of oncoproteins in tumor tissue]. Vopr Med Khim 1991; 37:53-9.
27. Lehrer S, O'Shaughnessy J, Song HK, et al. Activity of pp60c-src protein kinase in human breast cancer. Mt Sinai J Med 1989; 56:83-5.
28. Jacobs C, Rubsamen H. Expression of pp60c-src protein kinase in adult and fetal human tissue: high activities in some sarcomas and mammary carcinomas. Cancer Res 1983; 43:1696-702.
29. Shalloway D, Coussens PM, Yaciuk P. Overexpression of the c-src protein does not induce transformation of NIH 3T3 cells. Proc Natl Acad Sci U S A 1984; 81:7071-5.
30. Salomon DS, Brandt R, Ciardiello F, Normanno N. Epidermal growth factor-related peptides and their receptors in human malignancies. Crit Rev Oncol Hematol 1995; 19:183-232.
31. Scambia G, Benedetti-Panici P, Ferrandina G, et al. Epidermal growth factor, oestrogen and progesterone receptor expression in primary ovarian cancer: correlation with clinical outcome and response to chemotherapy. Br J Cancer 1995; 72:361-6.
32. Khazaie K, Schirrmacher V, Lichtner RB. EGF receptor in neoplasia and metastasis. Cancer Metastasis Rev 1993; 12:255-74.
33. Harris JR, Lippman ME, Veronesi U, Willett W. Breast cancer (3). N Engl J Med 1992; 327:473-80.
34. Luttrell DK, Luttrell LM. Not so strange bedfellows: G-protein-coupled receptors and Src family kinases. Oncogene 2004; 23:7969-78.
35. Sengupta S, Wang Z, Tipps R, Xu Y. Biology of LPA in health and disease. Semin Cell Dev Biol 2004; 15:503-12.

36. Mills GB, Moolenaar WH. The emerging role of lysophosphatidic acid in cancer. Nat Rev Cancer 2003; 3:582-91.
37. Boerner JL, Biscardi JS, Silva CM, Parsons SJ. Transactivating agonists of the EGF receptor require Tyr 845 phosphorylation for induction of DNA synthesis. Mol Carcinog 2005; 44:262-73.
38. Zhao Y, He D, Saatian B, et al. Regulation of lysophosphatidic acid-induced epidermal growth factor receptor transactivation and interleukin-8 secretion in human bronchial epithelial cells by protein kinase Cdelta, Lyn kinase, and matrix metalloproteinases. J Biol Chem 2006; 281:19501-11.
39. Shah BH, Baukal AJ, Shah FB, Catt KJ. Mechanisms of extracellularly regulated kinases 1/2 activation in adrenal glomerulosa cells by lysophosphatidic acid and epidermal growth factor. Mol Endocrinol 2005; 19:2535-48.
40. Buchanan FG, Wang D, Bargiacchi F, DuBois RN. Prostaglandin E2 regulates cell migration via the intracellular activation of the epidermal growth factor receptor. J Biol Chem 2003; 278:35451-7.
41. Pai R, Soreghan B, Szabo IL, Pavelka M, Baatar D, Tarnawski AS. Prostaglandin E2 transactivates EGF receptor: a novel mechanism for promoting colon cancer growth and gastrointestinal hypertrophy. Nat Med 2002; 8:289-93.
42. Zhang Q, Thomas SM, Xi S, et al. SRC family kinases mediate epidermal growth factor receptor ligand cleavage, proliferation, and invasion of head and neck cancer cells. Cancer Res 2004; 64:6166-73.
43. Kraus S, Naor Z, Seger R. Gonadotropin-releasing hormone in apoptosis of prostate cancer cells. Cancer Lett 2006; 234:109-23.
44. Grundker C, Emons G. Role of gonadotropin-releasing hormone (GnRH) in ovarian cancer. Reprod Biol Endocrinol 2003; 1:65.
45. Porcile C, Bajetto A, Barbieri F, et al. Stromal cell-derived factor-1alpha (SDF-1alpha/CXCL12) stimulates ovarian cancer cell growth through the EGF receptor transactivation. Exp Cell Res 2005; 308:241-53.
46. Hunyady L, Catt KJ. Pleiotropic AT1 receptor signaling pathways mediating physiological and pathogenic actions of angiotensin II. Mol Endocrinol 2006; 20:953-70.
47. Bagnato A, Tecce R, Di Castro V, Catt KJ. Activation of mitogenic signaling by endothelin 1 in ovarian carcinoma cells. Cancer Res 1997; 57:1306-11.
48. Bagnato A, Salani D, Di Castro V, et al. Expression of endothelin 1 and endothelin A receptor in ovarian carcinoma: evidence for an autocrine role in tumor growth. Cancer Res 1999; 59:720-7.
49. Spinella F, Rosano L, Di Castro V, Natali PG, Bagnato A. Endothelin-1-induced prostaglandin E2-EP2, EP4 signaling regulates vascular endothelial growth factor production and ovarian carcinoma cell invasion. J Biol Chem 2004; 279:46700-5.
50. Shah BH, Yesilkaya A, Olivares-Reyes JA, Chen HD, Hunyady L, Catt KJ. Differential pathways of angiotensin II-induced extracellularly regulated kinase 1/2 phosphorylation in specific cell types: role of heparin-binding epidermal growth factor. Mol Endocrinol 2004; 18:2035-48.
51. Filardo EJ. Epidermal growth factor receptor (EGFR) transactivation by estrogen via the G-protein-coupled receptor, GPR30: a novel signaling pathway with potential significance for breast cancer. J Steroid Biochem Mol Biol 2002; 80:231-8.
52. Vivacqua A, Bonofiglio D, Recchia AG, et al. The G protein-coupled receptor GPR30 mediates the proliferative effects induced by 17beta-estradiol and hydroxytamoxifen in endometrial cancer cells. Mol Endocrinol 2006; 20:631-46.
53. Sukocheva O, Wadham C, Holmes A, et al. Estrogen transactivates EGFR via the sphingosine 1-phosphate receptor Edg-3: the role of sphingosine kinase-1. J Cell Biol 2006; 173:301-10.
54. Shupnik MA. Crosstalk between steroid receptors and the c-Src-receptor tyrosine kinase pathways: implications for cell proliferation. Oncogene 2004; 23:7979-89.
55. Lange CA. Making sense of cross-talk between steroid hormone receptors and intracellular signaling pathways: who will have the last word? Mol Endocrinol 2004; 18:269-78.
56. Arnold SF, Vorojeikina DP, Notides AC. Phosphorylation of tyrosine 537 on the human estrogen receptor is required for binding to an estrogen response element. J Biol Chem 1995; 270:30205-12.
57. Barletta F, Wong CW, McNally C, Komm BS, Katzenellenbogen B, Cheskis BJ. Characterization of the interactions of estrogen receptor and MNAR in the activation of cSrc. Mol Endocrinol 2004; 18:1096-108.
58. Migliaccio A, Di Domenico M, Castoria G, et al. Steroid receptor regulation of epidermal growth factor signaling through Src in breast and prostate cancer cells: steroid antagonist action. Cancer Res 2005; 65:10585-93.

59. Yakar S, Leroith D, Brodt P. The role of the growth hormone/insulin-like growth factor axis in tumor growth and progression: Lessons from animal models. Cytokine Growth Factor Rev 2005; 16:407-20.
60. Chanson P, Salenave S. Diagnosis and treatment of pituitary adenomas. Minerva Endocrinol 2004; 29:241-75.
61. Billiau A, Heremans H, Vermeire K, Matthys P. Immunomodulatory properties of interferon-gamma. An update. Ann N Y Acad Sci 1998; 856:22-32.
62. Uribe JM, McCole DF, Barrett KE. Interferon-gamma activates EGF receptor and increases TGF-alpha in T84 cells: implications for chloride secretion. Am J Physiol Gastrointest Liver Physiol 2002; 283:G923-31.
63. Wiseman LR, Johnson MD, Wakeling AE, Lykkesfeldt AE, May FE, Westley BR. Type I IGF receptor and acquired tamoxifen resistance in oestrogen-responsive human breast cancer cells. Eur J Cancer 1993; 29A:2256-64.
64. Parisot JP, Hu XF, DeLuise M, Zalcberg JR. Altered expression of the IGF-1 receptor in a tamoxifen-resistant human breast cancer cell line. Br J Cancer 1999; 79:693-700.
65. Amos S, Martin PM, Polar GA, Parsons SJ, Hussaini IM. Phorbol 12-myristate 13-acetate induces epidermal growth factor receptor transactivation via protein kinase Cdelta/c-Src pathways in glioblastoma cells. J Biol Chem 2005; 280:7729-38.
66. Cabodi S, Calautti E, Talora C, Kuroki T, Stein PL, Dotto GP. A PKC-eta/Fyn-dependent pathway leading to keratinocyte growth arrest and differentiation. Mol Cell 2000; 6:1121-9.
67. Zhuang S, Schnellmann RG. H2O2-induced transactivation of EGF receptor requires Src and mediates ERK1/2, but not Akt, activation in renal cells. Am J Physiol Renal Physiol 2004; 286:F858-65.
68. Kevil CG, Okayama N, Alexander JS. H(2)O(2)-mediated permeability II: importance of tyrosine phosphatase and kinase activity. Am J Physiol Cell Physiol 2001; 281:C1940-7.
69. Tang H, Hao Q, Rutherford SA, Low B, Zhao ZJ. Inactivation of SRC family tyrosine kinases by reactive oxygen species in vivo. J Biol Chem 2005; 280:23918-25.
70. Boerner JL, Demory ML, Silva C, Parsons SJ. Phosphorylation of Y845 on the epidermal growth factor receptor mediates binding to the mitochondrial protein cytochrome c oxidase subunit II. Mol Cell Biol 2004; 24:7059-71.
71. Kloth MT, Laughlin KK, Biscardi JS, Boerner JL, Parsons SJ, Silva CM. STAT5b, a Mediator of Synergism between c-Src and the Epidermal Growth Factor Receptor. J Biol Chem 2003; 278:1671-9.
72. Brown GC, Borutaite V. Nitric oxide, cytochrome c and mitochondria. Biochem Soc Symp 1999; 66:17-25.
73. Yang WL, Iacono L, Tang WM, Chin KV. Novel function of the regulatory subunit of protein kinase A: regulation of cytochrome c oxidase activity and cytochrome c release. Biochemistry 1998; 37:14175-80.
74. Silva CM. Role of STATs as downstream signal transducers in Src family kinase-mediated tumorigenesis. Oncogene 2004; 23:8017-23.
75. Lin TS, Mahajan S, Frank DA. STAT signaling in the pathogenesis and treatment of leukemias. Oncogene 2000; 19:2496-504.
76. Yu CL, Jove R, Burakoff SJ. Constitutive activation of the Janus kinase-STAT pathway in T lymphoma overexpressing the Lck protein tyrosine kinase. J Immunol 1997; 159:5206-10.
77. Garcia R, Bowman TL, Niu G, et al. Constitutive activation of Stat3 by the Src and JAK tyrosine kinases participates in growth regulation of human breast carcinoma cells. Oncogene 2001; 20:2499-513.
78. Xi S, Zhang Q, Dyer KF, et al. Src kinases mediate STAT growth pathways in squamous cell carcinoma of the head and neck. J Biol Chem 2003; 278:31574-83.
79. Miyazaki T, Neff L, Tanaka S, Horne WC, Baron R. Regulation of cytochrome c oxidase activity by c-Src in osteoclasts. J Cell Biol 2003; 160:709-18.
80. Salvi M, Brunati AM, Bordin L, La Rocca N, Clari G, Toninello A. Characterization and location of Src-dependent tyrosine phosphorylation in rat brain mitochondria. Biochim Biophys Acta 2002; 1589:181-95.
81. Osherov N, Levitzki A. Epidermal-growth-factor-dependent activation of the src-family kinases. Eur J Biochem 1994; 225:1047-53.
82. Nishida K, Hirano T. The role of Gab family scaffolding adapter proteins in the signal transduction of cytokine and growth factor receptors. Cancer Sci 2003; 94:1029-33.

83. Gogg S, Smith U. Epidermal growth factor and transforming growth factor alpha mimic the effects of insulin in human fat cells and augment downstream signaling in insulin resistance. J Biol Chem 2002; 277:36045-51.
84. Fleming JM, Desury G, Polanco TA, Cohick WS. Insulin growth factor-1 and epidermal growth factor receptors recruit distinct upstream signaling molecules to enhance AKT activation in mammary epithelial cells. Endocrinology 2006; 147:6027-35.
85. Nishida K, Yoshida Y, Itoh M, et al. Gab-family adapter proteins act downstream of cytokine and growth factor receptors and T- and B-cell antigen receptors. Blood 1999; 93:1809-16.
86. Sato K, Gotoh N, Otsuki T, et al. Tyrosine residues 239 and 240 of Shc are phosphatidylinositol 4,5-bisphosphate-dependent phosphorylation sites by c-Src. Biochem Biophys Res Commun 1997; 240:399-404.
87. Blake RA, Broome MA, Liu X, et al. SU6656, a selective src family kinase inhibitor, used to probe growth factor signaling. Mol Cell Biol 2000; 20:9018-27.
88. Haynes MP, Li L, Sinha D, et al. Src kinase mediates phosphatidylinositol 3-kinase/Akt-dependent rapid endothelial nitric-oxide synthase activation by estrogen. J Biol Chem 2003; 278:2118-23.
89. Stephens LR, Anderson KE, Hawkins PT. Src family kinases mediate receptor-stimulated, phosphoinositide 3-kinase-dependent, tyrosine phosphorylation of dual adaptor for phosphotyrosine and 3-phosphoinositides-1 in endothelial and B cell lines. J Biol Chem 2001; 276:42767-73.
90. Kong M, Mounier C, Dumas V, Posner BI. Epidermal growth factor-induced DNA synthesis. Key role for Src phosphorylation of the docking protein Gab2. J Biol Chem 2003; 278:5837-44.
91. Hernandez-Sotomayor SM, Carpenter G. Epidermal growth factor receptor: elements of intracellular communication. J Membr Biol 1992; 128:81-9.
92. Thien CB, Langdon WY. Cbl: many adaptations to regulate protein tyrosine kinases. Nat Rev Mol Cell Biol 2001; 2:294-307.
93. Bao J, Gur G, Yarden Y. Src promotes destruction of c-Cbl: implications for oncogenic synergy between Src and growth factor receptors. Proc Natl Acad Sci U S A 2003; 100:2438-43.
94. Wilde A, Beattie EC, Lem L, et al. EGF receptor signaling stimulates SRC kinase phosphorylation of clathrin, influencing clathrin redistribution and EGF uptake. Cell 1999; 96:677-87.
95. Ware MF, Tice DA, Parsons SJ, Lauffenburger DA. Overexpression of cellular Src in fibroblasts enhances endocytic internalization of epidermal growth factor receptor. J Biol Chem 1997; 272:30185-90.
96. Ahn S, Kim J, Lucaveche CL, et al. Src-dependent tyrosine phosphorylation regulates dynamin self-assembly and ligand-induced endocytosis of the epidermal growth factor receptor. J Biol Chem 2002; 277:26642-51.
97. Couet J, Sargiacomo M, Lisanti MP. Interaction of a receptor tyrosine kinase, EGF-R, with caveolins. Caveolin binding negatively regulates tyrosine and serine/threonine kinase activities. J Biol Chem 1997; 272:30429-38.
98. Mineo C, Gill GN, Anderson RG. Regulated migration of epidermal growth factor receptor from caveolae. J Biol Chem 1999; 274:30636-43.
99. Lee H, Volonte D, Galbiati F, et al. Constitutive and growth factor-regulated phosphorylation of caveolin-1 occurs at the same site (Tyr-14) in vivo: identification of a c-Src/Cav-1/Grb7 signaling cassette. Mol Endocrinol 2000; 14:1750-75.
100. Playford MP, Schaller MD. The interplay between Src and integrins in normal and tumor biology. Oncogene 2004; 23:7928-46.
101. Schlaepfer DD, Mitra SK. Multiple connections link FAK to cell motility and invasion. Curr Opin Genet Dev 2004; 14:92-101.
102. Wu H, Parsons JT. Cortactin, an 80/85-kilodalton pp60src substrate, is a filamentous actin-binding protein enriched in the cell cortex. J Cell Biol 1993; 120:1417-26.
103. Kinley AW, Weed SA, Weaver AM, et al. Cortactin interacts with WIP in regulating Arp2/3 activation and membrane protrusion. Curr Biol 2003; 13:384-93.
104. Head JA, Jiang D, Li M, et al. Cortactin tyrosine phosphorylation requires Rac1 activity and association with the cortical actin cytoskeleton. Mol Biol Cell 2003; 14:3216-29.
105. Huang C, Liu J, Haudenschild CC, Zhan X. The role of tyrosine phosphorylation of cortactin in the locomotion of endothelial cells. J Biol Chem 1998; 273:25770-6.
106. Maa MC, Wilson LK, Moyers JS, Vines RR, Parsons JT, Parsons SJ. Identification and characterization of a cytoskeleton-associated, epidermal growth factor sensitive pp60c-src substrate. Oncogene 1992; 7:2429-38.

107. Nada S, Okada M, Aizawa S, Nakagawa H. Identification of major tyrosine-phosphorylated proteins in Csk-deficient cells. Oncogene 1994; 9:3571-8.
108. Parsons JT. Focal adhesion kinase: the first ten years. J Cell Sci 2003; 116:1409-16.
109. Moro L, Dolce L, Cabodi S, et al. Integrin-induced epidermal growth factor (EGF) receptor activation requires c-Src and p130Cas and leads to phosphorylation of specific EGF receptor tyrosines. J Biol Chem 2002; 277:9405-14.
110. Ignar-Trowbridge DM, Nelson KG, Bidwell MC, et al. Coupling of dual signaling pathways: epidermal growth factor action involves the estrogen receptor. Proc Natl Acad Sci U S A 1992; 89:4658-62.
111. Ignar-Trowbridge DM, Teng CT, Ross KA, Parker MG, Korach KS, McLachlan JA. Peptide growth factors elicit estrogen receptor-dependent transcriptional activation of an estrogen-responsive element. Mol Endocrinol 1993; 7:992-8.
112. Razandi M, Pedram A, Greene GL, Levin ER. Cell membrane and nuclear estrogen receptors (ERs) originate from a single transcript: studies of ERalpha and ERbeta expressed in Chinese hamster ovary cells. Mol Endocrinol 1999; 13:307-19.
113. Kato S, Endoh H, Masuhiro Y, et al. Activation of the estrogen receptor through phosphorylation by mitogen-activated protein kinase. Science 1995; 270:1491-4.
114. Bunone G, Briand PA, Miksicek RJ, Picard D. Activation of the unliganded estrogen receptor by EGF involves the MAP kinase pathway and direct phosphorylation. EMBO J 1996; 15:2174-83.
115. Migliaccio A, Di Domenico M, Castoria G, et al. Tyrosine kinase/p21ras/MAP-kinase pathway activation by estradiol-receptor complex in MCF-7 cells. EMBO J 1996; 15:1292-300.
116. Guo Z, Dai B, Jiang T, et al. Regulation of androgen receptor activity by tyrosine phosphorylation. Cancer Cell 2006; 10:309-19.
117. Kraus S, Gioeli D, Vomastek T, Gordon V, Weber MJ. Receptor for activated C kinase 1 (RACK1) and Src regulate the tyrosine phosphorylation and function of the androgen receptor. Cancer Res 2006; 66:11047-54.
118. Hanke JH, Gardner JP, Dow RL, et al. Discovery of a novel, potent, and Src family-selective tyrosine kinase inhibitor. Study of Lck- and FynT-dependent T cell activation. J Biol Chem 1996; 271:695-701.
119. Waltenberger J, Uecker A, Kroll J, et al. A dual inhibitor of platelet-derived growth factor beta-receptor and Src kinase activity potently interferes with motogenic and mitogenic responses to PDGF in vascular smooth muscle cells. A novel candidate for prevention of vascular remodeling. Circ Res 1999; 85:12-22.
120. Li Z, Hosoi Y, Cai K, et al. Src tyrosine kinase inhibitor PP2 suppresses ERK1/2 activation and epidermal growth factor receptor transactivation by X-irradiation. Biochem Biophys Res Commun 2006; 341:363-8.
121. Kim J, Eckhart AD, Eguchi S, Koch WJ. Beta-adrenergic receptor-mediated DNA synthesis in cardiac fibroblasts is dependent on transactivation of the epidermal growth factor receptor and subsequent activation of extracellular signal-regulated kinases. J Biol Chem 2002; 277:32116-23.
122. Hiscox S, Morgan L, Green TP, Barrow D, Gee J, Nicholson RI. Elevated Src activity promotes cellular invasion and motility in tamoxifen resistant breast cancer cells. Breast Cancer Res Treat 2006; 97:263-74.
123. Song L, Morris M, Bagui T, Lee FY, Jove R, Haura EB. Dasatinib (BMS-354825) selectively induces apoptosis in lung cancer cells dependent on epidermal growth factor receptor signaling for survival. Cancer Res 2006; 66:5542-8.
124. Evans TR, Yellowlees A, Foster E, et al. Phase III randomized trial of doxorubicin and docetaxel versus doxorubicin and cyclophosphamide as primary medical therapy in women with breast cancer: an anglo-celtic cooperative oncology group study. J Clin Oncol 2005; 23:2988-95.
125. Shah NP. Improving upon the promise of targeted therapy of human malignancy: chronic myeloid leukemia as a paradigm. Cancer Chemother Pharmacol 2006; 58 Suppl 7:49-53.
126. Angers-Loustau A, Hering R, Werbowetski TE, Kaplan DR, Del Maestro RF. SRC regulates actin dynamics and invasion of malignant glial cells in three dimensions. Mol Cancer Res 2004; 2:595-605.
127. Yamaguchi K, Richardson MD, Bigner DD, Kwatra MM. Signal transduction through substance P receptor in human glioblastoma cells: roles for Src and PKCdelta. Cancer Chemother Pharmacol 2005; 56:585-93.
128. Lund CV, Nguyen MT, Owens GC, et al. Reduced glioma infiltration in Src-deficient mice. J Neurooncol 2006; 78:19-29.

10 A Molecular Crosstalk between E-cadherin and EGFR Signaling Networks

Julie Gavard and J. Silvio Gutkind

Contents

INTRODUCTION
CADHERINS: ADHESIVE RECEPTORS
CADHERINS IN CANCER
CROSSTALK BETWEEN E-CADHERIN AND EGFR: ROLE IN CANCER
CONCLUSION
REFERENCES

Abstract

Classical cadherins are single-pass transmembrane glycoproteins engaged in homophilic calcium-dependent cell-cell adhesion complexes, a system highly conserved in all multicellular organisms. E-cadherin is one of these enthralling adhesive receptors, originally named uvomorulin, for its "glue" ability during the early stage of embryogenesis. Highly expressed in differentiated and polarized epithelial cells, the dynamic formation and disassembly of E-cadherin contacts participate in most developmental and pathological processes involving morphogenetic changes in the epithelium. E-cadherins bind through their extracellular region to E-cadherins expressed in adjacent cells and are linked through their intracytoplasmic tail to the cytoskeleton through a family of proteins collectively known as catenins, which also play an important role in E-cadherin-initiated intracellular signaling. E-cadherin is believed to act as a tumor- and metastasis-suppressor gene, as its expression and function are down-regulated or altered in many human cancers, and its re-expression decreases both the proliferative and invasive capacity of tumor cells. Recent evidence suggests the existence of a direct cross-talk between E-cadherin and EGF receptors (EGFR). Indeed, EGFR activation can cause the dismantling of cell-cell contacts by promoting the destabilization of E-cadherin/catenin adhesive complexes, the down-regulation of E-cadherin expression, and the endocytosis and subsequent degradation of pre-existing cell surface E-cadherins. On the other hand, the engagement of E-cadherin in newly formed cell contacts causes the rapid EGF-independent activation of EGFR, thereby triggering EGFR-initiated signaling pathways that enhance cell proliferation or survival through MAPK, PI3-Kinase and Rho GTPases. Further studies into the molecular mechanism underlying the interplay between E-Cadherin and EGFR in normal and tumoral epithelial cells may ultimately help to identify more effective EGFR-targeting strategies for cancer treatment.

Key Words: cell junction, cell adhesion, cadherin, catenin migration, EGFR, actin.

From: *Cancer Drug Discovery and Development: EGFR Signaling Networks in Cancer Therapy*
Edited by: J. D. Haley and W. J. Gullick, DOI: 10.1007/978-1-59745-356-1_10
© 2008 Humana Press, a part of Springer Science+Business Media, LLC

1. INTRODUCTION

The adhesive contacts between cells underlie many morphogenetic processes during embryonic development and the control of growth, turnover, and regeneration of adult tissues. Proteins involved in cell-cell and cell-matrix junctions define the molecular interactions between cells and their surrounding environment and neighboring cells. Among them, the adhesion molecules of the cadherin superfamily were initially described to serve as physical bridges between cells with the ability to regulate aggregation and sorting of cells (1). Since then, cadherins have been recognized to play a key role in the coordination of cell motility and cell fate decisions, due to their ability to transduce environment and cell-cell initiated signals into intracellular biochemical pathways controlling the expression and activity of molecules regulating cell motility, differentiation, and cell survival or death (2).

2. CADHERINS: ADHESIVE RECEPTORS

2.1. Adhesive Properties of Cadherins

The cadherins constitute a large superfamily of cell-cell adhesion molecules, as reflected by the presence of more than 200 genes encoding cadherins in the human genome. Most of our current knowledge on these cell surface molecules comes from studies on classical cadherins, which are Ca^{2+}-dependent, homophilic, cell-to-cell adhesion molecules expressed in nearly all cells within solid tissues. These molecules also participate in cell-cell recognition, a property that confers the ability of cells to aggregate with and ultimately sort their most physiologically relevant cell partners. For example, as illustrated in Fig. 10.1, only cells expressing the same type of cadherins may adhere to each other (3). The specificity of homophilic adhesion is conserved even throughout species, since orthologues of each cadherin class may preferentially bind to each other across species, instead of binding paralogues within the same species. The classical cadherins were originally named based on the tissue in which they are most prominently expressed. For example, E-cadherin is expressed primarily in epithelial cells, VE-cadherin in vascular endothelial cells and N-cadherin in nervous system and mesenchymal cells. It has become clear, however, that these expression patterns are not mutually exclusive, and most cadherins can be expressed at various levels in many different cells and tissues. Among these cadherins, E-cadherin is associated with the zonula adherens of the epithelial junctional complex, which helps the cells to form a tight, polarized cell layer that can perform barrier and transport functions (2). In general, classical cadherins form a core adhesion complex that consists of a cadherin dimer, binding through its extracellular region to another dimer of cadherins in adjacent cells, and an intracellular region, anchored to the plasma membrane and linked to the cytoskeleton through a family of proteins collectively known as catenins.

2.1.1. THE EXTRACELLULAR DOMAIN: HOMOPHILIC BINDING

The extracellular domain of the classical cadherin molecule consists of five cadherin-type repeats, called EC (extracellular cadherin) domains that are bound together by Ca^{2+} in a rod-like structure (4) (Fig. 10.2). The extracellular domain mediates the adhesive binding functions, which are regulated by the cytoplasmic region. Different models, however, have been proposed for the homophilic interactions within the extracellular domain, based on information obtained by the use of purified recombinant proteins containing either fragments or total ECs (2, 5). While the nature of the interactions involved in the formation of homophilic adhesion complexes is still a matter of debate, all the studies agree that EC dimers, either in *cis* or *trans,* represent the minimal cadherin adhesive functional unit. Moreover, calcium, which is required for cadherin function, rigidifies the protein structure, activates

Chapter 10 / A Molecular Crosstalk between E-cadherin and EGFR Signaling Networks

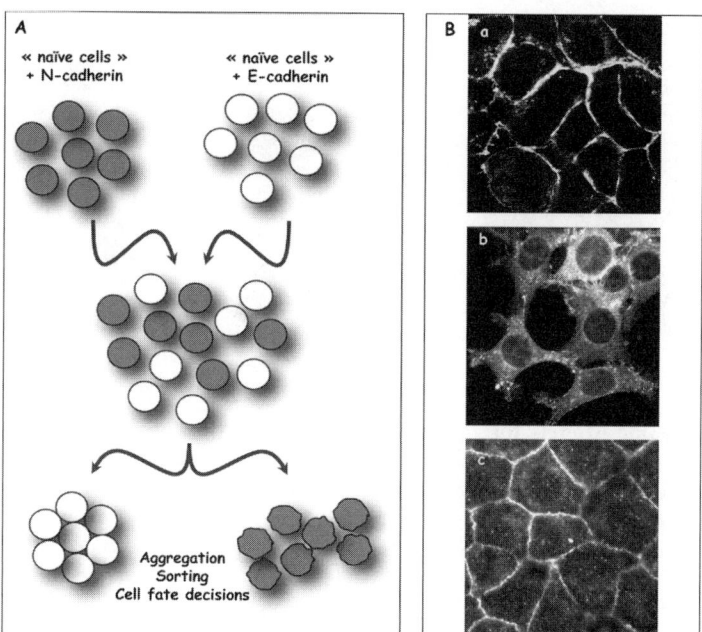

Fig. 10.1. Adhesive Properties of Cadherins: A Role in Aggregation, Segregation and Morphogenesis.
(A) Schematic representation of the seminal experiments demonstrating both aggregation and segregation properties of cadherins (adapted from (3)). Cells that do not express any cadherin (L cells, "naïve") do not adhere to each other. These cells were transfected with N-cadherin and labeled with a red dye (in gray); independently "naïve" cells were transfected with E-cadherin and labeled with a green dye (in white). Both cell types were then mixed and heterotypic contacts were forced. However, cells clearly associated and sorted with cells expressing the same type of cadherins, excluding the other cell type, leading to two distinct populations. (B) Immunofluorescence showing the heterogeneity of cadherin-based cell-cell contacts. An epithelial cell line (a, HaCaT) was stained for E-cadherin and showed a regularly aligned pattern; another epithelial cell line (b, HeLa) was stained for N-cadherin and exhibited weaker and loosely zones of cell-cell contacts. Endothelial cells (c, HUVEC) stained for VE-cadherin, harbor cell-cell junctions that are well defined but not as polarized as E-cadherin-expressing epithelial cells.

its adhesive properties, and imparts protease resistance (6). Early findings suggest that a histidine-alanine-valine (HAV) sequence in the first EC repeat (EC1) is required for homophilic interaction, but mutagenesis analysis unraveled that a tryptophane residue (W2) contributes also to an essential surface of interaction (7). Once engaged in homophilic interactions, the extracellular domains develop additional forces, strengthening the adhesive contacts while retaining the ability to associate-dissociate rapidly in response to dynamic changes in the cellular environment (8, 9).

2.1.2. THE INTRACELLULAR DOMAIN: THE ACTIN LINK

Classical cadherins are single-pass transmembrane proteins that interact with a number of different cytoplasmic partners to carry out their functions, which include cell-cell adhesion, cytoskeletal anchoring and signaling (Fig. 10.3). The cadherin-associated proteins, catenins, are universally present in classical cadherin complexes (10). In particular, β-catenin interacts with the distal part of the cadherin cytoplasmic domain and p120 catenin with a more proximal region. α-catenin does not bind directly to cadherin, but instead associates with β-catenin, and

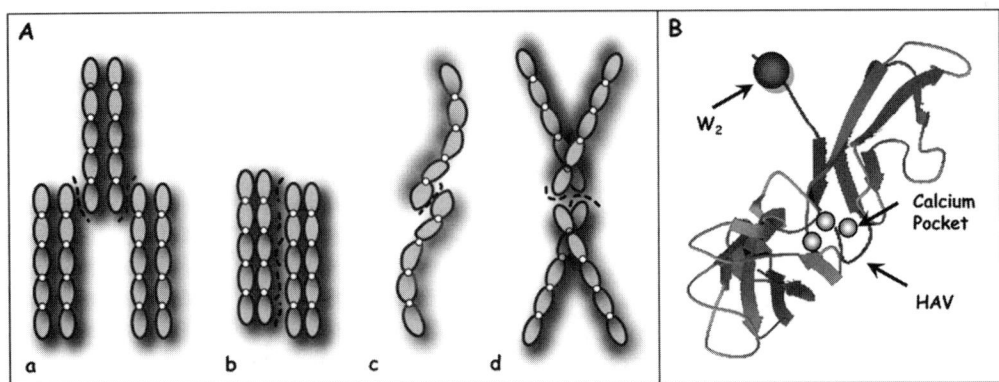

Fig. 10.2. **Molecular Models for the Homophilic Interaction of the Cadherin Extracellular Domain.** (A) Various models for the cadherin homophilic bond (adapted from (2)): (a) Linear zipper model composed of interdigitating Trp-mediated *cis* dimers. The *cis*-strand dimer results from the reciprocal insertion of the Trp2 residue (W) in the EC1 domain of one subunit into a hydrophobic pocket of the other subunit. The homophilic-binding (or *trans* interaction) occurs at a different site, which surrounds the HAV sequence. (b) This model invokes extensive overlap between Trp-mediated dimers and requires a role for EC1 and other EC domains in the formation of the homophilic bond. (c) This model implies a Ca^{2+}-dependent *cis* dimer, and intramolecular Trp2 binding to activate the adhesive binding interface. (d) Revised Trp-dimer model, in which Trp2 mediates the *trans*-homophilic bond rather than the cis dimer. Calcium ions are indicated by white circles, and the interaction surfaces are represented by dashed lines. (B) This panel shows the structure of the EC1 domain, as it can be configured at the adhesive dimer interface. The calcium pocket, the HAV sequence and the W2 are the proposed *trans* and *cis* dimerization sites.

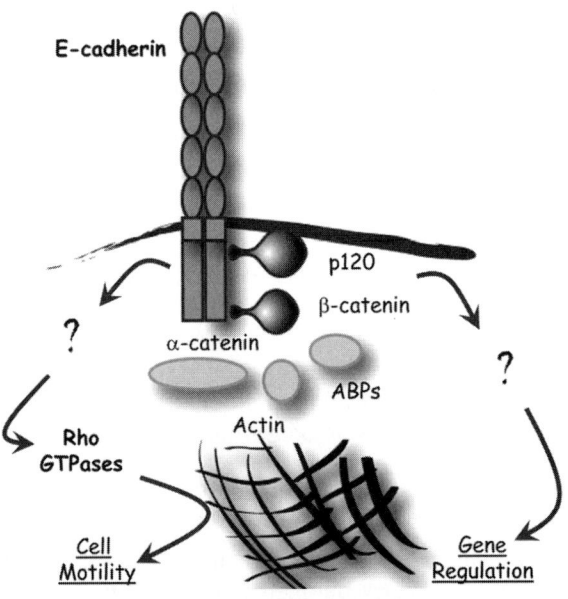

Fig. 10.3. **Organization of Cadherin Complexes at the Plasma Membrane: Initiation of Cell Signaling.** Cadherins are single-pass transmembrane glycoproteins, which function as a dimer. The extracellular part comprises five cadherin domain (EC) repeats conferring homophilic and calcium-dependent adhesive properties. The intracellular part can recruit the p120 catenin at the juxtamembrane

provides a physical link to the actin cytoskeleton, either by directly binding actin filaments or indirectly through other actin-binding proteins such as vinculin, β-actinin, and formins (11, 12), thus regulating actin polymerization, cross-linking, and dynamics at the cell-cell contact zones. On the other hand, p120 catenin seems to influence cadherin function by a variety of mechanisms, as detailed below (please see section 2.2.3).

2.2. Catenins

2.2.1. β-Catenin

β-catenin was biochemically identified based on its direct association with E-cadherin in a 1:1 stoichiometry in vertebrates, while independently isolated in a genetic screen in Drosophila for molecules involved in the Wnt pathway (13). β-catenin has 12 42-amino-acid armadillo repeats forming a superhelix. This central armadillo core binds to the cadherin tail (14). In addition, approximately 100 amino acids are present in each N- and C-terminal extension, which are the target of several serine/threonine and tyrosine phosphorylation events that can regulate the function, localization, and stability of β-catenin. The structures of β-catenin and of the cadherin/β-catenin complex, have been well established and provided the framework for our understanding of its key regulatory role in cadherin-mediated adhesion (14, 15). Moreover, biochemical data suggest that the localization of β-catenin at the plasma membrane or in the cytosol/nucleus is dictated by the regulation of distinct molecular forms of β-catenin with different binding properties (16).

The essential role of β-catenin in cadherin-based adhesion was revealed by the use of deletion mutants in the C-tail of E-cadherin (10, 17). Several studies suggest that the interaction of β-catenin with cadherin strengthens cell-cell contacts (18), although β-catenin may be substituted by γ-catenin in its adhesive function (19). The β-catenin/cadherin association appears to be initiated already in the endoplasmic reticulum, prior to E-cadherin shuttling to the plasma membrane, and may serve to fold the cadherin intracellular domain properly (15). In addition, the β-catenin phosphorylation status regulates the stability of the β-catenin/cadherin interaction, suggesting that many kinase/phosphatase cascades can modify the strength of the cell-cell adhesions through cadherins by regulating β-catenin (13). Finally, β-catenin may participate in signaling pathways initiated at the cell-cell contacts through its interaction with PI3-Kinase (20) or Rac signaling *via* IQGAP (21). The question as to whether or not the cadherin-bound pool of β-catenin can be released and made available for the Wnt signaling pathway, thereby controlling nuclear events, is still a matter of intense debate and will not be discussed here (13, 22).

2.2.2. α-Catenin

In contrast to β-catenin and p120 catenin, α-catenin is not directly bound to cadherin cytoplasmic domain and does not belong to the armadillo family. Its participation in cell-cell contacts is extensively demonstrated, however, as α-catenin is required for the

Fig. 10.3. (continued) region and β-catenin at the C-terminal portion. Both catenins can also participate in the regulation of gene expression upon shuttling to the nuclear compartment, through complex mechanisms. α-catenin participates in the anchoring of the cell membrane cadherin complexes by its interaction with β-catenin, while interacting with the actin cytoskeleton and many actin-binding proteins (ABP). Thus, α-catenin might regulate the actin dynamics at the area of cell-cell contacts. In addition, cadherins can directly control the activity of small Rho GTPases, thereby regulating the cytoskeleton organization and cell motility.

anchorage of the cadherin/β-catenin complex to the actin network at the cell-cell contact zone (23). Indeed, α-catenin possesses the ability to interact with the actin cytoskeleton and many actin-binding proteins, therefore regulating the actin dynamics, polymerization and cross-linking (11, 12). α-catenin, however, can be found in association with either β-catenin or the actin cytoskeleton. This mutually exclusive binding provides a dynamic link between the cadherin/catenin complexes at the plasma membrane and the actin cytoskeleton, thus participating in the formation, strengthening and remodeling of cell-cell contacts (24, 25) (Fig. 10.3).

2.2.3. p120 Catenin

Although p120 catenin was initially identified as a Src Kinase substrate (26), p120 belongs to the armadillo family, such as β-catenin, and displays a central core of armadillo repeats involved in the binding to the juxtamembrane domain of the cadherins. The modulatory role of p120 in cadherin-mediated cell adhesion relies on its multi-functional properties and the increasing number of molecular partners. For example, p120 is directly involved in the trafficking and turnover of cadherins at the plasma membrane (27), a property likely associated with the control of microtubule dynamics and transport (28, 29). In addition, p120 can regulate the activity of small Rho GTPases (30). Ultimately, p120 regulates cell motion by its ability to control both cell adhesion via regulating the availability of cadherins at the plasma membrane and the control of the actin cytoskeleton organization through the regulation of Rho GTPases signaling networks (31, 32). p120 also directly affects gene expression by repressing transcription through the scaffolding of a nuclear complex comprising the gene silencer, Kaiso (33). Moreover, the absence of p120 in the skin compartment induces hyperplasia and inflammation, concomitant with an increase of NFκB signaling (34).

2.2. Cadherin Adhesion Initiates Cell Signaling

Cadherins interact with numerous signaling molecules at the plasma membrane, such as tyrosine kinases, phosphatases, and proteases, and may be able to regulate nuclear signaling (13, 35-37). In addition, small Rho GTPases were found to be activated at the early stages during the assembly of cadherin-based adhesion, a process that is required for the appropriate cell-cell contact formation (35, 38). However, evidence suggesting that cadherin engagement upon homophilic binding triggers intracellular signaling events is experimentally limited by the fact that cadherins could function as both their own receptor and ligand. This technical limitation may be overcome artificially by the use of planar surfaces coated with purified cadherin extracellular domain, which acts as a ligand to stimulate cellular cadherin upon attachment (39, 40). Nonetheless, how and even whether cadherins transduce signals is still far from being understood, since no classical receptor activation mechanisms have been established. Thus, the current view is that cadherin-based adhesion may stabilize and/or re-organize sub-membranous adhesive and signaling scaffolds thereby regulating signal transmission.

3. CADHERINS IN CANCER

3.1. E-cadherin as a Tumor-suppressor and Metastasis-suppressor Gene

3.1.1. EMT and E-cadherin

Epithelial cell plasticity and dedifferentiation are hallmarks of carcinoma progression during the invasion of the adjacent tissues and the subsequent metastasis to the lymph nodes and distant organs. This process is frequently termed as EMT, for epithelial-mesenchymal transition, where the polarized and tightly organized epithelial cell layers acquire mesenchymal properties and morphology, which exhibit loose cell contacts and a highly motile phenotype (41). This process frequently involves the reduced expression of E-cadherin at the cell surface by a process that includes the inhibition of E-cadherin mRNA expression concomitant with the endocytic degradation of pre-existing E-cadherin molecules. While the former involves the activation of transcription factors acting as repressors onto the E-cadherin promoter, the latter is initiated by targeting E-cadherin to a lysosomal compartment (41).

3.1.2. Loss of E-cadherin Expression

The loss of E-cadherin adhesion may alter the overall organization of epithelial junctions, deregulating the normal growth and morphology of the epithelium and favoring a more invasive phenotype (Fig. 10.4). Indeed, it has been proposed that E-cadherin acts as a tumor- and invasive-suppressor gene (42, 43). Although rare, inactivating mutations in the E-cadherin gene, including splice site mutations and truncation caused by insertion, deletion and nonsense mutations have been reported in numerous cancers, such as gastric, colon, and breast tumors (44). Moreover, the E-cadherin promoter can be targeted by inhibitory signals that are elicited by growth factors and cell proliferation conditions (45). Forcing the re-expression of E-cadherin enhances cell-cell adhesion, while reducing tumorigenicty and invasiveness (46). The E-cadherin promoter is also sensitive to acetylation/deatecylation reactions, thus providing an epigenetic mechanism controlling E-cadherin expression in cancer cells that can be reversed by the use of histone deacytalases inhibitors, which can both restore E-cadherin expression and epithelial phenotype, while blocking cancer cell transformation (47, 48).

3.1.3. Loss of E-cadherin Adhesion

E-cadherin function can also be altered at the post-translational level (Fig. 10.4). Growth factors such as EGF, HGF, or IGF, which are locally produced in the tumor microenvironment, can promote the decrease of E-cadherin-mediated cell-cell contacts (49). Indeed, E-cadherin or β-catenin tyrosine phosphorylation can destabilize the membranous complexes (50), while the E-cadherin intracellular domain or its associated catenins can be a direct target of these receptor tyrosine kinases or non-receptor tyrosine kinases, such as c-Src, that can be activated by these receptors (36). An alternative and not exclusive mechanism involves the internalization of E-cadherin, which is then sequestred in a vesicular compartment or degraded in the lysosome (49). Finally, E-cadherin adhesion can be hijacked by proteins mimicking the cadherin extracellular domain involved in the homophilic interaction. These proteins can occupy cadherin receptors but lack the adhesive signal, as demonstrated for bacteria-host interactions (51) and in tumor cells expressing dysadherin (52).

3.2. Regulation of Cell Growth by E-cadherin

3.2.1. Contact Inhibition

Non-transformed primary and established cell lines are contact-inhibited when they reach confluence in monolayer tissue culture, leading to an arrest in the cell cycle progression. Although loss of contact inhibition is one of the classical hallmarks of transformation, the fact that intercellular adhesion may be part of this process was intuitive and was early defined as a "community effect" (53). Since E-cadherin expression is lost without mutations in its gene in many cancers, the transcriptional repression of the E-cadherin promoter may be a key component to relieve the growth constraints caused by contact inhibition. Transcription factors repressing E-cadherin expression include a family of zinc finger proteins of the Slug/Snail family, SIP1 from the Smad TGF -responsive family transcription factor, and the basic helix-loop-helix E12/E47 factors that interact with E-box sequences in the proximal E-cadherin promoter (48, 54-56). In this regard, it was reported that cell density regulates

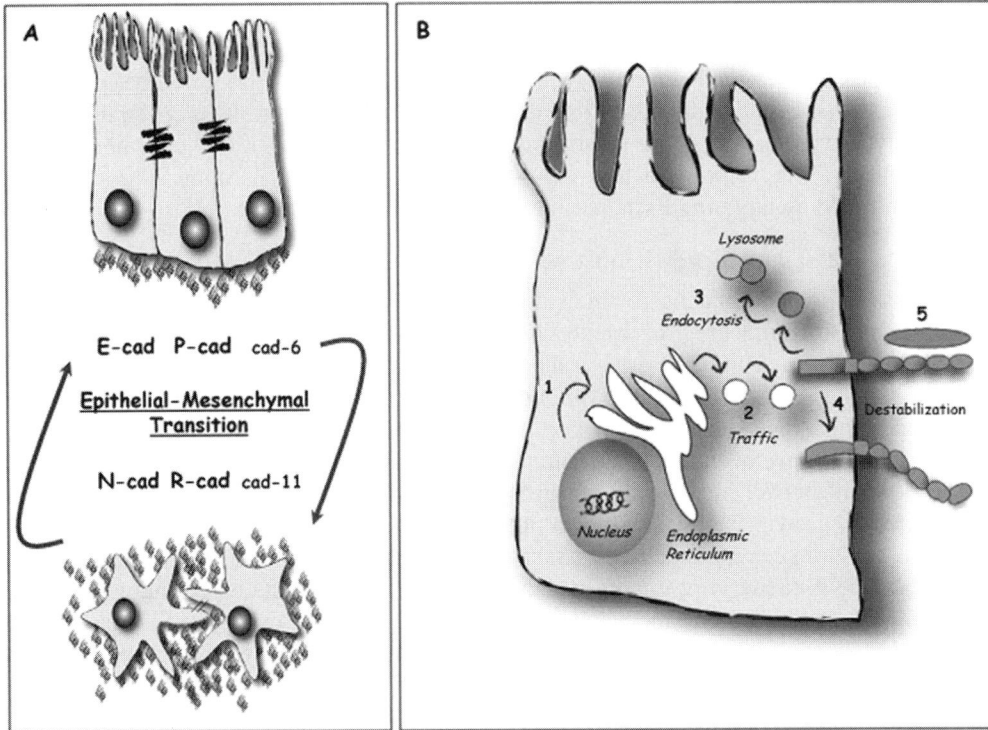

Fig. 10.4. **Cadherins and EMT: Multiple Mechanisms Regulate E-cadherin Expression and Function** (A) A profound remodeling of the epithelium occurs during epithelial-mesenchymal transition (EMT), where the highly polarized and organized epithelial cells acquired migratory and plastic phenotypes. This downregulation is accompanied by a switch in cadherin expression. E-cadherin, and to a lesser extend P-cadherin and cadherin-6, are substituted by N-cadherin, cadherin-11 and R-cadherin. (B) The loss of E-cadherin during normal or pathological EMT can be also regulated at different levels: 1- transcriptional repression and promoter hypermethylation, 2- alterations in the traffic of E-cadherin to the plasma membrane, 3- endocytosis and degradation of pre-existing E-cadherin, 4- destabilization of the adhesive complexes and, 5- disengagement of homophilic interactions by direct binding to the extracellular domain.

E-cadherin expression in colon cancer cells by a mechanism dependent on Slug repression downstream MAPK activation (57, 58). These observations raise the possibility that the growth suppressive and anti-migratory effects of E-cadherin can be overcome by oncogenes and growth factors acting through the MAPK signaling pathway.

3.2.2. THE CELL CYCLE CONTROL

E-cadherin re-expression is also associated with a switch from nuclear to membrane accumulation of β-catenin, thereby sequestering this potent cell proliferation transcription factor, most likely by a trapping mechanism rather than by an adhesion-dependent process (59-61). As such, enforced expression of E-cadherin in non-adherent mammary carcinoma cells inhibits cell proliferation, a process that appears to be dependent on the up-regulation of cyclin-dependent kinase inhibitors (43). Altogether, we have learned that the down-regulation of E-cadherin expression by cell growth signals may facilitate the transformation process, while overexpression of E-cadherin at the plasma membrane seems to be sufficient to suppress the unrestricted growth of cancer cells.

3.3. Regulation of Migration by E-cadherin

3.3.1. EXPRESSION OF INAPPROPRIATE CADHERINS

Without diminishing the levels of expression of E-cadherin, an inappropriate profile of cadherins is sufficient to modify the migratory behavior and the invasiveness properties of tumor cells (62). For example, N-cadherin, R-cadherin, and cadherin-11 expression in breast cancer cells promotes their motility and invasiveness (63-65). The cadherin extracellular domain seems to be involved in these dramatic changes, as suggested by studies using chimera between E-cadherin and N-cadherin (66, 67). However, rather than the adhesive function of N-cadherin, its signaling ability through the fibroblast growth factor receptor (FGFR) was suggested as a potential intervening mechanism (68).

3.3.2. PRO-MIGRATORY EFFECTS OF CADHERINS

The pro-migratory properties of certain cadherins may also result from their ability to stimulate Rho GTPase activation (38), lamellipodium formation (39, 40) and to regulate actin cytoskeleton dynamics through polymerization and mechanical tension (23, 69, 70), and microtubule polarity (71). Whereas the tumor-suppressor and metastatic-suppressor properties of E-cadherin are quite well established, their exact mechanism is less defined and may also involve a complex interplay at the translational and post-translational levels between cadherins, catenins, and their signaling partners.

4. CROSSTALK BETWEEN E-CADHERIN AND EGFR: ROLE IN CANCER

4.1. Cadherins and Tyrosine Kinase Receptors

In addition to their own signaling capacity, classical cadherins can also regulate the activity of other transmembrane receptors, including those exhibiting an intrinsic tyrosine kinase and phosphatase activity (36). In particular, work in our laboratory revealed that E-cadherin engagement can result in the EGF-independent activation of EGFR in epithelial cells (72). Similarly, VE-cadherin associates with VEGFR in endothelial cells (73), and N-cadherin interacts with FGFR in neurons and fibroblasts (68). Although the physical interaction between EGFR and E-cadherin at cell-cell contacts was early described (74), we have just begun to unravel the functional significance of the crosstalk between E-cadherin and EGFR in normal and cancer epithelial tissues. Ultimately, this EGFR/E-cadherin signaling axis can integrate information from the environment, such as cell density, availability of growth factors and nutrients, as well as the dynamic adhesive interactions with other cell types and the extracellular matrix, thereby controlling normal and aberrant cell growth.

4.2. Signaling from the EGFR to Cadherins

As described above, the activation of EGFR by its ligands generally results in the down-regulation of E-cadherin-mediated cell-cell adhesion, accompanying EGFR-dependent proliferation and migration of tumor cells (75). This organization can be achieved either by: 1) the destabilization of E-cadherin/catenin adhesive complexes, 2) E-cadherin endocytosis, or 3) the down-regulation of E-cadherin expression (Fig. 10.4). It is likely that these different mechanisms play a coordinated role in facilitating the dismantling of cell-cell contacts in response to EGFR stimulation.

4.2.1. DESTABILIZATION OF CADHERIN/CATENIN COMPLEXES

E-cadherin and catenins can be potential targets for the tyrosine-phosphorylating activity of EGFR and other receptor and non-receptor tyrosine kinases (36). The tyrosine-phosphorylation of cadherin and catenins decreases cadherin-adhesive functions, hence weakening the strength of cell-to-cell contacts (50, 76). For example, Src, a downstream target of EGFR, may phosphorylate directly E-cadherin or its associated catenins, resulting in conformational changes and destruction of the adhesive complexes (36, 77). Tyrosine phosphorylation, however, may also have a positive effect on E-cadherin-mediated cell-cell contact, particularly at the early steps of the assembly of adherens junctions (78, 79).

4.2.2. Cadherin Endocytosis

It has been observed that in response to EGF and other growth factors acting on receptor tyrosine kinases, E-cadherin complexes can be internalized by endocytosis (80-83). This process requires E-cadherin disengagement from cell-cell contacts at their extracellular region, as well as the reorganization and recruitment of specific molecular partners in their intracellular domain (49, 81). Specifically, it has been suggested that this mechanism relies on the clathrin-coated vesicular trafficking process (81, 84). This leads to degradation of cadherin/catenin complexes in the lysosomal compartment and/or by the ubiquitin-proteasome pathway (49, 83, 85). Alternatively, this endocytic process may be also transient, and cadherins may recycle back to the plasma membrane upon re-establishment of cell-cell contacts (80, 84).

4.2.3. EGFR Signaling to the E-cadherin Promoter

The down-regulation of E-cadherin by EGF activation may also occur also by diminishing its expression rate. For example, MAPK activation negatively regulates E-cadherin expression by a regulatory cell density-dependent mechanism (58). In tumor invasion models, EGF induces cell migration by the coordinated dismantlement of E-cadherin cell-cell contacts, endocytosis of pre-existing E-cadherin, and the reduction of E-cadherin expression (86). This three-prong mechanism leads to the up-regulation of β-catenin in the cytosol and the nucleus, which can contribute to the cell-cycle progression by controlling gene expression in the nucleus, as well as to cell migration and polarity through the formation of multimolecular complexes in the cytosol (13, 58, 86, 87).

4.3. Signaling from E-cadherin to the EGFR

4.3.1. Activation of EGFR Signaling by E-cadherin

The signaling capacity of E-cadherin has been approached by artificially mimicking the formation of cell-cell contacts (35). This approach enabled us and others to demonstrate that the engagement of E-cadherin in newly formed cell contacts activates intracellular signaling pathways such as MAPK and PI3-Kinase (72, 78), Rho GTPases (39, 88), and RTKs such as EGFR (20, 72, 89). Notably, EGFR activation by E-cadherin occurs shortly and transiently after the formation of cell-cell contacts. Indeed, E-cadherin can activate EGFR in the absence of its ligands, thereby triggering EGFR initiated signaling pathways (72, 90). E-cadherin-induced Rac activation is also a downstream event from this E-cadherin-dependent EGFR activation and contributes to the regulation of cell proliferation in epithelial cells (89). Thus, in newly formed contacts, E-cadherin can sensitize EGFR to low levels of EGF or even substitute for EGF to trigger EGFR-initiated pathways. E-cadherin may be also required for the proper EGFR signaling by regulating its localization or the local availability of signaling adapters (Fig. 10.5). In conclusion, E-cadherin engagement can trigger EGFR intracellular signaling cascades in a ligand-independent manner, thus enhancing cell proliferation or survival through MAPK, PI3-Kinase and Rac (72, 89, 90). However, the mechanism underlying E-cadherin-induced EGFR transactivation is still unclear. The E-cadherin extracellular domain appears to be required whereas the intracellular domain could play a regulatory function (90, 91). Because the co-localization and physical interaction of activated EGFR with E-cadherin is observed upon clustering of E-cadherin at the site of cell-cell contacts, it is also conceivable that the ability of E-cadherin to transduce signals through EGFR may depend on their physical association and/or the recruitment of other signaling and scaffolding systems (72). In this case, an intriguing scenario would involve the formation of higher order complexes between E-cadherin and EGFR, which could lead to a highly localized concentration of EGFR and its subsequent ligand-independent activation. In turn, the activation of EGFR in E-cadherin containing clusters may determine the nature, amplitude, and duration of the signals emanating from the cell-cell junctions.

4.3.2. REGULATION OF EPITHELIAL BIOLOGY BY THE E-CADHERIN/EGFR AXIS

The nascent cell-cell contacts and their associated signaling may recapitulate the status of poorly differentiated epithelia, such as during embryonic development, carcinogenesis, or morphogenesis (91-93). This mechanism may contribute to accelerate growth rates without a need for elevated levels of growth factors. One can postulate that, in a regulated process,

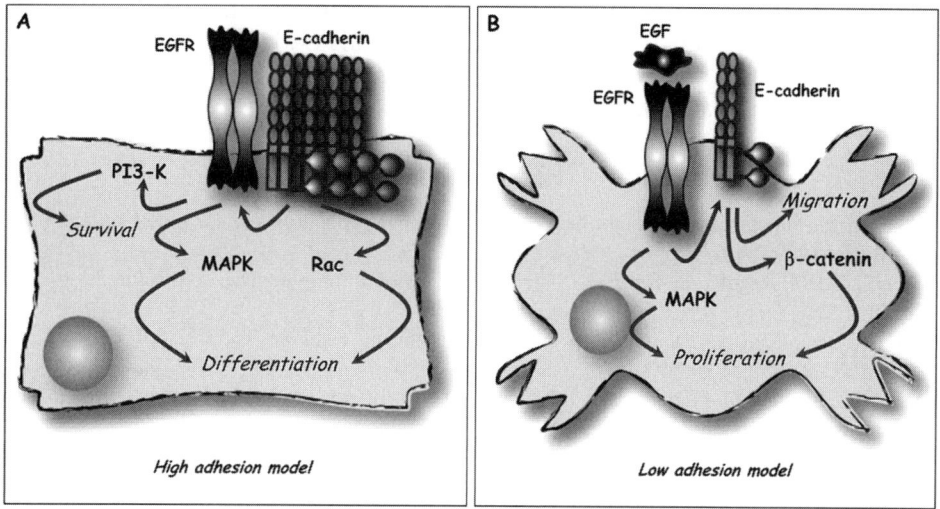

Fig. 10.5. The E-cadherin/EGFR Axis in the Epithelial Biology. The EGFR/E-cadherin signaling axis participates in the epithelial biology and might respond to environmental changes such as cell density and growth factors availability. (A) Under high cell density and high adhesion, E-cadherin complexes form stable complexes at the plasma membrane together with EGFR. In this case, the E-cadherin/EGFR complex can transduce intracellular signaling (MAPK, Rac, PI3-K) in the absence of EGFR ligands. This signaling cascade may promote differentiation and survival of the epithelium. (B) Under a low cell density situation, E-cadherin does not provide molecular scaffold enabling EGFR signaling. In contrast, the stimulation of EGFR by its ligand can trigger local phosphorylation cascades (MAPK), leading to cadherin destabilization and downregulation. Ultimately, β-catenin can be released and trigger cell cycle progression, in addition to proliferative signals initiated by the EGF/EGFR signaling pathway. The loss of E-cadherin adhesion contributes to EMT and the acquisition of a pro-migratory phenotype.

the stabilization of cell-cell contacts may subsequently switch-off the EGFR signaling by sequestering it in E-cadherin containing clusters (90, 94). This second level of E-cadherin/EGFR complexes may participate in the generation of survival and differentiation signals (95, 96) (Fig. 10.5). In this context of high adhesion and polarity of the epithelial cells, EGFR-ligand-based signal would lead to the destabilization of these E-cadherin/catenin/EGFR complexes and reinforcement of the proliferative and migratory potential of epithelial cells by reducing E-cadherin adhesion and releasing β-catenin (86). Ultimately, under physiological conditions this system is reversible and can still be turned-off by directing E-cadherin expression (58, 94).

5. CONCLUSION

E-cadherin is a major cell-cell adhesion molecule that regulates critical processes in the developmental morphogenesis of the epithelium in multicellular organisms, such as adhesion, polarity, differentiation, contact inhibition, and barrier function. Thus, subtle changes in E-cadherin expression, interactions, and localization have a broad impact as they can alter the overall physiology of the epithelium. E-cadherin function is indeed frequently altered in carcinoma and its reduced expression is frequently used as a diagnostic marker for cancer progression. It is not surprising that EGFR networks can modulate E-cadherin localization and expression, as well as the nature of its associated molecules. Emerging information, however, suggests that E-cadherin adhesive receptors can in turn initiate EGFR signaling, thus acting as a molecular sensor for cell density, polarity, migration, morphology, nutrient and growth factor availability. More extensive studies addressing the underlying molecular mechanisms are still required to assess the impact of EGFR/E-cadherin axis in tumor biology and cancer progression, which will surely help us to identify more effective EGFR-targeting strategies for cancer treatment.

REFERENCES

1. Takeichi M. Functional correlation between cell adhesive properties and some cell surface proteins. J Cell Biol 1977;75:464-74.
2. Gumbiner BM. Regulation of cadherin-mediated adhesion in morphogenesis. Nat Rev Mol Cell Biol 2005;6:622-34.
3. Nose A, Nagafuchi A, Takeichi M. Expressed recombinant cadherins mediate cell sorting in model systems. Cell 1988;54:993-1001.
4. Nagar B, Overduin M, Ikura M, Rini JM. Structural basis of calcium-induced E-cadherin rigidification and dimerization. Nature 1996;380: 360-4.
5. Leckband D, Prakasam A. MECHANISM AND DYNAMICS OF CADHERIN ADHESION. Annual Review of Biomedical Engineering 2006;8:259-87.
6. Pertz O, Bozic D, Koch AW, Fauser C, Brancaccio A, Engel J. A new crystal structure, Ca2+ dependence and mutational analysis reveal molecular details of E-cadherin homoassociation. Embo J 1999;18:1738-47.
7. Shapiro L, Fannon AM, Kwong PD, et al. Structural basis of cell-cell adhesion by cadherins. Nature 1995;374:327-37.
8. Chu YS, Thomas WA, Eder O, et al. Force measurements in E-cadherin-mediated cell doublets reveal rapid adhesion strengthened by actin cytoskeleton remodeling through Rac and Cdc42. J Cell Biol 2004;167:1183-94.
9. Perret E, Benoliel AM, Nassoy P, et al. Fast dissociation kinetics between individual E-cadherin fragments revealed by flow chamber analysis. Embo J 2002;21:2537-46.
10. Ozawa M, Baribault H, Kemler R. The cytoplasmic domain of the cell adhesion molecule uvomorulin associates with three independent proteins structurally related in different species. Embo J 1989;8:1711-7.
11. Mege RM, Gavard J, Lambert M. Regulation of cell-cell junctions by the cytoskeleton. Curr Opin Cell Biol 2006;18:541-8.

12. Kobielak A, Fuchs E. Alpha-catenin: at the junction of intercellular adhesion and actin dynamics. Nat Rev Mol Cell Biol 2004;5:614-25.
13. Nelson WJ, Nusse R. Convergence of Wnt, beta-catenin, and cadherin pathways. Science 2004;303:1483-7.
14. Huber AH, Weis WI. The Structure of the [beta]-Catenin/E-Cadherin Complex and the Molecular Basis of Diverse Ligand Recognition by [beta]-Catenin. Cell 2001;105(3):391.
15. Huber AH, Nelson WJ, Weis WI. Three-Dimensional Structure of the Armadillo Repeat Region of [beta]-Catenin. Cell 1997;90:871-82.
16. Gottardi CJ, Gumbiner BM. Distinct molecular forms of b-catenin are targeted to adhesive or transcriptional complexes. J Cell Biol 2004;167:339-49.
17. Sako Y, Nagafuchi A, Tsukita S, Takeichi M, Kusumi A. Cytoplasmic Regulation of the Movement of E-Cadherin on the Free Cell Surface as Studied by Optical Tweezers and Single Particle Tracking: Corralling and Tethering by the Membrane Skeleton. J Cell Biol 1998;140:1227-40.
18. Yap AS, Brieher WM, Gumbiner BM. Molecular and functional analysis of cadherin-based adherens junctions. Annu Rev Cell Dev Biol 1997;13:119-46.
19. Cattelino A, Liebner S, Gallini R, et al. The conditional inactivation of the b-catenin gene in endothelial cells causes a defective vascular pattern and increased vascular fragility. J Cell Biol 2003;162:1111-22.
20. Pece S, Chiariello M, Murga C, Gutkind JS. Activation of the Protein Kinase Akt/PKB by the Formation of E-cadherin-mediated Cell-Cell Junctions. EVIDENCE FOR THE ASSOCIATION OF PHOSPHATIDYLINOSITOL 3-KINASE WITH THE E-CADHERIN ADHESION COMPLEX. J Biol Chem 1999;274:19347-51.
21. Kuroda S, Fukata M, Nakagawa M, et al. Role of IQGAP1, a Target of the Small GTPases Cdc42 and Rac1, in Regulation of E-Cadherin- Mediated Cell-Cell Adhesion. Science 1998;281:832-5.
22. Gavard J, Mege RM. Once upon a time there was beta-catenin in cadherin-mediated signalling. Biol Cell 2005;97:921-6.
23. Vasioukhin V, Bauer C, Yin M, Fuchs E. Directed actin polymerization is the driving force for epithelial cell-cell adhesion. Cell 2000;100:209-19.
24. Drees F, Pokutta S, Yamada S, Nelson WJ, Weis WI. α-Catenin Is a Molecular Switch that Binds E-Cadherin-b-Catenin and Regulates Actin-Filament Assembly. Cell 2005;123:903-15.
25. Yamada S, Pokutta S, Drees F, Weis WI, Nelson WJ. Deconstructing the Cadherin-Catenin-Actin Complex. Cell 2005;123:889-911.
26. Kanner SB, Reynolds AB, Parsons JT. Tyrosine phosphorylation of a 120-kilodalton pp60src substrate upon epidermal growth factor and platelet-derived growth factor receptor stimulation and in polyomavirus middle-T-antigen-transformed cells. Mol Cell Biol 1991;11:713-20.
27. Reynolds AB, Roczniak-Ferguson A. Emerging roles for p120-catenin in cell adhesion and cancer. Oncogene 2004;23:7947-56.
28. Yanagisawa M, Kaverina IN, Wang A, Fujita Y, Reynolds AB, Anastasiadis PZ. A Novel Interaction between Kinesin and p120 Modulates p120 Localization and Function. J Biol Chem 2004;279:9512-21.
29. Chen X, Kojima S-i, Borisy GG, Green KJ. p120 catenin associates with kinesin and facilitates the transport of cadherin-catenin complexes to intercellular junctions. J Cell Biol 2003;163:547-57.
30. Anastasiadis PZ, Reynolds AB. Regulation of Rho GTPases by p120-catenin. Current Opinion in Cell Biology 2001;13:604-10.
31. Grosheva I, Shtutman M, Elbaum M, Bershadsky AD. p120 catenin affects cell motility via modulation of activity of Rho-family GTPases: a link between cell-cell contact formation and regulation of cell locomotion. J Cell Sci 2001;114:695-707.
32. Yanagisawa M, Anastasiadis PZ. p120 catenin is essential for mesenchymal cadherin-mediated regulation of cell motility and invasiveness. J Cell Biol 2006;174:1087-96.
33. Daniel JM, Reynolds AB. The Catenin p120ctn Interacts with Kaiso, a Novel BTB/POZ Domain Zinc Finger Transcription Factor. Mol Cell Biol 1999;19:3614-23.
34. Perez-Moreno M, Davis MA, Wong E, Pasolli HA, Reynolds AB, Fuchs E. p120-catenin mediates inflammatory responses in the skin. Cell 2006;124:631-44.
35. Yap AS, Kovacs EM. Direct cadherin-activated cell signaling: a view from the plasma membrane. J Cell Biol 2003;160:11-6.
36. Lilien J, Balsamo J. The regulation of cadherin-mediated adhesion by tyrosine phosphorylation/dephosphorylation of beta-catenin. Curr Opin Cell Biol 2005;17:459-65.
37. Marambaud P, Wen PH, Dutt A, et al. A CBP Binding Transcriptional Repressor Produced by the PS1/α-Cleavage of N-Cadherin Is Inhibited by PS1 FAD Mutations. Cell 2003;114:635-45.

38. Braga VMM, Yap AS. The challenges of abundance: epithelial junctions and small GTPase signalling. Current Opinion in Cell Biology 2005;17:466-74.
39. Kovacs EM, Ali RG, McCormack AJ, Yap AS. E-cadherin homophilic ligation directly signals through Rac and phosphatidylinositol 3-kinase to regulate adhesive contacts. J Biol Chem 2002;277:6708-18.
40. Gavard J, Lambert M, Grosheva I, et al. Lamellipodium extension and cadherin adhesion: two cell responses to cadherin activation relying on distinct signalling pathways. J Cell Sci 2004;117:257-70.
41. Thiery JP, Sleeman JP. Complex networks orchestrate epithelial-mesenchymal transitions. Nat Rev Mol Cell Biol 2006;7:131-42.
42. Vleminckx K, Vakaet L, Jr., Mareel M, Fiers W, van Roy F. Genetic manipulation of E-cadherin expression by epithelial tumor cells reveals an invasion suppressor role. Cell 1991;66:107-19.
43. St Croix B, Sheehan C, Rak JW, Florenes VA, Slingerland JM, Kerbel RS. E-Cadherin-dependent growth suppression is mediated by the cyclin-dependent kinase inhibitor p27(KIP1). J Cell Biol 1998;142:557-71.
44. Conacci-Sorrell M, Zhurinsky J, Ben-Ze'ev A. The cadherin-catenin adhesion system in signaling and cancer. J Clin Invest 2002;109:987-91.
45. Stemmler MP, Hecht A, Kinzel B, Kemler R. Analysis of regulatory elements of E-cadherin with reporter gene constructs in transgenic mouse embryos. Dev Dyn 2003;227:238-45.
46. Perl A-K, Wilgenbus P, Dahl U, Semb H, Christofori G. A causal role for E-cadherin in the transition from adenoma to carcinoma. Nature 1998;392:190-3.
47. Shi Y, Sawada J-i, Sui G, et al. Coordinated histone modifications mediated by a CtBP co-repressor complex. Nature 2003;422:735-8.
48. Peinado H, Ballestar E, Esteller M, Cano A. Snail mediates E-cadherin repression by the recruitment of the Sin3A/histone deacetylase 1 (HDAC1)/HDAC2 complex. Mol Cell Biol 2004;24:306-19.
49. Pece S, Gutkind JS. E-cadherin and Hakai: signalling, remodeling or destruction? Nat Cell Biol 2002;4: E72-4.
50. Roura S, Miravet S, Piedra J, de Herreros AG, Dunach M. Regulation of E-cadherin/Catenin Association by Tyrosine Phosphorylation. J Biol Chem 1999;274:36734-40.
51. Pizarro-Cerda J, Cossart P. Bacterial Adhesion and Entry into Host Cells. Cell 2006;124:715-27.
52. Ino Y, Gotoh M, Sakamoto M, Tsukagoshi K, Hirohashi S. Dysadherin, a cancer-associated cell membrane glycoprotein, down-regulates E-cadherin and promotes metastasis. PNAS 2002;99:365-70.
53. Holt CE, Lemaire P, Gurdon JB. Cadherin-mediated cell interactions are necessary for the activation of MyoD in Xenopus mesoderm. Proc Natl Acad Sci U S A 1994;91:10844-8.
54. Batlle E, Sancho E, Franci C, et al. The transcription factor snail is a repressor of E-cadherin gene expression in epithelial tumour cells. Nat Cell Biol 2000;2:84-9.
55. Cano A, Perez-Moreno MA, Rodrigo I, et al. The transcription factor snail controls epithelial-mesenchymal transitions by repressing E-cadherin expression. Nat Cell Biol 2000;2:76-83.
56. Comijn J, Berx G, Vermassen P, et al. The two-handed E box binding zinc finger protein SIP1 down-regulates E-cadherin and induces invasion. Mol Cell 2001;7:1267-78.
57. Takahashi K, Suzuki K. Density-dependent inhibition of growth involves prevention of EGF receptor activation by E-cadherin-mediated cell-cell adhesion. Exp Cell Res 1996;226:214-22.
58. Conacci-Sorrell M, Simcha I, Ben-Yedidia T, Blechman J, Savagner P, Ben-Ze'ev A. Autoregulation of E-cadherin expression by cadherin-cadherin interactions: the roles of {beta}-catenin signaling, Slug, and MAPK. J Cell Biol 2003;163:847-57.
59. Gottardi CJ, Wong E, Gumbiner BM. E-cadherin suppresses cellular transformation by inhibiting beta-catenin signaling in an adhesion-independent manner. J Cell Biol 2001;153:1049-60.
60. Wong AS, Gumbiner BM. Adhesion-independent mechanism for suppression of tumor cell invasion by E-cadherin. J Cell Biol 2003;161:1191-203.
61. Stockinger A, Eger A, Wolf J, Beug H, Foisner R. E-cadherin regulates cell growth by modulating proliferation-dependent b-catenin transcriptional activity. J Cell Biol 2001;154:1185-96.
62. Hazan RB, Qiao R, Keren R, Badano I, Suyama K. Cadherin switch in tumor progression. Ann N Y Acad Sci 2004;1014:155-63.
63. Islam S, Carey TE, Wolf GT, Wheelock MJ, Johnson KR. Expression of N-cadherin by human squamous carcinoma cells induces a scattered fibroblastic phenotype with disrupted cell-cell adhesion. J Cell Biol 1996;135:1643-54.
64. Nieman MT, Prudoff RS, Johnson KR, Wheelock MJ. N-Cadherin Promotes Motility in Human Breast Cancer Cells Regardless of their E-Cadherin Expression. J Cell Biol 1999;147:631-44.

65. Hazan RB, Phillips GR, Qiao RF, Norton L, Aaronson SA. Exogenous expression of N-cadherin in breast cancer cells induces cell migration, invasion, and metastasis. J Cell Biol 2000;148:779-90.
66. Kim J-B, Islam S, Kim YJ, et al. N-Cadherin Extracellular Repeat 4 Mediates Epithelial to Mesenchymal Transition and Increased Motility. J Cell Biol 2000;151:1193-206.
67. Fedor-Chaiken M, Meigs TE, Kaplan DD, Brackenbury R. Two Regions of Cadherin Cytoplasmic Domains Are Involved in Suppressing Motility of a Mammary Carcinoma Cell Line. J Biol Chem 2003;278:52371-8.
68. Suyama K, Shapiro I, Guttman M, Hazan RB. A signaling pathway leading to metastasis is controlled by N-cadherin and the FGF receptor. Cancer Cell 2002;2:301-14.
69. Kovacs EM, Goodwin M, Ali RG, Paterson AD, Yap AS. Cadherin-directed actin assembly: E-cadherin physically associates with the Arp2/3 complex to direct actin assembly in nascent adhesive contacts. Curr Biol 2002;12:379-82.
70. Vaezi A, Bauer C, Vasioukhin V, Fuchs E. Actin cable dynamics and Rho/Rock orchestrate a polarized cytoskeletal architecture in the early steps of assembling a stratified epithelium. Dev Cell 2002;3:367-81.
71. Chausovsky A, Bershadsky AD, Borisy GG. Cadherin-mediated regulation of microtubule dynamics. Nat Cell Biol 2000;2:797-804.
72. Pece S, Gutkind JS. Signaling from E-cadherins to the MAPK Pathway by the Recruitment and Activation of Epidermal Growth Factor Receptors upon Cell-Cell Contact Formation. J Biol Chem 2000;275:41227-33.
73. Carmeliet P, Lampugnani MG, Moons L, et al. Targeted deficiency or cytosolic truncation of the VE-cadherin gene in mice impairs VEGF-mediated endothelial survival and angiogenesis. Cell 1999;98:147-57.
74. Hoschuetzky H, Aberle H, Kemler R. Beta-catenin mediates the interaction of the cadherin-catenin complex with epidermal growth factor receptor. J Cell Biol 1994;127:1375-80.
75. Citri A, Yarden Y. EGF-ERBB signalling: towards the systems level. Nat Rev Mol Cell Biol 2006;7:505-16.
76. Ozawa M, Kemler R. Altered cell adhesion activity by pervanadate due to the dissociation of alpha-catenin from the E-cadherin.catenin complex. J Biol Chem 1998;273:6166-70.
77. Mariner DJ, Davis MA, Reynolds AB. EGFR signaling to p120-catenin through phosphorylation at Y228. J Cell Sci 2004;117:1339-50.
78. Pang JH, Kraemer A, Stehbens SJ, Frame MC, Yap AS. Recruitment of phosphoinositide 3-kinase defines a positive contribution of tyrosine kinase signaling to E-cadherin function. J Biol Chem 2005;280:3043-50.
79. Michalides R, Volberg T, Geiger B. Augmentation of adherens junction formation in mesenchymal cells by co-expression of N-CAM or short-term stimulation of tyrosine-phosphorylation. Cell Adhes Commun 1994;2:481-90.
80. Le TL, Yap AS, Stow JL. Recycling of E-cadherin: a potential mechanism for regulating cadherin dynamics. J Cell Biol 1999;146:219-32.
81. Paterson AD, Parton RG, Ferguson C, Stow JL, Yap AS. Characterization of E-cadherin endocytosis in isolated MCF-7 and chinese hamster ovary cells: the initial fate of unbound E-cadherin. J Biol Chem 2003;278:21050-7.
82. Kamei T, Matozaki T, Sakisaka T, et al. Coendocytosis of cadherin and c-Met coupled to disruption of cell-cell adhesion in MDCK cells--regulation by Rho, Rac and Rab small G proteins. Oncogene 1999;18:6776-84.
83. Palacios F, Schweitzer JK, Boshans RL, D'Souza-Schorey C. ARF6-GTP recruits Nm23-H1 to facilitate dynamin-mediated endocytosis during adherens junctions disassembly. Nat Cell Biol 2002;4: 929-36.
84. Gavard J, Gutkind JS. VEGF controls endothelial-cell permeability by promoting the beta-arrestin-dependent endocytosis of VE-cadherin. Nat Cell Biol 2006;8:1223-34.
85. Fujita Y, Krause G, Scheffner M, et al. Hakai, a c-Cbl-like protein, ubiquitinates and induces endocytosis of the E-cadherin complex. Nat Cell Biol 2002;4:222-31.
86. Lu Z, Ghosh S, Wang Z, Hunter T. Downregulation of caveolin-1 function by EGF leads to the loss of E-cadherin, increased transcriptional activity of b-catenin, and enhanced tumor cell invasion. Cancer Cell 2003;4:499-515.
87. Barth AIM, Nathke IS, Nelson WJ. Cadherins, catenins and APC protein: interplay between cytoskeletal complexes and signaling pathways. Current Opinion in Cell Biology 1997;9:683-90.
88. Anastasiadis PZ, Moon SY, Thoreson MA, et al. Inhibition of RhoA by p120 catenin. Nat Cell Biol 2000;2:637-44.

89. Betson M, Lozano E, Zhang J, Braga VM. Rac activation upon cell-cell contact formation is dependent on signaling from the epidermal growth factor receptor. J Biol Chem 2002;277:36962-9.
90. Qian X, Karpova T, Sheppard AM, McNally J, Lowy DR. E-cadherin-mediated adhesion inhibits ligand-dependent activation of diverse receptor tyrosine kinases. Embo J 2004;23:1739-48.
91. Fedor-Chaiken M, Hein PW, Stewart JC, Brackenbury R, Kinch MS. E-cadherin binding modulates EGF receptor activation. Cell Commun Adhes 2003;10:105-18.
92. Dumstrei K, Wang F, Shy D, Tepass U, Hartenstein V. Interaction between EGFR signaling and DE-cadherin during nervous system morphogenesis. Development 2002;129:3983-94.
93. Andl CD, Mizushima T, Nakagawa H, et al. Epidermal growth factor receptor mediates increased cell proliferation, migration, and aggregation in esophageal keratinocytes in vitro and in vivo. J Biol Chem 2003;278:1824-30.
94. Wilding J, Vousden KH, Soutter WP, McCrea PD, Del Buono R, Pignatelli M. E-cadherin transfection down-regulates the epidermal growth factor receptor and reverses the invasive phenotype of human papilloma virus-transfected keratinocytes. Cancer Res 1996;56:5285-92.
95. Singh AB, Harris RC. Epidermal growth factor receptor activation differentially regulates claudin expression and enhances transepithelial resistance in Madin-Darby canine kidney cells. J Biol Chem 2004;279:3543-52.
96. Lorch JH, Klessner J, Park JK, et al. Epidermal growth factor receptor inhibition promotes desmosome assembly and strengthens intercellular adhesion in squamous cell carcinoma cells. J Biol Chem 2004;279:37191-200.

11 Crosstalk Between Insulin-like Growth Factor (IGF) and Epidermal Growth Factor (EGF) Receptors

Marc A. Becker and Douglas Yee

CONTENTS

IGF & EGF SYSTEMS
IGF/EGF LIGANDS
IGF/EGF RECEPTORS
DOWNSTREAM SIGNALING
CO-TARGETING EGF/IGF
FUTURE PERSPECTIVES
REFERENCES

Abstract

Growth factors induce a multitude of responses integral to development and sustained physiological function in most normal tissues. Binding of growth factors to the epidermal growth factor (EGF) and insulin-like growth factor (IGF) transmembrane tyrosine kinase receptors activates downstream intracellular signaling pathways vital to both the normal and malignant cellular phenotype. Dysregulation of either one of these receptor-regulated pathways has been linked to aberrant modulations in proliferation, motility, and protection from apoptosis. More importantly, crosstalk between EGFR and IGF-IR has been implicated in a number of cancers and correlates with tumor grade and disease progression. The following review addresses the most recent findings involving EGF and IGF receptor crosstalk and how this interaction may impact clinical therapeutic efficacy.

Key Words: EGFR, IGF-IR, crosstalk, cancer, MAPK, PI3K.

1. IGF & EGF SYSTEMS

The insulin-like growth factor (IGF) system plays a vital role in normal physiological development and function in a host of tissues. This system is comprised of IGF ligands (insulin, IGF-I, IGF-II), receptors, binding proteins (IGF binding proteins 1–6), and binding-protein proteases (*1*). To date, numerous studies have shown that the IGF system possesses potent mitogenic and antiapoptotic properties and may therefore provide an important function in the pathophysiology of human disorders (*2–6*). IGF signaling is associated with the development and propagation of several aspects of tumor biology such as angiogenesis, proliferation, migration, invasion, and resistance to apoptosis. In the context of cancer, disruption of IGF signaling has antitumor properties in several distinct malignancies including mammary, prostate, hepatic, pancreatic, ovarian, colorectal and non-small cell lung cancer (NSCLC) to name a few (7–13). Therefore, targeting the IGF system through small molecule inhibitors and monoclonal antibodies would be a logical therapeutic approach. Inhibition of IGF signaling could cooperate and possibly synergize with other anti-cancer therapies, including cytotoxic chemotherapy, radiation, and other targeted drugs. This may in part result from a cooperative interplay between the IGF system and tyrosine kinase receptors sharing similar downstream signaling targets, namely the EGF system.

The type I IGF receptor (IGF-IR) is composed of two extracellular α-subunits responsible for ligand binding (IGF-I) and two membrane spanning β-subunits linked by disulfide bonds. When ligands bind the extracellular α-subunits, a conformational change occurs between the intracellular domains resulting in tyrosine kinase activity with resultant trans-autophosphorylation of the β-subunits at specific tyrosine residues. Phosphorylated receptor triggers the association of a multitude of intermediate docking proteins, including Shc, PI3K, Grb2, and various insulin receptor substrate isoforms (IRS-1, IRS-2). Subsequent activation of the mitogen-activated protein kinase (MAPK) cascade and phosphatidylinositol-3 kinase (PI3K) pathway ensues and alters cellular proliferation, metastatic behavior, as well as protects from apoptosis. A second receptor binds IGF-II with high affinity. This type II IGF receptor (IGF-IIR) does not appear to possess tyrosine kinase activity and will not be discussed here in great detail.

The epidermal growth factor (EGF) system also plays an important role in cell proliferation, survival, adhesion, migration, and differentiation (14). The system namely functions through four types of transmembrane tyrosine kinase receptors, including EGFR (HER1/ErbB1), HER2 (ErbB2/neu), HER3 (ErbB3) and HER4 (ErbB4) (15) (see also Chapter 2). Expression of the EGF receptor (EGFR) occurs in cells from the epithelial and mesenchymal lineages (16). Aberrant overexpression, mutation, and dysregulation of the EGF receptor (EGFR) occur frequently in a number of human malignancies. EGFR-positive tumors are reported in the majority of head and neck cancer cases, as well as in bladder, brain, breast, cervical, uterine, colon, esophageal, glioma, non-small-cell lung cancer (NSCLC), ovarian, pancreatic, and renal cell cancer (17–19) (see also Chapter 16).

EGFR activation initiates a myriad of intracellular signal transduction events frequently overlapping with those downstream of the IGF system, including the MAPK and PI3K pathways. Several studies have identified interactions between IGF-IR and EGFR that may affect cancer cell biology and serve as a point of therapeutic intervention.

2. IGF/EGF LIGANDS

Stimulation of receptor and downstream signaling components occurs primarily via the extracellular interaction between the IGF ligands and IGF-IR. Both IGF-I and IGF-II are abundantly present in the circulating blood of newborn infants and animal fetuses and levels directly correlate with birth size (20). During *in utero* development, fetal tissues are highly responsive to IGF stimulation and also express IGF-IR. After birth, hepatic expression of IGF-I is highly regulated by growth hormone and accounts for the linear growth of the skeleton during puberty, although IGF-I expression occurs ubiquitously throughout the body.

Just as IGF-IR regulates the growth and development of normal tissues, this receptor signaling system has been shown to play a key role in the development of the malignant phenotype. Signaling pathways emanating from the IGF-I/IGF-IR interaction affect cancer cell proliferation, adhesion, migration, and apoptosis (21–23). The downstream signaling components of the IGF-IR share several common targets related to EGFR (24, 25). Activation of both EGFR and IGF-IR can lead to the association of multiple adaptor molecules, including Shc, Grb-2, Sos, and p85. Upon association, adaptor proteins may lead to activation of

Ras/MAPK, Src/integrin crosstalk, JNK, and PI3K/Akt. In addition, EGF treatment increases the expression of IRS-1 and IRS-2 in breast carcinoma cell lines (26). Therefore, the mitogenic actions elicited by IGFs activation of IGF-IR activity could potentially influence EGF-mediated signaling and biology via activation of common pathways. Similarly, the EGF system may also influence components of the IGF system.

IGF and EGF ligands are essential for the growth of the mammary epithelium during development. In normal fibroblasts, EGF signaling requires a functional IGF-IR, suggesting a potential link between the two pathways (27). Mitogen-regulated cell cycle progression involves the induction of cyclin proteins that allow cells to transition through the G1 to S and G2 to M checkpoints. Unregulated proliferation and tumorigenesis can result from deregulated or overexpressed cyclins. Both IGF-I and EGF induce cyclin D1 in a number of normal and tumor cell lines (28–32). When combined with EGF, IGF-I treatment resulted in a synergistic promotion of DNA synthesis *in vitro* in mammary epithelial cells of C57Bl6/J mice cultured from the intact mammary gland (33). Furthermore, while both IGF and EGF were capable of inducing early G1 cyclins, presence of IGF-I was essential during the EGF-mediated progression of mammary epithelial cells into S phase in the intact mouse mammary gland.

Angiogenesis is required for tumor growth and cytokines and growth factors influence this process. IGF-II is highly expressed in tumors and has been recognized as an important angiogenic factor during solid tumor progression (34–36). EGF has also been linked to angiogenesis in a number of cancers, most notably in hepatocellular carcinoma (HCC) (37). When EGF and IGF-II were combined *in vivo*, angiogenic activity was synergistically increased as compared to IGF-II alone (38). Co-treatment of IGF-II and EGF resulted in a significant induction of functional new vessels as measured by Matrigel plug assay. Fibroblast growth factor (FGF) is another potent inducer of angiogenesis, and its expression was up-regulated in response to EGF/IGF-II cotreatment *in vivo*. In addition, EGF has been shown to down-regulate hypoxia-induced IGF-II binding protein-3 (IGFBP-3), a molecule responsible for binding to and inhibiting the action of IGF-II thereby preventing interaction and activation of IGF-IR (39). Thus, linked networks of growth factor action regulate several key aspects of tumor biology.

As previously mentioned, activation of IGF-IR by IGF initiates the association of the intracellular IRS signaling molecules to IGF-IR. With at least four IRS isoforms known to exist, studies involving IRS-1 and IRS-2 knockout mice greatly emphasize the impact of these two isoforms on normal physiologic function, as well as on tumor biology (40–42). Upon association with activated IGF-IR, IRS-1, and IRS-2 are rapidly phosphorylated at multiple tyrosine residues and present as docking sites for a multitude of Src homology 2 domain-containing proteins (Grb2, Nck/Crk, SHP2, Syp and the p85 regulatory subunit of PI3K) (43). The association of these proteins with IRS-1 and IRS-2 results in the activation of the EGFR-related Ras/Raf/MEK/MAPK and PI3K/Akt pathways, further suggesting that crosstalk may occur between the IGF/EGF systems.

The stimulation and duration of MAPK activation by various growth factors, including EGF and IGF, impact cellular proliferation, differentiation, and DNA synthesis (44–48). Previous work demonstrated that EGF and IGF differentially modulate Erk2 activation in mouse embryo derived 3T3-like cells when IGF-IR was homozygously deleted (R-) from wild-type cells (W) (49). Stimulation of quiescent normal cells with IGF-1, EGF or in combination induced both a maximal transient and a prolonged activation of ERK2 not seen in R- cells. R- Erk2 activation was restored to that of normal cells level upon reintroduction with wild-type human IGF-IR. This underlines the importance of not only a functional receptor, but suggests that a functional interplay may occur between EGF and IGF modulate and modulate downstream signaling activation.

3. IGF/EGF RECEPTORS

3.1. Receptor Co-expression/localization and Links to Disease Progression

Investigators have suggested that expression of the EGFR and IGFR are linked and that the EGFR/IGFR ratio may serve as a more sensitive prognostic indicator of tumor phenotype and therapeutic response than expression of single receptor alone (50). EGFR, HER2, and IGF-IR receptor are co-expressed in roughly 75% of colorectal tumor samples (51). While no statistical association was found between the expression or co-expression of total IGF-IR, EGFR, and HER2 and clinicopathological parameters or overall survival, further investigation of a wider spectrum of human tumors is warranted.

In a transgenic model, HK1.IGF-I mice overexpressing IGF-I in the epidermis via the human keratin 1 promoter displayed increases in the occurrence of skin tumors (52). Upon analysis of IGF-IR and EGFR activation, it was discovered that increased EGFR and IGF-IR tyrosine phosphorylation occurred in the epidermis suggesting cooperation between these two pathways in disease pathogenesis.

Both EGFR and IGF-IR correlate with the induction and progression of osteogenic and soft tissue sarcomas (STS) (53). Human sarcoma cells derived from surgical specimens of both primary and metastatic tumors were evaluated for the expression and function of EGFR and IGF-IR in order to establish a role for ligand-mediated receptor activation during sarcoma progression. A number of STS clones originating from an unclassified sarcoma lung metastasis, malignant fibrous histiocytoma lung metastasis, and dedifferentiated chondrosarcoma showed elevated steady-state levels of EGFR and IGF-IR mRNA transcripts and total protein. These increases correlated to receptor-specific tyrosine kinase activity and autophosphorylation in response to EGF and IGF-I ligand. Substantial increases in DNA synthesis and mitogenesis resulted from EGF treatment, while exposure to IGF-I showed a variable growth response that correlated with tumor origin. Recent findings reveal that IGF-1R expression is a common feature of highly malignant STS and a significant association was shown between high expression of IGF-1R and unfavorable outcome (54). These data support the involvement of EGFR and IGF-IR expression in the growth and metastasis of human soft tissue sarcoma.

Other studies suggest that the relationship between IGF-IR and EGFR expression is complex. A recent study evaluating the clinical relevance of IGF-IR expression within the context of patients following a trastuzumab-based therapy revealed that IGF-IR expression was not an accurate predictive measure for resistance to trastuzumab-based treatment in patients with HER2/neu overexpressing metastatic breast cancer (55). Neither IHC staining patterns nor intensity of tumor specimens from 72 patients receiving trastuzumab-based treatment identified an existing correlation between IGF-IR levels and biological tumor characteristics and/or clinical course of disease. However, the level of IGF-IR expression has not been linked to the biological function of this receptor, so it is uncertain whether levels of IGF-IR alone could serve a useful biomarker. In addition, the correlation between IGF-IR by immunohistochemical methods and number of cellular binding sites for the IGF ligands has not been established.

In addition to total expression, intracellular localization of the receptors is an important consideration in disease progression and severity. In the case of pancreatic cancer, both IGF-IR and EGFR have been shown to be frequently overexpressed and receptor localization mapped. Resected primary tumors from patients with primary invasive ductal pancreatic carcinoma were examined, and in lower-grade tumors from individuals diagnosed with a more favorable prognosis, EGFR predominantly localized to the membrane and IGF-IR to the cytoplasm. Analysis of higher-grade tumors from patients with a poor prognosis revealed a cytoplasm-dominant EGFR and membrane-dominant IGF-IR (56). An autopsy of hepatic metastatic tumors indicated that incidences of both IGF-IR and EGFR overexpression were significantly higher than in primary tumors alone.

Findings herein support the notion that tumor progression is not only a process involving aberrant regulation of gene expression, but that a dynamic interplay occurs between IGF-IR/EGFR levels and subcellular localization and fluctuations occur throughout the diseased state. These transient changes may further the link to tumor progression from a malignant to metastatic state.

3.2. EGFR/IGFR Crosstalk and Heterodimerization Contribute to Resistance

IGF-IR and EGFR act as regulators of a number of growth factor and mitogen-activated signaling pathways. While different molecules and downstream targets associate depending on receptor type, PI3K and MAPK are regarded as the primary signaling molecules of both pathways. Therefore, it is logical to postulate that EGFR and IGF-IR have the ability to develop a crosstalk that may contribute to the biological activity of a tumor.

Acquired resistance to tamoxifen is a common problem during the treatment of breast cancer. Recently, *in vitro* studies have suggested that signaling of the EGFR productively crosstalks to activate IGF-1R and in specific scenarios may activate estrogen receptor (ER) to alter the transcriptional activity through a number of key activating factor (AF-1) serine residues (57). These effects might facilitate an acquired resistance to tamoxifen.

Resistance to drug intervention may occur via a compensatory mechanism involving the non-targeted receptor, wherein either overexpression and/or activity may be altered. When EGFR/HER2 was targeted in breast cancer cells *in vitro* via administration of the antibody trastuzumab, resistance was induced as evidenced by increased signal transduction through ligand-dependent activation of IGF-IR (58). Furthermore, the ability of IGF-IR to confer resistance to trastuzumab involved targeting of p27Kip1, an inhibitor of cell cycle progression, to proteasomal-mediated degradation by ubiquitination. Targeting of p27Kip1 occurs through the up-regulation of the Skp2 ubiquitin ligase and predominantly activates the IGF-IR-linked PI3K leading to resistance. IGF-IR overexpression in HER2 sensitive cells resulted in interference with the antineoplastic action of trastuzumab and to a certain extent facilitated resistance (59). In MCF-7/HER2–18 cells, which overexpressed HER2/neu receptors and expressed IGF-IR receptors, trastuzumab inhibited proliferation (42%) only when IGF-IR signaling was nominal. When HER2 overexpressing SKBR3 cells (low IGF-IR levels) were treated with trastuzumab, proliferation was markedly reduced, regardless of IGF-I concentration. As expected, when these cells were genetically altered to overexpress IGF-IR and cultured with IGF-I, trastuzumab had no attenuating effects on proliferation.

The first evidence for crosstalk between the IGF-IR and EGFR was provided from studies investigating the effects of ZD1839, a selective inhibitor of EGFR tyrosine kinase activity, on MAPK- and PI3K-induced inhibition of the proapoptotic BH3 only protein BAD (60). It was suggested that IGF-I-induced activated IGF-IR was capable of transactivating EGFR in mammary epithelial cells to enhance BAD phosphorylation by MAPK and subsequently protect from apoptosis. Others have demonstrated that within C4HD epithelial breast cancer cells there exists a hierarchical interaction that occurs between IGF-IR and ErbB2 (61). Evidence of IGF-IR directing ErbB2/HER2 phosphorylation suggested that the hierarchical interaction involved a physical association of both receptors in order to result in the formation of a heteromeric complex capable of activating downstream signaling factors. Furthermore, when IGF-IR expression was suppressed by antisense oligodeoxynucleotides (ASODNs) a total loss of synthetic progestin medroxyprogesterone acetate (MPA)-induced HER2 phosphorylation was measured and suggested that HER2 activation required IGF-1R expression. In addition, *in vivo* C4HD breast cancer proliferation was directly inhibited by both intratumoral and intravenous delivery of IGF-IR antisense message (*62*). Not only was MAPK and PI3K activation blocked, but HER-2 tyrosine phosphorylation was abrogated. These results demonstrated for the first time that *in vivo* down-regulation of IGF-IR via antisense can inhibit breast cancer growth and further supports the strategy of dual-targeted therapy to disrupt the multiple cooperative signaling pathways associated with tumor pathology.

In SKBR3-derived trastuzumab-resistant cells HER2 uniquely interacted with IGF-IR, a phenomenon that was not seen in the parental trastuzumab-sensitive cells (*63*). IGF-I induced HER2 activation in resistant but not parental cells. Inhibition of IGF-IR kinase activity resulted in decreased HER2 phosphorylation in resistant cells. Moreover, EGFR/IGFR heterodimer disruption by the anti-IGF-IR antibody alpha-IR3 and anti-HER2 antibody pertuzumab restored sensitivity to trastuzumab in resistant breast cancer cells. Thus, IGF-IR may be a substrate for HER2 when cells are selected for resistance.

Resistance to TKIs in NSCLC is a common theme that may in part be mediated through the actions of IGF-IR. A number of NSCLC lines demonstrated increased EGFR/IGF-IR membrane-localized heterodimerization in response to prolonged treatment with the EGFR TKI erlotinib. In these cells, erlotinib treatment resulted in up-regulated IGF-IR activation as measured by analysis of downstream signaling components (*64*). In addition, acquired resistance to erlotinib stimulated *de novo* synthesis of EGFR and survivin through the translational activity of the downstream Akt target mammalian target of rapamycin (mTOR). When mTOR was suppressed, IGF-IR activation inhibited, or survivin expression knocked down, resistance to erlotinib was reversed and apoptosis of NSCLC cells was induced both *in vitro* and *in vivo*. These data suggest that the IGF-IR/HER2 heterodimer contribution to resistance justifies the need for further studies examining and targeting this complex as a potential therapeutic target in resistant tumors progressing during drug therapy.

4. DOWNSTREAM SIGNALING

Controlling the available level of IRS protein is one means by which a cell modulates IGF signal transduction. A negative feedback loop between the presence of IGF-I and IRS-1 protein degradation has been established in MCF-7 human breast carcinoma cells (*65*). Exposure to prolonged IGF-I results in the ligand-mediated degradation of IRS-1 via the ubiquitin-mediated 26S proteasome and a PI3K-dependent mechanism (*66*). IGF-1 treatment in prostate epithelial cells also targets IRS-1 to the proteasome for degradation. However, when EGF was present, IGF-I-mediated degradation of IRS-1 was prevented, thereby supporting the notion that EGFR activation enhances IGF-IR signaling by modulating protein levels of IRS-1 and may be an important consideration in tumors possessing activating mutations in EGFR.

Ligand activation of EGFR can also enhance IGF-IR signaling. In MCF-7 cells EGF increased IRS-1 protein levels in a MAPK-dependent but PI3K-dependent manner (*67*). As previously mentioned, induction of IRS expression via EGF extends to both IRS-1 and IRS-2 (*68*). EGF up-regulation of IRS-1 involved both extracellular signal-regulated kinase (MAPK) and c-Jun NH(2)-terminal kinase (JNK) signaling pathways. However, induction of IRS-2 expression by EGF was specifically mediated by JNK signaling. In addition to EGF-enhanced IGF-I-mediated tyrosine phosphorylation of IRS, inhibiting IRS-2 up-regulation ablated the EGF enhancement of cell motility. This suggests that increases in IRS-2 are important in the EGF regulation of breast cancer cell migration and may extend to additional malignant phenotypes.

5. CO-TARGETING EGF/IGF

Strategies to target the IGF system are predicated on the requirement of a ligand-receptor interaction to occur in order to trigger the signaling cascades that influence cancer biology. These strategies share some similarities with the EGF system, but differ in that inhibition of ligand production or ligand interaction with IGF-IR may be reasonable methods to disrupt signaling, while EGFR family members may be activated by overexpression alone, obviating a need for EGF ligands. Reducing the quantity of available IGFs and neutralization of IGF action by IGFBPs or antibodies may all be effective anti-IGF strategies, while ligand neutralization is less important in the EGF system. Disruption of receptor function through monoclonal antibodies, inhibition of receptor biochemical activity via small molecule tyrosine kinase inhibitors, antisense oligonucleotides, and targeting of downstream signaling pathways are strategies shared by the EGF and IGF systems (*69, 70*). Given the possibility of cooperativity and shared signaling pathways between the two systems, simultaneously targeting of the EGF and IGF systems may be more effective than targeting either system alone. Small molecule inhibitors and monoclonal antibodies that selectively inhibit either EGFR or IGF-IR have to date predominated as effective treatments in cotargeting strategies.

5.1. EGFR/IGFR Small Molecule Inhibitors

In malignant gliomas, EGFR overexpression is commonly observed and tumors that originate from glial tissue constitute some of the most aggressive and treatment-refractory tumors encountered in the clinic (*71, 72*). Blockade of EGF signaling at the level of the receptor enhanced apoptosis, attenuated metastatic behavior, and reduced angiogenic potential (*73–75*). Despite evidence of a similar anti-EGFR effect at the level of receptor as measured by phosphorylated EGFR, differing sensitivities to the EGFR inhibitor AG1478 was not dependent on the level of EGFR in glioblastoma multiforme (GBM) cells (*76*). Analysis revealed that GBM cells resistant to AG1478 responded to treatment by up-regulation of IGF-IR expression and a subsequent sustained increase in PI3K activity. This phenomenon was absent in AG1478-sensitive GBM cells. When IGF-IR and EGFR were co-targeted with AG1024 and AG1478, resistant cells experienced both spontaneous and radiation-induced apoptosis, as well as a reduction in the invasive potential.

Additional observations of a sensitization towards CD95L-induced cell death by combined EGFR/IGF-IR inhibition in human malignant glioma cells adds to the previous study reporting enhanced apoptotic effects of EGFR/IGF-IR co-inhibition in response to ionizing radiation and suggests that multiple death stimuli may be involved during sensitization (*77*). Detectable caspase 8 cleavage was enhanced following combined treatment of AG1478 and AG1024 in comparison to either inhibitor alone and the addition of crm-8, a potent caspase 8 inhibitor, abrogated cell death. As previously mentioned, activation of the PI3K-Akt-pathway is thought to play a key role during survival. However, wortmannin-induced PI3K inhibition did not sensitize LNT-229 and U87MG glioma cells to CD95L-induced apoptosis (*78*). Ribosomal protein S6 (RPS6), an important positive regulator of translation and survival, represents a target that is influenced by both the Akt and MAPK pathways, and while it was primarily phosphorylated through the PI3K/Akt/mTOR pathway, complete activation was facilitated through the MAPK pathway (*79*). Combining AG1478 and AG1024 resulted in a synergistic inhibition of RPS6 phosphorylation and in turn markedly increased apoptotic induction.

Phase II clinical trials employing the EGFR inhibitor gefitinib as a second- or third-line monotherapy in NSCLC and head and neck cancer patients revealed tumor response rates ranging between 9% and 19% (*80–83*). Unfortunately, gefitinib response rates in phase II clinical trials of advanced breast cancer patients elicited a measurable therapeutic response in fewer than 10% of patients (*84–86*). Influence from the IGF system may again be responsible for resistance to monotherapy. When AG1024 and gefitinib were combined to inhibit IGF-IR and EGFR activity *in vitro* in human breast cancer cell lines expressing similar levels of IGF-1R and varying levels of EGFR, an additive or synergistic response resulted as measured by growth inhibition and apoptosis (*87*). When MCF-7-derived tamoxifen resistant breast cancer cells were chronically exposed to a previously established effective inhibitory dose of gefitinib, a sustained growth inhibition (90%) resulted over a period of four months until surviving cells resumed proliferation (*88*). The tamoxifen/gefitinib resistant cell line (TAM/TKI-R) exhibited increased IGF activity as measured by increased IGF-IR, Akt, and protein kinase C (PKC) phosphorylation, increased growth inhibition in response to AG1024, and marked increases in migration in response to IGF-I and IGF-II treatment that was attenuated following AG1024 challenge. In addition, the EGFR-positive androgen-independent human prostate cancer cell line DU145 displayed comparably similar responses as compared with breast cancer cell line counterparts. These studies support the notion that increased activity of the EGF/IGF pathways may be responsible for acquired resistance to small molecule inhibitors targeting EGFR/IGFR and play a role in the proliferative and metastatic behavior associated with the malignant phenotype.

5.2. EGFR/IGFR Monoclonal Antibodies

Targeted therapies provide a new therapeutic approach in the treatment of cancer. Rather than eliminating both malignant and normal cells nonspecifically, these so-called "rational" therapies exploit second messenger proteins, ligands, and receptors that are known to be regulate the malignant phenotype in neoplastic cells (*89*). Monoclonal antibodies that specifically bind to EGFR and IGF-IR are emerging as a highly effective strategy in a wide variety of malignancies.

Breast cancer cells overexpressing HER2 respond favorably to the humanized anti-HER2 monoclonal antibody trastuzumab (Herceptin). Unfortunately, resistance is again an all-too-common adverse side effect to prolonged exposure and therapeutic options are narrowed as a result. Transfecting HER2/ErbB2-overexpressing MCF7HER18 breast cancer cells with an inducible dominant-negative form of IGF-IR severely limited downstream IGF signaling activation (*90*). More importantly, combining trastuzumab treatment with induction of dominant-negative IGF-IR expression potentiated growth inhibition *in vitro*. The humanized antibody h7C10 directed against IGF-IR significantly inhibited breast and NSCLC tumor cell proliferation both *in vitro* and *in vivo* (*91*). Decreased signal transduction, disruption of normal cell cycle progression, and receptor down-regulation may represent possible mechanisms that facilitate growth inhibition. In addition, when both the human and murine form of the antibody was combined with the EGFR targeting antibody 225, markedly enhanced antitumor activity resulted.

Overexpression of IGF-IR and its ligands occurs frequently in a number of human breast tumors and increases in IGF-I, reduced IGFBP-3, or an increased ratio of IGF-I to IGFBP-3 in the circulation has been linked with development of breast cancer (*92–94*). Recombinant human IGF binding protein 3 (rhIGFBP-3) acts as an antagonist of IGF-IR signaling by neutralizing IGF ligands (*95*). rhIGFBP-3 potentiated the activity of trastuzumab in both trastuzumab-resistant MCF-7/HER2-overexpressing human breast tumor cells *in vitro* and more importantly against advanced-stage MCF-7/HER2–18-transfected human breast cancer xenografts. In addition, the IGF-IR activation responsible for countering the early suppressive effect of trastuzumab on HER-2 signaling through Akt and MAPK was attenuated through rhIGFBP-3 administration. Loss of IGF-IR activation restored trastuzumab-induced reductions in Akt and MAPK phosphorylation *in vitro* and *in vivo*.

The therapeutic potential of monoclonal antibodies is promising due to specificity toward antigens pertaining to cancer cells. Efficacy is reduced by limited intrinsic cytotoxic activity and antibodies targeting tumors are most effective when used either in combination with another antibody or as an adjuvant to conventional chemotherapy regimens (96–100). Development of bispecific (BsAb) or multispecific antibodies targeting multiple tumor-associated antigens simultaneously may provide a novel and promising means of targeting multiple pathways concurrently (101). A BsAb that targets both the IGFR and EGFR was constructed using two neutralizing antibodies as building blocks (one directed against EGFR and the other against IGF-IR). The BsAb molecules were capable of binding to EGFR and IGFR to block the activation of downstream signaling molecules of both pathways as efficiently as the parental monospecific IgG antibodies. Actions of the BsAb were unique in that it was able to target two tumor-associated molecules (EGFR and IGF-IR) on single or adjacent tumor cells and simultaneously block activation of both receptors to enhance antitumor activity *in vitro* in a number of different cancer cell lines. Similarly, the recombinant human IgG-like BsAb, known as a Di-diabody, can be produced using the variable regions from two antagonistic antibodies of EGFR and IGF-IR that not only bind to both EGFR and IGF-IR, but effectively blocks *in vitro* EGF- and IGF-stimulated receptor activation and tumor cell proliferation (102). Finally, the Di-diabody triggered IGF-IR internalization and degradation, facilitated antibody-dependent cellular cytotoxicity (ADCC), and strongly inhibited the growth of human colorectal and pancreatic tumor xenografts in vivo.

6. FUTURE PERSPECTIVES

A number of significant advances have been made in the mechanistic elucidation of both the EGF and IGF system. As with many areas of investigation, these systems have been primarily studied in isolation. As noted, there are emerging data demonstrating the cooperation between these two systems in cancer cells. Certainly, both receptor systems activate similar signaling pathways related to tumor biology, and different model systems demonstrate that inhibition of either or both pathways can effectively inhibit tumor growth.

However, a number of questions remain regarding whether these pre-clinical observations have relevance to the low and often unpredictable response rates to therapies targeting only one system. Determining the specifics that guide EGFR/IGFR crosstalk during tumor cell initiation, progression and resistance is vital to further advancing strategies to target the EGF/IGF systems. Resistance to anti-EGFR therapy has emerged as a recurring theme in a number of cancers. In several model systems, resistance to EGFR family member inhibitors is due to activation of IGF-IR signaling events. Given the fact that these two receptors share similar signaling components, this was expected to a certain extent. In selected cases, tumor cells that are initially dependent upon EGFR modulate IGF-IR expression and activity when EGFR induction is no longer available. Since IGF-IR inhibitors are just now entering clinical trials, it will be important to see if IGF-IR resistance is due to activation of EGFR signaling. In any case, *de novo* or acquired resistance to a single inhibitor might be overcome by simultaneously blocking both pathways. Hopefully, further development of small molecule inhibitors, monoclonal antibodies, and other agents specifically targeting the EGF/IGF crosstalk network will lead to substantial improvements in therapeutic efficacy and improve patient outcome.

REFERENCES

1. Le Roith D. Seminars in medicine of the Beth Israel Deaconess Medical Center. Insulin-like growth factors. N Engl J Med 1997;336:633-40.
2. LeRoith D, Roberts CT. Insulin-like growth factors and their receptors in normal physiology and pathological states. J Pediatr Endocrinol 1993;6:251-255.
3. Lee AV, Hilsenbeck SG, Yee D. IGF system components as prognostic markers in breast cancer. Breast Cancer Res Treat 1998;47:295-302.

4. Hassan AB, Macaulay VM. The insulin-like growth factor system as a therapeutic target in colorectal cancer. Ann Oncol 2002;13:349-56.
5. Zofkova I. Pathophysiological and clinical importance of insulin-like growth factor-I with respect to bone metabolism. Physiol Res 2003;53:657-79.
6. Favoni RE, de Cupis A, Ravera F, Cantoni C, Pirani P, Ardizzoni A, Noonan D, Biassoni R. Expression and function of the insulin-like growth factor I system in human non-small-cell lung cancer and normal lung cell lines. Int J Cancer 1994;56:858-866.
7. Bonnette SG, Hadsell DL. Targeted disruption of the IGF-I receptor gene deceases cellular proliferation in mammary terminal end buds. Endocrinology 2001;142:4937-45.
8. Damon SE, Plymate SR, Carroll JM, Sprenger CC, Dechsukhum C, Ware JL, Roberts CT. Transcriptional regulation of insulin-like growth factor-I receptor gene expression in prostate cancer cells. Endocrinology 2001;142:21-7.
9. Alexia C, Fallot G, Lasfer M, Schweizer-Groyer G, Groyer A. An evaluation of the role of insulin-like growth factors (IGF) and of type-I IGF receptor signaling in hepatocarcinogenesis and in the resistance of hepatocarcinoma cells against drug-induced apoptosis. Biochem Pharmacol 2004;68:1003-15.
10. Stoeltzing O, Liu W, Reinmuth N, Fan F, Parikh AA, Bucana CD, Evans DB, Semenza GL, Ellis LM. Regulation of hypoxia-inducible factor-1alpha, vascular endothelial growth factor, and angiogenesis by an insulin-like growth factor-I receptor autocrine loop in human pancreatic cancer. Am J Pathol 2003;163:1001-11.
11. Bermont L, Fauconnet S, Lamielle F, Adessi GL. Cell-associated insulin-like growth factor-binding proteins inhibit insulin-like growth factor –I-induced endometrial cancer cell proliferation. Cell Mol Biol 2000;46:1173-82.
12. Hopfner M, Sutter AP, Huether A, Baradari V, Scherubi H. Tyrosine kinase of insulin-like growth factor receptor as target for novel treatment and prevention strategies of colorectal cancer. World J Gastroenterol 2006;12:5635-43.
13. Sueoka N, Lee HY, Wiehle S, Cristiano RJ, Fang B, Ji L, Roth JA, Hong WK, Cohen P, Kurie JM. Insulin-like growth factor binding protein-6 activates programmed cell death in non-small cell lung cancer cells. Oncogene 2000;19:4432-6.
14. Harari PM. Epidermal growth factor receptor inhibition strategies in oncology. Endocr Relat Cancer 2004;11:689-708.
15. Yarden Y, Sliwkowski MX. Untangling the ErbB signalling network. Nat Rev Mol Cell Biol 2001;2:127-37.
16. Wells A. EGF receptor. Int J Biochem Cell Biol 1999;31:637-43.
17. Nicholson RI, Gee JM, Harper ME. EGFR and cancer prognosis. Eur J Cancer 2001;37:S9-15.
18. Herbst RS. Targeted therapy in non-small-cell lung cancer. Oncology 2002 Sep;16:19-24.
19. Mendelsohn J, Baselga J. Status of epidermal growth factor receptor antagonists in the biology and treatment of cancer. J Clin Oncol 2003 15;21:2787-99.
20. Milner RD, Hill DJ. Fetal growth control: the role of insulin and related peptides. Clin Endocrinol (Oxf) 1984;21:415-33.
21. Ciampolillo A, De Tullio C, Giorgino F. The IGF-I/IGF-I receptor pathway: Implications in the Pathophysiology of Thyroid Cancer. Curr Med Chem 2005;12:2881-91.
22. Girnita L, Girnita A, Brodin B, Xie Y, Nilsson G, Dricu A, Lundeberg J, Wejde J, Bartolazzi A, Wiman KG, Larsson O. Increased expression of insulin-like growth factor I receptor in malignant cells expressing aberrant p53: functional impact. Cancer Res 2000;60:5278-83.
23. Tanno S, Tanno S, Mitsuuchi Y, Altomare DA, Xiao GH, Testa JR. AKT activation up-regulates insulin-like growth factor I receptor expression and promotes invasiveness of human pancreatic cancer cells. Cancer Res 2001;61:589-93.
24. Denley A, Cosgrove LJ, Booker GW, Wallace JC, Forbes BE. Molecular interactions of the IGF system. Cytokine Growth Factor Rev 2005;16:421-39.
25. Scaltriti M, Baselga J. The epidermal growth factor receptor pathway: a model for targeted therapy. Clin Cancer Res 2006;12:5268-72.
26. Cui X, Kim HJ, Kuiatse I, Kim H, Brown PH, Lee AV. Epidermal growth factor induces insulin receptor substrate-2 in breast cancer cells via c-Jun NH(2)-terminal kinase/activator protein-1 signaling to regulate cell migration. Cancer Res 2006;66:5304-13.

27. Coppola D, Ferber A, Miura M, Sell C, D'Ambrosio C, Rubin R, Baserga R. A functional insulin-like growth factor I receptor is required for the mitogenic and transforming activities of the epidermal growth factor receptor. Mol Cell Biol 1994;14:4588-95.
28. Yamamoto K, Hirai A, Ban T, Saito J, Tahara K, Terano T, Tamura Y, Saito Y, Kitagawa M. Thyrotropin induces G1 cyclin expression and accelerates G1 phase after insulin-like growth factor I stimulation in FRTL-5 cells. Endocrinology 1996;137:2036-42.
29. Furlanetto RW, Harwell SE, Frick KK. Insulin-like growth factor-I induces cyclin-D1 expression in MG63 human osteosarcoma cells in vitro. Mol Endocrinol 1994;8:510-7.
30. Perry JE, Grossmann ME, Tindall DJ. Epidermal growth factor induces cyclin D1 in a human prostate cancer cell line. Prostate 1998;35:117-24.
31. Kornmann M, Arber N, Korc M. Inhibition of basal and mitogen-stimulated pancreatic cancer cell growth by cyclin D1 antisense is associated with loss of tumorigenicity and potentiation of cytotoxicity to cisplatinum. J Clin Invest 1998;101:344-52.
32. Dupont J, Karas M, LeRoith D. The potentiation of estrogen on insulin-like growth factor I action in MCF-7 human breast cancer cells includes cell cycle components. J Biol Chem 2000;275:35893-901.
33. Stull MA, Richert MM, Loladze AV, Wood TL. Requirement for IGF-I in epidermal growth factor-mediated cell cycle progression of mammary epithelial cells. Endocrinology 2002;143:1872-9.
34. Kim KW, Bae SK, Lee OH, Bae MH, Lee MJ, Park BC. Insulin-like growth factor II induced by hypoxia may contribute to angiogenesis of human hepatocellular carcinoma. Cancer Res 1998;58:348-51.
35. Volpert O, Jackson D, Bouck N, Linzer DI. The insulin-like growth factor II/mannose 6-phosphate receptor is required for proliferin-induced angiogenesis. Endocrinology 1996;137:3871-6.
36. Bae MH, Lee MJ, Bae SK, Lee OH, Lee YM, Park BC, Kim KW. Insulin-like growth factor II (IGF-II) secreted from HepG2 human hepatocellular carcinoma cells shows angiogenic activity. Cancer Lett 1998;128:41-6.
37. Kornmann M, Arber N, Korc M. Inhibition of basal and mitogen-stimulated pancreatic cancer cell growth by cyclin D1 antisense is associated with loss of tumorigenicity and potentiation of cytotoxicity to cisplatinum. J Clin Invest 1998;101:344-52.
38. Lee YM, Bae MH, Lee OH, Moon EJ, Moon CK, Kim WH, Kim KW. Synergistic induction of in vivo angiogenesis by the combination of insulin-like growth factor-II and epidermal growth factor. Oncol Rep 2004;12:843-8.
39. Wraight CJ, Werther GA. Insulin-like growth factor-I and epidermal growth factor regulate insulin-like growth factor binding protein-3 (IGFBP-3) in the human keratinocyte cell line HaCaT. J Invest Dermatol 1995;105:602-7.
40. Tamemoto H, Kadowaki T, Tobe K, Yagi T, Sakura H, Hayakawa T, Terauchi Y, Ueki K, Kaburagi Y, Satoh S, et al. Insulin resistance and growth retardation in mice lacking insulin receptor substrate-1. Nature 1994;372:182-6.
41. Araki E, Lipes MA, Patti ME, Bruning JC, Haag B 3rd, Johnson RS, Kahn CR. Alternative pathway of insulin signalling in mice with targeted disruption of the IRS-1 gene. Nature 1994;372:186-90.
42. Withers DJ, Gutierrez JS, Towery H, Burks DJ, Ren JM, Previs S, Zhang Y, Bernal D, Pons S, Shulman GI, Bonner-Weir S, White MF. Disruption of IRS-2 causes type 2 diabetes in mice. Nature 1998;391:900-4.
43. White MF. The IRS-signaling system: a network of docking proteins that mediate insulin and cytokine action. Recent Prog Horm Res 1998;53:119-38.
44. Boulton TG, Nye SH, Robbins DJ, Ip NY, Radziejewska E, Morgenbesser SD, DePinho RA, Panayotatos N, Cobb MH, Yancopoulos GD. ERKs: a family of protein-serine/threonine kinases that are activated and tyrosine phosphorylated in response to insulin and NGF. Cell 1991;65:663-75.
45. Cahill AL, Perlman RL. Activation of a microtubule-associated protein-2 kinase by insulin-like growth factor-I in bovine chromaffin cells. J Neurochem 1991;57:1832-9.
46. Thomas G. MAP kinase by any other name smells just as sweet. Cell 1992;68:3-6.
47. Pages G, Lenormand P, L'Allemain G, Chambard JC, Meloche S, Pouyssegur J. Mitogen-activated protein kinases p42mapk and p44mapk are required for fibroblast proliferation. Proc Natl Acad Sci 1993;90:8319-23.
48. Marshall CJ. Specificity of receptor tyrosine kinase signaling: transient versus sustained extracellular signal-regulated kinase activation. Cell 1995;80:179-85.

49. Swantek JL, Baserga R. Prolonged activation of ERK2 by epidermal growth factor and other growth factors requires a functional insulin-like growth factor 1 receptor. Endocrinology 1999;140:3163-9.
50. van den Berg HW, Claffie D, Boylan M, McKillen J, Lynch M, McKibben B. Expression of receptors for epidermal growth factor and insulin-like growth factor I by ZR-75-1 human breast cancer cell variants is inversely related: the effect of steroid hormones on insulin-like growth factor I receptor expression. Br J Cancer 1996;73:477-81.
51. Cunningham MP, Essapen S, Thomas H, Green M, Lovell DP, Topham C, Marks C, Modjtahedi H. Coexpression of the IGF-IR, EGFR and HER-2 is common in colorectal cancer patients. Int J Oncol 2006;28:329-35.
52. Wilker E, Bol D, Kiguchi K, Rupp T, Beltran L, DiGiovanni J. Enhancement of susceptibility to diverse skin tumor promoters by activation of the insulin-like growth factor-1 receptor in the epidermis of transgenic mice. Mol Carcinog 1999;25:122-31.
53. Beech D, Pollock RE, Tsan R, Radinsky R. Epidermal growth factor receptor and insulin-like growth factor-I receptor expression and function in human soft-tissue sarcoma cells. Int J Oncol 1998;12:329-36.
54. Ahlen J, Wejde J, Brosjo O, von Rosen A, Weng WH, Girnita L, Larsson O, Larsson C. Insulin-like growth factor type 1 receptor expression correlates to good prognosis in highly malignant soft tissue sarcoma. Clin Cancer Res 2005;11:206-16.
55. Kostler WJ, Hudelist G, Rabitsch W, Czerwenka K, Muller R, Singer CF, Zielinski CC. Insulin-like growth factor-1 receptor (IGF-1R) expression does not predict for resistance to trastuzumab-based treatment in patients with Her-2/neu overexpressing metastatic breast cancer. J Cancer Res Clin Oncol 2006;132:9-18.
56. Ueda S, Hatsuse K, Tsuda H, Ogata S, Kawarabayashi N, Takigawa T, Einama T, Morita D, Fukatsu K, Sugiura Y, Matsubara O, Mochizuki H. Potential crosstalk between insulin-like growth factor receptor type 1 and epidermal growth factor receptor in progression and metastasis of pancreatic cancer. Mod Pathol 2006;19:788-96.
57. Gee JM, Robertson JF, Gutteridge E, Ellis IO, Pinder SE, Rubini M, Nicholson RI. Epidermal growth factor receptor/HER2/insulin-like growth factor receptor signalling and oestrogen receptor activity in clinical breast cancer. Endocr Relat Cancer 2005;12:S99-S111.
58. Lu Y, Zi X, Pollak M. Molecular mechanisms underlying IGF-I-induced attenuation of the growth-inhibitory activity of trastuzumab (Herceptin) on SKBR3 breast cancer cells. Int J Cancer 2004;108:334-41.
59. Lu Y, Zi X, Zhao Y, Mascarenhas D, Pollak M. Insulin-like growth factor-I receptor signaling and resistance to trastuzumab(Herceptin). J Natl Cancer Inst 2001;93:1852-7.
60. Gilmore AP, Valentijn AJ, Wang P, Ranger AM, Bundred N, O'Hare MJ, Wakeling A, Korsmeyer SJ, Streuli CH. Activation of BAD by therapeutic inhibition of epidermal growth factor receptor and transactivation by insulin-like growth factor receptor. J Biol Chem 2002;277:27643-50.
61. Balana ME, Labriola L, Salatino M, Movsichoff F, Peters G, Charreau EH, Elizalde PV. Activation of ErbB-2 via a hierarchical interaction between ErbB-2 and type I insulin-like growth factor receptor in mammary tumor cells. Oncogene 2001;20:34-47.
62. Salatino M, Schillaci R, Proietti CJ, Carnevale R, Frahm I, Molinolo AA, Iribarren A, Charreau EH, Elizalde PV. Inhibition of in vivo breast cancer growth by antisense oligodeoxynucleotides to type I insulin-like growth factor receptor mRNA involves inactivation of ErbBs, PI-3K/Akt and p42/p44 MAPK signaling pathways but not modulation of progesterone receptor activity. Oncogene 2004;23:5161-74.
63. Nahta R, Yuan LX, Zhang B, Kobayashi R, Esteva FJ. Insulin-like growth factor-I receptor/human epidermal growth factor receptor 2 heterodimerization contributes to trastuzumab resistance of breast cancer cells. Cancer Res 2005;65:11118-28.
64. Morgillo F, Woo JK, Kim ES, Hong WK, Lee HY. Heterodimerization of insulin-like growth factor receptor/epidermal growth factor receptor and induction of survivin expression counteract the antitumor action of erlotinib. Cancer Res 2006;66:10100-11.
65. Lee AV, Gooch JL, Oesterreich S, Guler RL, Yee D. Insulin-like growth factor I-induced degradation of insulin receptor substrate 1 is mediated by the 26S proteasome and blocked by phosphatidylinositol 3Î-kinase inhibition. Mol Cell Biol 2000;20:1489-96.

66. Zhang H, Hoff H, Sell C. Insulin-like growth factor I-mediated degradation of insulin receptor substrate-1 is inhibited by epidermal growth factor in prostate epithelial cells. J Biol Chem 2000;275: 22558-62.
67. Lassarre C, Ricort JM. Growth factor-specific regulation of insulin receptor substrate-1 expression in MCF-7 breast carcinoma cells: effects on the insulin-like growth factor signaling pathway. Endocrinology 2003;144:4811-9.
68. Cui X, Kim HJ, Kuiatse I, Kim H, Brown PH, Lee AV. Epidermal growth factor induces insulin receptor substrate-2 in breast cancer cells via c-Jun NH(2)-terminal kinase/activator protein-1 signaling to regulate cell migration. Cancer Res 2006;66:5304-13.
69. Zhang X, Yee D. The type I IGF receptor as a target for breast cancer therapy. Breast Dis 2003;17:115-24.
70. Woodburn JR. The epidermal growth factor receptor and its inhibition in cancer therapy. Pharmacol Ther 1999;82:241-50.
71. Chakravarti A, Delaney MA, Noll E, Black PM, Loeffler JS, Muzikansky A, Dyson NJ. Prognostic and pathologic significance of quantitative protein expression profiling in human gliomas. Clin Cancer Res 2001;7:2387-95.
72. Maher EA, Furnari FB, Bachoo RM, Rowitch DH, Louis DN, Cavenee WK, DePinho RA. Malignant glioma: genetics and biology of a grave matter. Genes Dev 2001;15:1311-33.
73. Bowers G, Reardon D, Hewitt T, Dent P, Mikkelsen RB, Valerie K, Lammering G, Amir C, Schmidt-Ullrich RK. The relative role of ErbB1-4 receptor tyrosine kinases in radiation signal transduction responses of human carcinoma cells. Oncogene 2001;20:1388-97.
74. Rubin Grandis J, Chakraborty A, Melhem MF, Zeng Q, Tweardy DJ. Inhibition of epidermal growth factor receptor gene expression and function decreases proliferation of head and neck squamous carcinoma but not normal mucosal epithelial cells. Oncogene 1997;15:409-16.
75. Milas L, Mason K, Hunter N, Petersen S, Yamakawa M, Ang K, Mendelsohn J, Fan Z. In vivo enhancement of tumor radioresponse by C225 antiepidermal growth factor receptor antibody. Clin Cancer Res 2000;6:701-8.
76. Chakravarti A, Loeffler JS, Dyson NJ. Insulin-like growth factor receptor I mediates resistance to anti-epidermal growth factor receptor therapy in primary human glioblastoma cells through continued activation of phosphoinositide 3-kinase signaling. Cancer Res 2002;62:200-7.
77. Steinbach JP, Eisenmann C, Klumpp A, Weller M. Co-inhibition of epidermal growth factor receptor and type 1 insulin-like growth factor receptor synergistically sensitizes human malignant glioma cells to CD95L-induced apoptosis. Biochem Biophys Res Commun 2004;321:524-30.
78. Wick W, Furnari FB, Naumann U, Cavenee WK, Weller M. PTEN gene transfer in human malignant glioma: sensitization to irradiation and CD95L-induced apoptosis. Oncogene 1999;18:3936-43.
79. Pende M, Um SH, Mieulet V, Sticker M, Goss VL, Mestan J, Mueller M, Fumagalli S, Kozma SC, Thomas G. S6K1(-/-)/S6K2(-/-) mice exhibit perinatal lethality and rapamycin-sensitive5Î-terminal oligopyrimidine mRNA translation and reveal a mitogen-activated protein kinase-dependent S6 kinase pathway. Mol Cell Biol 2004;24:3112-24.
80. Blackledge G, Averbuch S. Gefitinib ('Iressa', ZD1839) and new epidermal growth factor receptor inhibitors. Br J Cancer 2004;90:566-72.
81. Kris MG, Natale RB, Herbst RS, Lynch TJ Jr, Prager D, Belani CP, Schiller JH, Kelly K, Spiridonidis H, Sandler A, Albain KS, Cella D, Wolf MK, Averbuch SD, Ochs JJ, Kay AC. Efficacy of gefitinib, an inhibitor of the epidermal growth factor receptor tyrosine kinase, in symptomatic patients with non-small cell lung cancer: a randomized trial. JAMA 2003;290:2149-58.
82. Fukuoka M, Yano S, Giaccone G, Tamura T, Nakagawa K, Douillard JY, Nishiwaki Y, Vansteenkiste J, Kudoh S, Rischin D, Eek R, Horai T, Noda K, Takata I, Smit E, Averbuch S, Macleod A, Feyereislova A, Dong RP, Baselga J. Multi-institutional randomized phase II trial of gefitinib for previously treated patients with advanced non-small-cell lung cancer (The IDEAL 1 Trial) (corrected). J Clin Oncol 2003;21:2237-46.
83. Cohen EE, Rosen F, Stadler WM, Recant W, Stenson K, Huo D, Vokes EE. Phase II trial of ZD1839 in recurrent or metastatic squamous cell carcinoma of the head and neck. J Clin Oncol 2003;21:1980-7.
84. Baselga J, Albanell J, Ruiz A, Lluch A, Gascon P, Guillem V, Gonzalez S, Sauleda S, Marimon I, Tabernero JM, Koehler MT, Rojo F. Phase II and tumor pharmacodynamic study of gefitinib in patients with advanced breast cancer. J Clin Oncol 2005;23:5323-33.

85. Gee JM, Robertson JF, Gutteridge E, Ellis IO, Pinder SE, Rubini M, Nicholson RI. Epidermal growth factor receptor/HER2/insulin-like growth factor receptor signalling and oestrogen receptor activity in clinical breast cancer. Endocr Relat Cancer 2005;12:S99-S111.
86. von Minckwitz G, Jonat W, Fasching P, du Bois A, Kleeberg U, Luck HJ, Kettner E, Hilfrich J, Eiermann W, Torode J, Schneeweiss A. A multicentre phase II study on gefitinib in taxane- and anthracycline-pretreated metastatic breast cancer. Breast Cancer Res Treat 2005;89:165-72.
87. Camirand A, Zakikhani M, Young F, Pollak M. Inhibition of insulin-like growth factor-1 receptor signaling enhances growth-inhibitory and proapoptotic effects of gefitinib (Iressa) in human breast cancer cells. Breast Cancer Res 2005;7:R570-9.
88. Jones HE, Goddard L, Gee JM, Hiscox S, Rubini M, Barrow D, Knowlden JM, Williams S, Wakeling AE, Nicholson RI. Insulin-like growth factor-I receptor signalling and acquired resistance to gefitinib (ZD1839; Iressa) in human breast and prostate cancer cells. Endocr Relat Cancer 2004;11:793-814.
89. Johnson ML, Seidman AD. Emerging targeted therapies for breast cancer. Oncology 2005;19:611-8.
90. Camirand A, Lu Y, Pollak M. Co-targeting HER2/ErbB2 and insulin-like growth factor-1 receptors causes synergistic inhibition of growth in HER2-overexpressing breast cancer cells. Med Sci Monit 2002;8:BR521-6.
91. Goetsch L, Gonzalez A, Leger O, Beck A, Pauwels PJ, Haeuw JF, Corvaia N. A recombinant humanized anti-insulin-like growth factor receptor type I antibody(h7C10) enhances the antitumor activity of vinorelbine and anti-epidermal growth factor receptor therapy against human cancer xenografts. Int J Cancer 2005;113:316-28.
92. Jerome L, Shiry L, Leyland-Jones B. Deregulation of the IGF axis in cancer: epidemiological evidence and potential therapeutic interventions. Endocr Relat Cancer 2003;10:561-78.
93. Hankinson SE, Willett WC, Colditz GA, Hunter DJ, Michaud DS, Deroo B, Rosner B, Speizer FE, Pollak M. Circulating concentrations of insulin-like growth factor-I and risk of breast cancer. Lancet 1998;351:1393-6.
94. Li BD, Khosravi MJ, Berkel HJ, Diamandi A, Dayton MA, Smith M, Yu H. Free insulin-like growth factor-I and breast cancer risk. Int J Cancer 2001;91:736-9.
95. Jerome L, Alami N, Belanger S, Page V, Yu Q, Paterson J, Shiry L, Pegram M, Leyland-Jones B. Recombinant human insulin-like growth factor binding protein 3 inhibits growth of human epidermal growth factor receptor-2-overexpressing breast tumors and potentiates herceptin activity in vivo. Cancer Res 2006;66:7245-52.
96. Cheson B. Bexxar (Corixa/GlaxoSmithKline). Curr Opin Investig Drugs 2002;3:165-70.
97. Sievers EL, Linenberger M. Mylotarg: antibody-targeted chemotherapy comes of age. Curr Opin Oncol 2001;13:522-7.
98. Czuczman MS, Grillo-Lopez AJ, White CA, Saleh M, Gordon L, LoBuglio AF, Jonas C, Klippenstein D, Dallaire B, Varns C. Treatment of patients with low-grade B-cell lymphoma with the combination of chimeric anti-CD20 monoclonal antibody and CHOP chemotherapy. J Clin Oncol 1999;17:268-76.
99. Baselga J. Herceptin alone or in combination with chemotherapy in the treatment of HER2-positive metastatic breast cancer: pivotal trials. Oncology 2001;61:14-21.
100. Grillo-Lopez AJ. Zevalin: the first radioimmunotherapy approved for the treatment of lymphoma. Expert Rev Anticancer Ther. 2002;2:485-93.
101. Lu D, Zhang H, Ludwig D, Persaud A, Jimenez X, Burtrum D, Balderes P, Liu M, Bohlen P, Witte L, Zhu Z. Simultaneous blockade of both the epidermal growth factor receptor and the insulin-like growth factor receptor signaling pathways in cancer cells with a fully human recombinant bispecific antibody. J Biol Chem 2004;279:2856-65.
102. Lu D, Zhang H, Koo H, Tonra J, Balderes P, Prewett M, Corcoran E, Mangalampalli V, Bassi R, Anselma D, Patel D, Kang X, Ludwig DL, Hicklin DJ, Bohlen P, Witte L, Zhu Z. A fully human recombinant IgG-like bispecific antibody to both the epidermal growth factor receptor and the insulin-like growth factor receptor for enhanced antitumor activity. J Biol Chem 2005;280:19665-72.

12 Negative Regulation of Signaling by the EGFR Family

Kermit L. Carraway III, Lily Yen, Ellen Ingalla, and Colleen Sweeney

Contents

Introduction
Feedback Negative Regulation—Lessons from Flies
Mammalian ErbB Negative Regulation
ErbB Negative Regulatory Pathways—Degradation Mediated by E3 Ubiquitin Ligases
ErbB Negative Regulatory Pathways—Suppression of Receptor Activity
Conclusion
Acknowledgments
References

Abstract

Signaling through the EGFR or ErbB family of receptor tyrosine kinases must be precisely regulated to ensure the fidelity of tissue development and homeostasis, yet prevent tumor initiation and progression. The efficiency of receptor signaling in cells is tempered by a series of negative regulatory mechanisms that act directly on receptors to suppress their response to growth factor ligand. The past ten years have witnessed significant progress in the discovery of these pathways and the characterization of the mechanisms by which their loss in tumors might contribute to malignancy. These mechanisms include pathways that lead to receptor degradation, both in the absence and presence of activating ligand. The central components of such pathways are often E3 ubiquitin ligases, such as cbl or Nrdp1. Other mechanisms suppress the ability of receptors to respond to growth factor stimulation. Splice variants of ErbB receptor extracellular domains, proteins that contain leucine-rich repeats in their extracellular domains, and intracellular suppressor proteins such as RALT fall into this category. Here we review ErbB negative regulatory mechanisms, emphasizing what is known about the loss of these pathways in tumors, and highlighting the notion that pathway augmentation or restoration to tumor cells could ultimately be of therapeutic benefit to cancer patients.

Key Words: EGF receptor, ErbB2, feedback negative regulation, E3 ubiquitin ligase, breast cancer, transgenic mice.

From: *Cancer Drug Discovery and Development: EGFR Signaling Networks in Cancer Therapy*
Edited by: J. D. Haley and W. J. Gullick, DOI: 10.1007/978-1-59745-356-1_12
© 2008 Humana Press, a part of Springer Science+Business Media, LLC

1. INTRODUCTION

Growth factor receptor tyrosine kinases, such as the EGF receptor and its family members ErbB2, ErbB3, and ErbB4, play critical roles in specific developmental processes during embryogenesis and are essential for tissue maintenance in the adult. The fidelity of homeostatic processes in developed tissues requires very precise regulation of receptor activation. Insufficient receptor signaling can contribute to the suppression of cellular survival signals, leading to apoptosis and ultimately tissue atrophy and impairment of organ function. For example, mice conditionally lacking ErbB2 or ErbB4 in the mature heart develop dilated cardiomyopathy (1–3), underscoring the need for signaling through these receptors in cardiac tissue maintenance. On the other hand, hyper-signaling by receptors in differentiated tissues can lead to dysplasia, tumorigenesis, and tumor progression (4, 5). Overexpression of ErbB receptors, or their aberrant activation by mutation or by autocrine growth factor signaling, has been observed in various solid tumors. These events lead to constitutive receptor tyrosine phosphorylation and signaling, which in turn contribute to a variety of cellular events that can lead to the formation and progression of solid tumors. The necessity for signaling efficiency to fall within a relatively narrow range implies that sophisticated mechanisms have evolved to fine-tune receptor output, including positive regulatory mechanisms that ensure sufficient signaling to mediate homeostatic processes, and negative regulatory mechanisms that balance receptor activation by preventing the onset of oncogenic processes. The hyper-activation of positive pathways and the loss of negative pathways both have the potential to promote tumor progression.

Since the initial cloning of the ErbB receptors in the 1980s and early 1990s, major emphasis has been placed on understanding mechanisms of receptor activation and how activated receptors utilize signaling pathways to elicit cellular responses. These studies have led to the development of ErbB-directed antibody and small molecule inhibitors for the treatment of cancer patients whose tumors are driven by elevated ErbB activity. An increasing number of studies suggest, however, that a high proportion of tumors are either intrinsically refractory to such therapies, or develop resistance with prolonged treatment (6). These observations suggest that attacking ErbB receptor activity may not be the most effective means of suppressing the growth and progression of ErbB-dependent tumors. For example, a recent study has demonstrated that some tumors evade inhibition by ErbB-directed small molecule tyrosine kinase inhibitors by promoting the tyrosine phosphorylation of the kinase-inactive ErbB3 to augment its coupling to the PI 3-kinase pathway (7). Hence, a need is arising for the development of new strategies in therapeutically targeting ErbB-dependent tumors.

Over the past several years, a number of ErbB receptor negative regulatory pathways have been uncovered (8–11). Inhibitory mechanisms can employ either reversible or irreversible modes of action. Irreversible inhibition typically occurs via ubiquitin-mediated protein degradation of receptors and effectors. Reversible inhibition can interfere with receptor signaling at several key points. Compartmentalization of receptors away from their effectors and dephosphorylation of receptors and their effectors by tyrosine phosphatases are examples. Negative regulators can also function to blunt the entire scope of receptor signaling, or instead affect a specific signaling pathway. Negative regulators can be classified further still according to their temporal behavior. For example, inhibitors that are constitutively present in the cell are regulated primarily by the accessibility of receptors. Other inhibitors, those that function in feedback loops, are not constitutively present in the cell (or are present at very low, sub-optimal levels) and are transcriptionally induced or their proteins stabilized upon receptor activation. The action of these inhibitors is defined by the time it takes them to accrue to levels compatible with inhibition.

While the ErbB negative regulation field is still in its nascent stages, initial observations indicate that the key components of these negative regulatory pathways may be lost in a significant proportion of tumors. Thus, a possible novel avenue for thwarting ErbB-dependent tumors may involve the augmentation or restoration of suppressed negative regulatory pathways in tumor cells. Here we will review ErbB negative regulatory pathways, underscoring their potential role in cancer. It should be noted that numerous proteins have been identified that contribute to receptor negative regulation by generally influencing membrane protein trafficking and degradation. Moreover, negative regulators of the canonical signaling pathways downstream of ErbB receptors have been described, such as the dual specificity phosphatases (DUSPs) that suppress MAPK signaling and PTEN that suppresses PI3K signaling. Systemic targeting of such ubiquitous pathways could lead to deleterious side effects in patients, which may be avoided by more selectively targeting the ErbB receptors themselves. For these reasons our discussion here will focus on pathways that directly impinge on ErbB receptor function.

2. FEEDBACK NEGATIVE REGULATION—LESSONS FROM FLIES

In the 1990s, several labs employing genetic and biochemical approaches in the study of EGF receptor signaling in the fruit fly *Drosophila melanogaster* uncovered a series of novel negative regulatory genes (*12, 13*). The fly genome encodes a single ErbB family member, *Drosophila* EGF receptor (DER), which is acted upon by four different EGF-like ligands to mediate developmental events including oogenesis and wing and eye development (*14*). The timing and kinetics of DER activation are controlled in part by ligand activation, and in part by the negative regulatory proteins Argos and Kekkon-1 (*10*).

Argos is a secreted protein containing an atypical EGF-like domain with disrupted spacing of cysteine residues found in the activating EGF-like ligands. Early studies suggested that Argos acts as an antagonist of fly EGF receptor activity (*15–17*), binding to the receptor with modest affinity and inhibiting activation by growth factor. More recent studies indicate, however, that Argos actually binds to the activating growth factor Spitz, sequestering it from the receptor (*18, 19*) in a manner similar to IGF1 sequestration by members of the IGFBP family. While a human Argos homolog has not been identified, these observations raise the possibility that growth factor sequestration may similarly play a role in ErbB negative regulation.

Kekkon-1 (Kek1) is a transmembrane protein containing six leucine-rich repeats (LRRs) and an immunoglobulin (Ig) domain in its extracellular region, a single membrane spanning segment, and an intracellular domain with few distinguishing features. The leucine-rich repeat region of the Kek1 extracellular domain physically interacts with the extracellular domain of DER to suppress signaling (*20, 21*), possibly by interfering with growth factor binding or activation (*22*). Although there are five other Kek family members in Drosophila, only Kek1 inhibits DER signaling (*23*).

While Argos and Kek1 appear to inhibit DER function by disparate mechanisms, they are both transcriptionally induced by DER activation (*15, 20, 24*). Induction of receptor negative regulatory mechanisms then suppresses further receptor signaling, thus ensuring proper development. By extension, these observations suggest that feedback negative regulation may be a common theme in modulating the function of mammalian ErbB receptor family members.

3. MAMMALIAN ErbB NEGATIVE REGULATION

Since the strength of signaling output is dependent on the quantity of activated receptors, cells must maintain a narrow window of ErbB receptors at their surface. Sufficient numbers of receptors must be present to ensure the fidelity of tissue maintenance processes, but receptor overexpression must be prevented to suppress potential oncogenic events. Normal quantities are thought to be on the order of a few tens of thousands of receptors per cell. However, overexpression of ErbB receptors, particularly EGF receptor, ErbB2, and ErbB3, is common in numerous solid tumor types, and the overall quantity can reach a few million receptors per cell. Hence a key question concerns the mechanisms by which ErbB proteins are overexpressed in tumor cells. Conventional wisdom would suggest that events that lead to elevated receptor transcript levels are largely responsible, and it has been observed that some ErbB receptor genes are amplified in some tumor types. Recent evidence suggests, however, that gene amplification may not be sufficient; post-transcriptional mechanisms may also play major roles in regulating ErbB receptor levels in normal tissue. This point is best illustrated by the analysis of ErbB2 and ErbB3 overexpression in mammary tumors.

3.1. ErbB Receptors and Breast Cancer

Overexpression of three of the ErbB receptor family members has been repeatedly observed in breast tumors (4). Of particular note, ErbB2 overexpression has been observed in a significant proportion (25-30%) of breast cancer patient tumors, and is correlated with poor patient prognosis and shortened survival time (*25–27*). It is widely believed that the aberrant activation of ErbB2 protein tyrosine kinase activity through overexpression actively contributes to tumor progression by engaging cellular signaling pathways that promote tumor progression, such as proliferation, survival, motility, invasion, and resistance to chemotherapeutic agents (*28*). Thus, much emphasis has been placed on understanding the biochemical mechanisms by which ErbB2 and its relatives are activated in tumor cells, and on the development of ErbB antagonists that could function as anti-cancer agents. Indeed, Genentech's trastuzumab (Herceptin), a humanized antibody directed to the ErbB2 protein, is currently used in the treatment of ErbB2-positive patients. Significant proportions of ErbB2-positive tumors, however, either present as Herceptin-resistant or develop resistance within a year of the initiation of treatment (*6*). Moreover, Herceptin has been observed to induce potentially lethal cardiac myopathic side effects in some patients receiving this therapy in conjunction with anthracyclines (*29*). These observations validate the ErbB2 receptor as a target in the therapeutic intervention of breast cancer, but prompt questions as to whether more specific and efficient methods for interfering with ErbB2 signaling in breast tumors may be developed. In this regard, there is intense interest in developing alternate ErbB2-directed therapies.

While much effort over the past 15-20 years has gone into understanding the mechanisms by which ErbB2 overexpression and aberrant activation contribute to the cellular properties associated with malignancy, essentially no effort has been put into understanding how the protein becomes overexpressed in tumors in the first place. One of the original publications describing ErbB2 overexpression in breast tumors found a strong correlation between ErbB2 gene amplification and ErbB2 protein overexpression (*27*). This has since been confirmed by numerous studies, and it is generally accepted that the amplification of the ErbB2 gene by tumor cells, often up to 20-fold, leads to ErbB2 message overexpression and thus protein overexpression. The original study, however, documented a significant proportion of cases of ErbB2 protein overexpression in the absence of gene amplification, indicating that other mechanisms also contribute to ErbB2 protein accumulation in cells.

Another issue in ErbB2 oncogenic signaling concerns its heterodimerizing partner ErbB3. ErbB3 is also commonly overexpressed in breast tumors but no mutations or gene amplifications have been found (*30–32*). Reports of ErbB3 overexpression in breast cancer range from 17–52%, and overexpression is positively associated with lymph node metastases and histological grade. ErbB3 overexpression is an independent predictor of survival (*32*), but recent analyses have established a strong link between the coordinate overexpression and activation of ErbB2 and ErbB3 in breast tumor cell lines and in patient samples (*30, 31, 33, 34*). This is significant because the members of the ErbB receptor family undergo a network of homo- and heterodimerization events as part of

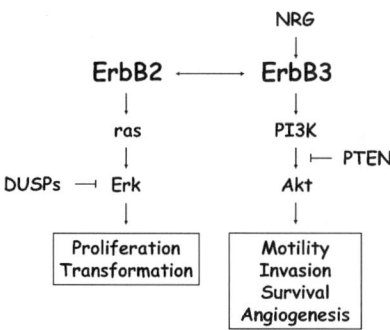

Fig. 12.1. The ErbB2/ErbB3 Oncogenic Unit. Overexpression or aberrant activation of ErbB2 in epithelial cells leads to tumorigenesis by promoting cellular proliferation and transformation through the ras/Erk pathway, while the accompanying phosphorylation of ErbB3 leads to tumor progression by promoting cellular survival, motility and invasion through the PI3K/Akt pathway. ErbB2 serves as the active kinase for the heterodimeric receptor species, while the kinase-inactive ErbB3 serves as the binding receptor for the NRG1 growth factor.

their activation mechanism. Particularly noteworthy is a strong propensity of ErbB2 to heterodimerize with and activate ErbB3 (*35–38*), especially when the two receptors are overexpressed. ErbB3 serves as a binding receptor for the EGF-like growth factor neuregulin-1 (NRG1 or heregulin; 39), but lacks intrinsic tyrosine kinase activity (*40*) and must necessarily heterodimerize with ErbB2 to signal (*35, 41*). On the other hand, no known diffusible growth factor binds to ErbB2; hence, it must heterodimerize with other ErbB family members to participate in growth factor-initiated signaling. Fig. 12.1 depicts a very simplistic model of ErbB2/ErbB3 heterodimer signaling in tumor cells. ErbB2 is uniquely suited to stimulate the ras/Erk pathway, leading to initial events in the tumorigenic process such as cellular transformation and proliferation, while ErbB3 is uniquely suited to engage the PI3 kinase pathway, leading to later events such as tumor cell survival and invasion. ErbB2 and ErbB3 synergize in promoting the growth and transformation of cultured fibroblasts (*42, 43*), and numerous studies demonstrate that the two receptors synergize in mediating increased proliferation (*44*) and invasiveness induced by the neuregulin-1 (NRG1) growth factor in breast tumor cell lines (*45–47*). Taken together, these observations suggest that there may be an advantage for both receptors to be present and activated in tumor cells to promote breast tumor growth and progression (*34, 44*). The ErbB2/ErbB3 heterodimer has thus been proposed to function as an "oncogenic unit," with ErbB3 as an essential partner in ErbB2-mediated proliferation (44). Genentech's second generation humanized anti-ErbB2 pertuzumab (Omnitarg), which inhibits ErbB2/ErbB3 dimerization but not ligand binding (*48*), is currently in phase II clinical trials (*49*).

3.2. ErbB2 Transgenic Model of Breast Cancer

Transgenic mouse models of breast cancer have led to considerable insight into the molecular and cellular mechanisms underlying breast cancer malignancy (*50*). Overexpression of ErbB2 in the mammary gland of transgenic mice using the murine mammary tumor virus (MMTV) promoter/enhancer gives rise to metastatic mammary tumors (*51*), underscoring the malignant potential of ErbB2 overexpression. However, tumors in this model develop with a significantly longer latency than in other oncogene models, suggesting that other processes must occur in addition to ErbB2 gene overexpression to drive tumorigenesis. In examining these animals, we, along with others, (*34, 52*) have observed that ErbB2 protein levels in non-tumor

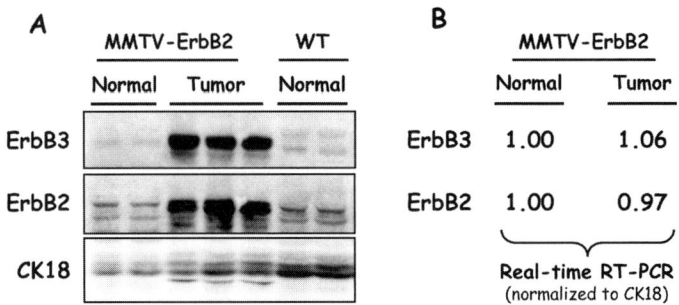

Fig. 12.2. ErbB2/ErbB3 Expression in ErbB2-induced Mouse Mammary Tumors. (A) Normal mammary tissue was harvested from two wild type (right two lanes) and two MMTV-ErbB2 (left two lanes) mice. Additionally, mammary tumor tissue was harvested from three transgenic animals (middle three lanes). Lysates from tissues were immunoblotted using antibodies to endogenous and transgene ErbB2, endogenous ErbB3, and cytokeratin 18 (CK18) to control for epithelial content. (B) Real-time RT-PCR analysis of ErbB2 and ErbB3 transcript levels was carried out on normal and tumor tissue from MMTV-ErbB2 mouse mammary glands, and levels were normalized to CK18.

mammary tissue from transgenic animals are similar to levels in wild-type (non-transgenic) animals, despite the increased transcript levels in transgenic animals (Fig. 12.2A). Hence, elevated ErbB2 transcript is not sufficient to produce elevated ErbB2 protein, suggesting that ErbB2 gene amplification may not be sufficient to drive ErbB2 overexpression in patients. ErbB2 protein, however, is dramatically overexpressed in tumors from transgenic animals compared with non-tumor tissue, even though tumor and uninvolved mammary tissue express similar levels of ErbB2 transcript as assessed by real-time RT-PCR (Fig. 12.2B). Even more striking is the expression of ErbB3 in this model. Normal mammary tissue from wild-type mice, normal tissue from transgenic mice, and tumors from transgenics all express comparable levels of endogenous ErbB3 transcript. Tumors from transgenics, however, express extremely high levels of ErbB3 protein compared to corresponding normal tissue from transgenics. IHC analysis has confirmed that both ErbB proteins in tumors are restricted to epithelial cells. Hence, these observations indicate that very potent post-transcriptional mechanisms exist that suppress ErbB protein expression in normal epithelial cells. These mechanisms could involve the selective suppression of ErbB synthesis, the selective augmentation of receptor degradation, or both. Such mechanisms probably evolved to prevent receptor overexpression, thus ensuring proper levels of signaling to mediate tissue development and maintenance without leading to dysplasia. Most importantly, these observations indicate that negative regulatory mechanisms are markedly suppressed in tumors, allowing ErbB receptors to accumulate to extraordinarily high levels. Indeed, since ErbB protein overexpression coincides with tumor onset, it is possible that the loss of these ErbB negative regulatory mechanisms is requisite for ErbB2-induced tumor formation.

4. ErbB NEGATIVE REGULATORY PATHWAYS—DEGRADATION MEDIATED BY E3 UBIQUITIN LIGASES

4.1. EGF Receptor Ubiquitination and Degradation

One of the primary mechanisms by which cells negatively regulate receptor tyrosine kinase activity is through receptor degradation (also see Chapter 4). For over a quarter century the EGF receptor has served as a prominent model for understanding how cell surface receptors undergo ligand-stimulated down-regulation and degradation. Studies over the past ten years point to a key role for ubiquitination in the down-regulation and degradation of a variety of plasma membrane proteins (*53, 54*), including receptor tyrosine kinases (*55*). Upon growth factor binding many receptor tyrosine kinases localize to clathrin-coated pits, become internalized, and are delivered to endosomes. Receptors are sorted in endosomes according to whether they are to be recycled to the cell surface or degraded in lysosomes based on their ubiquitination state. Ligand binding stimulates the multiple monoubiquitination of EGF receptor (*56*), and it has been demonstrated that monoubiquitination is sufficient to drive EGF receptor internalization and degradation (*57, 58*). Moreover, growth factor-stimulated monoubiquitination of endosomal sorting accessory proteins may regulate their function as ubiquitin receptors (*58, 59*), underscoring the central role of protein ubiquitination in receptor trafficking and degradation. Very recent evidence suggests that EGF also stimulates the K63 polyubiquitination of the EGF receptor (*60*) as well, although the function is unknown. Ubiquitination of EGF receptor is mediated, at least in part, by the RING finger E3 ubiquitin ligase cbl (*61*). cbl is recruited to the receptor in an activation-dependent manner by the binding of its tyrosine kinase binding (TKB) domain to phosphorylated tyrosine 1045 of the EGF receptor (*62–64*). Recruited cbl becomes tyrosine phosphorylated by the receptor, activating its ubiquitin ligase activity. cbl is then thought to ubiquitinate the receptor on kinase domain lysine residues (*60*) to promote receptor trafficking to lysosomes. Point mutation of Y1045 (*64*), or oxidant-induced receptor activation that does not result in Y1045 phosphorylation (*65*), suppresses EGF receptor down-regulation. Likewise, cbl mutants that are unable to mediate EGF receptor ubiquitination also promote receptor stability (*63, 64*). Overexpression of cbl augments EGF-stimulated receptor ubiquitination and degradation, and functional RING finger and phosphotyrosine binding domains are both required for enhanced degradation (*62, 63*). These studies, together with the characterization of an oncogenic cbl form that disrupts receptor ubiquitination (*64*), lead to the suggestion that the escape of RTKs from cbl-mediated down-regulation promotes cellular growth properties associated with oncogenesis (*66*). The cellular site(s) of cbl action toward the EGF receptor and its role in internalization are points of debate (*67, 68*). It is generally agreed, however, that cbl-mediated receptor ubiquitination targets endosomal receptors for degradation in the lysosome, while non-ubiquitinated receptors are routed back to the cell surface.

It is important to note that even in the absence of ligand binding, growth factor receptors undergo constant internalization and trafficking through endosomes. While most internalized receptors are returned to the cell surface, a fraction of unoccupied receptors is targeted for degradation. The competing processes of recycling and degradation establish an equilibrium that defines receptor half-life and hence steady-state levels of cell surface receptors (*69*). For example, in a normal epithelial cell a growth factor receptor may be recycled a dozen times prior to its degradation, resulting in a half-life of 12 hours. In a transformed cell, however, a smaller fraction of the trafficked receptors may be targeted for degradation, resulting in a markedly prolonged receptor half-life and elevated cell surface receptor levels. Hence, proteins involved in targeting receptors for ligand-independent degradation could play a significant role in suppressing tumor growth properties by suppressing endogenous receptor levels.

4.2. Other ErbB Degradation Mechanisms

While significant progress has been made in understanding EGF-induced EGFR receptor degradation, mechanisms that contribute to EGFR overexpression in the absence of growth factor remain to be explored. Moreover, very little is known about the degradation of the other members of the ErbB receptor family, either in the presence or absence of growth factor signaling. In this regard it is interesting that cbl has been reported not to be an efficient substrate of the other ErbB receptors under physiological conditions (*70*). These observations are consistent with reports suggesting that ErbB2, ErbB3, and ErbB4 do not undergo efficient ligand-induced down-regulation (*71*), and underscore the importance of other proteins or mechanisms in keeping these receptors in check.

One mechanism that has received significant attention is the regulation of ligand-independent ErbB2 levels by chaperone-mediated stability. Cytosolic molecular chaperones such as Hsp90 check and enable the correct folding of nascent polypeptides, and are additionally required for the refolding of mature proteins following their denaturation. Misfolded mature proteins that are not correctly refolded are degraded by proteasomes following ubiquitination by chaperone-associated E3 ubiquitin ligases. Hsp90 binds to the kinase domain of mature ErbB2 in a tyrosine phosphorylation-independent manner to promote receptor stability (*72*). Disruption of Hsp90/ErbB2 association with ansamycin antibiotics such as geldanamycin promotes ErbB2 degradation (*72, 73*). The chaperone-binding ubiquitin ligase CHIP (carboxy terminus of Hsc70 interacting protein) is characterized by a tetratricopeptide repeat (TPR) domain at its amino terminus responsible for interaction with Hsp90, and a U-box domain that binds to E2 ubiquitin conjugating enzymes. Its interaction with Hsp90 results in client substrate ubiquitination and subsequent degradation by the proteasome. Thus, CHIP tilts the folding-degradation machinery toward the degradative pathway (*74*). CHIP is highly expressed in heart, skeletal muscle, and brain tissues where ErbB signaling is critical for development and maintenance (*75–77*), and it efficiently ubiquitinates ErbB2 to mediate its degradation (*78, 79*). Together, these observations raise the possibility that CHIP-mediated ErbB2 degradation participates in the post-transcriptional suppression of ErbB2 levels in normal tissues. Chaperones such as Hsp90 are frequently overexpressed in tumors (*80*), and this overexpression may contribute to ErbB2 stability. This overexpression in turn points to the possibility that geldanamycin or similar chaperone-directed agents might be exploited for pharmacological intervention of ErbB2-overexpressing tumors. The clinical use of these drugs, however, may be complicated because Hsp90 inhibition activates the src tyrosine kinase, which in turn activates the kinase activity of ErbB2 (*81*).

Another E3 ubiquitin ligase, LNX1, has also been demonstrated to physically associate with ErbB2. LNX1 was originally characterized as a RING-type E3 ubiquitin ligase that targets the membrane-associated cell fate determinant Numb for ubiquitin-dependent degradation (*82*). A recent study suggests that LNX1 expression is inversely correlated with the responsiveness of neuromuscular junction perisynaptic Schwann cells to the growth factor NRG1, and that loss of LNX1 protein correlates with the appearance of ErbB2 protein upon denervation (*83*). While ligase activity toward ErbB2 has not yet been demonstrated, these observations suggest that LNX1 may be involved in the developmental suppression of ErbB2 protein in this cell type. Whether or not LNX1 is expressed in normal epithelia of tissue types susceptible to ErbB-induced tumor progression is a question of interest.

Our studies have demonstrated that Nrdp1 (Neuregulin receptor degradation protein-1), a RING finger domain-containing E3 ubiquitin ligase, is the central component of a novel protein degradation pathway that regulates the stability of ErbB3 (*84, 85*). Nrdp1 binds to this receptor independent of ligand stimulation through its unique carboxy terminal domain (*84, 86*), and promotes receptor ubiquitination through its RING finger domain. Overexpression of Nrdp1 in cultured breast cancer cells results in a loss of steady-state ErbB3 levels, while a dominant-negative form or shRNA-mediated knockdown of endogenous Nrdp1 augments receptor levels. These changes result in the corresponding inhibition and potentiation, respectively, of NRG1-induced cellular proliferation and motility (*52*), suggesting that Nrdp1 could play a key role in controlling ErbB-mediated developmental events by influencing steady-state receptor levels. Importantly, Nrdp1 protein levels in ErbB2-induced

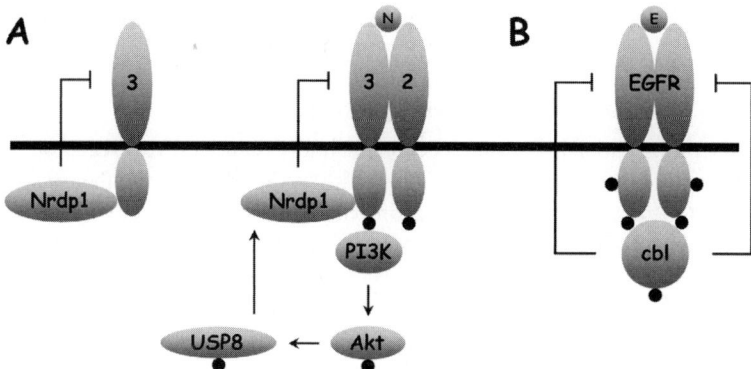

Fig. 12.3. **Feedback Negative Regulation of EGFR and ErbB3 by E3 Ubiquitin Ligases.**
(A) Cellular Nrdp1 governs steady-state ErbB3 levels in the absence of growth factor by ubiquitinating a fraction of the constitutively internalizing receptor to promote its delivery to lysosomes. Upon NRG1 stimulation, the ErbB3 complex recruits PI3K leading to the activation of Akt, which in turn phosphorylates (black dots) USP8 to promote the stabilization of Nrdp1. Elevated Nrdp1 then specifies that a greater fraction of ErbB3 is degraded upon internalization. (B) EGF stimulation of EGFR leads to Y1045 phosphorylation and the recruitment of cbl, which ubiquitinates the receptor to promote its lysosomal degradation.

tumors in transgenic mice are potently suppressed (52), which is consistent with the marked overexpression of ErbB3 protein in these tumors (Fig. 12.2A). Moreover, 57% of all primary tumors from breast cancer patients exhibit suppressed Nrdp1 protein levels (52). Our immunoblotting studies of patient-matched normal and tumor breast tissue indicate that 63% of tumors overexpress the ErbB3 protein, and of these almost 70% exhibit Nrdp1 protein loss. The strong correlation between ErbB3 overexpression and Nrdp1 loss in tumors points to the possibility that this ligase may play a central role in suppressing ErbB3 levels and signaling activity in normal breast tissue.

Since Nrdp1 levels could play a significant role in promoting tumor initiation or progression, a natural question concerns the mechanism(s) by which Nrdp1 protein levels are regulated. While the mechanism of Nrdp1 protein suppression in tumors is currently under investigation, our observations suggest that one of the mechanisms by which Nrdp1 is regulated in normal tissue is through autoubiquitination and proteasomal degradation (87). A key regulator of Nrdp1 stability is the deubiquitinating USP8, which removes ubiquitin from autoubiquitinated Nrdp1 to prevent its proteasomal degradation (87). Interestingly, USP8 appears to be regulated by growth factor stimulation (88), leading to the feedback negative regulatory loop illustrated in Fig. 12.3A. In this model, NRG1 stimulation of the ErbB2-ErbB3 heterodimer engages the PI3K-Akt signaling cascade, which mediates the phosphorylation of USP8 and the augmentation of its stabilizing activity toward Nrdp1, which in turn promotes ErbB3 degradation through its E3 ligase activity. In contrast with cbl, which acts on activated EGF receptors after ligand stimulation through its ability to couple to phosphorylated Y1045 (Fig. 12.3B), Nrdp1 acts on receptors independent of receptor activation and its accumulation in cells is stimulated by growth factor. In more general terms, these observations suggest that growth factor signaling is capable of augmenting mechanisms that keep basal receptors in check as a means of feedback negative regulation. As outlined above, other studies have suggested that ErbB2, ErbB3, and ErbB4 are incapable of ligand-induced down-regulation. It is possible, however, that the studies underlying these conclusions were carried out in cell types where ErbB negative regulatory pathways are either not present or have been lost.

5. ErbB NEGATIVE REGULATORY PATHWAYS—SUPPRESSION OF RECEPTOR ACTIVITY

5.1. ErbB Splice Variants

The second general mechanism by which cells negatively regulate ErbB receptors is through the use of modulator proteins that physically interact with receptors to dictate their response to ligand binding (10, 11). One class of naturally occurring negative modulators consists of splice variants encoding some or most of the extracellular portions of ErbB receptors. Herstatin is the product of an alternatively spliced human ErbB2 that leaves intron 8 in the message. The resulting expressed product encompasses half of the ErbB2 extracellular region along with 79 unique amino acids encoded by the retained intron (*89*). Herstatin binds with high affinity to EGFR, ErbB2, and ErbB4, suppresses receptor dimerization and activation without interfering with ligand binding (*90–92*), and appears to modulate signaling pathway usage by receptors to elicit cellular growth arrest (*91*). When co-expressed in ErbB2-expressing cells, Herstatin interacts with and sequesters wild-type ErbB2 in the endoplasmic reticulum to suppress cell surface delivery of the complex (*93*). Interestingly, the relative amount of intron 8-containing transcript and protein is very low in cell lines that overexpress full-length ErbB2 when compared with lines that express normal amounts of full-length ErbB2 (89), suggesting that the loss of this negative regulatory mechanism confers an advantage to ErbB2-dependent tumors. Given that Herstatin inhibits ErbBs activated both by ligand binding and by receptor overexpression, thus mimicking the properties of both Herceptin and Omnitarg, its therapeutic potential is quite promising. Indeed, transfected Herstatin inhibits the intracranial growth of EGFR-driven glioblastoma cells in nude mice (*94*), underscoring the potential clinical utility of this agent. EGFR-related peptide (ERRP), a 55 kDa variant of the EGFR extracellular domain (*95*), also inhibits basal and ligand-induced activation of ErbB family members (*96*). ERRP expression is high in benign colonic and gastric mucosa, as well as in the liver and pancreas, but low in the respective carcinomas of those tissues. Moreover, injection of recombinant protein inhibits tumor cell growth in xenograft models (*97*), underscoring the therapeutic potential of this agent. A similar splice variant of ErbB3 encoding most of the extracellular region followed by intron-encoded sequence may act as an inhibitor of cell growth by binding ligand to form non-productive ligand-receptor complexes (*98*). Collectively, these data suggest that cells utilize ErbB splice variants to suppress their signaling and raise the possibility that these agents may be employed therapeutically.

5.2. Ralt

Receptor-associated late transducer (RALT; also called gene33 or MIG-6) has received a lot of attention as a pan-ErbB inhibitor that is transcriptionally induced upon ErbB activation in a ras pathway-dependent manner (*99–102*). RALT expression suppresses ErbB-mediated mitogenesis (*101*), and its functional loss sensitizes cells to sub-optimal growth factor concentrations (*8, 103*). Moreover, induction of RALT expression by hypoxic conditions in cardiomyocytes may contribute to ischemic injury by suppressing cellular survival signaling through Akt and Erk pathways (*104*). Interestingly, RALT expression is suppressed in breast cancer cells exhibiting ErbB2 amplification, and reconstitution of RALT in these cells inhibits ErbB2-dependent mitogenesis and reverses Herceptin resistance (*103*). RALT overexpression in the skin of transgenic mice yields a phenotype similar to the Waved phenotype indicative of impaired EGF receptor signaling (*105*). RALT knockout in mice causes EGFR hyperactivation, induces some spontaneous tumors of various organs, and confers heightened susceptibility to chemically-induced skin tumors (*106, 107*). Missense and nonsense mutations in the RALT coding region, as well as transcriptional silencing, may give rise to the suppression of RALT protein in human tumors (107). Collectively, these findings suggest that loss of RALT may augment or cooperate with ErbB signaling to drive full oncogenic signaling.

5.3. LRR-containing Proteins

As outlined above, the Drosophila LRR/Ig protein Kekkon-1 is able to bind to and suppress the activities of mammalian ErbB receptors, suggesting that mammalian LRR proteins may possess similar functions. Indeed, decorin is a secreted proteoglycan containing nine leucine-richrepeats in its extracellular region that is frequently underexpressed in tumors. Decorin binds to mammalian ErbB receptors (*108*) to induce receptor down-regulation (*109, 110*), a property that may ultimately be exploited for therapeutic benefit. For example, inducible expression of decorin markedly suppresses both primary tumor growth and metastasis in an orthotopic mammary carcinoma model, and growth suppression correlates with a loss of ErbB2 (*111*). Moreover, intraperitoneal injection of recombinant decorin protein causes a significant and dose-dependent inhibition of squamous carcinoma xenograft growth (*112*). These observations raise the possibility that restoration of decorin to tumors could limit metastatic cancer in patients.

LRIG1 is a 140 kilodalton transmembrane protein containing 15 LRRs and 3 Ig domains expressed in most epithelial tissues, the endothelium, heart, skin, as well as smooth and striated muscle (*113, 114*). LRIG1 protein is particularly abundant in secretory epithelia, including breast and prostate (*115*). The LRIG1 gene is located at chromosome 3p14.3, an area frequently deleted in numerous tumor types, and its transcript is much less abundant in tumor cell lines derived from lung, prostate, and colon compared to normal tissue (*116*). We have observed that the majority of primary human breast tumors display decreased LRIG1 protein expression when compared to matched normal tissue (unpublished observations). In contrast, Ljuslinder et al. recently reported an increase in copy number at 3p14.3 in 39% of breast tumors, and a corresponding increase in protein expression in breast tumor lysates (*117*). Considering this discrepancy, a key question for future studies concerns the extent to which LRIG1 expression is dysregulated in breast tumors, and whether or not aberrant expression serves as a predictive or prognostic indicator.

LRIG1 deficient mice are normal with respect to viability and fertility, but exhibit an epidermal hyperplasia of the tail and face reminiscent of psoriasis (*114*). Interestingly, LRIG1 expression is also significantly down-regulated in psoriatic human skin. LRIG1 knockout keratinocytes are highly proliferative and display perturbed terminal differentiation (*114*), and very recent studies suggest that LRIG1 functions to maintain epidermal stem cells in a quiescent nondividing state (*118*). Since aberrant EGFR activation is commonly observed in human psoriasis, and transgenic mice overexpressing EGFR ligands display a psoriatic phenotype similar to LRIG1 knockout mice (*119, 120*), these observations suggest that LRIG1 may function as a Kek1-like EGFR negative regulator. Indeed, LRIG1 interacts with all four mammalian ErbB receptors to suppress signaling (*121, 122*). Interestingly, LRIG1 also acts as a negative regulator of the Met receptor tyrosine kinase (*123*), which has also been implicated in breast cancer malignancy. In contrast with Kek1, which interferes with growth factor binding to DER, LRIG1 appears to repress receptors by targeting them for degradation through enhanced ubiquitination. LRIG1 augments ligand-stimulated EGF receptor ubiquitination through its ability to bind directly to the cbl E3 ubiquitin ligase (*122*). This observation provides another mechanism for coupling EGF-stimulated EGFR to this ligase. However, LRIG1 also suppresses ErbB receptor levels independent of growth factor stimulation (*121, 122*). Our unpublished studies demonstrate that neither dominant-negative cbl nor dominant-negative Nrdp1 are able to interfere with LRIG1-induced basal loss of receptors, suggesting that another ubiquitin ligase is involved in this event. The molecular mechanisms by which LRIG1 mediates receptor degradation remain a very important issue because loss of this mechanism could contribute to ErbB receptor overexpression in tumors.

6. CONCLUSION

Because ErbB overexpression and aberrant activation is known to contribute to the malignancy of a variety of solid tumor types, much effort has been put into understanding the receptor-initiated pathways that contribute to cellular growth control. These efforts have led to the development of an array of antibody and small molecule ErbB-directed anti-cancer drugs that have either already received FDA approval or are currently in clinical trials (*124*). However, the emerging pattern of therapeutic resistance to ErbB-directed drugs by many tumor types prompts questions as to whether more effective strategies may be developed. The newly emerging field of ErbB negative regulation could uncover novel drug targets and offer new strategies in suppressing ErbB-dependent tumors. For example, rather than targeting the activity of overexpressed ErbB receptors in tumors, it may be possible to target the pathways that permit receptor overexpression. The observations outlined here point to the existence of several negative regulatory pathways that may play a central role in keeping cellular levels or activities of ErbB receptors in check. In addition to fine-tuning the extent and duration of ErbB signaling to ensure proper development and tissue maintenance, these pathways could act as endogenous suppressors of tumor cell growth and invasion. Thus, loss of pathway function could contribute to receptor overexpression associated with aggressive tumors. Likewise, restoration or augmentation of pathway function could offer novel means of suppressing ErbB activity in tumor cells.

In the future, it will be important to continue the discovery of novel ErbB negative regulatory pathways. Proteins involved in endocytosis and trafficking, proteins involved in localizing receptors to specific plasma membrane subdomains, protein tyrosine phosphatases that suppress receptor signaling, and proteins that interfere with growth factor binding and activation are all candidate negative regulators whose loss could contribute to ErbB-mediated tumor progression. In addition, it will be critical to determine the extent to which these pathways, both individually and collectively, are lost in ErbB-dependent human tumors, and whether pathway loss contributes to ErbB receptor overexpression or activation. If these pathways (or subsets of pathways) are commonly lost in tumors, it will additionally be important to understand the mechanisms underlying those losses. For example, loss of Nrdp1 pathway function could result from mutational disruption of either the Nrdp1 or the USP8 genes, silencing of those genes, or the disruption of the biochemical pathway leading to USP8 activation. Mouse models will provide important mechanistic insight into pathway function in tumors. For example, we would predict that transgenic mice overexpressing Nrdp1 or LRIG1 protein would be refractory to ErbB-induced tumors, while LRIG1 or Nrdp1 knockout mice would be particularly susceptible. A detailed understanding of the mechanisms underlying the loss of function of negative regulatory pathways in human tumors will in turn lead to the development of strategies to restore pathway function to tumor cells, hopefully leading to better treatments for patients with ErbB-positive tumors.

ACKNOWLEDGMENTS

Kermit Carraway is supported by NIH grants GM068994 and CA123541, and Colleen Sweeney is supported by NIH grant CA118384. Lily Yen is the recipient of a DoD Breast Cancer Research Program postdoctoral fellowship.

REFERENCES

1. Crone SA, Zhao YY, Fan L, Gu Y, Min amisawa S, Liu Y, Peterson KL, Chen J, Kahn R, Condorelli G, Ross J, Jr., Chien KR, Lee KF. ErbB2 is essential in the prevention of dilated cardiomyopathy. Nat Med 2002; 8:459-465.

2. Ozcelik C, Erdmann B, Pilz B, Wettschureck N, Britsch S, Hubner N, Chien KR, Birchmeier C, Garratt AN. Conditional mutation of the ErbB2 (HER2) receptor in cardiomyocytes leads to dilated cardiomyopathy. Proc Natl Acad Sci USA 2002; 99:8880-8885.
3. Garcia-Rivello H, Taranda J, Said M, Cabeza-Meckert P, Vila-Petroff M, Scaglione J, Ghio S, Chen J, Lai C, Laguens RP, Lloyd KC, Hertig CM. Dilated cardiomyopathy in Erb-b4-deficient ventricular muscle. Am J Physiol Heart Circ Physiol 2005;289:H1153-1160.
4. Holbro T, Civenni G, Hynes NE. The ErbB receptors and their role in cancer progression. Exp Cell Res 2003; 284:99-110.
5. Mosesson Y, Yarden Y. Oncogenic growth factor receptors: implications for signal transduction therapy. Semin Cancer Biol 2004; 14:262-270.
6. Nahta R, Yu D, Hung MC, Hortobagyi GN, Esteva FJ. Mechanisms of disease: understanding resistance to HER2-targeted therapy in human breast cancer. Nat Clin Pract Oncol 2006;3:269-280.
7. Sergina NV, Rausch M, Wang D, Blair J, Hann B, Shokat KM, Moasser MM. Escape from HER-family tyrosine kinase inhibitor therapy by the kinase-inactive HER3. Nature 2007;445:437-441.
8. Fiorini M, Alimandi M, Fiorentino L, Sala G, Segatto O. Negative regulation of receptor tyrosine kinase signals. FEBS Lett 2001; 490:132-141.
9. Dikic I, Giordano S. Negative receptor signalling. Curr Opin Cell Biol 2003; 15:128-135.
10. Sweeney C, Carraway KL, III. Negative regulation of ErbB family receptor tyrosine kinases. Br J Cancer 2004; 90:289-293.
11. Sweeney C, Miller JK, Shattuck DL, Carraway KL, III. ErbB receptor negative regulatory mechanisms: implications in cancer. J Mammary Gland Biol Neoplasia 2006; 11:89-99.
12. Perrimon N, McMahon AP. Negative feedback mechanisms and their roles during pattern formation. Cell 1999; 97:13-16.
13. Freeman M. Feedback control of intercellular signalling in development. Nature 2000; 408:313-319.
14. Shilo BZ. Signaling by the Drosophila epidermal growth factor receptor pathway during development. Exp Cell Res 2003; 284:140-149.
15. Schweitzer R, Howes R, Smith R, Shilo BZ, Freeman M. Inhibition of Drosophila EGF receptor activation by the secreted protein Argos. Nature 1995; 376:699-702.
16. Jin MH, Sawamoto K, Ito M, Okano H. The interaction between the Drosophila secreted protein argos and the epidermal growth factor receptor inhibits dimerization of the receptor and binding of secreted spitz to the receptor. Mol Cell Biol 2000; 20:2098-2107.
17. Vinos J, Freeman M. Evidence that Argos is an antagonistic ligand of the EGF receptor. Oncogene 2000; 19:3560-3562.
18. Klein DE, Nappi VM, Reeves GT, Shvartsman SY, Lemmon MA. Argos inhibits epidermal growth factor receptor signalling by ligand sequestration. Nature 2004; 430:1040-1044.
19. Alvarado D, Evans TA, Sharma R, Lemmon MA, Duffy JB. Argos mutants define an affinity threshold for spitz inhibition in vivo. J Biol Chem 2006; 281:28993-29001.
20. Ghiglione C, Carraway KL, III, Amundadottir LT, Boswell RE, Perrimon N, Duffy JB. The transmembrane molecule kekkon-1 acts in a feedback loop to negatively regulate the activity of the Drosophila EGF receptor during oogenesis. Cell 1999; 96:847-856.
21. Alvarado D, Rice AH, Duffy JB. Knockouts of Kekkon1 define sequence elements essential for Drosophila epidermal growth factor receptor inhibition. Genetics 2004; 166:201-211.
22. Ghiglione C, Amundadottir L, Andresdottir M, Bilder D, Diamonti JA, Noselli S, Perrimon N, Carraway, KL, III. Mechanism of inhibition of the Drosophila and mammalian EGF receptors by the transmembrane protein Kekkon 1. Development 2003; 130:4483-4493.
23. Alvarado D, Rice AH, Duffy JB. Bipartite inhibition of Drosophila epidermal growth factor receptor by the extracellular and transmembrane domains of Kekkon1. Genetics 2004; 167:187-202.
24. Golembo M, Schweitzer R, Freeman M, Shilo BZ. Argos transcription is induced by the Drosophila EGF receptor pathway to form an inhibitory feedback loop. Development 1996; 122:223-230.
25. Slamon DJ, Clark GM, Wong SG, Levin WJ, Ullrich A, McGuire WL. Human breast cancer: correlation of relapse and survival with amplification of the HER-2/neu oncogene. Science 1987; 235:177-182.
26. Berger MS, Locher GW, Saurer S, Gullick WJ, Waterfield MD, Groner B, Hynes NE. Correlation of c-erbB-2 gene amplification and protein expression in human breast carcinoma with nodal status and nuclear grading. Cancer Res 1988; 48:1238-1243.

27. Slamon DJ, Godolphin W, Jones LA, Holt JA, Wong SG, Keith DE, Levin WJ, Stuart SG, Udove J, Ullrich A, et al. Studies of the HER-2/neu proto-oncogene in human breast and ovarian cancer. Science 1989;244:707-712.
28. Zhou BP, Hung MC. Dysregulation of cellular signaling by HER2/neu in breast cancer. Semin Oncol 2003; 30:38-48.
29. Suter TM, Cook-Bruns N, Barton C. Cardiotoxicity associated with trastuzumab (Herceptin) therapy in the treatment of metastatic breast cancer. Breast 2004; 13:173-183.
30. Lemoine NR, Barnes DM, Hollywood DP, Hughes CM, Smith P, Dublin E, Prigent SA, Gullick WJ, Hurst HC. Expression of the ErbB3 gene product in breast cancer. Br J Cancer 1992; 66:1116-1121.
31. Naidu R, Yadav M, Nair S, Kutty MK. Expression of c-erbB3 protein in primary breast carcinomas. Br J Cancer 1998; 78:1385-1390.
32. Witton CJ, Reeves JR, Going JJ, Cooke TG, Bartlett JM. Expression of the HER1-4 family of receptor tyrosine kinases in breast cancer. J Pathol 2003; 200:290-297.
33. Rajkumar T, Gullick WJ. The type I growth factor receptors in human breast cancer. Breast Cancer Res Treat 1994; 29:3-9.
34. Siegel PM, Ryan ED, Cardiff RD, Muller WJ. Elevated expression of activated forms of Neu/ErbB-2 and ErbB-3 are involved in the induction of mammary tumors in transgenic mice: implications for human breast cancer. EMBO J 1999; 18:2149-2164.
35. Carraway KL, III, Cantley LC. A neu acquaintance for erbB3 and erbB4: a role for receptor heterodimerization in growth signaling. Cell 1994; 78:5-8.
36. Alroy I, Yarden Y. The ErbB signaling network in embryogenesis and oncogenesis: signal diversification through combinatorial ligand-receptor interactions. FEBS Lett 1997; 410:83-86.
37. Riese DJ, II, Stern DF. Specificity within the EGF family/ErbB receptor family signaling network. Bioessays 1998; 20:41-48.
38. Olayioye MA, Neve RM, Lane HA, Hynes NE. The ErbB signaling network: receptor heterodimerization in development and cancer. EMBO J. 2000; 19:3159-3167.
39. Carraway KL, III, Sliwkowski MX, Akita R, Platko JV, Guy PM, Nuijens A, Diamonti AJ, Vandlen RL, Cantley LC, Cerione RA. The erbB3 gene product is a receptor for heregulin. J Biol Chem 1994; 269:14303-14306.
40. Guy PM, Platko JV, Cantley LC, Cerione RA, Carraway KL, III. Insect cell-expressed p180erbB3 possesses an impaired tyrosine kinase activity. Proc Natl Acad Sci U S A 1994; 91:8132-8136.
41. Sliwkowski MX, Schaefer G, Akita RW, Lofgren JA, Fitzpatrick VD, Nuijens A, Fendly BM, Cerione RA, Vandlen RL, Carraway KL, III. Coexpression of erbB2 and erbB3 proteins reconstitutes a high affinity receptor for heregulin. J Biol Chem 1994; 269:14661-14665.
42. Carraway KL, III, Soltoff SP, Diamonti AJ, Cantley LC. Heregulin stimulates mitogenesis and phosphatidylinositol 3-kinase in mouse fibroblasts transfected with ErbB2/neu and ErbB3. J Biol Chem 1995; 270:7111-7116.
43. Alimandi M, Romano A, Curia MC, Muraro R, Fedi P, Aaronson SA, Di Fiore PP, Kraus MH. Cooperative signaling of ErbB3 and ErbB2 in neoplastic transformation and human mammary carcinomas. Oncogene 1995; 10:1813-1821.
44. Holbro T, Beerli RR, Maurer F, Koziczak M, Barbas CF, III, Hynes NE. The ErbB2/ErbB3 heterodimer functions as an oncogenic unit: ErbB2 requires ErbB3 to drive breast tumor cell proliferation. Proc Natl Acad Sci USA. 2003; 100:8933-8938.
45. Xu FJ, Stack S, Boyer C, O'Briant K, Whitaker R, Mills GB, Yu YH, Bast RC, Jr. Heregulin and agonistic anti-p185(c-erbB2) antibodies inhibit proliferation but increase invasiveness of breast cancer cells that overexpress p185(c-erbB2): increased invasiveness may contribute to poor prognosis. Clin Cancer Res 1997; 3:1629-1634.
46. Tan M, Grijalva R, Yu D. Heregulin beta1-activated phosphatidylinositol 3-kinase enhances aggregation of MCF-7 breast cancer cells independent of extracellular signal-regulated kinase. Cancer Res 1999; 59:1620-1625.
47. Hijazi MM, Thompson EW, Tang C, Coopman P, Torri JA, Yang D, Mueller SC, Lupu R. Heregulin regulates the actin cytoskeleton and promotes invasive properties in breast cancer cell lines. Int J Oncol 2000; 17:629-641.
48. Agus DB, Akita RW, Fox WD, Lewis GD, Higgins B, Pisacane PI, Lofgren JA, Tindell C, Evans DP, Maiese K, Scher HI, Sliwkowski MX. Targeting ligand-activated ErbB2 signaling inhibits breast and prostate tumor growth. Cancer Cell 2002; 2:127-137.

49. Walshe JM, Denduluri N, Berman AW, Rosing DR, Swain SM. A phase II trial with trastuzumab and pertuzumab in patients with HER2-overexpressed locally advanced and metastatic breast cancer. Clin Breast Cancer 2006; 6:535-539.
50. Cardiff RD, Wellings SR. The comparative pathology of human and mouse mammary glands. J Mammary Gland Biol Neoplasia 1999;4:105-122.
51. Guy CT, Webster MA, Schaller M, Parsons TJ, Cardiff RD, Muller WJ. Expression of the neu protooncogene in the mammary epithelium of transgenic mice induces metastatic disease. Proc Natl Acad Sci U S A 1992; 89:10578-10582.
52. Yen L, Cao Z, Wu X, Ingalla ER, Baron C, Young LJ, Gregg JP, Cardiff RD, Borowsky AD, Sweeney C, Carraway KL, III. Loss of Nrdp1 enhances ErbB2/ErbB3-dependent breast tumor cell growth. Cancer Res. 2006; 66:11279-11286.
53. Hicke L. Gettin' down with ubiquitin: turning off cell-surface receptors, transporters and channels. Trends Cell Biol 1999; 9:107-112.
54. Katzmann DJ, Odorizzi G, Emr SD. Receptor downregulation and multivesicular-body sorting. Nat Rev Mol Cell Biol 2002; 3:893-905.
55. Shtiegman K, Yarden Y. The role of ubiquitylation in signaling by growth factors: implications to cancer. Semin Cancer Biol 2003; 13:29-40.
56. Haglund K, Sigismund S, Polo S, Szymkiewicz I, Di Fiore PP, Dikic I. Multiple monoubiquitination of RTKs is sufficient for their endocytosis and degradation. Nat Cell Biol 2003; 5:461-466.
57. Mosesson Y, Shtiegman K, Katz M, Zwang Y, Vereb G, Szollosi J, Yarden Y. Endocytosis of receptor tyrosine kinases is driven by monoubiquitylation, not polyubiquitylation. J Biol Chem 2003; 278:21323-21326.
58. Di Fiore PP, Polo S, Hofmann K. When ubiquitin meets ubiquitin receptors: a signalling connection. Nat Rev Mol Cell Biol 2003; 4:491-497.
59. Haglund K, Di Fiore PP, Dikic I. Distinct monoubiquitin signals in receptor endocytosis. Trends Biochem Sci 2003; 28:598-603.
60. Huang F, Kirkpatrick D, Jiang X, Gygi S, Sorkin A. Differential regulation of EGF receptor internalization and degradation by multiubiquitination within the kinase domain. Mol Cell 2006; 21:737-748.
61. Thien CB, Langdon WY. Cbl: many adaptations to regulate protein tyrosine kinases. Nat Rev Mol Cell Biol 2001; 2:294-307.
62. Levkowitz G, Waterman H, Zamir E, Kam Z, Oved S, Langdon WY, Beguinot L, Geiger B, Yarden Y. c-Cbl/Sli-1 regulates endocytic sorting and ubiquitination of the epidermal growth factor receptor. Genes Dev 1998; 12:3663-3674.
63. Lill NL, Douillard P, Awwad RA, Ota S, Lupher ML, Jr., Miyake S, Meissner-Lula N, Hsu VW, Band H. The evolutionarily conserved N-terminal region of Cbl is sufficient to enhance down-regulation of the epidermal growth factor receptor. J Biol Chem 2000; 275:367-377.
64. Levkowitz G, Waterman H, Ettenberg SA, Katz M, Tsygankov AY, Alroy I, Lavi S, Iwai K, Reiss Y, Ciechanover A, Lipkowitz S, Yarden Y. Ubiquitin ligase activity and tyrosine phosphorylation underlie suppression of growth factor signaling by c-Cbl/Sli-1. Mol Cell 1999; 4:1029-1040.
65. Ravid T, Sweeney C, Gee P, Carraway KL, III, Goldkorn T. Epidermal growth factor receptor activation under oxidative stress fails to promote c-Cbl mediated down-regulation. J Biol Chem 2002; 277:31214-31219.
66. Peschard P, Park M. Escape from Cbl-mediated downregulation: a recurrent theme for oncogenic deregulation of receptor tyrosine kinases. Cancer Cell 2003; 3:519-523.
67. de Melker AA, van der Horst G, Calafat J, Jansen H, Borst J. c-Cbl ubiquitinates the EGF receptor at the plasma membrane and remains receptor associated throughout the endocytic route. J Cell Sci 2001; 114:2167-2178.
68. Duan L, Miura Y, Dimri M, Majumder B, Dodge IL, Reddi AL, Ghosh A, Fernandes N, Zhou P, Mullane-Robinson K, Rao N, Donoghue S, Rogers RA, Bowtell D, Naramura M, Gu H, B and V, B and H. Cbl-mediated ubiquitinylation is required for lysosomal sorting of epidermal growth factor receptor but is dispensable for endocytosis. J Biol Chem 2003; 278:28950-28960.
69. Wiley HS. Trafficking of the ErbB receptors and its influence on signaling. Exp Cell Res 2003; 284:78-88.
70. Levkowitz G, Klapper LN, Tzahar E, Freywald A, Sela M, Yarden Y. Coupling of the c-Cbl protooncogene product to ErbB-1/EGF-receptor but not to other ErbB proteins. Oncogene 1996; 12:1117-1125.

71. Baulida J, Kraus MH, Alimandi M, Di Fiore PP, Carpenter G. All ErbB receptors other than the epidermal growth factor receptor are endocytosis impaired. J Biol Chem 1996; 271:5251-5257.
72. Xu W, Mimnaugh E, Rosser MF, Nicchitta C, Marcu M, Yarden Y, Neckers L. Sensitivity of mature ErbB2 to geldanamycin is conferred by its kinase domain and is mediated by the chaperone protein Hsp90. J Biol Chem 2001;276:3702-3708.
73. Citri A, Alroy I, Lavi S, Rubin C, Xu W, Grammatikakis N, Patterson C, Neckers L, Fry DW, Yarden Y. Drug-induced ubiquitylation and degradation of ErbB receptor tyrosine kinases: implications for cancer therapy. EMBO J 2002;21:2407-2417.
74. McDonough H, Patterson C. CHIP: a link between the chaperone and proteasome systems. Cell Stress Chaperones 2003;8:303-308.
75. Gassmann M, Lemke G. Neuregulins and neuregulin receptors in neural development. Curr Opin Neurobiol 1997;7:87-92.
76. Falls DL. Neuregulins and the neuromuscular system: 10 years of answers and questions. J Neurocytol 2003;32:619-647.
77. Negro A, Brar BK, Lee KF. Essential roles of Her2/erbB2 in cardiac development and function. Recent Prog Horm Res 2004;59:1-12.
78. Xu W, Marcu M, Yuan X, Mimnaugh E, Patterson C, Neckers L. Chaperone-dependent E3 ubiquitin ligase CHIP mediates a degradative pathway for c-ErbB2/Neu. Proc Natl Acad Sci USA 2002;99:12847-12852.
79. Zhou P, Fernandes N, Dodge IL, Reddi AL, Rao N, Safran H, DiPetrillo TA, Wazer DE, Band V, Band H. ErbB2 degradation mediated by the co-chaperone protein CHIP. J Biol Chem 2003;278:13829-13837.
80. Isaacs JS, Xu W, Neckers L. Heat shock protein 90 as a molecular target for cancer therapeutics. Cancer Cell 2003; 3:213-217.
81. Xu W, Yuan X, Beebe K, Xiang Z, Neckers L. Loss of Hsp90 association up-regulates Src-dependent ErbB2 activity. Mol Cell Biol. 2007; 27:220-228.
82. Nie J, McGill MA, Dermer M, Dho SE, Wolting CD, McGlade CJ. LNX functions as a RING type E3 ubiquitin ligase that targets the cell fate determinant Numb for ubiquitin-dependent degradation. EMBO J 2002;21:93-102.
83. Young P, Nie J, Wang X, McGlade CJ, Rich MM, Feng G. LNX1 is a perisynaptic Schwann cell specific E3 ubiquitin ligase that interacts with ErbB2. Mol Cell Neurosci 2005;30:238-248.
84. Diamonti AJ, Guy PM, Ivanof C, Wong K, Sweeney C, Carraway KL, III. An RBCC protein implicated in maintenance of steady-state neuregulin receptor levels. Proc Natl Acad Sci USA 2002; 99:2866-2871.
85. Qiu XB, Goldberg AL. Nrdp1/FLRF is a ubiquitin ligase promoting ubiquitination and degradation of the epidermal growth factor receptor family member, ErbB3. Proc Natl Acad Sci USA 2002; 99:14843-14848.
86. Bouyain S, Leahy DJ. Structure-based mutagenesis of the substrate-recognition domain of Nrdp1/FLRF identifies the binding site for the receptor tyrosine kinase ErbB3. Protein Sci 2007;16:654-661.
87. Wu X, Yen L, Irwin L, Sweeney C, Carraway KL, III. Stabilization of the E3 ubiquitin ligase Nrdp1 by the deubiquitinating enzyme USP8. Mol Cell Biol. 2004; 24:7748-7757.
88. Cao Z, Wu X, Yen L, Sweeney C, Carraway KL, III. Neuregulin-induced ErbB3 downregulation is mediated by a protein stability cascade involving the E3 ubiquitin ligase Nrdp1. Mol Cell Biol 2007; 27:2180-2188.
89. Doherty JK, Bond C, Jardim A, Adelman JP, Clinton GM. The HER-2/neu receptor tyrosine kinase gene encodes a secreted autoinhibitor. Proc Natl Acad Sci USA 1999; 96:10869-10874.
90. Azios NG, Romero FJ, Denton MC, Doherty JK, Clinton GM. Expression of herstatin, an autoinhibitor of HER-2/neu, inhibits transactivation of HER-3 by HER-2 and blocks EGF activation of the EGF receptor. Oncogene 2001; 20:5199-5209.
91. Justman QA, Clinton GM. Herstatin, an autoinhibitor of the human epidermal growth factor receptor 2 tyrosine kinase, modulates epidermal growth factor signaling pathways resulting in growth arrest. J Biol Chem 2002; 277:20618-20624.
92. Jhabvala-Romero F, Evans A, Guo S, Denton M, Clinton GM. Herstatin inhibits heregulin-mediated breast cancer cell growth and overcomes tamoxifen resistance in breast cancer cells that overexpress HER-2. Oncogene 2003; 22:8178-8186.

93. Hu P, Zhou T, Qian L, Wang J, Shi M, Yu M, Yang Y, Zhang X, Shen B, Guo N. Sequestering ErbB2 in endoplasmic reticulum by its autoinhibitor from translocation to cell surface: an autoinhibition mechanism of ErbB2 expression. Biochem Biophys Res Commun 2006; 342:19-27.
94. Staverosky JA, Muldoon LL, Guo S, Evans AJ, Neuwelt EA, Clinton GM. Herstatin, an autoinhibitor of the epidermal growth factor receptor family, blocks the intracranial growth of glioblastoma. Clin Cancer Res 2005; 11:335-340.
95. Yu Y, Rishi AK, Turner JR, Liu D, Black ED, Moshier JA, Majumdar AP. Cloning of a novel EGFR-related peptide: a putative negative regulator of EGFR. Am J Physiol Cell Physiol 2001; 280: C1083-1089.
96. Xu H, Yu Y, Marciniak D, Rishi AK, Sarkar FH, Kucuk O, Majumdar AP. Epidermal growth factor receptor (EGFR)-related protein inhibits multiple members of the EGFR family in colon and breast cancer cells. Mol Cancer Ther 2005; 4:435-442.
97. Majumdar AP. Therapeutic potential of EGFR-related protein, a universal EGFR family antagonist. Future Oncol 2005; 1:235-245.
98. Lee H, Akita RW, Sliwkowski MX, Maihle NJ. A naturally occurring secreted human ErbB3 receptor isoform inhibits heregulin-stimulated activation of ErbB2, ErbB3, and ErbB4. Cancer Res 2001; 61:4467-4473.
99. Fiorentino L, Pertica C, Fiorini M, Talora C, Crescenzi M, Castellani L, Alema S, Benedetti P, Segatto O. Inhibition of ErbB-2 mitogenic and transforming activity by RALT, a mitogen-induced signal transducer which binds to the ErbB-2 kinase domain. Mol Cell Biol 2000; 20:7735-7750.
100. Hackel PO, Gishizky M, Ullrich A. Mig-6 is a negative regulator of the epidermal growth factor receptor signal. Biol Chem 2001; 382:1649-1662.
101. Anastasi S, Fiorentino L, Fiorini M, Fraioli R, Sala G, Castellani L, Alema S, Alimandi M, Segatto O. Feedback inhibition by RALT controls signal output by the ErbB network. Oncogene 2003; 22 4221-4234.
102. Xu D, Makkinje A, Kyriakis JM. Gene 33 is an endogenous inhibitor of epidermal growth factor (EGF) receptor signaling and mediates dexamethasone-induced suppression of EGF function. J Biol Chem 2005; 280:2924-2933.
103. Anastasi S, Sala G, Huiping C, Caprini E, Russo G, Iacovelli S, Lucini F, Ingvarsson S, Segatto O. Loss of RALT/MIG-6 expression in ERBB2-amplified breast carcinomas enhances ErbB-2 oncogenic potency and favors resistance to Herceptin. Oncogene 2005; 24:4540-4548.
104. Xu D, Patten RD, Force T, Kyriakis JM. Gene 33/RALT is induced by hypoxia in cardiomyocytes, where it promotes cell death by suppressing phosphatidylinositol 3-kinase and extracellular signal-regulated kinase survival signaling. Mol Cell Biol 2006; 26:5043-5054.
105. Ballaro C, Ceccarelli S, Tiveron C, Tatangelo L, Salvatore AM, Segatto O, Alema S. Targeted expression of RALT in mouse skin inhibits epidermal growth factor receptor signalling and generates a Waved-like phenotype. EMBO Rep 2005; 6:755-761.
106. Ferby I, Reschke M, Kudlacek O, Knyazev P, Pante G, Amann K, Sommergruber W, Kraut N, Ullrich A, Fassler R, Klein R. Mig6 is a negative regulator of EGF receptor-mediated skin morphogenesis and tumor formation. Nat Med 2006; 12:568-573.
107. Zhang YW, Staal B, Su Y, Swiatek P, Zhao P, Cao B, Resau J, Sigler R, Bronson R, Vande Woude GF. Evidence that MIG-6 is a tumor-suppressor gene. Oncogene 2007; 26:269-276.
108. Iozzo RV, Moscatello DK, McQuillan DJ, Eichstetter I. Decorin is a biological ligand for the epidermal growth factor receptor. J Biol Chem 1999; 274:4489-4492.
109. Csordas G, Santra M, Reed CC, Eichstetter I, McQuillan DJ, Gross D, Nugent MA, Hajnoczky G, Iozzo RV. Sustained down-regulation of the epidermal growth factor receptor by decorin. A mechanism for controlling tumor growth in vivo. J Biol Chem 2000; 275:32879-32887.
110. Santra M, Eichstetter I, Iozzo RV. An anti-oncogenic role for decorin. Down-regulation of ErbB2 leads to growth suppression and cytodifferentiation of mammary carcinoma cells. J Biol Chem 2000; 275:35153-35161.
111. Reed CC, Waterhouse A, Kirby S, Kay P, Owens RT, McQuillan DJ, Iozzo RV. Decorin prevents metastatic spreading of breast cancer. Oncogene 2005; 24:1104-1110.
112. Seidler DG, Goldoni S, Agnew C, Cardi C, Thakur ML, Owens RT, McQuillan DJ, Iozzo RV. Decorin protein core inhibits in vivo cancer growth and metabolism by hindering epidermal growth factor receptor function and triggering apoptosis via caspase-3 activation. J Biol Chem 2006; 281:26408-26418.

113. Nilsson J, Vallbo C, Guo D, Golovleva I, Hallberg B, Henriksson R, Hedman H. Cloning, characterization, and expression of human LIG1. Biochem Biophys Res Commun 2001; 284:1155-1161.
114. Suzuki Y, Miura H, Tanemura A, Kobayashi K, Kondoh G, Sano S, Ozawa K, Inui S, Nakata A, Takagi T, Tohyama M, Yoshikawa K, Itami S. Targeted disruption of LIG-1 gene results in psoriasiform epidermal hyperplasia. FEBS Lett 2002; 521:67-71.
115. Nilsson J, Starefeldt A, Henriksson R, Hedman H. LRIG1 protein in human cells and tissues. Cell Tissue Res 2003; 312:65-71.
116. Hedman H, Nilsson J, Guo D, Henriksson R. Is LRIG1 a tumour suppressor gene at chromosome 3p14.3? Acta Oncol 2002; 41:352-354.
117. Ljuslinder I, Malmer B, Golovleva I, Thomasson M, Grankvist K, Hockenstrom T, Emdin S, Jonsson Y, Hedman H, Henriksson R. Increased copy number at 3p14 in breast cancer. Breast Cancer Res 2005; 7:R719-727.
118. Jensen KB, Watt FM. Single-cell expression profiling of human epidermal stem and transit-amplifying cells: Lrig1 is a regulator of stem cell quiescence. Proc Natl Acad Sci USA 2006; 103:11958-11963.
119. Vassar R, Fuchs E. Transgenic mice provide new insights into the role of TGF-alpha during epidermal development and differentiation. Genes Dev 1991; 5:714-727.
120. Cook PW, Piepkorn M, Clegg CH, Plowman GD, DeMay JM, Brown JR, Pittelkow MR. Transgenic expression of the human amphiregulin gene induces a psoriasis-like phenotype. J Clin Invest 1997; 100:2286-2294.
121. Laederich MB, Funes-Duran M, Yen L, Ingalla E, Wu X, Carraway KL, III, Sweeney C. The leucine-rich repeat protein LRIG1 is a negative regulator of ErbB family receptor tyrosine kinases. J Biol Chem 2004; 279:47050-47056.
122. Gur G, Rubin C, Katz M, Amit I, Citri A, Nilsson J, Amariglio N, Henriksson R, Rechavi G, Hedman H, Wides R, Yarden Y. LRIG1 restricts growth factor signaling by enhancing receptor ubiquitylation and degradation. EMBO J 2004; 23:3270-3281.
123. Shattuck DL, Miller JK, Laederich M, Funes M, Petersen H, Carraway KL, III, Sweeney C. LRIG1 is a novel negative regulator of the Met receptor and opposes Met and Her2 synergy. Mol Cell Biol 2007; 27:1934-1946.
124. Arteaga CL. ErbB-targeted therapeutic approaches in human cancer. Exp Cell Res 2003; 284:122-130.

13 Nuclear ErbB Receptors: Pathways and Functions

Hong-Jun Liao and Graham Carpenter

CONTENTS
    INTRODUCTION
    CONVENTIONAL ERBB PATHWAYS
    MECHANISM OF ERBB TRANSLOCATION TO THE NUCLEUS
    NUCLEAR FUNCTIONS FOR ERBB
    CONCLUSION
    REFERENCES

Abstract

Accumulating evidence suggests a new mode of ErbB receptor signaling in which intact or fragmented ErbB receptors traffic from the cell surface to the nucleus following the addition of a cognate ligand. In the nucleus, ErbB receptors have a role, probably indirect, in modulating gene expression. Following the addition of growth factor, ErbB1 is sorted from the cell surface to the endoplasmic reticulum where it interacts with the Sec61 translocon and is retrotranslocated from the endoplasmic reticulum to cytoplasm. This is a precursor step for subsequent nuclear localization of the receptor and the induction of cyclin D by EGF. In the case of ErbB4, the receptor is processed by two membrane-localized proteases to produce a soluble cytoplasmic domain fragment that translocates to the nucleus. Nuclear ErbB1 and ErbB4 have been detected in the tissue of cancer patients and may portend a poorer prognosis. Less understood are mechanisms that provoke nuclear localization of ErbB2 and ErbB3, which have been described in cell culture systems.

Key Words: ErbB, Epidermal Growth Factor, Epidermal Growth Factor Receptor, Nucleus, Signal Transduction.

1. INTRODUCTION

The epidermal growth factor (EGF) receptor family includes the EGF receptor (ErbB1/HER1) and three other family members: ErbB2 (HER2), ErbB3 (HER3), and ErbB4 (HER4). ErbB1 and ErbB2 play key roles in the tumorogenesis of epithelial-derived cancers and are attractive candidates for the development of target-based treatments. ErbB receptor activation and signaling are known to depend on growth factor induced homo- and heterodimerization with the subsequent activation of tyrosine kinase activity. Co-incident with the activation of signaling pathways, ErbB receptors are subjected to internalization and intracellular trafficking. The role of trafficking in signaling and cellular response to growth factors is beginning to be elucidated.

From: *Cancer Drug Discovery and Development: EGFR Signaling Networks in Cancer Therapy*
Edited by: J. D. Haley and W. J. Gullick, DOI: 10.1007/978-1-59745-356-1_13
© 2008 Humana Press, a part of Springer Science+Business Media, LLC

Though older reports of nuclear ErbB1 and ErbB2 exist (1), recent and more rigorous data have renewed interest in this topic. Accumulating evidence shows the growth factor-dependent translocation of ErbB1 and ErbB4 to the nucleus and that these nuclear receptors have roles in gene expression. The scope of this review is to describe available data that describe the different and novel mechanisms of intracellular trafficking of these two receptors to the nucleus. Also, addressed are the known functions of nuclear ErbB1 and ErbB4.

2. CONVENTIONAL ErbB PATHWAYS

2.1. ErbB Receptor Signaling

ErbB receptor tyrosine kinases are Type I transmembrane molecules positioned at the cell surface to detect the presence of cognate growth factors produced into the extracellular milieu by neighboring cells. This recognition event activates the intrinsic tyrosine kinase activity of each ErbB receptor and initiates a network of signaling pathways that relay information from cell surface to the nucleus, as well as other points in the cell (2, 3). Sequentially acting components, such as those of the Ras/MAP kinase pathway, or single component systems, such as the STAT pathway, are considered to constitute the mechanisms by which this intracellular transfer of biochemical information is mediated. Current thinking is that the combinatorial information provided by these signal transduction pathways can explain the biological responses of cells to growth factors.

2.2. ErbB Receptor Trafficking

Growth factor: receptor tyrosine kinase complexes formed at the plasma membrane are neither stagnant nor restricted to the cell surface. That the complexes are rapidly internalized through clathrin-coated pits into an endocytic pathway has been recognized for a number of years. Subsequent to internalization, receptor complexes remain active but are eventually sorted either to the lysosome and degraded or recycled back to the cell surface (4, 5).

One report indicates that the full-length ErbB1, subsequent to activation by EGF, translocates from cell surface to the mitochondria and associates with cytochrome oxidase subunit II (Cox II) (6). This interaction is dependent on phosphorylation of Y845 of ErbB1. This is not, however, an autophosphorylation site, but rather a site phosphorylated by Src (7). The functional consequence of ErbB1 mitochondrial translocation is anti-apoptosis; however, the mechanism for ErbB1 mitochondrial translocation is not clear. Interestingly, the cell death response to production of the ErbB4 intracellular domain fragment (ICD) is also associated with the translocation of this ICD to mitochondria (8, 9).

Evidence has also begun to accumulate that the endocytic pathway is a site for the generation of signal transduction to the nucleus. An endosomal compartment bearing Rab5 and APPL acts as an intermediate in signaling between the plasma membrane and the nucleus (10). The GTPase Rab5 is present on distinct intracellular organelles: plasma membrane, clathrin-coated vesicles, and early endosomes. APPL1 and 2, two Rab5 effectors, reside on a subpopulation of endosomes. Following EGF stimulation, Rab5 is recruited to the plasma membrane and EEA1-positive early endosomes by activated ErbB1. This allows for efficient ErbB1 internalization and subsequent transport to multivesicular bodies, late endosomes, and lysosomes. APPL1 and APPL2 bind to active Rab5 and then translocate from the endosome membrane to the nucleus by an unknown mechanism. In the nucleus, APPL1or 2 interacts with the nucleosome remodeling and histone deacetylase multiprotein complex NuRD/MeCP1, which is an established regulator of chromatin structure and gene expression. Both APPL1 and 2 are essential for cell proliferation and their function requires Rab5 binding. In this mechanism ErbB1 containing endosomes are required for the nuclear localization APPL1 and 2; however, nuclear translocation of ErbB1 was not reported in this study.

3. MECHANISIM OF ErbB TRANSLOCATION TO THE NUCLEUS

Published data describe ErbB receptor in the nucleus in two forms - either the intact molecule (ErbB1,-2,-3) or an intracellular cytoplasmic domain fragment (ErbB4). The means by which an intact receptor is translocated from the plasma membrane to the nucleus is relatively recent (see below). The mechanism for fragment formation and translocation, however, is known and supported by precedents of other cell surface transmembrane molecules.

3.1. ErbB Fragments and the Protease-Dependent Route

Earlier data showed that the Notch transmembrane receptor (a non-receptor tyrosine kinase) is cleaved following ligand binding by the sequential action of two distinct membrane-localized proteases and that an ICD fragment is produced and translocates to the nucleus (11, 12). A similar scenario has been described for proteolytic processing of the Alzheimer's Precursor Protein (APP). This mechanism has now been extended to ErbB4 (13, Fig. 13.1), and several other cell-surface molecules, as shown in Table 13.1

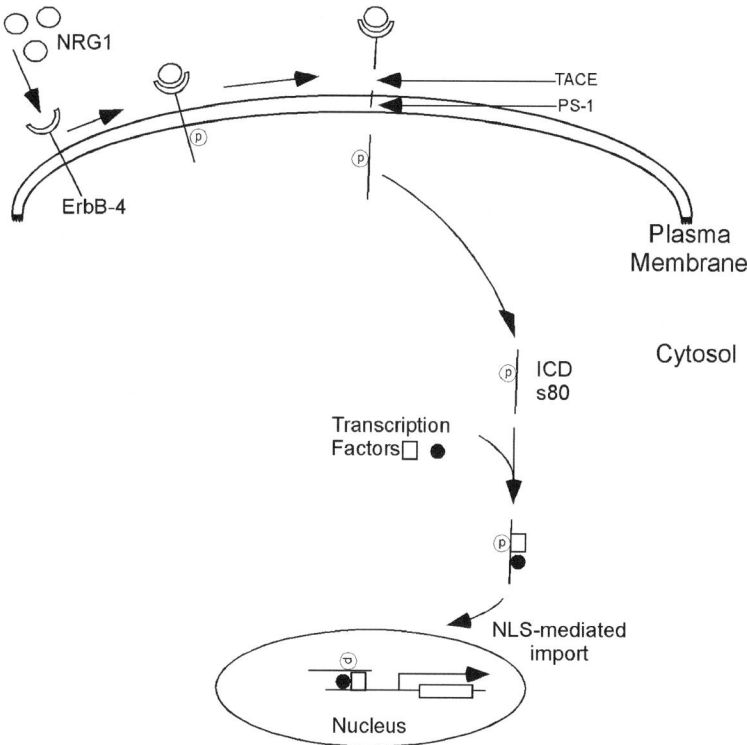

Fig. 13.1. Pathways for the ErbB4 from the cell surface to the nucleus. Following ligand binding, ErbB4 receptor is subjected a two-step sequential cleavage. The first cleavage is executed by TACE in extracellular juxtamembrane region, rel eases the ectodomain and produces a cell-associated transmembrane(TM)-ICD fragment. The TM-ICD is then cleaved by λ-secratase activity within the TM domain and produces a soluble cytoplasmic tyrosine kinase domain designated ICD or soluble 80 kDa fragment (s80). The ICD interacts with the cytosolic transcription factors and chaperones these into the nucleus to effect gene expression.

Table 13.1
Cell Surface Proteins Translocation into the Nucleus and Their Possible Functions

Cell Surface Protein	Basal/ Stimulated	Holoreceptor/ ICD Fragment	Evidence of Nuclear Function	Reference
ErbB1	EGF, radiation	Holo	Yes	29, 31, 32
ErbB2	Basal	Holo	Yes	33, 34
ErbB3	Basal	Holo	No	35
ErbB4	Heregulin, TPA	ICD	Yes	13
FGFR	FGF-2	Holo	Yes	36, 54
c-met	Basal	ICD	Yes	39
Notch	Delta	ICD	Yes	12
APP	Basal	ICD	Yes	13
p75 Neruotrophin Receptor	Nerutrophins	ICD	Yes	55
CD44	TPA, Ionomycin	ICD	Yes	56, 57
E-cadherin	Staurosporine	ICD	Yes	58
Low-Density Lipoprotein Receptor-Related Protein	TPA	ICD	No	59
Calcium channel $Ca_v1.2$	Calcium	ICD	Yes	60
Endothelin Receptor	Endothelin	Holo	No	62
Angiotension I Receptor	Angiotension	Holo	No	63
Bradykinin B2 Receptor	Bradykinin	Holo	No	63
Apelin Receptor	Apelin	Holo	No	63

The binding of ligand to ErbB4 (14) or the activation of protein kinase C by TPA (15) provokes ectodomain cleavage that releases a 120 kDa ectodomain fragment into the extracellular milieu and generates a membrane-associated 80 kDa fragment that includes the receptor's tyrosine kinase function. This cleavage requires metalloprotease activity and is the initial and rate-limiting step in agonist-dependent ErbB4 processing and eventual nuclear translocation. There is a low but detectable basal level of ErbB4 ectodomain cleavage in various cells (16), but how it is controlled, if at all, is not known. This constitutive cleavage of ErbB4 is analogous to the cleavage of the APP, which has no known ligand.

Based on the fact that TPA fails to stimulate ErbB4 ectodomain cleavage in TACE (Tumor Necrosis Factor Alpha Converting Enzyme) null cells (17) and the general role of TACE (ADAM 17) or closely related ADAMs in mediating cell surface shedding of numerous membrane molecules (18), it is clear that TACE participates in ErbB4 ectodomain cleavage. That TACE executes this cleavage event has not been demonstrated, however. TACE and its related ADAMs are single transmembrane molecules that have a metalloprotease active site within their ectodomain (18).

While TPA or heregulin stimulate this initial cleavage of ErbB4, the mechanisms seem to be distinct (14). For example, a general protein kinase C inhibitor blocks the TPA-induced cleavage, but not that induced by heregulin. Additionally, the evidence suggests that heregulin-induced cleavage is associated with ErbB4 endocytosis, while TPA is not. Ligand-induced proteolytic cleavage of Notch is clearly associated with endocytosis (12). It should be mentioned that TPA induces cleavage of ErbB4 in all cell backgrounds; however, heregulin-induced cleavage is only detectable in a subset of cell lines (14). The meaning of this is unclear. That the ectodomain cleavage of ErbB4 has biologic significance is suggested by the fact that a non-cleavable isoform of ErbB4 has been characterized in mouse tissues (19) and human tumor specimens (20, 21). This isoform is apparently generated by the use of alternate exons to alter the ErbB4 coding sequence in the stalk region of the receptor's ectodomain, the known site of TACE-induced cleavage. ErbB4 isoforms are reviewed elsewhere (22).

There is evidence that at least one of the products derived from ErbB4 ectodomain cleavage is functional. Than the cell-associated 80 kDa fragment remains an active tyrosine kinase (16) is not surprising, as there is evidence for several receptor tyrosine kinases that loss of the ectodomain activates tyrosine kinase activity. Importantly, this membrane-associated 80 kDa ErbB4 fragment is a substrate for additional protease systems. With time the fragment is ubiquitinated and degraded by proteosome activity (16). However, this fragment also serves as a substrate for γ-secretase activity (16, 23), which typically cleaves a membrane protein within its transmembrane domain and thereby provokes release of the intracellular cytoplasmic domain or ICD into the cytosol (12). γ-Secretase activity converts the membrane-associated 80 kDa ErbB4 fragment to a soluble or ICD fragment. The action of γ-secretase on transmembrane proteins, including ErbB4, requires preceding ectodomain cleavage for reasons that are not known (12).

Treatment of ErbB4 expressing cells with heregulin or TPA provokes release of the ICD into the cytoplasm and the fragment is then rapidly detected in the nucleus (13). Expression of a GFP tagged ErbB4 cytoplasmic domain fragment in recipient cells also shows significant accumulation in the nucleus, particularly if Leptomycin B, an inhibitor of nuclear export, is present. Putative nuclear import and export sequences in this ErbB4 fragment have been identified (13, 23), but have not been mutated. Interestingly, immunohistochemical studies of human tissues have noted the presence of nuclear ErbB4 (24-26). In breast tumor tissue, nuclear ErbB4 is on some studies correlated with a slightly poorer prognosis.

There are two well established precedents for this cleavage mechanism: the Notch receptor and the APP, neither of which are receptor tyrosine kinases. In both instances, the released cytoplasmic domain fragments are translocated to the nucleus and function to regulate transcription (11, 12). That this pathway may be more widespread is indicated by analogous cleavage events reported for other cell surface protein (Table 13.1). TPA-induced ectodomain shedding has also been reported for several additional recaptor tyrosine kinases (CSF-1, c-Kit, MGF, Axl, TrkA, Met, Tie-1), and ligand-induced ectodomain cleavage has been reported for TrkA (27) and the discoidin domain-1 receptor (28). Whether any of these or other receptor tyrosine kinases are also processed by γ-secretase activity remains to be seen, though such processing seems likely in the case of the CSF-1 receptor.

3.2. Holoreceptors in the Nucleus

Several recent papers have added substantially to previously published data reporting the presence of full-length receptor tyrosine kinases in the nucleus. In the case of ErbB1, addition of the cognate ligand is required for nuclear localization and, in fact, the ligand:receptor complex has been characterized as present in the nucleus (29). Recent reports indicate that following exposure to oxidative stress ErbB1 undergoes perinuclear trafficking (30), resembling the endoplasmic reticulum, and that radiation induces ErbB1 translocation into the nucleus (31, 32).

Intact ErbB2 has been detected in the nucleus of cultured cells, as well as primary tumor tissues (33). Nuclear ErbB2 was found to associate (directly or indirectly) with multiple genomic targets in vivo, including the COX-2 gene promoter. ErbB2 nuclear localization involves interaction with importin ß1 and nuclear pore protein Nup358 (34). Knocking down importin ß1 with siRNA or inactivation of the GTPase Ran, by expression of a dominant-negative mutant, abrogates nuclear localization of ErbB2. Mutation of a putative nuclear localization signal in ErbB2 presents interaction with importin ß1 and arrests nuclear translocation, while inactivation of the nuclear export receptor CRM1 provokes accumulation of ErbB2 within the nucleus. Additionally, blocking receptor internalization by a dominant-negative mutant of dynamin halts its nuclear localization. Thus, the cell membrane-embedded

ErbB2, through endocytosis using the endocytic vesicle as a vehicle, interacts with importin β1 and Nup358 in order to translocate from the cell surface to the nucleus.

A third receptor tyrosine kinase ErbB3, which binds the growth factor heregulin was reported to be constitutively present in an uncleaved form in nucleus, while addition of its ligand influenced the receptor's distribution between the nucleus and cytosol (35). When ErbB3 expressing cells were grown on filters to induce epithelial polarity, ErbB3 was concentrated in nucleoli. Nuclear localization of the full-length fibroblast growth factor receptor-I (FGFR-I) is promoted by the addition of FGF to cells (36, 37) and appears to involve interaction of this receptor with importin-β (38). Depletion of cellular ATP not only augmented the FGF-dependent nuclear accumulation of FGFR-I but was also sufficient to promote nuclear accumulation in the absence of FGF. The authors' conclusion is that ATP depletion results in an increased level of cytoplasmic importin, which facilitates nuclear localization of this receptor tyrosine kinase. Lastly, nuclear localization of c-met, the receptor for hepatocyte growth factor, has been reported recently (39).

The available reports suggest that these nuclear receptor tyrosine kinases are not found in the nuclear envelope but rather are present in the nucleoplasm in a non-membranous environment. In the cases of ErbB1 and FGFR-I, nuclear localization is ligand-dependent and involves endocytosis together with an unknown mechanism to traffic these receptor tyrosine kinases to the nucleus. Hence, the main complication would seem to be a mechanism to remove the intact receptor from a membrane bilayer, either at the cell surface or within an intracellular compartment, such as the endosome (1).

Recently a mechanism for this mode of intracellular receptor trafficking has been reported and involves ErbB1 translocation to the endoplasmic reticulum (ER) and extraction of intact transmembrane proteins into the cytoplasm and subsequent transport to the nucleus. This mechanism is described in the following section.

3.3. The Sec61 Pathway to the Nucleus

Following the addition of EGF, cell surface activated ErbB1 is trafficked to the ER where it associates with Sec61β, a component of the Sec61 translocon, and is retrotranslocated from the ER to the cytoplasm. Abrogation of Sec61β expression prevents EGF-dependent localization of ErbB1 to the nucleus. This result indicates that ErbB1 is trafficked from the ER to the nucleus by a novel pathway that involves the Sec61 translocon. This pathway is described in more detail in the following paragraphs.

The overall mechanism is depicted in Fig. 13.2 and describes a new route of intracellular trafficking not only for the activated ErbB1 but for any hormone receptor. However, this pathway from the cell surface to the ER is known for certain toxins (40) and for the SV40 virus (41). Toxins, such as cholera toxin, are internalized primarily, but not exclusively, from caveolae and trafficked first to the Golgi and then retrogradely transported to ER. Transport to the cytosolic site and toxin targets is mediated by the Sec61 translocon. SV40 is internalized from caveolae at the cell surface and via intracellular vesicles, termed caveosomes, trafficked to the ER. It is not known how virus particles exit the ER, but interruption of the pathway blocks virus replication, which requires nuclear localization. Preliminarily, it has been reported that translocons in the ER mediate virus penetration to the cytosol (42). These systems show that, in addition to their role in protein synthesis and quality control, translocons in the ER facilitate the mechanism of action of biological agents.

While intracellular trafficking of ErbB1 to the ER has not been previously reported, recent data show that ErbB1 is slowly trafficked from the cell surface to the ER (43). At three or six hours following the addition of EGF, about 10% or 25%, respectively, of the total cell surface ErbB1 receptor is present in the ER. Therefore, EGF receptor trafficking from the cell surface to the ER is relatively slow and involves, in the first hour, a small pool of internalized receptor.

As most published trafficking studies of the EGF receptor have focused on events within one hour following growth factor addition, it seems likely that the ER pool was too small to be considered significant in previous investigations. Interestingly, trafficking of SV40 and cholera toxin from the cell surface to the ER is also on the order of 2-3 hours (41, 44).

In terms of a mechanism of trafficking of the ErbB1 from the cell surface to the ER, little is known, including whether the Golgi is an intermediate. Others (45) have reported that the receptor-mediated endocytosis and importin β are required for nuclear localization of the ErbB1, which is consistent with trafficking to the ER following coated-pit internalization, as depicted in Fig. 13.2.

A major obstacle in understanding trafficking to the nucleus is reconciling a known mechanism with the fact that the nuclear EGF receptor is a transmembrane domain-containing molecule in a non-membranous environment (29). The ER-localized Sec61 translocon provides a mechanism to extract the receptor from its lipid bilayer. As part of the ER-associated degradation (ERAD) pathway, Sec61 retrotranslocates malfolded transmembrane proteins to the cytosol for proteosomal degradation. Retrotranslocation requires lumenal ER and cytoplasmic chaperones (46). HSP70 seems to be required for ErbB1 retrotranslocation and may simply function to prevent receptor aggregation in the cytosol (43).

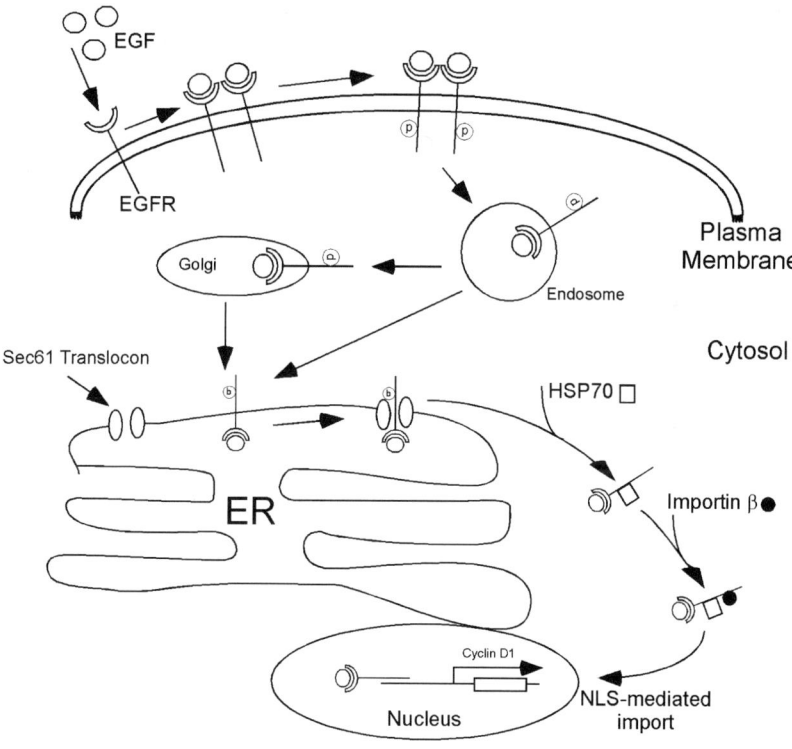

Fig. 13.2. Pathways for ErbB1 from cell surface to the nucleus. EGF binds to ErbB1 on the cell surface and induces ErbB1 dimerization and tyrosine kinase activation. Activated ErbB1 then is internized into endosomes. Endosomal ErbB1 translocates to ER directly or indirectly via the Golgi. ErbB1 interacts with the Sec 61 trasnlocon. Subsequently, ErbB1 is retrotranslocated by Sec 61 from the ER into cytosol and associates with HSP70. The cytoplasmic ErbB1 then interacts with importin β and translocates into nucleus, which it may associate (perhaps indirectly) with the *Cyclin* D1 promotor to modulate *Cyclin* D1 expression. Also, nuclear ErbB1 may phosphorylate substrates such as PCNA, in the nucleus.

Efficient proteosomal degradation of retrotranslocated glycoproteins, as part of the ERAD pathway, requires the removal of N-linked oligosaccharides by peptide-N-glycanase (47). Glycoprotein substrates in the ERAD system contain only high-mannose chains and peptide-N-glycanase exhibits a strong preference for high-mannose oligosaccharide-containing substrates. Therefore, the cell surface-derived ErbB1, which contains mostly complex oligosaccharides, should be a poor substrate for proteosomal degradation and this may indirectly promote receptor translocation to the nucleus. As discussed earlier, ErbB1 has been reported to associate with mitochondria (6) and mitochondria could be another trafficking site for retrotranslocated receptor.

The high-resolution structures of bacterial Sec61 orthologs suggest that the α and γ components are essential channel components, while the more peripheral β protein has a less clear functional role (48). This observation may suggest that knockdown of Sec61β may be more tolerable than other Sec61 subunits, particularly regarding interference with EGF receptor biosynthesis. Transient knockdown of Sec61β substantially depletes the intracellular pool of Sec61β protein and mRNA, but does not attenuate the level of ErbB1 protein nor EGF-induced ErbB1 phosphorylation (43). However, receptor in the nuclear fraction is significantly reduced in Sec61 β depleted cells, which indicates that Sec 61β is necessary for the nuclear localization of the ErbB1.

4. NUCLEAR FUNCTIONS FOR ErbB

The physiologic importance of receptor tyrosine kinase nuclear localization has been established, in a few cases, by identifying putative promoter targets and demonstrating that these targets are required for a growth factor cellular response. In the case of ErbB4, proteolytic processing, an initial study showed that γ-secretase inhibition blocked heregulin-dependent growth inhibition of T47 cells (13). While the inhibitor could have other unknown effects, it did not influence EGF-dependent growth stimulation in the same cells.

It has been demonstrated that nuclear signaling by ErbB4 ICD inhibits the responsiveness of precursors to astrocyte differentiation factors while maintaining their neurogenic potential (49). Upon neuregulin-induced activation and presenilin-dependent cleavage of ErbB4, the ICD forms a complex with TAB2 and the corepressor N-CoR. This complex undergoes nuclear translocation and binds to promoters of astrocytic genes repressing their expression. Consistent with this observation, astrogenesis occurs precociously in ErbB4 knockout mice.

In studies of mammary differentiation, the ErbB4 ICD chaperones cytoplasmic transcription factors, such as STAT5, into the nucleus and thereby promotes gene expression. Whether the ICD has an additional function at the promoter is unclear. CHIP experiments reveal the STAT5 promoter in association with the ICD, though this is not necessarily a direct association. One report (50) shows that ErbB4 ICD is required for tyrosine phosphorylation of Mdm2, a protein that is predominantly localized in the nucleus and that regulates p53 levels. When the ErbB4 ICD fragment was expressed in H1299 cells, it promoted Hdm2 ubiquitination and increased the levels of p53 and p21, a transcriptional target of p53. Another report (51) shows that ErbB4 ICD in the nucleus interacts with Eto2, a transcriptional co-repressor that is involved in erythrocyte differentiation and is also implicated in human breast cancer. Expression of ICD blocks Eto2-mediated transcriptional repression of a heterologous promoter.

Evidence for an ErbB1 role in transcription includes an in vitro demonstration of ErbB1 binding to a specific DNA sequence designated ARTS (29). Subsequent experiments in vivo showed the EGF-dependent stimulation of a reporter construct containing the ARTS sequence and a chromatin immunoprecipitation assay demonstrated ErbB1 bound to the cyclin D1 promoters, which contain an ARTS sequence. Sec61 β depletion experiments (43) demonstrated that the EGF induction of cyclin D1, but not c-fos, is significantly diminished in MDA-MB-468 and HeLa cells. HeLa cells do not overexpress ErbB1 and express 20-fold fewer receptors than MDA-MB-468 cells. These results indicate that Sec61 is required not only for nuclear localization of the ErbB1, but also for the receptor's capacity to act as a transcriptional co-activator.

Another report (52) has shown that ErbB1 physically interacts with STAT3 in the nucleus, leading to transcriptional activation of inducible nitric oxide synthase (iNOS). In case of radiation-induced ErbB1 translocation to the nucleus (31, 32), C225, an ErbB1 monoclonal antibody, abolished ErbB1 import into the nucleus and radiation-induced activation of DNA-PK, which is essential for repair of DNA-strand breaks. In contrast, the chromatin-bound proliferating cell nuclear antigen (PCNA) protein, which is required for maintaining its function on chromatin, is phosphorylated at Tyr 211 by nuclear ErbB1 (53). These results identify a novel nuclear mechanism linking tyrosine kinase receptor function with the regulation of the PCNA sliding clamp on chromatin.

The capacity of FGF-2 to induce the expression of c-jun or cyclin D1 mRNA was demonstrated to be sensitivity to the presence or absence of an artificial nuclear localization sequence incorporated into a transfected FGFR-I (38). One study has provided evidence that FGFR-I acts as a transcription factor at the FGF-2 promoter (54).

5. CONCLUSION

Obviously, these new observations raise provocative ideas about the trafficking and signaling mechanisms of receptor tyrosine kinases. The nuclear localization of other cell surface molecules or their cytoplasmic domain fragments are parallel examples of a direct communication mechanism between these two cellular compartments. It seems logical to expect that additional examples, including other receptor tyrosine kinases, will be added in the near future.

REFERENCES

1. Wells A, Marti U. Signalling shortcuts: cell-surface receptors in the nucleus? Nature Rev 2002; 3:1-6.
2. Schlessinger J. Cell signaling by receptor tyrosine kinases. Cell 2000; 103:211-221.
3. Brivanlou AH, Darnell JE Jr. Signal transduction and the control of gene expression. Science 2002, 295:813-818.
4. Carpenter G. The EGF receptor: a nexus for trafficking and signaling. BioEssays 2000, 22:697-707.
5. Sorkin A, von Zastro M: Signal transduction and endocytosis: close encounters of many kinds. Nature Rev 2002, 3:600-614.
6. Boerner JL, Demory ML, Silva C, Parsons SJ. Phosphorylation of Y845 on the epidermal growth factor receptor mediates binding to the mitochondrial protein cytochrome c oxidase subunit II. Mol Cell Biol 2004; 24:7059-7071.
7. Biscardi JS, Maa MC, Tice DA, et al. c-Src-mediated phosphorylation of the epidermal growth factor receptor on Tyr845 and Tyr1101 is associated with modulation of receptor function. J Biol Chem 1999; 274:8335-8343.
8. Muraoka-Cook RS, Sandahl M, Husted C et al. The intracellular domain of ErbB4 induces differentiation of mammary epithelial cells. Mol Biol Cell 2006; 17:4118-4129.
9. Naresh A, Long W, Vidal GA, et al. The ERBB4/HER4 intracellular domain 4ICD is a BH3-only protein promoting apoptosis of breast cancer cells. Cancer Res. 2006; 66:6412-6420.
10. Miaczynska M, Christoforidis S, Giner A, et al. APPL proteins link Rab5 to nuclear signal transduction via an endosomal compartment. Cell 2004; 116:445-456.
11. Ebinu JO, Yankner BA: A RIP tide in neuronal signal transduction. Neuron 2002; 34: 499-502.
12. Fortini ME: γ-Secretase-mediated proteolysis in cell-surface-receptor signalling. Nature Rev 2002; 3: 673-684.
13. Ni C-Y, Murphy MP, Golde TE, Carpenter G. γ-Secretase cleavage and nuclear localization of ErbB-4 receptor tyrosine kinase. Science 2001; 294:2179-2181.

14. Zhou W, Carpenter G. Heregulin-dependent trafficking and cleavage of ErbB-4. J Biol Chem 2000; 275:34737-34743.
15. Vecchi M, Baulida J, Carpenter, G. Selective cleavage of the heregulin receptor erbB-4 by protein kinase C activation. J Biol Chem 1996; 271:18989-18995.
16. Vecchi M, Carpenter G. Constitutive proteolysis of the ErbB-4 receptor tyrosine kinase by a unique, sequential mechanism. J Cell Biol 1997; 139:995-1003.
17. Rio C, Buxbaum JD, Peschon JJ, Corfas G: Tumor necrosis factor-α-converting enzyme is required for cleavage of erbB4/HER4. J Biol Chem 2000; 275:10379-10387.
18. Blobel CP. Remarkable roles of proteolysis on and beyond the cell surface. Curr Opin Cell Biol 2000; 12:606-612.
19. Elenius K, Corfas G, Paul S, Choi CJ, et al. A novel juxtamembrane domain isoform of HER4/ErbB4. Isoform-specific tissue distribution and differential processing in response to phorbol ester. J Biol Chem 1997; 272:26761-26768.
20. Gilmour LMR, Macleod KG, McCaig A, et al. Expression of erbB-4/HER-4 growth factor receptor isoforms in ovarian cancer. Cancer Res 2001; 61:2169-2176.
21. Gilbertson R, Hernan R, Pietsch T, et al. Novel ErbB4 juxtamembrane splice variants are frequently expressed in childhood medulloblastoma. Genes, Chromosomes Cancer 2001; 31:288-294.
22. Juntilla TT, Sundvall M, Määttä JA, Elenius K. ErbB4 and its isoforms. Selective regulation of growth factor responses by naturally occurring receptor variants. Trends Cardivasc Med 2000; 10:304-310.
23. Lee H-J, Jung K-M, Huang YZ, et al. Presenilin-dependent γ-secretase-like intramembrane cleavage of ErbB4. J Biol Chem 2002; 277:6318-6323.
24. Srinivasan R, Gillett CE, Barnes DM, Gullick WJ. Nuclear expression of the c-erbB-4/HER-4 growth factor receptor in invasive breast cancers. Cancer Res 2000; 60:1483-1487.
25. Zhang M, Ding D, Salvi R. Expression of heregulin and ErbB/Her receptors in adult chinchilla cochlear and vestibular sensory epithelium. Hearing Res 2002; 169:56-68.
26. Srinivasan R, Benton E, McCormick F, et al. Expression of the c-erbB-3/HER-3 and c-erbB-4/HER-4 growth factor receptors and their ligands, neuregulin-1α, neuregulin-1β, and betacellulin, in normal endometrium and endometrial cancer. Clin Cancer Res 1999; 5:2877-2883.
27. Cabrera N, Díaz-Rodríguez E, Becker E, et al. TrkA receptor ectodomain cleavage generates a tyrosine-phosphorylated cell-associated fragment. J Cell Biol 1996; 132:427-436.
28. Vogel WF. Ligand-induced shedding of discoidin domain receptor 1. FEBS Lett 2002; 514; 175-180.
29. Lin S-Y, Makino K, Xia W, et al. Nuclear localization of EGF receptor and its potential new role as a transcription factor. Nature Cell Biol 2001; 3:802-808.
30. Khan EM, Heidinger JM, Levy M, et al. Epidermal growth factor receptor exposed to oxidative stress undergoes Src- and caveolin-1-dependent perinuclear trafficking. J Biol Chem 2006; 281:14486-14493.
31. Dittmann K, Mayer C, Rodemann HP. Inhibition of radiation-induced EGFR nuclear import by C225 (Cetuximab) suppresses DNA-PK activity. Radiother Oncol. 2005; 76:157-161.
32. Dittmann K, Mayer C, Fehrenbacher B, et al. Radiation-induced epidermal growth factor receptor nuclear import is linked to activation of DNA-dependent protein kinase. J Biol Chem. 2005; 280:31182-31189.
33. Wang SC, Lien HC, Xia W, et al. Binding at and transactivation of the COX-2 promoter by nuclear tyrosine kinase receptor ErbB-2. Cancer Cell 2004; 6:251-261.
34. Giri DK, Ali-Seyed M, Li LY, et al. Endosomal transport of ErbB-2:mechanism for nuclear entry of the cell surface receptor. Mol Cell Biol 2005; 25:11005-11018.
35. Offterdinger M, Schöfer C, Weipoltshammer K, Grunt TW. C-erbB-3: a nuclear protein in mammary epithelial cells. J Cell Biol 2002; 157:929-939.
36. Maher PA. Nuclear translocation of fibroblast growth factor (FGF) receptors in response to FGF-2. J Cell Biol 1996; 134:529-536.
37. Stachowiak MK, Maher PA, Joy A, et al. Nuclear accumulation of fibroblast growth factor receptors is regulated by multiple signals in adrenal medullary cells. Mol Biol Cell 1996; 7:1299-1317.
38. Reilly JF, Maher PA: Importin -mediated nuclear import of fibroblast growth factor receptor: role in cell proliferation. J Cell Biol 2001; 152:1307-1312.
39. Pozner-Moulis S, Pappas DJ, Rimm DL. Met, the hepatocyte growth factor receptor, localizes to the nucleus in cells at low density. Cancer Res 2006; 66:7976-7982.

40. Sandvig K, van Deurs B. Entry of ricin and Shiga toxin into cells: molecular mechanisms and medical perspectives. EMBO J 2000; 19:5943-5950.
41. Pelkmans L, Kartenbeck J, Helenius A. Caveolar endocytosis of simian virus 40 reveals a new two-step vesicular-transport pathway to the ER. Nat Cell Biol. 2001; 3:473-483.
42. Marsh M, Helenius A. Virus entry: open sesame. Cell 2006; 124:729-740.
43. Liao H.-J, and Carpenter G. The role of Sec61 translocon in EGF receptor intracellular trafficking to the nucleus and gene expression. Mol Biol Cell 2007;18:1064-1072.
44. FujinagaY, Wolf, A.A., Rodighiero, C, et al. Gangliosides that associate with lipid rafts mediate transport of cholera and related toxins from the plasma membrane to the endoplasmic reticulum. Mol Cell Biol 2003; 14:4783-4793.
45. Lo, H.-W, Ali-Seyed, M, Wu, Y, et al. Nuclear-cytoplasmic transport of EGFR involves receptor endocytosis, importin, β1 and CRM1. J. Cell. Biochem 2006; 98:1570-1583.
46. Römisch, K. Endoplasmic reticulum-associated degradation. Annu. Rev Cell Dev. Biol. 2005; 21: 435-456.
47. Hirsch C, Blom D, Ploegh HL. A role for N-glycanase in the cytosolic turnover of glycoproteins. EMBO J 2003; 22:1036-1046.
48. van den Berg B, Clemons WM, Jr, Collinson I., et al. X-ray structure of a protein-conducting channel. Nature 2003; 42:36-44.
49. Sardi SP, Murtie J, Koirala S, et al. Presenilin-dependent ErbB4 nuclear signaling regulates the timing of astrogenesis in the developing brain. Cell. 2006; 127:185-197.
50. Arasada RR, Carpenter G. Secretase-dependent tyrosine phosphorylation of Mdm2 by the ErbB-4 intracellular domain fragment. J Biol Chem. 2005; 280:30783-30787.
51. Linggi B, Carpenter G. ErbB-4 s80 intracellular domain abrogates ETO2-dependent transcriptional repression. J Biol Chem. 2006; 281:25373-25380.
52. Lo HW, Hsu SC, Ali-Seyed M, Gunduz M, Xia W, Wei Y, Bartholomeusz G, Shih JY, Hung MC. Nuclear interaction of EGFR and STAT3 in the activation of the iNOS/NO pathway. Cancer Cell. 2005; 7:575-589.
53. Wnag S-C, Nakajima Y, Yu Y-L, et al. Tyrosine phosphorylation controls PCNA function through protein stability. Nat Cell Biol 2006; 8:1359-1368.
54. Peng H, Moffett J, Myers J, et al. Novel nuclear signaling pathway mediates activation of fibroblast growth factor-2 gene by type 1 and type 2 angiotensin II receptors. Mol Biol Cell 2001, 12:449-462.
55. Frade JM. Nuclear translocation of the p75 neurotrophin receptor cytoplasmic domain in response to neurotrophin binding. J Neurosci 2005; 25:1407-1411.
56. Okamoto I, Kawano Y, Murakami D, et al. Proteolytic release of CD44 intracellular domain and its role in the CD44 signaling pathway. J Cell Biol 2001; 155:755-762.
57. Lammich S, Okochi M, Takeda M, et al. Presenilin dependent intramembrane proteolysis of CD44 leads to the liberation of its intracellular domain and the secretion of an Aβ-like peptide. J Biol Chem 2002; 277:44754-44759.
58. Marambaud P, Shioi J, Serban G, et al. A presenilin-1/γ-secretase cleavage releases the E-cadherin intracellular domain and regulates disassembly of adherens junctions. EMBO J 2002; 21:1948-1956.
59. My P, Reddy YK, Herz J. Proteolytic processing of low density lipoprotein receptor-related protein mediates regulated release of its intracellular domain. J Biol Chem 2002; 277:18736-18743.
60. Gomez-Ospina N, Tsuruta F, Barreto-Chang O, et al. The C terminus of the L-type voltage-gated calcium channel Ca(V)1.2 encodes a transcription factor. Cell 2006; 127:591-606.
61. Boivin B, Chevalier D, Villeneuve LR, et al. Functional endothelin receptors are present on nuclei in cardiac ventricular myocytes. J Biol Chem. 2003; 278:29153-29163.
62. Lee DK, Lanca AJ, Cheng R, et al. Agonist-independent nuclear localization of the Apelin, angiotensin AT1, and bradykinin B2 receptors. J Biol Chem. 2004; 279:7901-7908.

14 Temporal Dynamics of EGF Receptor Signaling by Quantitative Proteomics

Blagoy Blagoev, Irina Kratchmarova, Jesper V. Olsen, and Matthias Mann

CONTENTS

    INTRODUCTION
    QUANTITATIVE CHARACTERIZATION OF THE ErbB RECEPTOR
        FAMILY INTERACTOME
    GLOBAL COMPARISON OF DIVERGENT RTK SIGNALING NETWORKS
    TEMPORAL DYNAMICS OF THE EGFR TYROSINE PHOSPHOPROTEOME
    GLOBAL, SITE-SPECIFIC PHOSPHORYLATION DYNAMICS IN THE
        EGFR SIGNALING CASCADES
    CONCLUSION
    REFERENCES

Abstract

    The ability to respond to divergent stimuli by inducing a multitude of signaling pathways is one of the most fundamental functions of a living cell. Investigation of the highly complex and dynamic processes initiated by growth factors that activate receptors on the cell surface has been greatly facilitated by the recent developments in the field of mass spectrometry-based proteomics. In particular, quantitative mass spectrometry approaches such as Stable Isotope Labeling by Amino acids in Cell culture (SILAC) have provided new insights into cellular signaling by compiling a global view of the temporal dimension of signaling cascades. In this chapter, we focus on the characterization of the interaction networks and the creation of dynamic phosphorylation profiles initiated by the epidermal growth factor receptor and its family members using SILAC-based quantitative proteomic approaches.

    Key Words: Protein quantitation, SILAC, dynamics, mass spectrometry, phosphorylation, stable isotope labeling.

1. INTRODUCTION

    In multi-cellular organisms a variety of growth factors serve as messengers transmitting signals between cells. These hormones bind specifically to receptors on the cell surface, thereby inducing a series of events ultimately leading to specific biological outcomes. Signaling initiated by the attachment of polypeptide growth factors to receptor tyrosine kinases

From: *Cancer Drug Discovery and Development: EGFR Signaling Networks in Cancer Therapy*
Edited by: J. D. Haley and W. J. Gullick, DOI: 10.1007/978-1-59745-356-1_14
© 2008 Humana Press, a part of Springer Science+Business Media, LLC

(RTKs) is mediated via complex and diverse protein networks involving a plethora of different molecules with a multitude of cellular responses (*1–3*). The impact that a growth factor has on a given cell can be as dramatic as inducing a cell's growth, its entry into or withdraw from the cell cycle, control of cell death and survival or directing the processes of development and differentiation. Investigation of cell-signaling cascades and in particular the signaling initiated by growth factors has been an ongoing task for several decades. The epidermal growth factor receptor (EGFR) pathway is one of the most extensively studied over the years. The EGF signaling network includes adaptor and scaffold molecules, kinases, phosphatases and other types of enzymes and it is capable of modulating most if not all of the major cellular processes. Inappropriate activation of those molecules due to mutation or overexpression often leads to development of diseases, in particular a large number of cancers (*4*). The EGFR has been found overexpressed, deregulated or mutated in many malignancies and the EGFR activation is important in the processes of tumor growth and progression (see Chapters 16 and 17).

A large part of signaling research has focused on obtaining comprehensive information for the mechanism of action of the receptor tyrosine kinase EGFR (ErbB1) and its three closely related family members (ErbB2/HER2, ErbB3/HER3 and ErbB4/HER4). As signaling cascades are highly dynamic, it is very important to follow the space and time-ordered sequence of events that occur as a result of growth factor stimulation. However, the investigation of cell signaling dynamics in a global comprehensive manner has been a major challenge for several decades. Very recently, this research has obtained a major stimulus by the fast development in the field of quantitative proteomics (*5, 6*) where a combination of technical advances and method development has resulted in the accumulation of a critical mass of tools and data that will ultimately lead to better understanding of the cellular function.

At present, proteomics in general can be defined as large-scale studies that compare proteomes, either qualitatively or quantitatively, in order to better define and understand a specific biological process or entity (*5*). From the large field of proteomics, quantitative mass spectrometry (MS)-based proteomics is having a tremendous impact on cell-signaling research. Quantitative MS-based proteomics is a rapidly emerging area that is becoming indispensable for investigation of signaling networks and creation of dynamic interaction maps of the signaling cascades (*6–9*). It is also opening up the possibilities for in depth and highly specific characterization of protein interaction networks as a basis for systems biology. Furthermore, it allows addition of another dimension to the signaling studies – the temporal and spatial order of the dynamic signaling events following growth factor stimulation. In this chapter we will focus on the investigation of cell signaling via the EGFR and its related family members using quantitative MS-based proteomics.

2. QUANTITATIVE CHARACTERIZATION OF THE ErbB RECEPTOR FAMILY INTERACTOME

Classical MS-based strategies have been successfully used for identification of interaction partners involved in various RTK networks. In a prototypical study by Pandey et al. (*10*), several components of the EGFR signaling pathway were identified using antibodies for enrichment of tyrosine-phosphorylated proteins followed by analysis by matrix-assisted laser desorption/ionization (MALDI) and nanoelectrospray tandem mass spectrometry (nanoESI-MS/MS). Among the identified proteins were Vav-2, a recently discovered guanosine nucleotide exchange factor that was confirmed as a direct substrate for EGFR and a novel protein containing a phosphotyrosine binding (PTB) domain (*10–12*). This strategy, which basically made use of the high sensitivity and specificity of mass spectrometry to sequence low amounts of proteins, has been used for routine identification of downstream effectors of RTKs, resulting in the discovery of a number of novel proteins such as STAM2 (signal transducing adaptor molecule 2) and Odin (also called ankyrin repeat and SAM domain-containing protein 1A) that were not previously known or associated with growth factor signaling (*11, 13, 14*).

In recent years, quantitative MS-based approaches have allowed accurate quantitation of proteins in complex mixtures containing hundreds or even thousands of proteins (*6*). These methods greatly aid the investigation of RTK interaction networks. For example, a long-standing problem when performing classical interaction studies by biochemical approaches involves distinguishing genuine interaction partners from background contaminant binders. We have addressed this major challenge for the investigation of functional protein-protein interactions by applying the SILAC quantitative proteomics method in a novel functional format (*15, 16*). The essence of SILAC lies in the incorporation of a stable isotope labeled amino acid (non-radioactive isotopes) into all proteins of a given cellular population until the entire proteome becomes encoded either with the normal ('light') or stable isotope substituted ('heavy') version of the same amino acid. This encoding is accomplished by expanding cells in the labeling media for a defined number of population doublings after which their proteomes are fully metabolically labeled, making them easily distinguishable by mass spectrometry (Fig. 14.1) (*16*). After complete labeling, the 'light' and 'heavy' cells are pooled together in equal proportions and changes in protein abundance between the two cell populations are determined from the isotope ratios of peptides derived by enzymatic digestion of the enriched protein populations. Importantly, in the SILAC procedure, any sample manipulation such as protein purification, fractionation, interaction assay etc. is performed on the already combined protein sample, which results in minimized quantitation errors (*6, 7*). The intrinsic accuracy and flexibility has made SILAC an increasingly popular method to studying variety of biological processes. Depending on the experimental setup, SILAC allows determination of specific protein-protein interactions and functional protein complexes (*15, 17, 18*), characterization of post-translational modifications (*19, 20*), quantitative comparison between distinct signaling pathways (*21*) and temporal phosphorylation dynamics of signaling molecules (*22–24*).

The strength of SILAC to discriminate true protein-protein interactors from a large access of background contaminants was fully utilized to characterize functional protein complexes associated with activated EGFR (*15*). Light and heavy-labeled cells were either stimulated with EGF or left untreated, and their combined lysates were affinity-purified using the SH2 domain of the adapter protein Grb2. Of the 228 identified proteins, 28 displayed differential enrichment ratios that indicated them as specific members of the activated EGFR complexes. They included plectin, epiplakin, the glycosylphosphatidylinositol (GPI)-anchored molecule CD59, and two novel proteins (*15*). This study showed the great potential of functional quantitative proteomic approaches in protein interaction studies and the general scheme was easily modified to identify other specific protein-protein, protein-domain, or protein-peptide motive interactions (*17, 25*).

Using pairs of phosphorylated and non-phosphorylated synthetic peptides for pull-down experiments, an essentially identical experimental approach was utilized to determine the interaction partners to all cytosolic tyrosine residues of the four members of the ErbB receptor family (*25*). Characteristic subsets of binding partners were identified for each receptor and most of the interacting proteins had multiple docking sites on the respective receptor. The ErbB3 receptor had six binding sites for phosphatidylinositol 3-kinase (PI3K), whereas several binding sites for Grb2 were found for EGFR and ErbB4. These results demonstrate that the members of the EGFR family clearly differ in their preferred interaction partners indicating distinct roles in cellular signaling. The ErbB receptor family phosphotyrosine-dependent interactome has also been probed in vitro by an alternative proteomic approach using protein microarrays consisting of nearly all SH2 and PTB domains in the human genome (*26*). The results suggested that, as opposed to ErbB3, the changes in EGFR and ErbB2 networks become more promiscuous with an increasing protein concentration or receptor expression levels and this effect may contribute to the oncogenic potential of these two receptors.

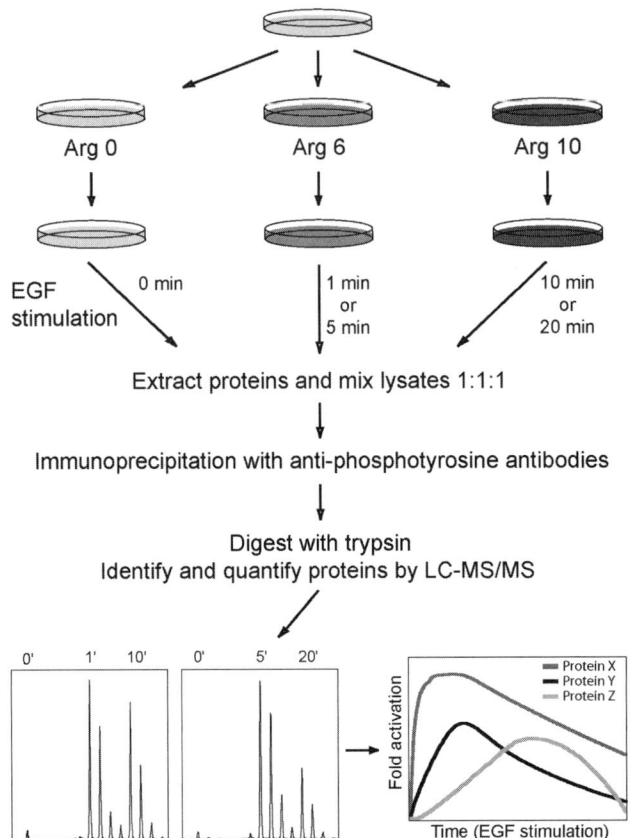

Fig. 14.1. **SILAC Approach for Temporal Analysis of EGFR Signaling Network** Cells growing in standard media are seeded into SILAC-labeling media containing "light" (Arg0), "medium" (Arg6) or "heavy" (Arg10) versions of arginine and expanded in the corresponding media until full metabolic incorporation of the amino acid. Each population is stimulated for a different length of time with EGF and then lysed. Protein extracts are mixed in equal proportions according to their protein concentration and tyrosine phosphorylated proteins are immuno-affinity purified followed by trypsin digestion and analysis by LC-MS/MS. Mass spectra show distinct triplets of peptides that represent the same peptide from the three cell populations. The observed peptide ratios reflect the level of activation of the identified protein by EGF at the corresponding time point. Five time-point activation profiles are generated by combining data from two experiments with an overlapping time point.

3. GLOBAL COMPARISON OF DIVERGENT RTK SIGNALING NETWORKS

Binding of growth factors to their respective RTKs triggers a cascade of phosphorylation events on tyrosine residues of the receptor and subsequently on downstream effector molecules, thereby inducing parallel signaling pathways. The initial flow of tyrosine phosphorylations is a tightly regulated process, and it is the determining factor in RTK signaling. Various growth factor receptors, such as EGF and platelet-derived growth factor (PDGF) receptors, often activate universal signaling pathways. Activation of these receptors, however, can lead to distinct or even opposite biological effects. For example, the osteoblast differentiation of human mesenchymal stem cells was found to be greatly enhanced by EGF but not PDGF (*21*). A combination of SILAC and anti-phosphotyrosine immunoprecipitation was used to comprehensively and quantitatively compare the total phosphotyrosine-dependent networks of EGFR and PDGFR in these cells. Although 90% of all 113 activated signaling proteins were utilized by both ligands, all regulatory and catalytic subunits of the PI3K were detected only in the cells stimulated with PDGF. This intriguing difference could therefore account for the differential effects of the two growth factors on the mesenchymal stem cells conversion to osteoblasts. Indeed, treatment of the cells with PDGF in combination with specific PI3K inhibitors led to an enhanced differentiation effect similar to the one induced by EGF (*21*). In addition to the biological and clinical significance of this finding, this work demonstrated the ability of quantitative MS-based proteomics to compare entire signaling networks and to discover critical control points that can influence the cell fate.

In a study by Wolf-Yadlin et al., a similar strategy using a chemical labeling method, iTRAQ, was utilized to compare EGF and heregulin (HRG) signaling in normal and ErbB2-overexpressing mammary epithelial cells (*27*). These investigators found that EGF stimulated cell migration of ErbB2-overexpressing cells involved multiple signaling pathways, whereas HRG treatment promoted the phosphorylation of only a small subset of those proteins, in particular Src, FAK, paxillin, and p130Cas. Furthermore, self-organizing maps were created based on the phosphoproteomics data, which allowed determination of specific modules involved in the control of cellular proliferation and migration.

4. TEMPORAL DYNAMICS OF THE EGFR TYROSINE PHOSPHOPROTEOME

Numerous advances made in quantitative MS-based proteomics in the last several years have provided the necessary tools to follow the highly dynamic changes occurring in the cell in a global and unbiased manner, in contrast to looking only at isolated snap shots of the signaling cascades. The first dynamic map of the entire phosphotyrosine-dependent signaling network induced by EGF was generated using a SILAC-based quantitative proteomic approach (*22*). The proteomes of three cell populations were encoded with different forms of arginine, and each cell population was stimulated with EGF for a different time. The phosphorylated proteins and tightly associated binding partners were captured using anti-phosphotyrosine antibodies, digested with trypsin and identified by mass spectrometry (Fig. 14.1). Two experimental datasets were combined, yielding five-point dynamic profiles of 81 signaling proteins that included virtually all known EGFR substrates and 31 novel effectors. The diverse protein activation profiles observed by MS reflected the precise temporal involvement of the corresponding proteins in the signaling cascades. For example, the chronological order of events from EGFR via adaptors and guanine exchange factors to the mitogen-activated protein kinases was easily followed through their dynamic profiles, whereas proteins involved in the regulation of the actin cytoskeleton showed an intriguing oscillatory kinetics (*22*). Moreover, five novel proteins were identified in the study, and their activation curves suggested their functional position in the signaling network. Swiprosin 1, for example, was connected with actin rearrangements by shared kinetics, while TOM1-like protein 2 was linked to endosomal trafficking. In this way, time course activation profiles provide additional information and insights into the signaling cascade initiated by EGF. They also serve as constraints in systems biology modeling of the EGFR network (*28*).

Several other MS-based proteomic studies have also focused on the dynamic aspects of EGFR signaling. A combination of affinity enrichment of tyrosine phosphorylated peptides and iTRAQ labeling led to the identification and temporal profiling over four time points of EGF stimulation of 104 phosphotyrosine-containing peptides derived from 76 proteins (*29*). The same enrichment strategy was later combined with improved mass spectrometric analyses and resulted in generation of temporal phosphorylation profiles of 222 tyrosine phosphorylated peptides across seven time points following stimulation with EGF (*30*).

In the studies described above, the earliest time point was at least 30 seconds after growth factor addition due to technical difficulties commonly associated with large-scale approaches. However, a novel quantitative proteomics experimental set-up was recently described, which allows accurate analysis of the phosphorylation events occurring almost instantly in cells treated with EGF (23). With this method, named qPACE (quantitative Proteomic Assessment of very early Cellular signaling Events), SILAC-labeled cells were first pumped through a continuous quench-flow system to assure efficient trapping of temporal signaling states on a timescale of seconds. The qPACE system was used to analyze the phosphorylation of EGFR and its direct substrates Shc and PLC-γ after 1, 5, 10 and 60 seconds of EGF treatment. Multiple phosphorylation sites were identified on the receptor, as well as on these two signaling proteins. It was demonstrated that EGFR autophosphorylation occurs as early as one second after addition of the growth factor, and it is followed immediately by Shc phosphorylation, which suggests very close proximity of the receptor and the adaptor. Therefore, qPACE not only permits determination of the very early phosphorylation events but also enables us to distinguish molecules acting as sensors from downstream signal transducers.

5. GLOBAL, SITE-SPECIFIC PHOSPHORYLATION DYNAMICS IN THE EGFR SIGNALING CASCADES

Signaling by RTKs is a sequence of reverse phosphorylation events that are a function of stimulus, time and localization. The initial flow of tyrosine phosphorylation is an essential step that triggers consequent downstream cascades of mainly threonine and serine phosphorylation events on various proteins that may have positive as well as negative effects on the signaling initiated by a RTK. The cellular outcome of any given signaling cascade is entirely dependent on the series of induced phosphorylation both on tyrosine and serine/threonine residues as it is integrated with internal state information and other signals that the cell receives. Therefore, a creation of global phosphorylation profiles of growth factor induced changes is an essential step toward understanding the mechanism of regulation of these signaling cascades. Although still quite challenging technically, recently a general mass spectrometric strategy for identification and quantitation of phosphorylation sites has been developed (Fig. 14.2) (24).

Using a workflow consisting of SILAC-labeled cells, protein fractionation and phosphopeptide enrichment followed by high-resolution mass spectrometric analysis, over 6,000 phosphorylation sites on more than 2,200 proteins were detected after stimulation with EGF (24). Most importantly, about 14% of the phosphorylation sites were regulated at least two-fold by EGF, highlighting them as functionally relevant in this particular signaling network. The majority of the proteins that became phosphorylated contained multiple phosphorylation sites with different dynamic profiles indicating their differential regulation by the applied stimulus over time. For example, all of the tyrosine autophosphorylation sites on EGFR showed immediate activation profiles, while its serine/threonine sites displayed delayed phosphorylation kinetics consistent with negative feedback regulation from downstream kinases. Furthermore, 26 different transcription factors with 34 regulated phosphopeptides and 20 transcriptional co-regulators with EGF-dependent phosphorylation sites were identified in addition to numerous sites on various kinases, ubiquitin ligases, guanine nucleotide exchange factors etc (Fig. 14.2). This dataset revealed that the EGF signal spreads to at least 46 transcriptional regulators, of which only a subset has previously been known to be involved in growth factor signaling. The global quantitative investigation of phosphoproteomes opens the perspective of direct access to 'RTK systems biology' and adds another layer of understanding of the complex and dynamic EGFR signaling networks.

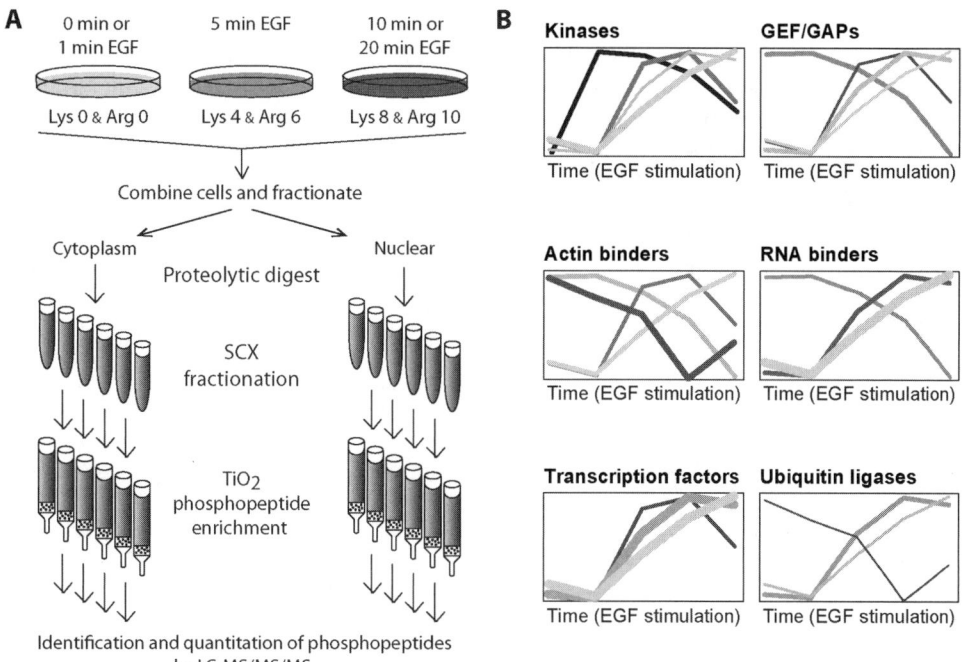

Fig. 14.2. **Site-specific Phosphorylation Dynamics of EGFR Signaling Cascades** (**A**) Three cell populations are encoded with "light," "medium" or "heavy" forms of arginine and lysine. The SILAC-encoded cells are stimulated with EGF for different periods of time, subsequently combined and fractionated to nuclear and cytoplasmic extracts. Following proteolytic digest, the peptides are fractionated by strong cation exchange (SCX) chromatography, and phosphopeptides are enriched using TiO_2. The resulting phosphopeptide mixtures are then subjected to quantitative LC-MS/MS/MS analysis. (**B**) Dynamic profiles of different functional protein categories representing the phosphorylation-dependent signaling network of EGFR. For each category, the kinetic curves of the proteins are drawn in proportion to the number of phosphopeptides with the corresponding regulation profile.

6. CONCLUSION

In summary, studying the combinatorial action of different signals coming from the cell surface and defining the outcome for the cells represents a definite challenge to the biological and biomedical sciences. Signaling of RTKs is one of the fundamental mechanisms controlling cellular fate, and aberrations at any given point in the signaling cascades can have serious if not lethal consequences for the entire organism. In this regard, the EGFR signaling network is probably the most studied and well understood. The protein interaction networks, however, are not simple static systems but highly dynamic processes of tightly regulated and time-ordered events. In the last few decades of extensive research, many individual proteins and specific protein-protein interactions that are involved in RTK pathways have been identified. Nevertheless, it has also become apparent that signaling cascades do not operate in a simple linear fashion, but rather as complex interactive networks, allowing cross-talk between different pathways. We still know only very little about their global makeup and regulation and especially about their dynamics. In recent years, the fast developments in the field of quantitative MS-based proteomics have started to allow in-depth and unambiguous "dissection" of signaling cascades. Combination with different methodologies and techniques like cDNA microarrays, RNAi interference or live-cell imaging will provide further integrated information and critical new insights into the distinct biological functions of the members of the EGFR family. This will ultimately lead to determining possible points of perturbation in the signaling cascades and the development of more specific and better targeted drugs that improve treatment for growth factor associated diseases and disorders.

REFERENCES

1. Hunter T. Signaling--2000 and beyond. Cell 2000;100:113-27.
2. Pawson T, Nash P. Assembly of cell regulatory systems through protein interaction domains. Science 2003;300:445-52.
3. Schlessinger J. Cell signaling by receptor tyrosine kinases. Cell 2000;103:211-25.
4. Blume-Jensen P, Hunter T. Oncogenic kinase signalling. Nature 2001;411:355-65.
5. Aebersold R, Mann M. Mass spectrometry-based proteomics. Nature 2003;422:198-207.
6. Ong SE, Mann M. Mass spectrometry-based proteomics turns quantitative. Nat Chem Biol 2005; 1:252-62.
7. Blagoev B, Mann M. Quantitative proteomics to study mitogen-activated protein kinases. Methods 2006;40:243-50.
8. Cheng X. Understanding signal transduction through functional proteomics. Expert Rev Proteomics 2005;2:103-16.
9. Schmelzle K, White FM. Phosphoproteomic approaches to elucidate cellular signaling networks. Curr Opin Biotechnol 2006;17:406-14.
10. Pandey A, Podtelejnikov AV, Blagoev B, Bustelo XR, Mann M, Lodish HF. Analysis of receptor signaling pathways by mass spectrometry: identification of vav-2 as a substrate of the epidermal and platelet-derived growth factor receptors. Proc Natl Acad Sci U S A 2000; 97:179-84.
11. Pandey A, Blagoev B, Kratchmarova I, et al. Cloning of a novel phosphotyrosine binding domain containing molecule, Odin, involved in signaling by receptor tyrosine kinases. Oncogene 2002;21:8029-36.
12. Tamas P, Solti Z, Bauer P, et al. Mechanism of epidermal growth factor regulation of Vav2, a guanine nucleotide exchange factor for Rac. J Biol Chem 2003;278:5163-71.
13. Kristiansen TZ, Nielsen MM, Blagoev B, Pandey A, Mann M. Mouse embryonic fibroblasts derived from Odin deficient mice display a hyperproliiferative phenotype. DNA Res 2004;11:285-92.
14. Pandey A, Fernandez MM, Steen H, et al. Identification of a novel immunoreceptor tyrosine-based activation motif-containing molecule, STAM2, by mass spectrometry and its involvement in growth factor and cytokine receptor signaling pathways. J Biol Chem 2000;275:38633-9.
15. Blagoev B, Kratchmarova I, Ong SE, Nielsen M, Foster LJ, Mann M. A proteomics strategy to elucidate functional protein-protein interactions applied to EGF signaling. Nat Biotechnol 2003;21:315-8.
16. Ong SE, Blagoev B, Kratchmarova I, et al. Stable isotope labeling by amino acids in cell culture, SILAC, as a simple and accurate approach to expression proteomics. Mol Cell Proteomics 2002; 1:376-86.
17. Trinkle-Mulcahy L, Andersen J, Lam YW, Moorhead G, Mann M, Lamond AI. Repo-Man recruits PP1 gamma to chromatin and is essential for cell viability. J Cell Biol 2006;172:679-92.
18. Jin J, Li GJ, Davis J, et al. Identification of Novel Proteins Associated with Both {alpha}-Synuclein and DJ-1. Mol Cell Proteomics 2007;6:845-59.
19. Ibarrola N, Molina H, Iwahori A, Pandey A. A novel proteomic approach for specific identification of tyrosine kinase substrates using [13C]tyrosine. J Biol Chem 2004;279:15805-13.
20. Ong SE, Mittler G, Mann M. Identifying and quantifying in vivo methylation sites by heavy methyl SILAC. Nat Methods 2004;1:119-26.
21. Kratchmarova I, Blagoev B, Haack-Sorensen M, Kassem M, Mann M. Mechanism of divergent growth factor effects in mesenchymal stem cell differentiation. Science 2005;308:1472-7.
22. Blagoev B, Ong SE, Kratchmarova I, Mann M. Temporal analysis of phosphotyrosine-dependent signaling networks by quantitative proteomics. Nat Biotechnol 2004;22:1139-45.
23. Dengjel J, Akimov V, Olsen JV, et al. Quantitative proteomic assessment of very early cellular signaling events. Nat Biotechnol 2007;25:566-8.
24. Olsen JV, Blagoev B, Gnad F, et al. Global, in vivo, and site-specific phosphorylation dynamics in signaling networks. Cell 2006;127:635-48.

25. Schulze WX, Deng L, Mann M. Phosphotyrosine interactome of the ErbB-receptor kinase family. Mol Syst Biol 2005;1:2005 0008.
26. Jones RB, Gordus A, Krall JA, MacBeath G. A quantitative protein interaction network for the ErbB receptors using protein microarrays. Nature 2006;439:168-74.
27. Wolf-Yadlin A, Kumar N, Zhang Y, et al. Effects of HER2 overexpression on cell signaling networks governing proliferation and migration. Mol Syst Biol 2006;2:54.
28. Kholodenko BN. Cell-signalling dynamics in time and space. Nat Rev Mol Cell Biol 2006; 7:165-76.
29. Zhang Y, Wolf-Yadlin A, Ross PL, et al. Time-resolved mass spectrometry of tyrosine phosphorylation sites in the epidermal growth factor receptor signaling network reveals dynamic modules. Mol Cell Proteomics 2005;4:1240-50.
30. Wolf-Yadlin A, Hautaniemi S, Lauffenburger DA, White FM. Multiple reaction monitoring for robust quantitative proteomic analysis of cellular signaling networks. Proc Natl Acad Sci U S A 2007; 104:5860-5.

15 Computational and Mathematical Modeling of the EGF Receptor System

Colin G. Johnson, Emmet McIntyre, and William Gullick

CONTENTS

  WHY MODEL AND SIMULATE?
  METHODS FOR MODELING AND SIMULATION
  IMPLEMENTING INDIVIDUAL BASED METHODS
  EXAMPLES OF SIMULATIONS
  PROSPECTS
  REFERENCES

Abstract

This chapter gives an overview of computational models and simulations of the EGF receptor system. It begins with a survey of motivations for producing such models and then describes the main approaches that are taken to carrying out such modeling, with respect to differential equations and individual-based modeling. Finally, a number of projects that apply modeling and simulation techniques to various aspects of the EGF receptor system are described.

Key Words: EGF receptor, computational models, mathematical models.

1. WHY MODEL AND SIMULATE?

By *modeling* we mean the construction of some computer program or mathematical description that describes some aspect of a system. *Simulation* is the running of a computer implementation of that model, i.e., setting parameters in and the initial state of a model, after which the state of that model is modified a number of times to represent the system changing in time.

There are a number of motivations for developing such models. At the simplest level, models can be used as informal tools to develop intuitions and ideas about the functioning of a system. By attempting to build a formal model that incorporates existing knowledge about the system, the less-well understood components of the system can become clearer; furthermore conjectures can be made, and tested for plausibility, about mechanisms that might explain those components. This process is, in general, referred to as synthetic biology. It is an attempt to gain an understanding of a system by building it.

From: *Cancer Drug Discovery and Development: EGFR Signaling Networks in Cancer Therapy*
Edited by: J. D. Haley and W. J. Gullick, DOI: 10.1007/978-1-59745-356-1_15
© 2008 Humana Press, a part of Springer Science+Business Media, LLC

Such a model, however, cannot confirm anything positive about a system. Typically, it will be used to inspire further experimental work, by providing a *prima facie* case that some experiment might produce results of interest. Another function of such a system is to demonstrate that a particular mechanism cannot explain a particular behavior, by showing that an implementation of that mechanism in simulation produces different behavior (either at a qualitative or quantitative level) to an observed system.

More formally, models can be used to integrate together a number of aspects of a system that are individually well understood, yet where the interactions between those aspects are not. In such an approach, we build a number of computer programs or mathematical systems, each of which describes the individually well-understood subsystem and which has inputs and outputs that allow it to interact with other components of the system. Provided that such models are complete, and that their inclusion in a wider system does not produce additional effects or ill-understood non-linear interactions, such a system can produce accurate predictions about the behavior of the system. Such an approach, however, is limited by our lack of such complete understanding of many biological systems (a situation which contrasts, for example, with models in physics, where many subsystems are well understood).

More rigorous uses of modeling and simulation will attempt to combine the model with experimental or observational data. In such an approach, the model typically represents a hypothesis about how the system works. Typically, a hypothesis is tested by 'bringing the data to the hypothesis;' that is, data is measured or transformed so that it can be directly compared with the hypothesis. Simulation can 'take the hypothesis' (part of the way) to the data. A model is constructed, based on a hypothesis about the functioning of the system, and this model is then simulated by implementing it as a computer program and measuring those aspects of the simulation that correspond to the experimental data. These measurements can be compared to the experimental or observational data.

There are a number of issues with this approach, two of which we shall explore. The first is that a typical model will have unknown parameters, which can affect both the qualitative and quantitative results that are measured. One approach to this issue is to use parameter fitting where the model is viewed as a parameterized space of models, and some optimization technique used to find an (heuristically) optimal setting for those parameters that maximizes fit with the data. One of the advantages of this approach is that it gives an estimate for those parameters as part of the process; however, it should be noted that for many model/dataset pairs, many different possible parameter sets can give rise to behavior compatible with the data.

A final view of such models is that they represent hypothesis-driven combinations of attributes, which can be used as inputs to systems for prediction and classification problems. Typically, a statistical/computational model for prediction is produced by a supervised learning technique (*1*). That is, we have a set of experimental or observational data, including one attribute of the system that we would like to be able to predict in the future (referred to as the class). For example, a medical dataset might consist of a list of patients: for each patient a list of symptoms is recorded, and an expert diagnosis carried out. Supervised learning is any technique that takes such a dataset and produces a statistical/computational model that will make a prediction of the class; well-known examples are naïve Bayes methods (see e.g., (*2*)) and decision tree induction (*3*). In our example, the model would take a list of symptoms and make a diagnosis.

Typically, such systems work using the raw data as inputs to the training process, that is, the process by which a generic predictive model is adjusted to generalize from the particular set of data being used. In some situations, however, constructed attributes can be used: that is, attributes from the data are combined to form new data attributes (*4*). Typically, such constructions are simple and based on a basic search process for useful combinations. One way to view simulations is as hypothesis-driven attribute construction methods; that is, a simulation provides a new source of data for making predictions about a model, which is based on some hypothesis about the functioning of the system. In such a situation the final test of value is simply whether the addition of the new data source from the simulation adds to the accuracy of the simulation, measured on a previously unseen set of test data.

2. METHODS FOR MODELING AND SIMULATION

There are a number of methods for modeling and simulating cellular systems. In this section we discuss the various methods, focusing on differential equation-based and individual-based methods.

2.1. Differential Equation Methods

One approach is to develop a set of differential equations that describe the system (5, 6). That is, the various interactions and reactions between entities in the system are described in terms of rates of exchange between different quantities (a classic example is the Michaelis-Menten equation for enzyme kinetics (7)). In such a system, when an amount of some substance is transformed in some way, the quantity of the original substance is reduced and that of the outcome of the transformation increased. So, for example, a phosphorylation event on molecule X would consist of reducing the amount of X in the system, and increasing the amount of phosphorylated-X.

This is a powerful approach to modeling the basic levels of each substance of interest, and it has an advantage over some other methods in that many methods exist to get some analytic understanding of the problem (i.e., to understand some general properties and overall dynamics of the system), as well as to simulate it for a particular set of parameters and initial conditions.

There are disadvantages to this kind of modeling, however. In particular, there are issues concerned with scaling and with representing space. Differential equation models provide a succinct summary of the interactions between a small number of molecule-types. However, when a system contains many types of molecules, accounting for the different types while retaining a comprehensible model, it eventually becomes intractable. In terms of spatial distribution, differential equation models are better used when dealing with a small number of components where the free-mixing assumption can be made (i.e., that any molecule can interact with any other). In systems where genuine spatial distribution is important, this can be modeled by partial differential equations; however, dealing with complex interactions between different molecule types across a space is difficult, and many of the mathematical techniques for getting a qualitative understanding of the model break down in such situations.

2.2. Individual Based Methods

The second main approach to modeling is individual-based modeling. In such a model, each entity in the system is represented by a separate entity in the computer, which contrasts with differential equation models that keep track of aggregate counts of objects over time. This approach has a number of advantages. Two particularly significant advantages are that models of systems with many different kinds of components can be readily built and that a full spatial model can be readily incorporated.

In order to generate such a model, four aspects of the system need to be specified. First, a list of the kinds of entities found in the system needs to be compiled. For a cell-biology model, these will typically be lists of molecules found in the system. Second, the kinds of interactions between those entities need to be defined: most importantly, if two entities meet, do they bind? With what probability? Third, the movement of the entities is defined: for example, Brownian motion, or flow through a region at a certain rate. Finally, a set of initial conditions needs to be specified.

Commonly, not all of the information required to set up such a model is known in advance. As a result, a typical "model" is not a single model, but a parameterized space of possible models, i.e., there are a number of unknown parameters in the model, and setting these parameters to a particular value specifies a particular model. Sometimes, such models can be used as part of a process to estimate the unknown parameters. For example, a model might represent a process that is too small to observe directly experimentally; however, this process might give rise to a phenomenon that can be directly observed. By finding a parameter setting within that space of models that reproduces the observed behavior, we can conclude that the parameters (which will include properties of the unobservable behavior) are a feasible set of parameters for the real system.

Typically, this search through the parameter space will be carried out using some optimization heuristic (8), which will search for values of the parameters that maximize the fit between experimentally observable features of the system in simulation and in reality.

An alternative approach is to use qualitative reasoning methods (9, 10). This approach consists of running a simulation using qualitative features about the objects in the simulation, rather than particular values: is a quantity positive or negative, is a relationship proportional, negative-proportional, threshold, etc.? This approach can give a broad understanding of a model, even in the absence of concrete parameter settings.

3. IMPLEMENTING INDIVIDUAL BASED METHODS

Individual based methods are typically implemented using an object-oriented programming technique (11) such as Java or C++. In order to create a program in such a language, the programmer first creates types of objects known as classes, specifying the information that is stored within an object of that class and how objects of that class interact with other objects. The simulation then progresses by the creation and interaction of individual objects, each of which belongs to (and has its behavior defined by) one of the classes. There are a number of different ways in which to manage the interactions between these objects; therefore, the programmer of a simulation has to make a number of choices before writing the simulation program.

The first of these decisions is whether the model will be implemented in an event-based or timestep-based fashion. An event-based simulation (12) is one where the program maintains a list of events that change the state of the system, and the simulation is carried out by processing an event (such as an interaction between two molecules), calculating whether this generates any new events (e.g., a molecule dissociating from a complex, which might lead to a new interaction for that molecule), and then moving forward in time to the next event. This works well for systems where the "next event" can be readily calculated. In many biochemical models, however, this calculation is not easy due to processes such as Brownian motion, which can rapidly introduce a new potential interaction where there was none before. As a result, time-step-based methods, which move in a regular time-step and calculate all activity within that time-step, are commonly used in such situations.

A second decision is the level of detail that the model will use. Different questions/hypotheses will require different levels of detail in the model. Ultimately, the model needs to be a useful abstraction from reality—incorporating those features that are needed for the question at hand, while ignoring features that are irrelevant. There are also practical concerns in the decision. In particular, very detailed models can be time consuming to compute (up to the point where computation might be infeasible), or else not admit the kind of analytical techniques that can be used on simpler models.

A third decision is whether the calculations will be stochastic (i.e. incorporating some randomness in the events) or deterministic. Given that all models at the cellular level will have some element of randomness in them when viewed at that level (Brownian motion and probability of two molecules binding are two examples), the stochastic modeling approach seems immediately more appropriate. When many objects are interacting, however, these individual interactions are often somewhat irrelevant. Instead, these large numbers of random events can be approximated by a deterministic rate of occurrence. Stochastic models are of most interest when the individual actions of molecules that exist in small numbers can have significant consequences for the system as a whole, as discussed by Andrews and Bray (*13*) and Lemerle et al. (*14*).

A final decision concerns how space is handled within the model. The simplest model of space is to assume that all of the components of the system interact within a single space, which is referred to as complete mixing. The next simplest model is that there are a number of components in the model (for example, within and outside the cell) with some communication or exchange going on between these components, representing exchange of molecules between the domains or communication through transmembrane proteins. Models that have a further level of detail have a spatial position for each component of the system, either represented as an approximation on a grid or as a position given by decimal-number coordinates. This level of detail is important for some models (for example, studying the structure of receptor clusters or the formation of signaling complexes); however, for other models the complete mixing assumption is sufficient.

4. EXAMPLES OF SIMULATIONS

Computational and mathematical models have been used for understanding a number of aspects of the EGF receptor system. Most simulations have concentrated on aspects of the intracellular signaling cascade; however, other approaches have addressed the oligomerization behavior on the cell surface. As note by Gullick et al. (*15*, *16*), there are three main processes in the EGF receptor system. First, the liganding of the extracellular domain; secondly, the dimerization and oligomerization of these receptors; and finally the intracellular signaling cascade set off by this dimerization. The majority of effort in this area has focused on the intracellular signaling cascade, using differential equation models, which is where we begin our survey. Later in this section we discuss models of the cell-surface behavior, integrated models that examine multiple stages, and systems that introduce formal languages for the description of interactions and that take steps toward integrating models into broader systems biology projects.

4.1. Differential Equation Models of Intracellular Signaling Cascades

The largest amount of work on simulation of the EGF receptor system has focused on differential equation models of the intracellular signaling cascade. These models have been surveyed by Wiley et al. (*17*) and Orton et al. (*18*).

The core of such a model is a list of the various proteins involved in the signaling process and a list of differential equations that specify the reaction rates between these proteins. These models are then simulated by the used of a numerical method, either from a generic mathematical software package such as Mathematica (*19*) or Matlab (*20*), or by software specifically designed for sets of biochemical interactions such as Gepasi (*21*).

The main parameters in such models are rate constants for the various reactions in the system. Typically, these parameters are derived from existing experimental work; if they are missing, a sensitivity analysis can sometimes be performed to check whether or not the particular value of the parameter is having a significant impact on the phenomenon of interest.

A typical "experiment" using such a model will be to develop a model that introduces some new mechanism or interaction which, it is hypothesized, produces a particular experimentally-observed behavior and therefore produces a viable hypothesis to explain the mechanism underlying that behavior. In the remainder of this section we give a number of examples of such models.

A detailed example of such a model is given by Suresh Babu et al. (*22*). This paper begins by detailing a set of differential equations that represent the various reactions in the system. At the end of this process, a parameterized space of models has been created, where the parameters represent the various rate constants for the reactions in the model. They then realize a particular model by inserting rate constants found in the literature. They then test the accuracy of the model by a number of comparisons between experimental and computational work: plotting time-courses of Raf, MEK, and ERK activation levels and comparing the latter two against Western blot analyses of wet lab experiments with the same setup; studying the effects of over-expression of proteins in the model and comparisons with known experimental effects of overexpression; studying time courses of phosphorylation and dephosphorylation; and, carrying out a sensitivity analysis of the system. This work shows that an accurate model of the cascade can be produced; however, they do not apply their simulation to testing any specific new hypotheses about the functioning of the system.

One example of the application of computational methods to a specific problem in their area is the work of Brightman and Fell (*23*). This paper describes a model of the MAP kinase cascade using the simulation system Gepasi (*21*), and applies this to form hypotheses for the difference in behavior when the cascade is stimulated by EGF (in this case, the cascade is activated for a short time) and by NGF (in which case the cascade is stimulated for a sustained period of time). The simulation is used to narrow down where in the system a change will produce the effects seen in experimental work. In particular, it is shown that mechanisms that simply affect the intensity of signaling at the cell surface, or mechanisms that influence the phosphatase activity in the cascade are unlikely to produce the differences in effect observed in the experimental system. By contrast, the simulation of variations in the negative feedback regulation in the cascade do demonstrate a variety of differences in cascade persistence consistent with the experimental observations. Therefore, they conclude that this final mechanism is the most likely candidate mechanism to explain the differences.

Hendricks et al. (*24*) also apply simulations to help make a differentiation between two competing hypotheses to explain a particular observed phenomenon. The phenomenon is the localization of dephosphorylation activity in the ErbB-triggered signaling cascade. They simulate two hypotheses concerning this: the first, that the activity is localized in the cell surface plasma membrane; the second, that intracellular, endosomal regions are the focus for it. By comparing these simulations with experimental data, they show that the former localization is more likely to explain the observed phenomenon.

Shvartsmann et al. (*25*) use a simulation to show that a proposed hypothesis is sufficient to explain an experimentally observed phenomenon. The phenomenon in question is the development of a single-peaked input into a pattern with two peaks, which is needed to show how the development of paired organs during development occurs. The computational model shows the ranges of parameters that would be required to generate the phenomenon in question, which could be seen as refinement of an initial qualitative hypothesis into more quantitative terms. Maly et al. (*26*) also carry out a simulation focused on feasibility. They demonstrate that a particular arrangement of feedback loops in an autocrine-signaling system is capable of generating and maintaining cell polarity.

4.2. Other Modeling Methods for the Intracellular Signaling Cascade

Techniques other than differential equations have been used to model the signaling cascade. For example, Hlavacek et al. (*27*) have developed a system called BioGenNet that is based on lists of rewriting rules, i.e., rules that describe how parts of one structure can be transformed into another. This system allows hierarchies of reaction rules to be created, which eliminates the need to specify each rule individually, as in the differential equation-based systems discussed above. In addition, such systems of rules permit new analytic methods such as model checking, which is a system for checking whether a set of rules is consistent with a formal description of how parts of a system will change with time.

Blinov et al. (*28*) apply similar methods to reproduce and extend the earlier model of Kholodenko et al. (*29*), incorporating a larger number of reactions including proteins not incorporated into the Kholodenko model.

Another method that has been used to model the signaling cascade is Petri nets (*30*). This method is a visually intuitive way of constructing and simulating systems, which can be readily visualized while the simulation is running.

Schamel and Dick (*31*) have proposed an analogy between the signal transduction process and the Parallel Distributed Processing model used in modeling neural networks. Rather than representing a way to implement simulations, however, this model remains at the conceptual level.

An alternative approach to modeling is given by Pawson and Linding (*32*), which takes an approach sometimes known as a synthetic biology approach to the problem. In this approach, signaling networks are reverse engineered from known components. By carrying out such a reconstruction, the developer of the simulation is required to think carefully about the functional role of each of the components, and therefore develops a better understanding of the role that each component plays and the possible ways in which they can interact.

4.3. Modeling Behavior on the Cell Surface in the EGF Receptor System

The process of dimerization and higher-level clustering of EGF receptors on the cell surface is the subject of a paper by Goldman et al. (*33*). This model consists of an object-oriented individual-based model, where receptors move under Brownian motion on a model of the cell surface, are able to be liganded, and which form clusters by binding with other receptors using a probabilistic model with parameters that can be specified by the user.

A model using similar techniques has been developed to model the diffusion of ligands in the intercellular medium, and thus help to understand juxtacrine and paracrine signaling (*34*).

4.4. Modeling the Overall System

Recently, attempts have been made to combine models of various aspects of the system. For example, Hendriks et al (*35*) have developed a differential equation model that combines a model of dimerization of liganded receptors with a model of the consequent intracellular signaling cascade. This model has been applied to model hypotheses concerning differences in the behavior between ErbB1 receptors that are sensitive to the drug getfitinib (IRESSA), and those that are not.

4.5. Higher Level Models for Intracellular Signaling Cascades

Each piece of work described so far has consisted of a single modeling technique being applied to some particular problem. Recent papers by Calder et al. (*18, 36*) take a different approach. The approach taken is to describe the MAP kinase cascade in a mathematical language known as process algebra, which is a formal description of the various interactions within the system. This high-level description can be automatically converted into both a deterministic, differential equation-based system that can be simulated using numerical methods and automatically converted into a stochastic model that can be simulated using an individual-based model. If the model is robust, both of these techniques should produce a similar outcome; however, sometimes artifacts from the particular simulation/numerical analysis method used can distort the solution.

Calder et al. (*36*) use a comparison between the two models, derived from the process algebra description, to show such an artifact in the earlier paper of Schoberl et al. (*37*), which underestimates the peak concentration of Ras-GTP in the system by a factor of two.

Descriptions such as the process algebra have two main advantages. First, they can be automatically converted into simulations of different types, thus showing up problems with a particular simulation technique for a particular problem. Second, they have the potential advantage that models can be analyzed for qualitative features, as well as being converted into executable models. Some general issues concerned with models of this kind are discussed by Kolch et al. (*38*).

4.6. Integration with Larger System Biology Software Systems

It has been noted by Hornberg et al. (*39*) that cancer is a canonical systems biology disease: if we want to understand cancer, we need to understand how information flows between many different parallel systems of chemical interactions. Other discussions of the impact of systems biology on signal transduction are given by Citri and Yarden (*40*) and Suresh Babu et al. (*41*). In recent years, attempts have been made to create software and description languages that allow the sharing and combining of models of biochemical systems. One of the most important of these languages is the Systems Biology Markup Language (SBML) (*42*). The aim of this language is to provide a common set of formal notation for the recording of diagrams of biochemical interactions, so that models can be shared between different software packages and combined into larger integrated models (for example the E-Cell project (*43*)).

Recently, some early efforts have been made to give an SBML description of the EGF receptor system and its associated signaling cascade (*44*). A more general discussion of this kind of notation is given by Kitano (*45*), Blinov (*28*), and Cary et al. (*46*).

High-throughput techniques for data collection, such as microarrays, are often associated with systems biology approaches, as they can provide the detailed data needed to complete a systems biology model. Studies such as that of Jones et al. (*47*) show how large-scale protein networks can be studied and reaction rates quantified, which provide valuable input for simulations.

5. PROSPECTS

Mathematical and computational models have proven useful in testing various hypotheses about the functioning of the EGF receptor system and in providing a precise language for the expression of such hypotheses. In the future, we can see four new important directions for work of this type:

- The use of such methods in combination with data gained from experiment.
- The integration of these models into a wider set of tools for systems biology, leading to the integration of multiple models.
- The use of languages to describe these systems that can be realized in a number of different ways, and have a number of different analytical tools applied to them.
- The simulation of the activity of drugs on the system and the use of computational search techniques to discover new targets for drug discovery (as illustrated by the work of Haugh et al. (*48*)).

Breitling and Hoeller (*49*) also discuss future directions for such models. They outline four main directions for future applications of modeling of the EGF system: modeling of endosomal compartmentalization, developing more sophisticated models of the protein interaction network, spatial modeling, and including feedback loops and crosstalk in models.

REFERENCES

1. Mitchell TM (1997) Machine learning. McGraw-Hill, Boston.
2. Witten IH, Frank E (2005) Data mining: practical machine learning tools and techniques. Elsevier, Amsterdam.
3. Quinlan R (1992) C4.5: programs for machine learning. Morgan Kaufmann, San Francisco.
4. Rendell L, Seshu R. Learning hard concepts through constructive induction: framework and rationale. Computational Intelligence, 1995;6:247–270.
5. Fall CP, et al. (2002) Computational cell biology. Springer-Verlag, Berlin.
6. Murray JD. (2004) Mathematical biology: I. an introduction, 3rd ed. Springer-Verlag, Berlin.
7. Nelson DL, Cox MM. (2004) Lehninger principles of biochemistry. Palgrave-Macmillan, London.
8. Michalewicz Z, Fogel DB. (2004) How to solve it: Modern Heuristics, 2nd ed. Berlin: Springer-Verlag.
9. Kuipers B. (1994) Qualitative reasoning: modeling and simulation with incomplete knowledge. MIT Press, Cambridge.
10. Kuipers B. (2001) Qualitative simulation. In: Meyers RA (ed), Encyclopedia of physical science and technology, 2nd ed. Academic Press.
11. Johnson CG, Goldman JP, Gullick WJ. Simulating complex intracellular processes using object-oriented computational modelling. Progress in Biophysics and Molecular Biology, 2004;86:379–406.
12. Law AM. (2006) Simulation, modeling and analysis, 4th ed. McGraw-Hill, New York.
13. Andrews SS, Bray D. Stochastic simulation of chemical reactions with spatial resolution and single molecule detail Physical Biology 2005;1:137-151.
14. Lemerle C, Di Ventura B, Serrano L. Space as the final frontier in stochastic simulations of biological systems. FEBS Letters, 2005;559:1789–1794.
15. Gullick WJ. The type 1 growth factor receptors and their ligands considered as a complex system. Endocrine-Related Cancer 2001;8:75–82.
16. Bazley LA, Gullick WJ. The epidermal growth factor receptor family. Endocrine-Related Cancer 2005;12(S17–S27).
17. Wiley HS, Shvartsman SY, Lauffenburger DA. Computational modeling of the EGF-receptor system: a paradigm for systems biology. TRENDS in Cell Biology, 2003;13(1):43–50.
18. Orton RJ, Sturm OE, Vyshemirsky V, et al. Computational modelling of the receptor-tyrosine-kinase-activated MAPK pathway. Biochemistry Journal, 2005;392:249–261.
19. Wolfram S. (2004) The *Mathematica* book (5th ed). Wolfram Media, Champaign.
20. Higham DJ, Higham NJ. Matlab guide. (2005) Society for Industrial and Applied Mathematics, Philadelphia.
21. Mendes P. Biochemistry by numbers: simulation of biochemical pathways with Gepasi 3. *Trends in Biochemical Science,* 1997; 22:361–363.
22. Suresh Babu CV, Yoon S, Nam H-S, Yoom YS. Simulation and sensitivity analysis of phophorylation of EGFR signal transduction pathway in PC12 cell model. Systems Biology, 2004;1(2):213–221.
23. Brightman FA, Fell DA. Differential feedback regulation of the MAPK cascade underlies the quantitative differences in EGF and NGF signalling in PC12 cells. FEBS Letters, 2000;482:169–174.
24. Hendricks BS, et al. Computational modelling of ErbB family phosphorylation dynamics in response to transforming growth factor alpha and heregulin indicates spatial compartmentalisation of phosphatase activity. IEE Proceedings—Systems Biology, 2006;153(1): 22–33.
25. Shvartsman SY, Muratov CB, Lauffenburger DA. Modelling and computational analysis of EGF receptor-mediated cell communication in *Drosophila* oogenesis. Development, 2002;129:2577–2589.
26. Maly IV, Wiley SH, Lauffenburger DA. Self-organizations of polarized cell signalling via autocrine circuits: computational model analysis. Biophysical Journal, 2004; 86:10–22.
27. Hlavacek WS, Faeder JR, Blinov ML, et al. (2006) Rules for modelling signal-transduction systems. Science's STKE.
28. Blinov ML, Yang J, Faeder JR, Hlavacek W. Depicting signaling cascades. Nature Biotechnology, 2006;24(2):137–138.
29. Kholodenko BN, Demin OV, Moehren G, Hoek JB. Quantification of short term signalling by the epidermal growth factor receptor. Journal of Biological Chemistry, 1999;274:30169–30181.
30. Lee D-Y, Zimmer R, Lee SY, Park S. Colored Petri net modeling and simulation of signal transduduction pathways. Metabolic Engineering,2006; 8:112–122.

31. Schamel WWA, Dick TP. Signal transduction: specificity of growth factors explained by parallel distributed processing. Medical Hypotheses,1996; 47:249–255.
32. Pawson T, Linding R. Synthetic Modular Systems—reverse engineering of signal transduction. FEBS Letters, 2005;579:1808–1814.
33. Goldman JP, Gullick WJ, Johnson CG. Individual-based simulation of the clustering behaviour of epidermal growth factor receptors. Scientific Programming, 2004;12(1):25–43.
34. Walker D, Wood S, Southgate J, Holcombe M, Smallwood R. An integrated agent-mathematical model of the effect of intercellular signalling via the epidermal growth factor receptor on cell proliferations. Journal of Theoretical Biology, 2006;242(3):774–789.
35. Hendricks BS, et al. Decreased internalisation of ErbB1 mutants in lung cancer is linked with a mechanism conferring sensitivity to getfitinib. IEE Proceedings—Systems Biology, 2006;153(6):457–466.
36. Calder M, Duguid A, Gilmore S, Hillston J. (2006) Stronger computational modelling of signalling pathways using both continuous and discrete-state methods. In: Priami C (Ed.), Proceedings of the Fourth International Workshop on Computational Methods in Systems Biology. Springer-Verlag (Lecture Notes in Computer Science vol. 4210), Berlin.
37. Schoeberl B, Eichler-Jonsson C, Gilles ED, Muller G. Computational modeling of the dynamics of the MAP kinase cascade activated by surface and internalised EGF receptors. Nature Biotechnology, 2002;20:370–275.
38. Kolch W, Calder M, Gilbert D. When kinases meet mathematics: the systems biology of MAPK signalling. FEBS Letters, 2005;579:1891–1895.
39. Hornberg JJ, Bruggeman FJ, Westerhoff HV, Lankelma J. Cancer: a systems biology disease. BioSystems, 2005;83:81–90.
40. Citri A Yarden Y. EGF-ERBB signalling: towards the systems level. Nature Reviews Molecular Cell Biology, 2006;7:505–515.
41. Suresh Babu CV, Song EJ, Yoo YS. Modeling and simulation in signal transduction pathways: a systems biology approach. Biochemie, 2006;88(3–4):277–83.
42. Hucka M, Finney A, Sauro HM, et al. The Systems Biology Markup Language (SBML): A Medium for Representation and Exchange of Biochemical Network Models. Bioinformatics, 2003; 19(4):524-531.
43. Tomita M, Hasimoto K, Takahashi K, et al. E-CELL: software environment for whole-cell simulation. Bioinformatics, 1999;15(1):72-84.
44. Oda K, et al. A comprehensive pathway map of epidermal growth factor receptor signaling. Molecular Systems Biology, 2005;1, doi:10.1038/msb4100014.
45. Kitano H, Funahashi A, Matsuoka Y, Oda K. Using process diagrams for the graphical representation of biochemical networks. Nature Biotechnology, 2005;23:961–966.
46. Cary MP, Bader GD, Sander C. Pathway information for systems biology. FEBS Letters, 2005;579:1815–1820.
47. Jones RB, Gordus A, Krall JA, MacBeath G. A quantitative protein interaction network for the ErbB receptors using protein microarrays. Nature, 2006;439(7073):168–174.
48. Haugh JM, Wells A, Lauffenburger DA. Mathematical modeling of epidermal growth factor receptor signalling through the phospholipase pathway: mechanistic insights and predictions for molecular interventions. Biotechnology and Bioengineering, 2000;70(2):225–238.
49. Breitling R, Hoeller D. Current challenges in quantitative modelling of epidermal growth factor receptor signalling. FEBS Letters, 2005;579:6289–6294.

Section II
EGFR in Tumorigenesis and EGFR Tyrosine Kinase Inhibitors in Cancer Therapy

16 Expression and Prognostic Significance of the EGFR in Solid Tumors

Nicola Normanno, Caterina Bianco, Antonella De Luca, Luigi Strizzi, Marianna Gallo, Mario Mancino, and David S. Salomon

CONTENTS

INTRODUCTION
EXPRESSION OF ErbB RECEPTORS AND COGNATE LIGANDS
  IN HUMAN CARCINOMAS
CONCLUSION
REFERENCES

Abstract

The epidermal growth factor receptor (EGFR) is expressed in the majority of human carcinomas, where it regulates proliferation and survival of cancer cells. Clinical studies have failed, however, to demonstrate a direct correlation between expression of this receptor and prognosis of cancer patients. In this regard, pre-clinical studies suggest that the transforming ability of the EGFR depends on the levels of expression of EGFR ligands and that it is greatly enhanced when different ErbB receptors are co-expressed. Indeed, co-expression of different ErbB receptors and EGF-like growth factors has been demonstrated to occur in several human carcinomas. This observation leads to hypothesize that the growth of human tumors might be regulated by a network of receptors and ligands of the EGFR family. Therefore, the global levels of expression of these proteins should be determined for prognostic and therapeutic applications. Finally, recent findings suggest that the EGFR system might regulate the functions of the tumor microenvironment that are important for tumor progression such as neo-angiogenesis and osteoclast activation.

Key Words: EGFR, ErbB2, ErbB3, ErbB4, EGF-like growth factors, cancer, prognosis.

1. INTRODUCTION

A number of preclinical studies have demonstrated the involvement of the epidermal growth factor receptor (EGFR) signaling in tumor pathogenesis. Indeed, overexpression of EGFR is able to induce in vitro transformation in presence of appropriate levels of specific ligands (*1*). In addition, the role of EGFR in the autonomous proliferation of carcinoma cells has been formally demonstrated by using different approaches such as retroviral antisense expression vectors, antisense oligonucleotides, or neutralizing antibodies. In fact, blockade of EGFR results in a significant inhibition of the in vitro and in vivo growth of several different cell lines derived from human carcinoma of various histological types (2). Transgenic mice studies have shown that overexpression of the EGFR might lead to transformation of the mammary gland, but not of other tissues (1, 3). In addition, the observation that mammary carcinomas arise only after pregnancy also suggests that overexpression of the EGFR by itself is not able to induce in vivo transformation, and that other events such as activation of protooncogenes or inactivation of tumor suppressor genes are required for this phenomenon to occur (1, 3). In agreement with these results, evidence suggests that the transforming ability of the EGFR is greatly enhanced when different ErbB receptors are co-expressed. In this regard, Kokai and co-workers (4) demonstrated that co-expression of rodent p185c-neu and EGFR in NIH-3T3 cells was necessary to induce full transformation of these cells. In addition, Cohen et al. (5) have shown that in vitro transformation of a NIH-3T3 clone devoid of detectable endogenous ErbB receptors occurred preferentially when two different ErbB receptors were expressed in presence of an appropriate ligand. Any combination of ErbB receptors was able to induce in vitro transformation. However, the EGFR/ErbB2 heterodimer was the only receptor pair able to efficiently induce in vivo transformation (i.e., a tumorigenic phenotype).

Therefore, overexpression of ErbB2 appears to be an amplifier of the signaling stimuli that are carried by other ErbB receptors. The importance of the cooperation of ErbB2 and other ErbB receptors in inducing in vivo transformation is indeed suggested by different observations. For example, mammary tumors derived from transgenic mice engineered to overexpress the mouse ErbB2 homologue *neu* are also characterized by expression of high levels of endogenous EGFR (6). Similarly, transgenic mice carrying an activated *neu* show high levels of tyrosine phosphorylation of both *neu* and ErbB3 (7). The *neu* proto-oncogene and transforming growth factor-α (TGF-α), the main EGFR ligand, have also shown a synergistic interaction in inducing transformation in the mammary epithelium of transgenic mice (8). Bitransgenic female mice co-expressing TGF-α and *neu* developed multifocal mammary tumors with significantly shorter latency period as compared with either parental strain alone. Finally, treatment of ErbB2 transgenic mice with an EGFR tyrosine kinase inhibitor such as gefitinib efficiently prevents the formation of mammary tumors (9).

These findings emphasize that the EGFR, together with the other ErbB receptors and growth factors of the EGF-family, form an integrated system in which a signal that impinges upon an individual receptor type is often transmitted to other receptors of the same family (Fig. 16.1). This mechanism leads to amplification and diversification of the initial signal, a phenomenon that is important for cell transformation. In addition, recent findings suggest that the response of tumor cells to anti-EGFR therapies might be significantly affected by the expression of other ErbB-receptors and of EGFR ligands in cancer cells and in the tumor microenvironment (1). In fact, activation of these receptors is dependent on the levels of EGF-like growth factors that are produced by either cancer cells or in the surrounding stromal cells. Therefore, the role of EGFR expression and activation in human tumors cannot be discussed without taking in account the complex interactions existing within the ErbB family of receptors and their ligands (see also Chapter 2).

2. EXPRESSION OF ErbB RECEPTORS AND COGNATE LIGANDS IN HUMAN CARCINOMAS

2.1. EGFR

Expression of the EGFR protein and/or mRNA has been found in the majority of carcinoma types. The frequency of expression of the EGFR in human carcinomas is generally high, with some tumors such as head and neck carcinomas having been reported to express the EGFR

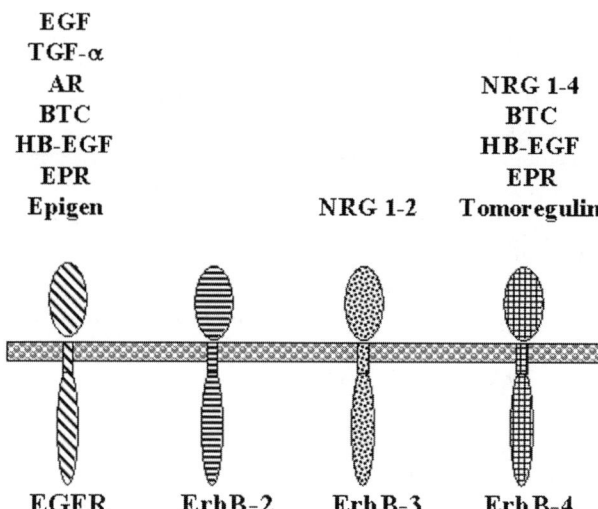

Fig. 16.1. The ErbB receptors an their cognate ligands. Abbreviations: EGF, epidermal growth factor; TGF-α, transforming growth factor-α; AR, amphiregulin; BTC, betacellulin, HB-EGF, heparin binding-EGF; EPR, epiregulin; NRG, neuregulin.

Table 16.1
Expression of ErbB Receptors in Human Carcinomas

ErbB Receptors	Breast	Lung	Colon	Ovary	Head & Neck
EGFR	14-91%	40-80%	25-77%	35-70%	36-100%
ErbB2	9-39%	18-60%	11-20%	8-32%	17-53%
ErbB3	22-90%	25-85%	65-89%	85%	81%
ErbB4	82%	NA*	NA	93%	28-69%

*NA: not assessed

in up to 100% of the cases (*1, 2, 10*). As shown in Table 16.1, the frequency of expression of the EGFR in carcinomas has a wide range. For example, in breast carcinomas expression of the EGFR has been reported in 14% to 91% of human tumors with an average of approximately 50%. Several reasons could explain such variability. In fact, different techniques have been employed to assess the levels of expression of the EGFR protein in primary tumors, i.e. radioimmunoassays western blotting and immunohistochemistry. The cut off values to discriminate positive and negative samples differ in each study. Furthermore, different antibodies have been used to detect the expression of the EGFR in tumor tissues. Finally, some studies have measured the overexpression of the EGFR in the tumor as compared with normal mucosa, and they have assessed as negative the tumor samples expressing EGFR levels similar to normal mucosa (*10*). Recent results from pre-clinical and clinical studies with anti-EGFR agents suggest that tumors with low levels of expression of the EGFR might respond to these agents (*11*). Therefore, it is essential to define standardized, highly sensitive techniques for the detection of EGFR expression in primary tumors that should represent a tool to select patients to treat with anti-EGFR agents.

Overexpression of EGFR is sometimes associated with EGFR gene amplification (*10*). This phenomenon is not frequent in human carcinomas, however, and overexpression of the EGFR in the absence of gene amplification has been found. Mutations of the EGFR have been also described to occur in human tumors. The most frequent EGFR mutation is the EGFR vIII form, that is characterized by a large deletion of the extracellular domain of the receptor (12). This mutation is frequent in gliomas and it has been described to occur in carcinomas, such as breast, ovarian and lung cancers (12). However, the frequency of this mutation and the percentage of tumor cells carrying the mutated EGFR in tumors other than gliomas need to be addressed in larger studies. More recently, small in frame deletions or point mutations occurring in the tyrosine kinase domain of the EGFR have been found in approximately 10% of non-small-cell lung cancer (NSCLC) (3) (see also Chapter 20). These mutations are associated with an increased response to EGFR tyrosine kinase inhibitors. The EGFR mutations were highly frequent in female non-smoker patients with adenocarcinoma, most notably in the Asian population. The growth of this type of tumor seems to be strictly dependent on the activation of the EGFR pathway, which might represent the leading pathway in inducing cellular transformation in these selected patients.

Several studies have addressed the prognostic significance of the EGFR in cancer patients without reaching a definitive conclusion. For example, discordant results on the correlation between the level of expression of this receptor and outcome of breast cancer patients have been reported. The major drawback of these studies is that different techniques have been employed to assess the expression of EGFR in breast cancer specimens, including ligand-binding assays, autoradiography, immunohistochemistry (IHC), immunoenzymatic assays (ELISA), measurement of EGFR transcripts by using different techniques, or EGFR associated phosphotyrosine kinase activity. Furthermore, different cutpoints have been used to distinguish negative and positive samples, resulting in a wide spectrum for assigning a positive status. Finally, multivariate analysis has been applied in a minority of these studies, making it difficult to interpret these results. In order to analyze the prognostic role of the EGFR in breast cancer, we have selected 29 studies in which at least 100 patients (range 107-1029) have been analyzed for EGFR expression by using different techniques. Original studies and reviews summarizing results of different studies have been used as data-source and are cited in this chapter (13–24). The percentage of EGFR positive tumors in these studies ranged between 20% and 91%. The majority of these studies were retrospective. The type of adjuvant therapy that patients received following surgery was not specified in all the studies. A minority of the patients in early studies were not treated after surgery. However, the majority of the patients received either hormonal therapy or chemotherapy, or both treatments. It has long been suggested that the EGFR might represent a marker for early relapse of breast cancer (10). For this reason, we analyzed separately the correlations existing between EGFR expression, Relapse Free Survival (RFS) and Overall Survival (OS). By univariate analysis, a significant correlation between expression of the EGFR and RFS was demonstrated in 15/25 retrospective studies. In contrast, a significant association between EGFR levels and OS was demonstrated only in five studies. By multivariate analysis, the correlation between EGFR and RFS was confirmed in eight studies, whereas two studies have demonstrated a significant correlation between expression of the EGFR and OS. The correlation between EGFR expression and both RFS and OS was also analyzed in four prospective studies (14, 17, 18, 24). The univariate analysis demonstrated a positive correlation between EGFR levels and both RFS and OS in 2/4 studies. Multivariate analysis, however, confirmed these findings in one study. Taken together, these results suggest that the expression of the EGFR in breast cancer might be useful to identify a subgroup of early relapsing tumors, whereas it is of little utility for assessing survival probability.

In agreement with these findings, a recent study has shown that long-term survival for NSCLC correlates with low levels of EGFR mRNA expression (25). However, other studies have suggested no correlation between EGFR expression and patient prognosis in NSCLC, or prognostic significance only when combined with ErbB2 (26, 27). A recent study has demonstrated that expression of the EGFR is an independent prognostic factor in stage II colon carcinoma (28). In agreement with these findings, survival of colorectal cancer patients with increased tumor EGFR levels as measured with ^{125}I-EGF-binding techniques was significantly reduced in comparison to patients with low tumor EGFR levels (29). Expression of EGFR, however, was not found to correlate with patient outcome in a different study in which the receptor was determined by using immunohistochemistry (30). Interestingly, significant differences between results obtained with immunocytochemistry or radioreceptor assay were observed by Kopp and co-workers (29).

2.2. ErbB2

The expression of ErbB2 in primary human carcinomas is generally more restricted as compared with the EGFR (Table 16.1) (2,10). The role of ErbB2 in the transformation of mammary epithelial cells has been formally proven, whereas the involvement of this receptor in the pathogenesis and/or progression of other tumor types needs to be further experimentally addressed. Over expression of ErbB2 is frequently associated with gene amplification, although overexpression in absence of gene amplification has been described (2, 10). The ErbB2 gene is not usually mutated in carcinomas. A recent study, however, demonstrated the occurrence of in frame insertion or missense substitutions in the kinase domain of the ErbB2 receptor (31). ErbB2 mutations were initially detected in NSCLC patients with adenocarcinoma with a frequency close to 10% (5/51), and were more frequent in current or ex-smokers. However, a more recent study found mutations of the ErbB2 tyrosine kinase domain in 1.6% of 671 NSCLC (32). These mutations were more frequent in patients with adenocarcinoma, female and non-smoker, i.e., the same phenotype of patients carrying EGFR mutations. Interestingly, ErbB2 mutations were found in patients that did not carry mutations of EGFR. However, the kinase activity and the transforming potential of this mutated form of ErbB2 have not yet been evaluated. Finally, both EGFR and ErbB2 mutations were found in patients that did not carry ras mutations, suggesting that these proteins are involved in different processes of transformation. Mutations of K-ras have been shown to be associated with resistance to the EGFR tyrosine kinase inhibitors gefitinib and erlotinib in NSCLC (33).

It is difficult to summarize the available data on the prognostic role of ErbB2 in breast cancer. In fact, a MEDLINE search using the key words breast cancer, ErbB2 and prognosis retrieves over 1500 articles. ErbB2 expression or gene amplification has been assessed in approximately 30% of these studies. Different techniques have been employed to detect ErbB2 overexpression or gene amplification in primary tumors: IHC, ELISA, FISH, Southern blot or dot blot, Western blot. The tumors that were positive for ErbB2 overexpression or gene amplification ranged between 9 and 39%. The majority of the studies were retrospective, and different cutpoints and stratification of patients have been employed for analysis. Still, more uniform results have been obtained in studies on ErbB2 expression as compared with the EGFR.

We selected 74 studies in which at least 100 breast cancer patients (range 100-1576) have been analyzed for ErbB2 overexpression or gene amplification by using different techniques. Sixty-four studies that we have analyzed are listed in a review article by Ross and co-workers (34). Ten articles were from the above mentioned MEDLINE search (22, 23, 35–42). Of these studies, only seven were prospective (35, 38–40, 43–45). The majority of the above referenced studies have analyzed the correlation of ErbB2 with prognosis in both node-positive and node-negative subgroups. In 20 retrospective studies, however, this subgroup analysis was not performed. Since the majority of these studies, as well as studies run in node-positive patients alone, resulted in positive findings, we have grouped their results together, whereas we have analyzed separately the results obtained in the node-negative patients cohorts (studies specific for node-negative patients, or results of analysis of the node-negative subgroup in studies which enrolled both negative and positive patients).

By univariate analysis, 51/53 retrospective studies have shown a significant association of ErbB2 overexpression or gene amplification with RFS and/or OS in unselected patients and/or in node-positive subgroups. Multivariate analysis was run in 47 of these studies, with 40 analyses confirming this association. For node-negative patients, 19/33 retrospective studies have demonstrated a significant correlation between ErbB2 overexpression or gene amplification and prognosis at univariate analysis. However, multivariate analysis confirmed such association only in 14/19 studies. Of the seven prospective studies, only two regarded node-positive patients, for which a significant association of ErbB2 with prognosis was demonstrated by both univariate and multivariate analysis (17, 35). Node-negative patients were analyzed in six prospective studies, with 5/6 studies showing a prognostic role of ErbB2 by univariate analysis, which was confirmed by multivariate analysis only in four studies (17, 38, 39, 43–45). It is important to note that in these prospective studies different techniques have been employed (ELISA, IHC, PCR, Slot blot, Southern Blot), and this might explain in part the uneven results that have been obtained. However, taken together, these results suggest that ErbB2 overexpression or gene amplification is an important prognostic factor in node-positive patients, whereas the prognostic value of this marker in node-negative patients is still unclear. In this respect, analysis of a large homogenous cohort of patients in which ErbB2 expression has been assessed with standard techniques is required to address this issue. Indeed, a recent report suggested that ErbB2 gene amplification but not protein expression is a prognostic factor in node-negative breast cancer patients (46).

Prognostic value of ErbB2 in NSCLC patients has also been assessed. High levels of ErbB2 expression are associated with an unfavourable outcome of lung carcinoma patients (47). These findings have been more recently confirmed by Brabender and co-workers (27). Interestingly, patients with high levels of expression of both ErbB2 and EGFR transcripts showed a worse prognosis as compared with patients expressing a single receptor.

2.3. ErbB3 and ErbB4

The frequency of ErbB3 expression in human carcinomas has been recently reviewed (Table 16.1) (2). The levels and the frequency of expression of ErbB3 in human carcinomas are generally comparable to EGFR. The prognostic role of this receptor in human carcinomas is still debated. For example, ErbB3 expression has been associated in breast cancer patients with either adverse prognostic factors such as lymph node metastasis or with the prognostically-favorable estrogen receptor positive phenotype (48–50). However, expression of ErbB3 seems to be associated with a worse prognosis in bladder, oral squamous cell and pancreatic cancer patients (51–53). Immunoreactive ErbB4 or specific transcripts have been found in different tumors, such as breast, ovarian, squamous cell, esophageal, bladder, and pancreatic cancer (Table 16.1) (2). In breast cancer, expression of this receptor is generally associated with a better outcome, with a more differentiated phenotype and with expression of the estrogen receptor (48, 50).

2.4. EGF-like Growth Factors

The majority of human carcinomas express EGF-like growth factors (Table 16.2). TGF-α expression occurs in all carcinoma types, with many tumors showing overexpression of this protein as compared with normal tissue (54). In some tumor types expression of TGF-α correlates with a less differentiated phenotype. For example, in breast cancer cell lines, higher levels of expression of TGF-α have been found in estrogen receptor negative tumors as compared with estrogen receptor positive carcinomas (55). TGF-α expression has also been found in pre-malignant lesions such as in situ breast carcinomas or colon adenomas, suggesting a potential role of this growth factor in the early phases of tumorigenesis (10, 54). However, various studies failed to demonstrate a significant correlation between TGF-α expression and patient outcome. The lack of correlation between expression of TGF-α and patient prognosis might be due to the co-expression of

Table 16.2
Expression of EGF-like Peptides in Human Carcinomas

EGF-like proteins	Breast	Lung	Colon	Ovary	Head & Neck
TGF-α	40-70%	60-100%	50-90%	55-100%	40-100%
AR	37-80%	11-78%	50-77%	18-76%	NA
HRG/NRG	25-30%	NA	NA	77-87%	NA
HB-EGF	72%	0%	28%	56%	NA

*NA: not assessed

several EGF-like peptides in the majority of human carcinomas. In this respect, expression of amphiregulin (AR) has also been demonstrated in different carcinoma types (10, 54). In contrast with TGF-α, expression of AR is generally associated with a more differentiated phenotype. In fact, a strong correlation between AR and estrogen receptor expression has been shown in a subset of human primary breast carcinomas that were examined for AR mRNA expression by Northern blot analysis (56). In colon carcinomas, a correlation between AR expression and a more differentiated phenotype has also been demonstrated (57). More recently, we found that AR is preferentially expressed in ovarian carcinomas with lower proliferative activity and low grade (58). Finally, expression of AR frequently occurs in normal tissues, whereas loss of expression has been demonstrated in the tissues surrounding both colon and breast carcinomas (57, 59, 60). These observations suggest that loss of AR expression might be involved in the early phases of cancerogenesis that are associated with loss of differentiation. Interestingly, AR overexpression has been found to be an independent prognostic factor in NSCLC (61). In this regard, a recent report demonstrated that AR activates a mechanism that inhibits apoptosis through an insulin like growth factor-1 (IGF-1)-dependent survival pathway in NSCLC cells (62).

Heparin binding-EGF (HB-EGF) is expressed in 72% of human breast carcinomas but only marginally in normal mammary glands (63). Interestingly, the expression of HB-EGF is inversely related to the biological aggressiveness of the tumors. HB-EGF is not expressed in lung carcinomas (64). However, HB-EGF protein and/or transcripts have been detected in hepatocellular, gastric, ovarian and colon carcinomas (65–68). The frequency of expression of HB-EGF is higher in colon adenomas as compared with carcinomas, suggesting a role of this growth factor in the early phases of colon tumorigenesis.

The expression of proteins of the neuregulin (NRG) or heregulin (HRG) subfamily in human carcinomas is generally more restricted. HRG expression has been mainly investigated in breast carcinomas. HRG mRNA expression has been detected in about 25-30% of human primary breast carcinomas (56, 69). Expression of different proteins of the HRG family has also been demonstrated in breast cancers by immunocytochemical staining (70). Expression of NRG-1 α and NRG-1 β proteins were detected by immunohistochemistry in 46 of 53 (87%) and 41 of 53 (77%) ovarian carcinomas, respectively. NRG mRNA was also detected by RT-PCR in 20 of 24 (83%) ovarian carcinomas and eight of nine (89%) ovarian cancer cell lines (71).

2.5. Co-expression of ErbB Receptors and Ligands in Tumors

It is important to underline that due to the high frequency of expression of individual ErbB receptor types in different types of human carcinomas, co-expression of different receptors occurs in the majority of tumors. As we have discussed above, this phenomenon might be important for tumor pathogenesis. Indeed, tumors that co-express different ErbB receptors are often associated with a more aggressive phenotype and a worse prognosis. For example, an elegant paper by DiGiovanna et al. (*72*) demonstrated EGFR expression in only 15% of 807 invasive breast cancers. However, the majority of EGFR-positive tumors (87%) were found to co-express ErbB2. More importantly, almost all tumors that expressed the phosphorylated form of ErbB2, co-expressed EGFR. Expression of phosphorylated ErbB2 or co-expression of ErbB2 and EGFR was associated with the shortest survival in cancer patients. In contrast, patients with tumors that were negative for all three markers, or that expressed only EGFR or only non-phosphorylated ErbB2 had a relatively good outcome. Taken together, these data clearly establish a link in vivo between expression of EGFR and activation of ErbB2 in breast cancer patients.

In agreement with these findings, co-expression of EGFR, ErbB2, and ErbB3 has a negative synergistic effect on patient outcome, independent of tumor size or lymph node status, in a cohort of 242 patients with invasive breast carcinomas with a median 15-year follow-up (*73*). A direct correlation was found between the number of ErbB receptors expressed within the tumor and patients' outcome. Breast cancer patients whose tumors co-expressed ErbB2 and ErbB3, as well as those whose tumors co-expressed EGFR, ErbB2, and ErbB4, showed an unfavorable outcome as compared with other groups, while combined ErbB3 and ErbB4 expression was associated with a better outcome (*42*). Interestingly, Brabender et al. (*27*) found that NSCLC patients with high levels of expression of transcripts for both ErbB2 and EGFR have a worse prognosis as compared with patients expressing a single receptor. Additional studies have shown that co-expression of different ErbB receptors is associated with worse outcome as compared with expression of a single receptor in colon carcinoma, transitional cell carcinoma of the urinary bladder and oral squamous cell carcinoma patients (*52, 53, 74*).

The redundancy of expression in human carcinomas is not limited to the ErbB receptors. In fact, a number of studies have demonstrated that co-expression of different EGF-like peptides occurs in a majority of human carcinomas. For example, we have demonstrated that TGF-α, AR and/or NRG are expressed in human colon, breast, lung, ovarian and gastric carcinomas, suggesting that co-expression of different EGF-like growth factors is a common phenomenon in human carcinogenesis (*54*). In this respect, both tumor cells and surrounding stromal cells might represent a source of ErbB ligands.

2.6. Expression and Function of the EGFR in Non-tumor Cells of the Neoplastic Environment

The majority of studies have been focused on the assessment of the expression and function of the EGFR and related proteins in tumor cells. However, expression of the EGFR occurs in all non-transformed cell types with the exception of mature hemopoietic cells. In this regard, pre-clinical data suggest that activation of the EGFR in at least two non-tumor cell populations might play an important role in tumor progression. Several reports have demonstrated the expression of the EGFR in the endothelial cells of the tumor microenvironment (*75*). In addition, it has been established that EGF like growth factors such as EGF, TGFα, and AR have a pro-angiogenic activity (*76, 77*). More recently, it has been demonstrated that EGFR tyrosine kinase inhibitors have a direct effect on the migration of microvascular endothelial cells (*78*). In this regard, expression and activation of EGFR in endothelial cells of tumor expressing EGFR ligands has also been shown (*79*). Anti-EGFR agents have also been shown to selectively produce a reduction in the levels of EGFR phosphorylation in endothelial cells within bone metastases (*80*). Taken together, these observations suggest that the EGFR and its ligands might be involved in tumor progression by directly stimulating neo-angiogenesis.

In addition, we have recently demonstrated that stromal cells of the bone marrow microenvironment express a functional EGFR (*81*). These cells play an important role in the pathogenesis of bone metastases. In fact, although it has been shown that cancer cells can directly resorb bone, the main mechanism responsible for bone destruction in cancer patients is tumor-mediated stimulation of osteoclastic bone resorption (82). Two main factors are involved in osteoclast activation and formation: macrophage colony stimulating factor (M-CSF), which induces proliferation and differentiation of pre-osteoclast cells, and receptor activator of NF-kB ligand (RANKL) that is involved in fusion and activation of these cells (83). Tumor cells synthesize growth factors and cytokines that lead to the activation of osteoclasts by binding to accessory cells of the bone marrow microenvironment and stimulating the production of pro-osteoclastogenic factors such as M-CSF and RANKL (82). In this regard, we have shown that blockade of the EGFR in bone marrow stromal cells significantly affects their ability to produce M-CSF and RANKL and to sustain the differentiation of osteoclast precursors (81). Since expression of EGF-like peptides has been demonstrated in a majority of human carcinomas, these data suggest that activation of the EGFR in bone marrow stromal cells might represent an important mechanism through which tumor cells can establish bone metastases.

3. CONCLUSION

The data summarized in this chapter clearly support the hypothesis that the ErbB receptors and their ligands are involved in the pathogenesis of different types of human carcinomas, and that therefore they represent suitable targets for novel therapeutic approaches. However, the observation that human carcinomas co-express different ErbB receptors and ligands, strongly support the hypothesis that a network formed by these molecules sustains the growth, survival and metastasis of cancer cells. In this regard, the type and the amount of receptors and ligands expressed on tumor cells and within the tumor environment might affect both the "quality" and the "quantity" of ErbB signaling within each individual cancer. This observation might be important for prognostic assessment and therapeutic intervention. In fact, evidence suggests that the prognosis of human carcinoma might be related to the global levels of expression of the different ErbB receptors and ligands within the tumor. Analogously, several studies have demonstrated that response to anti-EGFR agents is not related to the levels of expression of the target receptor. This phenomenon is not surprising, since low levels of EGFR can be sufficient to turn on other receptors such as ErbB2. In this respect, it is possible that response to anti-EGFR agents might depend on the levels of other ErbB receptors and ligands expressed in each tumor. In addition, co-expression of different receptors and growth factors in carcinomas, suggest that a more efficient blockade of tumor growth might be obtained by using combinations of agents directed against different targets. Indeed, we demonstrated that treatment of tumor cells with combinations of antisense oligonucleotides directed against different growth factors results in a synergistic anti-tumor effects in different tumor types (84–87). More recently, we showed that combined treatment of breast cancer cells with the EGFR tyrosine kinase inhibitor gefitinib and the anti-ErbB2 monoclonal antibody herceptin produces a synergistic anti tumor effect (88). These results have been confirmed by different groups and contributed to develop a novel therapeutic approach of human carcinoma. However, the prognostic and predictive value of EGFR needs to be addressed in the context of the complex molecular alterations that are present in each individual tumor. In this respect, important information is arising from studies with high throughput technologies. For example, in breast cancer a gene signature that identifies the "basal" phenotype has been found (89). This group of tumors has a high frequency of expression of EGFR as compared with other sub-types of breast carcinomas. Studies focused in this cohort of patients might help to define the role of the EGFR in the pathogenesis and progression of breast cancer. Finally, the observation that the EGFR regulates in non-tumor cells of the neoplastic environment mechanisms that are involved in tumor progression, opens a new field for the treatment of cancer patients (90).

REFERENCES

1. Normanno N, Bianco C, Strizzi L, Mancino M, Maiello MR, De Luca A, Caponigro F, Salomon DS: The erbb receptors and their ligands in cancer: An overview. Curr Drug Targets 2005;6:243-257.
2. Normanno N, Bianco C, De Luca A, Maiello MR, Salomon DS: Target-based agents against erbb receptors and their ligands: A novel approach to cancer treatment. Endocr Relat Cancer 2003;10:1-21.
3. Normanno N, De Luca A, Bianco C, Strizzi L, Mancino M, Maiello MR, Carotenuto A, De Feo G, Caponigro F, Salomon DS: Epidermal growth factor receptor (egfr) signaling in cancer. Gene 2006;366:2-16.
4. Kokai Y, Myers JN, Wada T, Brown VI, LeVea CM, Davis JG, Dobashi K, Greene MI: Synergistic interaction of p185c-neu and the egf receptor leads to transformation of rodent fibroblasts. Cell 1989;58:287-292.
5. Cohen BD, Kiener PA, Green JM, Foy L, Fell HP, Zhang K: The relationship between human epidermal growth-like factor receptor expression and cellular transformation in nih3t3 cells. J Biol Chem 1996;271:30897-30903.
6. DiGiovanna MP, Lerman MA, Coffey RJ, Muller WJ, Cardiff RD, Stern DF: Active signaling by neu in transgenic mice. Oncogene 1998;17:1877-1884.
7. Siegel PM, Ryan ED, Cardiff RD, Muller WJ: Elevated expression of activated forms of neu/erbb-2 and erbb-3 are involved in the induction of mammary tumors in transgenic mice: Implications for human breast cancer. Embo J 1999;18:2149-2164.
8. Muller WJ, Arteaga CL, Muthuswamy SK, Siegel PM, Webster MA, Cardiff RD, Meise KS, Li F, Halter SA, Coffey RJ: Synergistic interaction of the neu proto-oncogene product and transforming growth factor alpha in the mammary epithelium of transgenic mice. Mol Cell Biol 1996;16:5726-5736.
9. Lu C, Speers C, Zhang Y, Xu X, Hill J, Steinbis E, Celestino J, Shen Q, Kim H, Hilsenbeck S, Mohsin SK, Wakeling A, Osborne CK, Brown PH: Effect of epidermal growth factor receptor inhibitor on development of estrogen receptor-negative mammary tumors. J Natl Cancer Inst 2003;95:1825-1833.
10. Salomon DS, Brandt R, Ciardiello F, Normanno N: Epidermal growth factor-related peptides and their receptors in human malignancies. Crit Rev Oncol Hematol 1995;19:183-232.
11. Campiglio M, Locatelli A, Olgiati C, Normanno N, Somenzi G, Vigano L, Fumagalli M, Menard S, Gianni L: Inhibition of proliferation and induction of apoptosis in breast cancer cells by the epidermal growth factor receptor (egfr) tyrosine kinase inhibitor zd1839 ('iressa') is independent of egfr expression level. J Cell Physiol 2004;198:259-268.
12. Pedersen MW, Meltorn M, Damstrup L, Poulsen HS: The type iii epidermal growth factor receptor mutation. Biological significance and potential target for anti-cancer therapy. Ann Oncol 2001;12:745-760.
13. Fox SB, Harris AL: The epidermal growth factor receptor in breast cancer. J Mammary Gland Biol Neoplasia 1997;2:131-141.
14. Bolla M, Chedin M, Colonna M, Marron-Charriere J, Rostaing-Puissant B, Pasquier D, Panh MH, Winckel P, Chambaz EM: Lack of prognostic value of epidermal growth factor receptor in a series of 229 t1/t2, n0/n1 breast cancers, with well defined prognostic parameters. Breast Cancer Res Treat 1994;29:265-270.
15. Sainsbury JR, Farndon JR, Needham GK, Malcolm AJ, Harris AL: Epidermal-growth-factor receptor status as predictor of early recurrence of and death from breast cancer. Lancet 1987;1:1398-1402.
16. Gohring UJ, Ahr A, Scharl A, Weisner V, Neuhaus W, Crombach G, Holt JA: Immunohistochemical detection of epidermal growth factor receptor lacks prognostic significance for breast carcinoma. J Soc Gynecol Investig 1995;2:653-659.
17. Seshadri R, McLeay WR, Horsfall DJ, McCaul K: Prospective study of the prognostic significance of epidermal growth factor receptor in primary breast cancer. Int J Cancer 1996;69:23-27.
18. Hawkins RA, Tesdale AL, Killen ME, Jack WJ, Chetty U, Dixon JM, Hulme MJ, Prescott RJ, McIntyre MA, Miller WR: Prospective evaluation of prognostic factors in operable breast cancer. Br J Cancer 1996;74:1469-1478.
19. Schroeder W, Biesterfeld S, Zillessen S, Rath W: Epidermal growth factor receptor-immunohistochemical detection and clinical significance for treatment of primary breast cancer. Anticancer Res 1997;17:2799-2802.

20. Ferrero JM, Ramaioli A, Largillier R, Formento JL, Francoual M, Ettore F, Namer M, Milano G: Epidermal growth factor receptor expression in 780 breast cancer patients: A reappraisal of the prognostic value based on an eight-year median follow-up. Ann Oncol 2001;12:841-846.
21. Tsutsui S, Ohno S, Murakami S, Hachitanda Y, Oda S: Prognostic value of epidermal growth factor receptor (egfr) and its relationship to the estrogen receptor status in 1029 patients with breast cancer. Breast Cancer Res Treat 2002;71:67-75.
22. Tolgay Ocal I, Dolled-Filhart M, D'Aquila TG, Camp RL, Rimm DL: Tissue microarray-based studies of patients with lymph node negative breast carcinoma show that met expression is associated with worse outcome but is not correlated with epidermal growth factor family receptors. Cancer 2003;97:1841-1848.
23. Bieche I, Onody P, Tozlu S, Driouch K, Vidaud M, Lidereau R: Prognostic value of erbb family mrna expression in breast carcinomas. Int J Cancer 2003;106:758-765.
24. Koenders PG, Beex LV, Kienhuis CB, Kloppenborg PW, Benraad TJ: Epidermal growth factor receptor and prognosis in human breast cancer: A prospective study. Breast Cancer Res Treat 1993;25:21-27.
25. Volm M, Koomagi R, Mattern J, Efferth T: Expression profile of genes in non-small cell lung carcinomas from long-term surviving patients. Clin Cancer Res 2002;8:1843-1848.
26. Rusch V, Klimstra D, Venkatraman E, Pisters PW, Langenfeld J, Dmitrovsky E: Overexpression of the epidermal growth factor receptor and its ligand transforming growth factor alpha is frequent in resectable non-small cell lung cancer but does not predict tumor progression. Clin Cancer Res 1997;3:515-522.
27. Brabender J, Danenberg KD, Metzger R, Schneider PM, Park J, Salonga D, Holscher AH, Danenberg PV: Epidermal growth factor receptor and her2-neu mrna expression in non-small cell lung cancer is correlated with survival. Clin Cancer Res 2001;7:1850-1855.
28. Resnick MB, Routhier J, Konkin T, Sabo E, Pricolo VE: Epidermal growth factor receptor, c-met, beta-catenin, and p53 expression as prognostic indicators in stage ii colon cancer: A tissue microarray study. Clin Cancer Res 2004;10:3069-3075.
29. Kopp R, Rothbauer E, Ruge M, Arnholdt H, Spranger J, Muders M, Pfeiffer DG, Schildberg FW, Pfeiffer A: Clinical implications of the egf receptor/ligand system for tumor progression and survival in gastrointestinal carcinomas: Evidence for new therapeutic options. Recent Results Cancer Res 2003;162:115-132.
30. Khorana AA, Ryan CK, Cox C, Eberly S, Sahasrabudhe DM: Vascular endothelial growth factor, cd68, and epidermal growth factor receptor expression and survival in patients with stage ii and stage iii colon carcinoma: A role for the host response in prognosis. Cancer 2003;97:960-968.
31. Stephens P, Hunter C, Bignell G, Edkins S, Davies H, Teague J, Stevens C, O'Meara S, Smith R, Parker A, Barthorpe A, Blow M, Brackenbury L, Butler A, Clarke O, Cole J, Dicks E, Dike A, Drozd A, Edwards K, Forbes S, Foster R, Gray K, Greenman C, Halliday K, Hills K, Kosmidou V, Lugg R, Menzies A, Perry J, Petty R, Raine K, Ratford L, Shepherd R, Small A, Stephens Y, Tofts C, Varian J, West S, Widaa S, Yates A, Brasseur F, Cooper CS, Flanagan AM, Knowles M, Leung SY, Louis DN, Looijenga LH, Malkowicz B, Pierotti MA, Teh B, Chenevix-Trench G, Weber BL, Yuen ST, Harris G, Goldstraw P, Nicholson AG, Futreal PA, Wooster R, Stratton MR: Lung cancer: Intragenic erbb2 kinase mutations in tumours. Nature 2004;431:525-526.
32. Shigematsu H, Takahashi T, Nomura M, Majmudar K, Suzuki M, Lee H, Wistuba, II, Fong KM, Toyooka S, Shimizu N, Fujisawa T, Minna JD, Gazdar AF: Somatic mutations of the her2 kinase domain in lung adenocarcinomas. Cancer Res 2005;65:1642-1646.
33. Pao W, Wang TY, Riely GJ, Miller VA, Pan Q, Ladanyi M, Zakowski MF, Heelan RT, Kris MG, Varmus HE: Kras mutations and primary resistance of lung adenocarcinomas to gefitinib or erlotinib. PLoS Med 2005;2:e17.
34. Ross JS, Fletcher JA, Linette GP, Stec J, Clark E, Ayers M, Symmans WF, Pusztai L, Bloom KJ: The her-2/neu gene and protein in breast cancer 2003: Biomarker and target of therapy. Oncologist 2003;8:307-325.
35. Tsuda H, Sakamaki C, Tsugane S, Fukutomi T, Hirohashi S: A prospective study of the significance of gene and chromosome alterations as prognostic indicators of breast cancer patients with lymph node metastases. Breast Cancer Res Treat 1998;48:21-32.
36. Bohn U, Aguiar J, Bilbao C, Murias A, Vega V, Chirino R, Diaz-Chico N, Diaz-Chico JC: Prognostic value of the quantitative measurement of the oncoprotein p185(her-2/neu) in a group of patients with breast cancer and positive node involvement. Int J Cancer 2002;101:539-544.

37. Tsutsui S, Ohno S, Murakami S, Kataoka A, Kinoshita J, Hachitanda Y: Prognostic significance of the coexpression of p53 protein and c-erbb2 in breast cancer. Am J Surg 2003;185:165-167.
38. Schlotter CM, Vogt U, Bosse U, Mersch B, Wassmann K: C-myc, not her-2/neu, can predict recurrence and mortality of patients with node-negative breast cancer. Breast Cancer Res 2003; 5:R30-36.
39. Zemzoum I, Kates RE, Ross JS, Dettmar P, Dutta M, Henrichs C, Yurdseven S, Hofler H, Kiechle M, Schmitt M, Harbeck N: Invasion factors upa/pai-1 and her2 status provide independent and complementary information on patient outcome in node-negative breast cancer. J Clin Oncol 2003;21:1022-1028.
40. Volpi A, Nanni O, De Paola F, Granato AM, Mangia A, Monti F, Schittulli F, De Lena M, Scarpi E, Rosetti P, Monti M, Gianni L, Amadori D, Paradiso A: Her-2 expression and cell proliferation: Prognostic markers in patients with node-negative breast cancer. J Clin Oncol 2003;21:2708-2712.
41. Bianchi S, Palli D, Falchetti M, Saieva C, Masala G, Mancini B, Lupi R, Noviello C, Omerovic J, Paglierani M, Vezzosi V, Alimandi M, Mariani-Costantini R, Ottini L: Erbb-receptors expression and survival in breast carcinoma: A 15-year follow-up study. J Cell Physiol 2006;206:702-708.
42. Abd El-Rehim DM, Pinder SE, Paish CE, Bell JA, Rampaul RS, Blamey RW, Robertson JF, Nicholson RI, Ellis IO: Expression and co-expression of the members of the epidermal growth factor receptor (egfr) family in invasive breast carcinoma. Br J Cancer 2004;91:1532-1542.
43. Gaci Z, Bouin-Pineau MH, Gaci M, Daban A, Ingrand P, Metaye T: Prognostic impact of cathepsin d and c-erbb-2 oncoprotein in a subgroup of node-negative breast cancer patients with low histological grade tumors. Int J Oncol 2001;18:793-800.
44. Volpi A, De Paola F, Nanni O, Granato AM, Bajorko P, Becciolini A, Scarpi E, Riccobon A, Balzi M, Amadori D: Prognostic significance of biologic markers in node-negative breast cancer patients: A prospective study. Breast Cancer Res Treat 2000;63:181-192.
45. Andrulis IL, Bull SB, Blackstein ME, Sutherland D, Mak C, Sidlofsky S, Pritzker KP, Hartwick RW, Hanna W, Lickley L, Wilkinson R, Qizilbash A, Ambus U, Lipa M, Weizel H, Katz A, Baida M, Mariz S, Stoik G, Dacamara P, Strongitharm D, Geddie W, McCready D: Neu/erbb-2 amplification identifies a poor-prognosis group of women with node-negative breast cancer. Toronto breast cancer study group. J Clin Oncol 1998;16:1340-1349.
46. Schmidt M, Lewark B, Kohlschmidt N, Glawatz C, Steiner E, Tanner B, Pilch H, Weikel W, Kolbl H, Lehr HA: Long-term prognostic significance of her-2/neu in untreated node-negative breast cancer depends on the method of testing. Breast Cancer Res 2005;7:R256-266.
47. Tateishi M, Ishida T, Mitsudomi T, Kaneko S, Sugimachi K: Prognostic value of c-erbb-2 protein expression in human lung adenocarcinoma and squamous cell carcinoma. Eur J Cancer 1991;27:1372-1375.
48. Pawlowski V, Revillion F, Hebbar M, Hornez L, Peyrat JP: Prognostic value of the type i growth factor receptors in a large series of human primary breast cancers quantified with a real-time reverse transcription-polymerase chain reaction assay. Clin Cancer Res 2000;6:4217-4225.
49. Naidu R, Yadav M, Nair S, Kutty MK: Expression of c-erbb3 protein in primary breast carcinomas. Br J Cancer 1998;78:1385-1390.
50. Knowlden JM, Gee JM, Seery LT, Farrow L, Gullick WJ, Ellis IO, Blamey RW, Robertson JF, Nicholson RI: C-erbb3 and c-erbb4 expression is a feature of the endocrine responsive phenotype in clinical breast cancer. Oncogene 1998;17:1949-1957.
51. Friess H, Yamanaka Y, Kobrin MS, Do DA, Buchler MW, Korc M: Enhanced erbb-3 expression in human pancreatic cancer correlates with tumor progression. Clin Cancer Res 1995;1:1413-1420.
52. Chow NH, Chan SH, Tzai TS, Ho CL, Liu HS: Expression profiles of erbb family receptors and prognosis in primary transitional cell carcinoma of the urinary bladder. Clin Cancer Res 2001;7:1957-1962.
53. Xia W, Lau YK, Zhang HZ, Xiao FY, Johnston DA, Liu AR, Li L, Katz RL, Hung MC: Combination of egfr, her-2/neu, and her-3 is a stronger predictor for the outcome of oral squamous cell carcinoma than any individual family members. Clin Cancer Res 1999;5:4164-4174.
54. Normanno N, Bianco C, De Luca A, Salomon DS: The role of egf-related peptides in tumor growth. Front Biosci 2001;6:D685-707.
55. Salomon DS, Kim N, Saeki T, Ciardiello F: Transforming growth factor-alpha: An oncodevelopmental growth factor. Cancer Cells 1990;2:389-397.

56. Normanno N, Kim N, Wen D, Smith K, Harris AL, Plowman G, Colletta G, Ciardiello F, Salomon DS: Expression of messenger rna for amphiregulin, heregulin, and cripto-1, three new members of the epidermal growth factor family, in human breast carcinomas. Breast Cancer Res Treat 1995;35:293-297.
57. Saeki T, Stromberg K, Qi CF, Gullick WJ, Tahara E, Normanno N, Ciardiello F, Kenney N, Johnson GR, Salomon DS: Differential immunohistochemical detection of amphiregulin and cripto in human normal colon and colorectal tumors. Cancer Res 1992;52:3467-3473.
58. D'Antonio A, Losito S, Pignata S, Grassi M, Perrone F, De Luca A, Tambaro R, Bianco C, Gullick WJ, Johnson GR, Iaffaioli VR, Salomon DS, Normanno N: Transforming growth factor alpha, amphiregulin and cripto-1 are frequently expressed in advanced human ovarian carcinomas. Int J Oncol 2002;21:941-948.
59. Qi CF, Liscia DS, Normanno N, Merlo G, Johnson GR, Gullick WJ, Ciardiello F, Saeki T, Brandt R, Kim N, et al.: Expression of transforming growth factor alpha, amphiregulin and cripto-1 in human breast carcinomas. Br J Cancer 1994;69:903-910.
60. De Angelis E, Grassi M, Gullick WJ, Johnson GR, Rossi GB, Tempesta A, De Angelis F, De Luca A, Salomon DS, Normanno N: Expression of cripto and amphiregulin in colon mucosa from high risk colon cancer families. Int J Oncol 1999;14:437-440.
61. Fontanini G, De Laurentiis M, Vignati S, Chine S, Lucchi M, Silvestri V, Mussi A, De Placido S, Tortora G, Bianco AR, Gullick W, Angeletti CA, Bevilacqua G, Ciardiello F: Evaluation of epidermal growth factor-related growth factors and receptors and of neoangiogenesis in completely resected stage i-iiia non-small-cell lung cancer: Amphiregulin and microvessel count are independent prognostic indicators of survival. Clin Cancer Res 1998;4:241-249.
62. Hurbin A, Dubrez L, Coll JL, Favrot MC: Inhibition of apoptosis by amphiregulin via an insulin-like growth factor-1 receptor-dependent pathway in non-small cell lung cancer cell lines. J Biol Chem 2002;277:49127-49133.
63. Ito Y, Takeda T, Higashiyama S, Noguchi S, Matsuura N: Expression of heparin-binding epidermal growth factor-like growth factor in breast carcinoma. Breast Cancer Res Treat 2001;67:81-85.
64. Chong IW, Lin SR, Lin MS, Huang MS, Tsai MS, Hwang JJ: Heparin-binding epidermal growth factor-like growth factor and transforming growth factor-alpha in human non-small cell lung cancers. J Formos Med Assoc 1997;96:579-585.
65. Ito Y, Higashiyama S, Takeda T, Okada M, Matsuura N: Bimodal expression of heparin-binding egf-like growth factor in colonic neoplasms. Anticancer Res 2001;21:1391-1394.
66. Miyamoto S, Hirata M, Yamazaki A, Kageyama T, Hasuwa H, Mizushima H, Tanaka Y, Yagi H, Sonoda K, Kai M, Kanoh H, Nakano H, Mekada E: Heparin-binding egf-like growth factor is a promising target for ovarian cancer therapy. Cancer Res 2004;64:5720-5727.
67. Inui Y, Higashiyama S, Kawata S, Tamura S, Miyagawa J, Taniguchi N, Matsuzawa Y: Expression of heparin-binding epidermal growth factor in human hepatocellular carcinoma. Gastroenterology 1994;107:1799-1804.
68. Naef M, Yokoyama M, Friess H, Buchler MW, Korc M: Co-expression of heparin-binding egf-like growth factor and related peptides in human gastric carcinoma. Int J Cancer 1996;66:315-321.
69. Bacus SS, Gudkov AV, Zelnick CR, Chin D, Stern R, Stancovski I, Peles E, Ben-Baruch N, Farbstein H, Lupu R, et al.: Neu differentiation factor (heregulin) induces expression of intercellular adhesion molecule 1: Implications for mammary tumors. Cancer Res 1993;53:5251-5261.
70. Dunn M, Sinha P, Campbell R, Blackburn E, Levinson N, Rampaul R, Bates T, Humphreys S, Gullick WJ: Co-expression of neuregulins 1, 2, 3 and 4 in human breast cancer. J Pathol 2004; 203:672-680.
71. Gilmour LM, Macleod KG, McCaig A, Sewell JM, Gullick WJ, Smyth JF, Langdon SP: Neuregulin expression, function, and signaling in human ovarian cancer cells. Clin Cancer Res 2002;8:3933-3942.
72. DiGiovanna MP, Stern DF, Edgerton SM, Whalen SG, Moore D, 2nd, Thor AD: Relationship of epidermal growth factor receptor expression to erbb-2 signaling activity and prognosis in breast cancer patients. J Clin Oncol 2005;23:1152-1160.
73. Wiseman SM, Makretsov N, Nielsen TO, Gilks B, Yorida E, Cheang M, Turbin D, Gelmon K, Huntsman DG: Coexpression of the type 1 growth factor receptor family members her-1, her-2, and her-3 has a synergistic negative prognostic effect on breast carcinoma survival. Cancer 2005;103: 1770-1777.

74. Lee JC, Wang ST, Chow NH, Yang HB: Investigation of the prognostic value of coexpressed erbb family members for the survival of colorectal cancer patients after curative surgery. Eur J Cancer 2002;38:1065-1071.
75. van Cruijsen H, Giaccone G, Hoekman K: Epidermal growth factor receptor and angiogenesis: Opportunities for combined anticancer strategies. Int J Cancer 2005;117:883-888.
76. Schreiber AB, Winkler ME, Derynck R: Transforming growth factor-alpha: A more potent angiogenic mediator than epidermal growth factor. Science 1986;232:1250-1253.
77. Ma L, Gauville C, Berthois Y, Millot G, Johnson GR, Calvo F: Antisense expression for amphiregulin suppresses tumorigenicity of a transformed human breast epithelial cell line. Oncogene 1999;18:6513-6520.
78. Hirata A, Ogawa S, Kometani T, Kuwano T, Naito S, Kuwano M, Ono M: Zd1839 (iressa) induces antiangiogenic effects through inhibition of epidermal growth factor receptor tyrosine kinase. Cancer Res 2002;62:2554-2560.
79. Baker CH, Kedar D, McCarty MF, Tsan R, Weber KL, Bucana CD, Fidler IJ: Blockade of epidermal growth factor receptor signaling on tumor cells and tumor-associated endothelial cells for therapy of human carcinomas. Am J Pathol 2002;161:929-938.
80. Weber KL, Doucet M, Price JE, Baker C, Kim SJ, Fidler IJ: Blockade of epidermal growth factor receptor signaling leads to inhibition of renal cell carcinoma growth in the bone of nude mice. Cancer Res 2003;63:2940-2947.
81. Normanno N, De Luca A, Aldinucci D, Maiello MR, Mancino M, D'Antonio A, De Filippi R, Pinto A: Gefitinib inhibits the ability of human bone marrow stromal cells to induce osteoclast differentiation: Implications for the pathogenesis and treatment of bone metastasis. Endocr Relat Cancer 2005; 12:471-482.
82. Roodman GD: Biology of osteoclast activation in cancer. J Clin Oncol 2001;19:3562-3571.
83. Boyle WJ, Simonet WS, Lacey DL: Osteoclast differentiation and activation. Nature 2003;423:337-342.
84. Normanno N, Bianco C, Damiano V, de Angelis E, Selvam MP, Grassi M, Magliulo G, Tortora G, Bianco AR, Mendelsohn J, Salomon DS, Ciardiello F: Growth inhibition of human colon carcinoma cells by combinations of anti-epidermal growth factor-related growth factor antisense oligonucleotides. Clin Cancer Res 1996;2:601-609.
85. De Luca A, Casamassimi A, Selvam MP, Losito S, Ciardiello F, Agrawal S, Salomon DS, Normanno N: Egf-related peptides are involved in the proliferation and survival of mda-mb-468 human breast carcinoma cells. Int J Cancer 1999;80:589-594.
86. De Luca A, Arra C, D'Antonio A, Casamassimi A, Losito S, Ferraro P, Ciardiello F, Salomon DS, Normanno N: Simultaneous blockage of different egf-like growth factors results in efficient growth inhibition of human colon carcinoma xenografts. Oncogene 2000;19:5863-5871.
87. Casamassimi A, De Luca A, Agrawal S, Stromberg K, Salomon DS, Normanno N: Egf-related antisense oligonucleotides inhibit the proliferation of human ovarian carcinoma cells. Ann Oncol 2000;11:319-325.
88. Normanno N, Campiglio M, De LA, Somenzi G, Maiello M, Ciardiello F, Gianni L, Salomon DS, Menard S: Cooperative inhibitory effect of zd1839 (iressa) in combination with trastuzumab (herceptin) on human breast cancer cell growth. Ann Oncol 2002;13:65-72.
89. Brenton JD, Carey LA, Ahmed AA, Caldas C: Molecular classification and molecular forecasting of breast cancer: Ready for clinical application? J Clin Oncol 2005;23:7350-7360.
90. Normanno N, Gullick WJ: Epidermal growth factor receptor tyrosine kinase inhibitors and bone metastases: Different mechanisms of action for a novel therapeutic application? Endocr Relat Cancer 2006;13:3-6.

17 Signaling by the EGF Receptor in Human Cancers: Accentuate the Positive, Eliminate the Negative

Haley L. Bennett, Tilman Brummer, Paul Timpson, Kate I. Patterson, and Roger J. Daly

CONTENTS

ONCOGENIC CHANGES IN SIGNAL TRANSDUCERS
PERTUBATION OF FEEDBACK CONTROL OF EGFR SIGNALING
ATTENUATION OF EGFR DOWN-REGULATION AND ITS ROLE IN HUMAN CANCERS
FUTURE PERSPECTIVES
REFERENCES

Abstract

As described in accompanying chapters, enhanced EGF receptor (EGFR) signaling in human cancers can occur due to receptor overexpression or mutational activation. However, it may also arise from perturbations in the signal transduction pathways that function downstream of the receptor or the regulatory processes that tune the magnitude and duration of their output (Fig. 17.1). In this chapter we focus on the latter two aspects of oncogenic EGFR signaling. Specifically, we address: cancer-related changes that occur in the expression and/or activity of key signal relay molecules; pertubation of feedback control mechanisms; and attenuation of receptor down-regulation as a mechanism for signal amplification. We also discuss the impact of these changes on cellular sensitivity to EGFR-directed therapies, and how they inform more effective use of such therapies, alone or in combination with other signal transduction inhibitors, in a clinical setting.

Key Words: Src, Ras, Raf, Erk, PI3-kinase, PTEN, feedback loops, c-Cbl, endocytosis, EGFR inhibitors.

1. ONCOGENIC CHANGES IN SIGNAL TRANSDUCERS

Ligand binding to the EGFR promotes receptor dimerization and kinase activation, leading to autophosphorylation of particular tyrosine residues within its cytoplasmic domain (*1, 2*). These phosphorylated residues provide binding sites for specific src homology (SH)2 and

From: *Cancer Drug Discovery and Development: EGFR Signaling Networks in Cancer Therapy*
Edited by: J. D. Haley and W. J. Gullick, DOI: 10.1007/978-1-59745-356-1_17
© 2008 Humana Press, a part of Springer Science+Business Media, LLC

phosphotyrosine binding (PTB) domain-containing cytoplasmic proteins that include adaptors, non-receptor tyrosine kinases and enzymes that regulate the production of lipid second messengers (*3–5*) (Fig. 17.2). Adaptors such as Grb2 and Shc promote the formation of

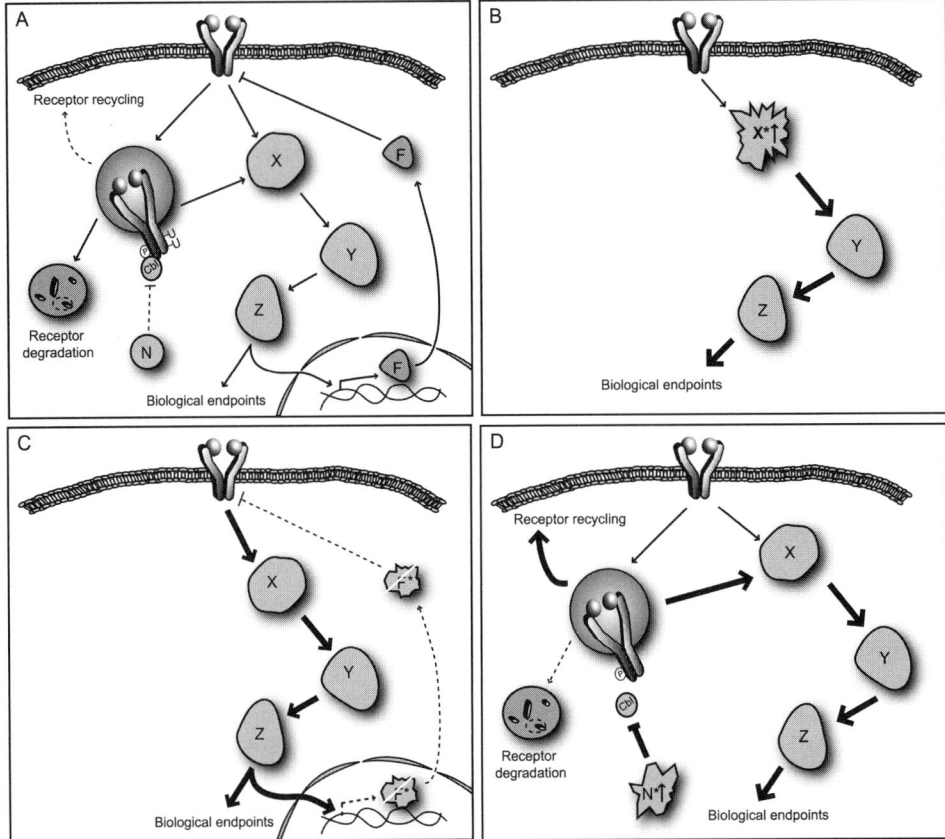

Fig. 17.1. **Mechanisms Contributing to Amplification of EGFR Signaling in Human Cancer. A. EGFR Signaling in a Normal Cell.** Ligand stimulation of the receptor activates a signaling pathway consisting of the components X, Y and Z. In addition to promoting biological endpoints such as proliferation and survival, this pathway induces transcription of a delayed negative feedback regulator (F) that attenuates receptor signaling. A further mechanism for signal termination is provided by postendocytic degradation of the receptor in lysosomes, which is promoted by c-Cbl-catalysed receptor ubiquitylation. The expression of a negative regulator of c-Cbl (N) is low, so that receptor degradation, rather than recycling, is favored. **B. Oncogenic Signaling Due to Mutation or Overexpression of Signal Transducer X.** This amplifies signaling from X and may reduce the EGFR-dependency of this pathway. The latter effect will dampen the effect of negative feedback regulator F. **C. Sustained Signaling Due to Loss of Negative Feedback Control.** This may occur due to an inactivating mutation in F, and/or deletion/epigenetic silencing of the corresponding gene. **D. Sustained Signaling Due to Attenuation of Receptor Down-regulation.** Increased expression or mutational activation of N leads to inhibition of EGFR/c-Cbl coupling. The reduced ubiquitylation of the receptor promotes receptor recycling and further rounds of receptor activation and signaling. In addition, the receptor may be retained in a signaling-competent endosomal compartment, allowing continued activation of X. Note that since enhanced signaling is normally counteracted by negative feedback loops, mechanism C will cooperate with mechanisms B and D to amplify signaling. For all panels, asterisks indicate mutation, vertical arrows overexpression, and diagonal lines loss of expression.

signaling complexes that contain catalytic relay molecules, leading to the activation of downstream effectors. In the case of proteins with enzymatic activity, for example phospholipase C (PLC)γ and c-Src, receptor binding, membrane recruitment and/or tyrosine phosphorylation leads to their activation (*3-5*). It is now clear that altered expression and/or mutation of both non-catalytic signaling proteins (i.e., those of the adaptor or docking protein class) and enzymatic signal transducers can occur in cancer cells and amplify EGFR signaling (Fig. 17.1 and 17.2). Therefore, this first section will focus on the key signaling pathways downstream of the EGFR and describe how they are subject to such oncogenic deregulation.

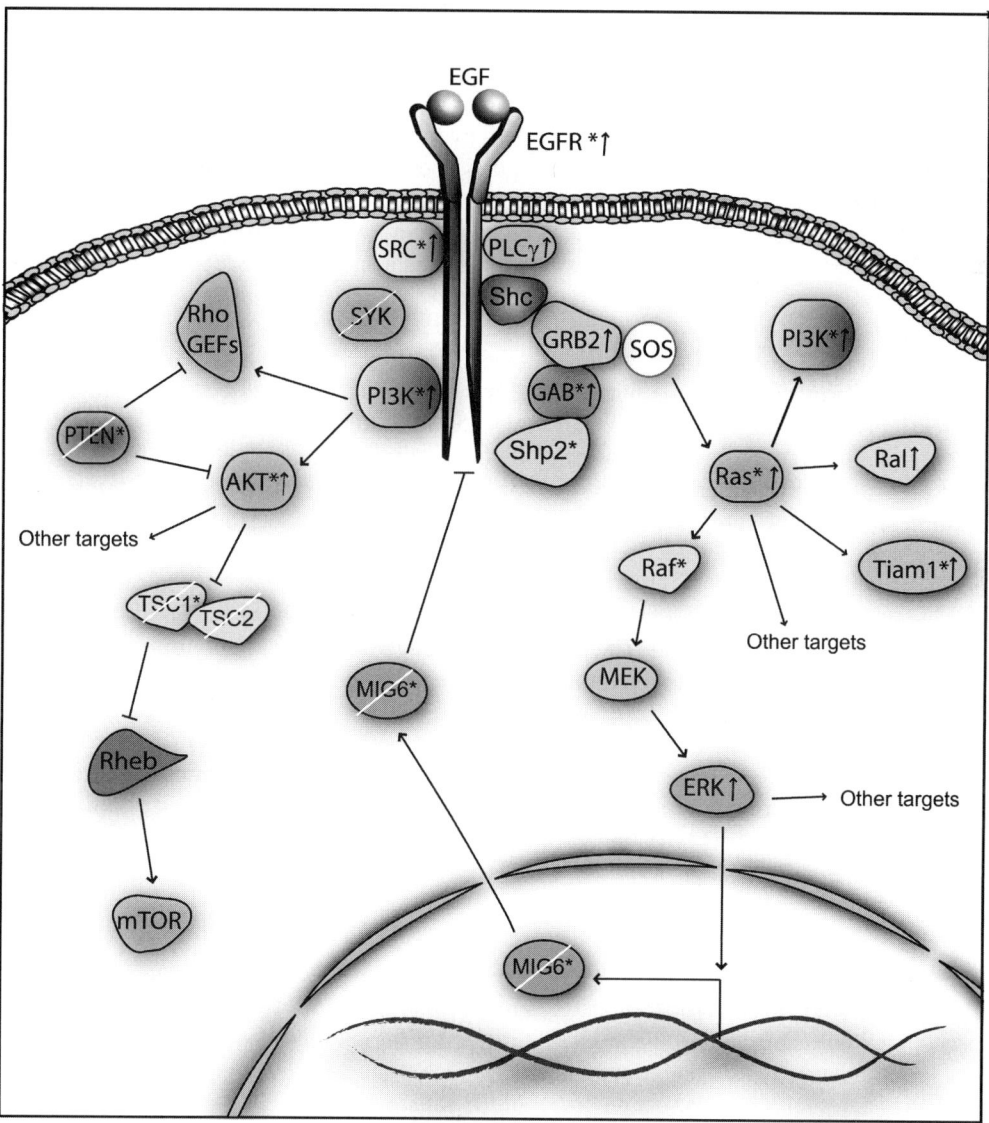

Fig. 17.2. Pertubations in EGFR Signaling Pathways in Human Cancers. The schematic highlights known alterations that occur in epithelial malignancies. For simplicity, the only negative feedback loop included is that involving MIG-6. Asterisks indicate mutation, vertical arrows overexpression, and diagonal lines loss of expression. For full details please refer to text.

1.1. Non-receptor Tyrosine Kinases

The cytoplasmic tyrosine kinase and proto-oncogene product c-Src plays an important role in signal propagation, amplification, and diversification downstream of the EGFR. Signaling interplay between c-Src and the EGFR is bi-directional, since c-Src binds to the activated receptor leading to stimulation of c-Src catalytic activity, and c-Src also phosphorylates the EGFR on Y845 within the receptor activation loop, triggering downstream signaling events that include Stat5b tyrosine phosphorylation and activation (6). As described in Chapter 9, c-Src activation can also enhance EGFR signaling by attenuating receptor down-regulation. Although the transforming activity of c-Src is low, when overexpressed c-Src cooperates with the EGFR to promote tumor formation in nude mice (7). This is significant given that c-Src exhibits increased expression and/or activity in many malignancies that express the EGFR, including those of the breast, colon, ovary, lung, esophagus, stomach, and pancreas (8). Activation of c-Src in human cancers may result from altered expression of proteins that normally act to negatively (e.g., C-terminal Src kinase, (9)) or positively (eg PTP1b, (10)) regulate this enzyme. Furthermore, a truncating mutation in c-Src that leads to enhanced catalytic activity has been detected in a subset of late-stage colon cancer patients (11), although this mutation does not appear to be a common mode of oncogenic deregulation for this kinase.

A variety of intracellular targets are regulated by c-Src, including PLCγ-1, phosphatidylinositol (PI)3-kinase and focal adhesion kinase, and as a result, c-Src influences multiple aspects of cancer cell behavior, including proliferation, survival, invasion and angiogenesis (8, 12, 13). Indeed, in a recent study, blocking c-Src activation in MCF-7 breast cancer cells via expression of a dominant negative mutant reduced cell proliferation and migration in vitro and tumorigenesis in nude mice (14). Given these pleiotropic effects, c-Src represents a potential cancer drug target, and small molecule inhibitors that target either the kinase or SH2 domain have been developed, with some undergoing clinical trials (15). The impact of elevated Src activity on sensitivity to therapies targeted against the EGFR is an important question. In a recent study, expression of active Src in gallbladder adenocarcinoma cells conferred resistance to the selective EGFR kinase inhibitor gefitinib that was associated with increased activation of Akt and Erk (16). Also, the Src inhibitor AZD0530 and gefitinib were additive when examined for their ability to inhibit the motility and invasion of tamoxifen-resistant breast cancer cells (17). The latter findings suggest that Src inhibitors could be used in combination with EGFR-targeted therapies to treat particular cancers.

In contrast to c-Src, expression of Syk is reduced during progression of breast and gastric cancer and in some reports, has been associated with metastatic disease (18). Expression of Syk in breast cancer cells suppresses proliferation in vitro and tumorigenicity in nude mice and promotes aberrant cytokinesis (18). In the context of EGFR signaling, it is noteworthy that Syk suppresses EGFR tyrosine phosphorylation in the immortalized human mammary epithelial cell line MCF-10A (19) and c-Src activation in BT-549 breast cancer cells (20), but the underlying mechanisms are unclear.

1.2. Pathways Upstream and Downstream of Ras GTPases

Binding of Grb2 to the EGFR, either directly or indirectly via Shc, leads to membrane recruitment of the Ras guanine nucleotide exchange factor (GEF) Sos and subsequent activation of Ras proteins and their downstream effector pathways (3-5). The latter include the serine/threonine kinase Raf, the p110 catalytic subunit of class I PI3-kinase and RalGDS (Fig. 17.2) (21).

Increased levels of Grb2 or Shc have been detected in breast and prostate cancers (22-25) and while overexpression of either protein in the mammary glands of transgenic mice is insufficient to promote tumor development, both accelerate tumor growth when individually co-expressed with a mutant form of polyomavirus middle T antigen (26). Thus, Grb2 and Shc may cooperate with other oncogenes to promote tumorigenesis by increasing the sensitivity of the cancer cell to growth factor signals. Furthermore, an increase in Shc tyrosine phosphorylation, rather than expression, has also been reported in human cancers, with the p46 and p52 isoforms being implicated as positive mediators of receptor signaling (27, 28). Ascertaining the role of the p66 isoform has been more challenging. While one study suggests that this may be inhibitory, a positive association with metastatic progression has also been reported (28, 29).

In addition to Sos, Grb2 also recruits the docking proteins Grb2-associated binder (Gab)1 and Gab2 to the EGFR, and these act to amplify EGF-induced Ras/Erk activation via their binding to the protein tyrosine phosphatase (PTP) Shp2 (Fig. 17.2) (30, 31). Gab2 is overexpressed in a subset of breast cancer cell lines and primary breast cancers (32), which partially reflects amplification of the *GAB2* gene (33). Functional analyses have revealed that Gab2 overexpression in MCF-10A cells enhances proliferation and EGF-independent acinar morphogenesis in 3D Matrigel cultures (31). Also, when co-expressed with erbB2 in this system, Gab2 promotes the formation of multiacinar, invasive structures, and Gab2 accelerates mammary tumorigenesis induced by activated erbB2 in transgenic mice (33). Since the *GAB2* gene localizes to chromosome 11q13, a region amplified in cancers of the lung, liver, esophagus, bladder and head and neck, as well as those of the breast (34), it will be interesting to determine whether Gab2 enhances EGF-induced signaling in other malignancies. Also, recent studies have revealed that the Gab/Shp2 pathway may be deregulated in EGFR-expressing cancers by gene mutation. First, a recent study identified mutations in the coding region of the *GAB1* gene in a subset of breast cancer patients (35), although the functional consequences of these alterations are unclear. Second, Shp2 mutations occur at a low frequency in colon and lung cancers (36).

The Ras family of low molecular weight GTPases comprises three closely-related members with contrasting signaling potential: H-, K- and N-Ras (21). Activating mutations in these proteins have been detected in a variety of human malignancies, although the incidence and family members involved varies. From a signaling perspective, these mutations decrease the intrinsic GTPase activity of these proteins and lock them in a GTP-bound state, leading to constitutive activation of their effector pathways and induction of autocrine loops involving EGFR ligands (see also Chapter 7). Of relevance to this review, K-Ras mutations are particularly prevalent in adenocarcinoma of the pancreas (90% of patients), colon (50%) and lung (30%) (37). In breast cancer, the incidence of Ras mutations is rare (<5% of cancers), although overexpression of the wild-type protein occurs (38). In non-small cell lung cancer (NSCLC), K-Ras mutations and activating EGFR mutations tend to be mutually exclusive (39, 40), and mutated K-Ras is associated with resistance to the small molecule EGFR inhibitors erlotinib and gefitinib (39, 41, 42). Furthermore, in colorectal cancer, the presence of mutated K-Ras is predictive of poor response to the anti-EGFR mAb cetuximab (43).

Raf proteins activate a evolutionarily-conserved kinase cascade consisting of the dual-specificity kinase MEK and the serine/threonine kinases Erk1 and Erk2, which, via phosphorylation of cytoplasmic (eg myosin light chain kinase) and nuclear (e.g., p62 TCF/Elk1) targets, regulate a variety of processes including cell proliferation, differentiation, motility and invasion (44). Oncogenic mutations in B-Raf are common in certain cancers, with the V600E substitution predominating. Of note in the context of EGFR-expressing malignancies, 30% of ovarian and 5-20% of colorectal cancers harbor this mutation (45). Since the occurrence of activating Ras mutations and B-Raf V600E seems to be mutually exclusive (46), and K-Ras mutations affect responsiveness of colorectal cancers to cetuximab (43), it will be important to determine whether the presence of B-Raf mutations also affects sensitivity to EGFR targeted therapies, as it might be possible to use the mutational status of both K-Ras and B-Raf to select patients for optimal treatment strategies. Finally, overexpression of the downstream MAP kinases (MAPKs) Erk1 and Erk2 has been detected in several human cancers, including breast and hepatocellular carcinomas (47, 48). This may also modulate sensitivity to EGFR inhibitors, since expression of an activated form of Erk2 in MCF-10A cells results in a 2-3 fold increase in the IC50 for gefitinib (49).

When considering Ras effector pathways and their role in human cancer, the Ras/Raf/Erk cascade and PI3-kinase, which is discussed in the next section, have been studied in the most detail. However, attention has been drawn recently to other pathways, since genetically-modified mice deficient in the Ras effectors RalGDS, Tiam1 or phospholipase Cε are resistant to the development of Ras-induced skin tumors (50-52). RalGDS is a GEF for the small GTPases RalA and RalB, and studies using Ras effector domain mutants, combined with gain/loss-of-function analyses of these GTPases, indicate that they are required for Ras-induced transformation of human epithelial cells and contribute to the proliferation and survival of human cancer cells (53). Interestingly, the RalB-Sec5 effector pathway, which had previously only been considered in the context of the exocyst complex and hence secretory vesicle trafficking, recruits and activates the atypical IκB kinase family member TBK1 and hence promotes cancer cell survival (54). To date, studies on the Ral effector arm in human cancers are limited, although overexpression of Ral has been detected in nasopharyngeal carcinomas (55). Tiam1, a GEF for the low molecular weight GTPase Rac, is overexpressed in high-grade prostatic intraepithelial neoplasia and prostate carcinomas relative to benign epithelium, and is an independent predictor of decreased disease-free survival for patients with prostate cancer (56). Furthermore, an activating mutation in Tiam1 occurs in approximately 12% of primary renal cell carcinomas and cell lines derived from this malignancy (57). It is expected that studies on these and other 'alternative' Ras effectors in human cancers will be a fertile area for future research.

1.3. Phospholipid Hydrolysis and Signaling

EGF-induced tyrosine phosphorylation of PLCγ, coupled with binding of its pleckstrin homology (PH) domain to phosphatidylinositol 3,4,5 trisphosphate (PIP3) generated in response to growth factor treatment, stimulates its hydrolysis of phosphatidylinositol 4,5 bisphosphate (PIP2) to the second messengers inositol 1,4,5 trisphosphate (IP3) and diacylglycerol (DAG) (3). PIP2 hydrolysis releases sequestered actin-binding proteins such as gelsolin, while DAG and IP3 activate specific protein kinase C isoforms and trigger the release of calcium from intracellular stores, respectively. These signaling events enhance the synthesis of new actin filaments and regulate adhesion turnover and acto-myosin contractility (58). Consistent with these effects, PLCγ is required for EGF-induced cell motility (59) and inhibition of PLCγ catalytic activity reduces invasion of glioblastoma cells and prostate, breast, bladder and head and neck cancer cells in either in vitro or animal models (58, 60). Interestingly, PLCγ is overexpressed in breast and head and neck carcinomas (60, 61), indicating that this enzyme represents a potential target for anti-metastatic therapeutics.

The PI3K family of lipid kinases phosphorylate the 3' hydroxyl group of specific phosphoinositides and is divided into three classes based on modes of activation, substrate specificities and structure (62). A member of Class Ia PI3Ks, p110α, and its associated subunit, p85, are strongly implicated in human cancers. This enzyme is activated downstream of the EGFR by binding of p85 in a SH2 domain-dependent manner to erbB3, a heterodimerization partner of the EGFR, or to Gab family docking proteins, in combination with direct activation of p110α by binding to GTP-loaded Ras (63). Phosphorylation of PIP2 by p110α generates the second messenger PIP3, which binds to the PH domain of specific effectors, such as the serine/threonine kinase Akt and particular Rho family GEFs (Fig. 17.2). Recruitment of Akt to the plasma membrane leads to its activation and the phosphorylation of targets that regulate cell proliferation (eg the cyclin-dependent kinase inhibitor p27), survival (e.g., the

Bcl2 family member Bad), growth (e.g., tuberous sclerosis (TSC)2, which regulates the mammalian target of rapamycin (mTOR) pathway and hence protein synthesis) and motility (e.g., girdin). It is now evident that the three Akt isoforms (Akt1-3) possess both redundant and distinct functional roles, the latter presumably reflecting differences in expression profile, subcellular targeting and substrate specificity (64).

The PI3K isoform p110α is encoded by *PIK3CA*, which is one of the most commonly mutated genes in cancer, with up to 40% of breast and 32% of colon cancers harboring a somatic mutation (65). These mutations tend to be single amino acid substitutions, and over 80% cluster in the helical and catalytic domains (66-69). Studies on the two common p110α mutants E545K and H1047R reveal that the mutations confer p110α with enhanced kinase activity, and expression of the mutant proteins in MCF-10A cells leads to anchorage-independent growth and protection from anoikis (70). Furthermore, these mutants can cooperate with expression of hTERT, inactivation of the p53 and Rb tumor suppressor pathways and c-Myc overexpression to transform primary human mammary epithelial cells (71). Interestingly, mutations in the gene encoding p85α, *PIK3R1*, which can also lead to activation of PI3K signaling have been reported in ovarian and colon cancers (72). Furthermore, amplification of *PIK3CA* leading to protein overexpression has been detected in numerous malignancies, including cancers of the ovary, esophagus, and head and neck (73-75).

Analysis of expression profiles of Akt isoforms in human cancers has identified Akt2 as the most commonly deregulated enzyme (76), which likely reflects its transforming activity (77) and ability to enhance cell migration and invasion (78, 79). Amplification and/or overexpression of *AKT2* has been reported in ovarian, breast, pancreatic, colorectal and hepatocellular cancers (80-84). *AKT1* or *AKT3* amplification is not a common occurrence in cancer, although overexpression of these genes has been detected in subsets of breast cancer patients, with elevated *AKT3* mRNA being associated with estrogen receptor negativity (85, 86). Furthermore, a recent study has detected a low frequency of somatic mutations affecting the kinase domain of Akt2 in gastric and lung cancers, while no mutations were found in Akt1 or 3 (87).

A further mechanism for deregulation of PI3K signaling in human cancers is *via* mutation and/or loss of expression of the tumor suppressor gene product phosphatase and tensin homolog deleted on chromosome ten (PTEN), which dephosphorylates PIP3 on the D3 position, thereby terminating activation of PI3K effectors (Fig. 17.2) (63). Germline mutations in *PTEN* underlie Cowden syndrome, an inherited disorder characterized by the development of hamartomas in multiple tissues and associated with an increased risk of breast and other cancers (88). Mutations in *PTEN* occur at a relatively high frequency in sporadic glioblastoma (20-45% of patients), endometrial cancer (40-50%) and to a lesser extent, prostate cancer (13%), and loss of heterozygosity (LOH) at the *PTEN* locus also occurs at a high frequency (30-80%) in these malignancies. In other cancer types such as those of the colon, breast and lung, *PTEN* mutations are relatively rare, but LOH and loss of gene expression occur at significant frequencies (88-90). In breast cancer, *PIK3CA* mutations and *PTEN* silencing are mutually exclusive, indicating that more than half of all breast cancers exhibit upregulated PI3-kinase signaling (91). Importantly, deletion of *pten* in genetically-modified mouse models has confirmed its tumor suppressor activity in tissues such as the prostate, mammary gland and endometrium (88).

Finally, it should be noted that downstream of Akt is an additional tumor suppressor, in this case the TSC1/TSC2 heterodimer. This complex functions as a Rheb GTPase-activating protein and hence inhibits mTOR activation in the absence of Akt-mediated phosphorylation of TSC2 (Fig. 17.2). Germline mutations in *TSC1* and *TSC2* are associated with the hamartoma syndrome TSC, and although somatic mutations in these genes in sporadic cancers are rare and to date appear to be limited to *TSC1* in bladder cancers (92, 93), loss of TSC1 and/or TSC2 expression has been reported in breast (94) and pancreatic cancers (95).

Importantly, activation of PI3-kinase signaling by PIK3CA mutation or PTEN loss is emerging as a marker of insensitivity to EGFR kinase inhibitors. In gefitinib-sensitive NSCLC cell lines, the EGFR activates PI3-kinase via heterodimerization with ErbB3, and inhibition of cell proliferation by gefitinib correlates with down-regulation of PI3-kinase/Akt signaling (*96*). Expression of the constitutively active PIK3CA mutant E545K in the gefitinib-sensitive NSCLC cell line HCC827 leads to a significant reduction in gefitinib-induced apoptosis, indicating that EGFR-independent PI3-kinase signaling is sufficient to confer decreased sensitivity to this drug (*97*). As mentioned previously, this pathway can also be upregulated by loss of PTEN. In glioblastoma patients, the presence of the EGFR vIII variant and PTEN was associated with clinical response to gefitinib or erlotinib, and expression of these two proteins in the glioblastoma cell line U87MG, which is PTEN-deficient, enhanced the sensitivity of the cells to proliferation-arrest by erlotinib. Furthermore, expression of PTEN in the PTEN-null glioblastoma cell line SF295 increased apoptosis induced by the EGFR kinase inhibitor PKI-166 (*98*). Studies in vitro indicate that the sensitivity of breast (*99, 100*) and prostate (*101*) cancer cells to gefitinib is also promoted by the presence of functional PTEN. These findings have important implications in terms of patient selection for treatment with EGFR inhibitors. Furthermore, they inform the rational design of combination therapies. In support of this concept, the mTOR inhibitor rapamycin enhances the sensitivity of PTEN-deficient glioblastoma cells to erlotinib in vitro (*102*). The interactions of PI-3 kinase and EGFR are further discussed in detail in Chapter 8.

2. PERTUBATION OF FEEDBACK CONTROL OF EGFR SIGNALING

In recent years, the importance of feedback loops for the fine-tuning of intracellular signaling pathways has been increasingly recognized (*5, 103*). Here, we focus on positive feedback loops involved in signal amplification, and negative feedbacks that attenuate signaling. Intracellular feedback loops can be grouped into two categories: immediate/early feedback loops, which occur within seconds or minutes after signal initiation and usually involve the post-translational modification of a key element within the signal transduction pathway, and delayed feedbacks that require the *de novo* synthesis of a regulatory protein, e.g., an autocrine growth factor such as heparin-binding (HB)-EGF, or a phosphatase involved in signal termination. Feedback loops are relevant to human cancer for two reasons. First, perturbations in these control mechanisms are associated with human malignancies. Indeed, loss of negative feedback regulation may be required early in tumorigenesis to avoid oncogene-induced senescence (*104*). Second, the characterization of these negative feedback loops is of particular importance in the identification and validation of drug targets that reside within intracellular signaling pathways, since inhibition of a downstream kinase may prolong the activation of upstream signal relay molecules that would be otherwise negatively regulated by a negative feedback loop, and in addition, may result in 'signal overflow' into other pathways. For example, use of mTOR inhibitors can relieve negative feedback regulation of IRS-1 by mTOR and thus enhance Akt-mediated survival signaling. This may attenuate the clinical efficacy of such drugs (*105*).

2.1. Immediate/early Feedback Loops

These can be found at many levels in the EGFR signaling network. The EGFR itself is a substrate for several serine/threonine kinases that are activated upon EGF-stimulation, including the Erks (*106*). As these phosphorylation events are associated with decreased tyrosine kinase activity of the receptor and enhanced receptor down-regulation, it is generally accepted that they represent a classical negative feedback mechanism. Although deletion of one of the negative regulatory sites contributes to the transforming potential of the v-erbB oncoprotein (*107*), mutation of the targeted residues in human cancers has not been reported.

Such feedback loops, however, may be attenuated by indirect mechanisms. For example, the docking protein SNT-2/FRS2β/FRS3 suppresses EGFR signaling by recruiting Erk2 to the receptor, and is down-regulated in cell lines derived from lung cancers and brain tumors, malignancies where the EGFR is known to play an important role (*108*).

In addition to the EGFR, several important downstream signaling proteins are subject to immediate/early feedback regulation, such as Raf-1 and Gab2 (*109, 110*). Interestingly, feedback-phosphorylated and consequently inactivated Raf-1 serves as a substrate of the phosphorylation-dependent prolyl isomerase Pin1 that, in cooperation with the Ser/Thr-phosphatase PP2A, recycles Raf-1 to the activation competent state (*109*). As Pin-1 is often overexpressed in human cancers, including those of the breast, prostate, ovary, and lung (*111*), one mechanism whereby this protein may contribute to tumorigenesis is by enhancing the reversal of phosphorylation events at negative regulatory sites.

2.2. Delayed Negative Feedbacks

Delayed negative feedback control of EGFR signaling can occur via diverse mechanisms, and several of these are altered in human cancers. Genetic analyses of receptor tyrosine kinase signaling pathways in *Drosophila* have identified two types of growth factor-inducible negative regulator in the products of the *Sprouty* (*Spry*) and *Kekkon* genes. Vertebrates contain four Spry homologs, which each contain a N-terminal tyrosine phosphorylation site and a conserved C-terminal cysteine-rich domain (*112*). Consistent with a role as repressors of Ras/Raf/Erk signaling, Spry1 and Spry2 are downregulated in breast and prostate cancers (*113*). The function of specific Spry proteins, however, is context-dependent, and while attenuation of EGF-induced Erk activation has been reported for Spry2 (*114*), this protein can also enhance EGFR signaling by sequestering the E3 ubiquitin ligase c-Cbl from the receptor and inhibiting CIN85-mediated clustering of c-Cbl molecules (*112*). Consequently, the impact of Spry loss on EGFR signaling in human cancer requires further investigation.

Recently, three distant relatives of the *Drosophila* Kekkon proteins have been identified in vertebrates and named LRIG1-3 (*115*). Like Kekkon proteins, LRIG1 is an EGF-inducible, transmembrane protein. It contains 15 leucine-rich repeats and 3 immunoglobulin domains in its extracellular region, and interacts with all four erbB family members. LRIG1 downregulates EGFR signaling by recruiting c-Cbl, which in turn triggers the poly-ubiquitylation and subsequent degradation of both LRIG1 and the EGFR (*115*). Furthermore, disruption of the murine *lrig1* gene causes epidermal hyperplasia and psoriasiform lesions (*116*), a phenotype that is often observed upon loss of negative control of EGFR activity in the epidermis. Interestingly, the human *LRIG1* and *LRIG2* genes are localised on chromosome 3p14 and 1p13 respectively, which are regions commonly deleted in various human cancers, e.g., carcinomas of the breast, lung, and kidney (*117, 118*).

Another delayed feedback regulator of all ErbB family members is the MIG-6 protein (also known as RALT or Gene 33), expression of which is induced upon activation of the Erk pathway or dexamethasone treatment (*119-121*). Although its mode of action remains to be fully characterized, MIG-6 directly binds the EGFR and inhibits its autophosphorylation via a MIG-6 domain that exhibits homology to activated Cdc42-associated kinase-1 (Ack-1). This leads to attenuated activation of the Erk, Akt and JNK pathways (*121*). Following its induction, MIG-6 is polyubiquitylated then degraded by the proteasome (*119*). Thus, like LRIG1, the expression level of this protein is tightly controlled by opposing transcriptional and post-translational regulatory mechanisms. Importantly, gene-targeting experiments in mice have recently identified MIG-6 as a pivotal negative regulator of the ErbB signaling network in a physiological setting. MIG-6-deficient mice exhibit an epidermal phenotype characteristic of EGFR hyperactivation, with enhanced proliferation and impaired differentiation of keratinocytes, and an increased susceptibility to carcinogen-induced skin tumors.

Both the skin defects and tumors are sensitive to gefitinib treatment (*122*). Also, the gene knock-out mice develop spontaneous tumors in organs such as the lungs, stomach, gall bladder and bile-duct (*122, 123*). Interestingly, *MIG-6* expression is reduced in skin, breast, pancreatic and ovarian carcinomas (*122*), and *MIG-6* missense and nonsense mutations, as well as transcriptional silencing, occur in human cancer cell lines (*123*). Furthermore, the *MIG-6* gene maps to human chromosome 1p36, a locus displaying a high frequency of allelic loss in several human cancers, including those of the lung and breast. Clearly, this protein may prove a useful marker of responsiveness to therapies targeted to erbB receptors, and in support of this hypothesis, reconstitution of MIG-6 expression in erbB2-overexpressing breast cancer cells enhanced sensitivity to herceptin in vitro (*124*).

MAPK phosphatases (MKPs) are classified as dual specificity phosphatases (DUSPs) because they inactivate MAPKs by dephosphorylating both the phosphotyrosine and phosphothreonine residues within the pTXpY motif of the MAPK activation loop (*125*). Many DUSPs are expressed in an inducible manner, providing a tightly controlled feedback mechanism for the attenuation of mitogenic signaling. For example, DUSP1/MKP1/CL100 is induced upon activation of the EGFR (*126*). Also, increased expression of DUSP6/MKP3 is observed in immortalized human bronchial epithelial cells upon expression of EGFRs harboring mutations detected in NSCLC patients, and this appears to counteract Erk1/2 activation in these cells (*127*).

The role played by DUSPs in EGFR-expressing malignancies appears complex. DUSP1 is down-regulated in a subset of hepatocellular carcinomas, and its expression is significantly associated with increased survival (*128*). Similarly, DUSP6/MKP3 expression is down-regulated in invasive pancreatic cancer (*129*). Although DUSP1 is overexpressed in NSCLC, DUSP1-positivity represents an independent predictor of improved survival (*130*). DUSP1 is also overexpressed in early-stage prostate, colon and bladder cancers, but there is a loss of expression in higher histological grade cancers and metastases (*131*). The above findings are consistent with an inhibitory function of the particular DUSPs during tumor progression. DUSP1 overexpression in pancreatic cancers, however, may promote cancer cell proliferation and tumorigenicity (*132*). Also, although there is a progressive loss of expression of DUSP1 during ovarian cancer development and progression (*133*), DUSP1-positivity in this disease has been identified as an independent prognostic marker for decreased progression-free survival (*134*). Furthermore, in a study of malignant effusions from patients with serous ovarian carcinoma, high expression of DUSP2 was positively correlated with a worse overall survival (*135*). In order to interpret these findings, it is necessary to consider the diverse stimuli that modulate DUSP expression in cancer cells, the different cellular responses these enzymes regulate, and the roles these enzymes play in integrating signaling pathways. For example, DUSPs may be induced by inflammatory cytokines or by chemotherapeutic agents (*134*). Also, while DUSP1 can suppress cell proliferation (*133*), it also inhibits JNK-induced apoptosis (*136, 137*). Finally, DUSPs may enhance activation of upstream signaling proteins within a network by dephosphorylating the MAPKs that would otherwise mediate negative feedback regulation.

2.3. Delayed Positive Feedbacks

An example of this type of regulation is the induction of autocrine loops involving growth factors that mediate mitogenic or pro-survival effects. For example, chronic Erk activation resulting from the expression of oncogenic Ras or Raf proteins induces the production of the EGFR ligands HB-EGF, transforming growth factor-α and amphiregulin (*138*). Importantly, activating an autocrine loop permits an oncoprotein to elicit biological responses that lie outside of its normal 'portfolio'. For example, MCF-10A cells expressing an activated Raf-1 protein are protected from anoikis due to induction of an autocrine loop that acts via the EGFR to activate PI3-kinase (*138*).

3. ATTENUATION OF EGFR DOWN-REGULATION AND ITS ROLE IN HUMAN CANCERS

In addition to negative feedback loops, two other mechanisms act to terminate EGFR signaling: dephosphorylation of the receptor by specific PTPs, and internalization of ligand-activated receptors by endocytosis and their subsequent degradation in lysosomes, a process termed receptor down-regulation. Interestingly, the receptor PTP DEP-1, a candidate tumor suppressor in colon, breast and lung cancers, dephosphorylates the receptor post-internalization, indicating a partial overlap between these two processes (*139, 140*). In this section, we describe how the process of endocytic down-regulation is subject to oncogenic subversion at multiple steps, leading to sustained signaling (Fig. 17.3).

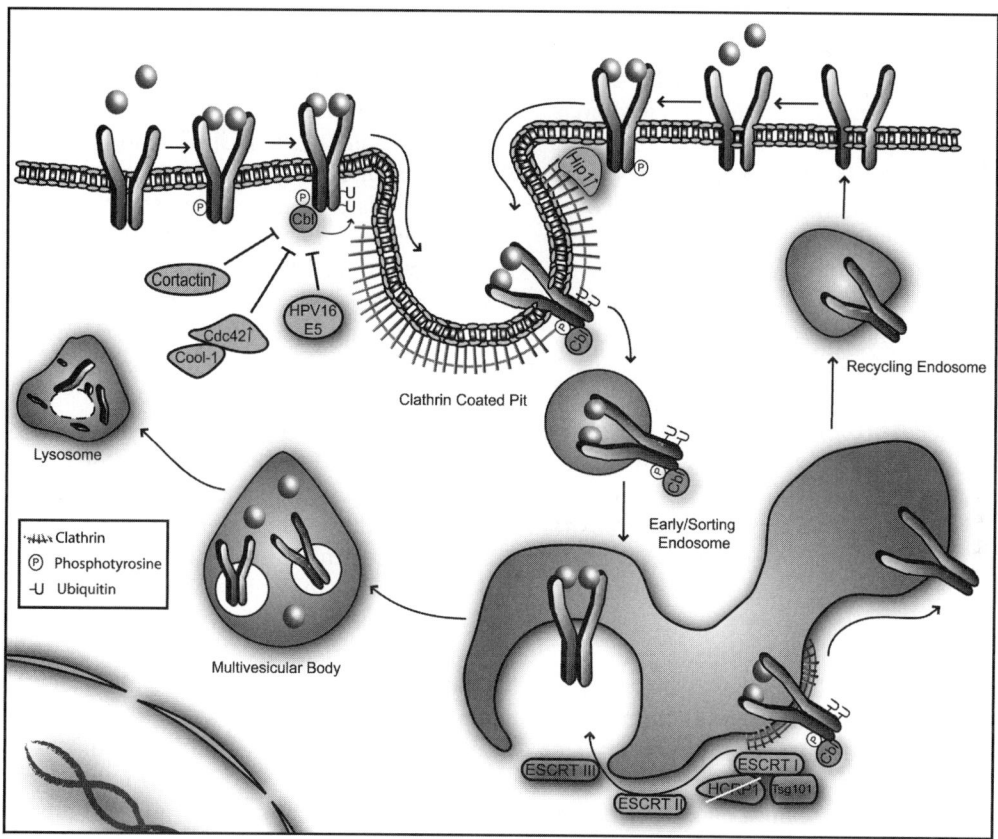

Fig. 17.3. Mechanisms Underlying Attenuation of EGFR Down-regulation in Human Cancers. The schematic illustrates the steps involved in receptor endocytosis, recycling and down-regulation, and the sites subject to oncogenic pertubation. Vertical arrows indicate overexpression, and diagonal lines, loss of expression. Following activation, the EGFR recruits c-Cbl, leading to receptor ubiquitylation. This modification ultimately promotes sorting of the receptor to lysosomes for degradation. As indicated, several proteins implicated in epithelial cancers can inhibit EGFR/c-Cbl coupling. The receptor is internalized *via* clathrin-coated pits, and Hip1 may be involved in cargo recruitment into these sites. Following uncoating, the endocytic vesicle fuses with the early endosome, and the ubiquitylated receptor is sorted into a bilayered clathrin coat. The ESCRT complexes then sort the receptor into intraluminal vesicles of the endosome, which terminates signaling. Two components of ESCRT-I, Tsg101 and HCRP1, are aberrantly expressed in particular human cancers. A multivesicular body is formed which finally fuses with a lysosome, where the receptor is degraded. For full details please refer to text.

3.1. Inhibition of c-Cbl Function

The E3 ubiquitin ligase c-Cbl plays two roles in EGFR down-regulation. First, it promotes receptor endocytosis by linking the EGFR to the scaffolding proteins CIN85 and CD2AP, which in turn associate with endophilin, a protein that induces negative curvature of the plasma membrane *(141-143)*. Second, c-Cbl-mediated receptor ubiquitylation tags the EGFR for lysosomal degradation *(144)* (see also Chapter 4). Interestingly, alterations to c-Cbl function and recruitment have been observed in many experimental models of cancer *(145)*. Although the N-terminal truncation found in v-Cbl, or point mutations in the α-helix linking the SH2 and RING finger domains of c-Cbl render this protein oncogenic *(146)*, such alterations in c-Cbl are not common in human epithelial malignancies *(145)*. However, consistent with the observation that an EGFR mutant lacking the direct binding site for c-Cbl (Y1045) elicits enhanced mitogenic signaling *(147)*, several EGFR variants exhibiting enhanced transforming potential have lost the ability to associate with c-Cbl. For example, the EGFRvV mutant identified in a subset of human glioblastomas exhibits a truncation at position 958 and therefore lacks Y1045, and the constitutively active EGFRvIII mutant, which has been detected in glioblastomas as well as lung, ovarian and breast cancers, exhibits reduced c-Cbl binding *(148-150)*. Also, c-Cbl recruitment to the EGFR is modulated by co-expression with other members of the erbB family. ErbB2, the preferred heterodimerization partner of the EGFR, is poorly coupled to c-Cbl and is overexpressed in several human cancers, including those of the breast, lung, pancreas, colon and ovary *(5)*. Heterodimerization of the EGFR with ErbB2 impairs c-Cbl recruitment to the EGFR resulting in enhanced receptor recycling to the cell surface and sustained receptor signaling *(151-153)*.

Interestingly, c-Cbl is itself regulated by a number of proto-oncogenes implicated in cancers that express the EGFR. Phosphorylation of c-Cbl by the cytoplasmic tyrosine kinase c-Src promotes auto-ubiquitylation and the destruction of c-Cbl in a proteasome-dependent manner. This results in impaired ligand-induced down-regulation of the EGFR, ultimately leading to increased recycling of the receptor *(154)*. A further mechanism whereby Src family kinases may antagonize c-Cbl function towards the EGFR is by tyrosine phosphorylation of Spry2, leading to Spry2/c-Cbl complex formation *(112)*. Also, another non-receptor tyrosine kinase, c-Abl, has recently been shown to inhibit EGFR internalization via phosphorylation of the receptor on Y1173, and to uncouple the EGFR from c-Cbl-mediated down-regulation *(155)*. Since increased expression and/or activity of Src and Abl family kinases has been detected in epithelial malignancies, including those of the breast and colon, the above effects on receptor down-regulation may lead to cooperation between these non-receptor tyrosine kinases and the EGFR during disease progression *(6, 156, 157)*.

The Rho family GTPase Cdc42 is activated downstream of the EGFR *(158)* and is overexpressed in breast cancers *(159)*. It is also required for Ras-induced transformation, and fibroblasts expressing Cdc42-V12 exhibit anchorage-independent growth and form tumors in nude mice *(160)*. Recently, a novel mechanism underlying the transforming potential of Cdc42 has been described, in which Cdc42-GTP associates with c-Cbl via the adaptor protein Cool-1/β-Pix and inhibits the coupling of c-Cbl to the EGFR. The subsequent impairment of receptor ubiquitylation and degradation sustains EGFR signaling and enhances cellular transformation *(161)*. Consistent with these findings, suppression of Cdc42 in breast cancer cells decreases EGFR expression *(162)*. Interestingly, EGF-induced tyrosine phosphorylation of Cool-1, which is mediated by a pathway involving c-Src and FAK, enhances its activity as a Cdc42 GEF and promotes its binding to both active Cdc42 and c-Cbl *(158)*. Thus, both Cdc42 and c-Src function in a positive feedback loop on the EGFR that may be exploited in cancer cells to amplify signaling.

Two other proteins implicated in human malignancies also impair c-Cbl function towards the EGFR, although the underlying mechanisms are unclear. First, the E5 protein of human papillomavirus type 16 (HPV16) inhibits the association of c-Cbl with the EGFR and decreases ubiquitylation of the receptor (*163*). Interestingly, HPV16 E5 also promotes receptor recycling by inhibiting late endosome acidification, and delays trafficking from the early to late endosome, indicating that it modulates down-regulation at multiple steps. These effects may contribute to the overexpression of the EGFR in cervical cancer, an HPV16-associated disease (*163*). The second protein that perturbs c-Cbl function is cortactin. This protein functions as an adaptor that links the actin-related protein (Arp)2/3 complex to a variety of regulatory proteins that bind its C-terminal SH3 domain (*164*). One cellular role for cortactin is to bridge the Arp2/3 complex and CD2AP and thereby regulate EGFR endocytosis (*143*). The gene encoding cortactin localizes to chromosome 11q13, which as described in Section 1.2, is a region commonly amplified in several human cancers (*34*). Interestingly, recent studies have demonstrated that cortactin overexpression inhibits ligand-induced EGFR down-regulation leading to sustained mitogenic signaling, and these effects are associated with reduced coupling of the EGFR to c-Cbl (*165*). Thus, in addition to directly promoting cancer cell motility and invasion through its effects on the cortical actin cytoskeleton, cortactin may regulate endpoints such as proliferation and survival via amplification of EGFR signaling.

3.2 Pertubation of Endocytic Down-regulation at Other Sites

In addition to these effects on c-Cbl, additional endocytic and sorting proteins are deregulated in human cancers (Fig. 17.3). Hip1 is a mammalian homologue of the yeast endocytic protein Sla2p and interacts with AP-2, clathrin and specific phosphoinositides (*166*). Overexpression of Hip1 impairs EGFR down-regulation, which has been attributed to reduced levels of clathrin at the plasma membrane, and induces cell transformation (*167*). Moreover, elevated levels of Hip1 have been detected in breast, colon and prostate cancers (*167, 168*). Furthermore, two components of the Endosomal Sorting Complex Required for Transport (ESCRT-I), which sorts the EGFR into intraluminal vesicles of the multivesicular body for degradation, have been implicated as tumor suppressors. Specifically, antisense-mediated suppression of tumor susceptibility gene 101 (Tsg101) leads to cell transformation, and aberrant splicing of *TSG101* transcripts have been detected in breast cancers (*169*). Also, the gene encoding hepatocellular carcinoma-related protein (HCRP)1/hVps37A localizes to chromosome 8p22, a region commonly deleted in hepatocellular carcinoma and other cancers, and lowering the expression of this protein impairs EGFR degradation and enhances cell proliferation (*170, 171*).

3.3. Receptor Down-regulation and Sensitivity to EGFR Inhibitors

Although largely unexplored, alterations in receptor endocytic trafficking and down-regulation may influence cellular sensitivity to EGFR-directed therapies by direct or indirect mechanisms. Evidence for the former has recently been provided by studies on gefitinib-resistant NSCLC cells (*172*). These cells exhibit increased internalization of ligand-activated EGFRs, leading the authors to speculate that this leads to enhanced dissociation of the EGFR-gefitinib complex in the low pH of intracellular vesicles. A different group reported, however, that gefitinib resistance in a panel of NSCLC cell lines was associated with decreased EGFR internalization rates (*173*). This resistance may reflect an indirect mechanism, whereby endocytic down-regulation of other receptor tyrosine kinases in addition to the EGFR is attenuated, and this reduces cellular dependency on EGFR-derived proliferative and survival signals. Further studies are warranted in this area, as it may lead to novel or improved therapeutic strategies.

4. FUTURE PERSPECTIVES

The previous two decades have seen the detailed characterization of the EGFR- signaling network, and as detailed here, how it is perturbed in epithelial malignancies. Although further validation is required, this has enabled the identification of candidate markers of clinical resistance to EGFR-directed therapies, and as cancer genome projects gather pace, it is likely that additional mutations in signaling components will be identified that can be used to improve patient stratification. Importantly, our understanding of this network and its crosstalk with other signaling systems is also leading to the rational design of therapeutic modalities involving combinations of signal transduction inhibitors that are predicted to exhibit synergistic interactions (*174*). As recently highlighted (*5*), the application of mathematical modeling and a systems biology approach to this signaling network is expected to reveal additional therapeutic opportunities (see also Chapters 14 and 15).

REFERENCES

1. Burgess AW, Cho HS, Eigenbrot C, et al. An open-and-shut case? Recent insights into the activation of EGF/ErbB receptors. Mol Cell 2003;12:541-552.
2. Zhang X, Gureasko J, Shen K, Cole PA, Kuriyan J. An allosteric mechanism for activation of the kinase domain of epidermal growth factor receptor. Cell 2006;125:1137-1149.
3. Schlessinger J. Cell signaling by receptor tyrosine kinases. Cell 2000;103:211-225.
4. Hynes NE, Lane HA. ERBB receptors and cancer: the complexity of targeted inhibitors. Nat Rev Cancer 2005;5:341-354.
5. Citri A, Yarden Y. EGF-ERBB signalling: towards the systems level. Nat Rev Mol Cell Biol 2006;7:505-516.
6. Ishizawar R, Parsons SJ. c-Src and cooperating partners in human cancer. Cancer Cell 2004;6:209-214.
7. Maa MC, Leu TH, McCarley DJ, Schatzman RC, Parsons SJ. Potentiation of epidermal growth factor receptor-mediated oncogenesis by c-Src: implications for the etiology of multiple human cancers. Proc Natl Acad Sci U S A 1995;92:6981-6985.
8. Irby RB, Yeatman TJ. Role of Src expression and activation in human cancer. Oncogene 2000;19:5636-5642.
9. Cam WR, Masaki T, Shiratori Y, et al. Reduced C-terminal Src kinase activity is correlated inversely with pp60(c-src) activity in colorectal carcinoma. Cancer 2001;92:61-70.
10. Bjorge JD, Pang A, Fujita DJ. Identification of protein-tyrosine phosphatase 1B as the major tyrosine phosphatase activity capable of dephosphorylating and activating c-Src in several human breast cancer cell lines. J Biol Chem 2000;275:41439-41446.
11. Irby RB, Mao W, Coppola D, et al. Activating SRC mutation in a subset of advanced human colon cancers. Nat Genet 1999;21:187-190.
12. Zhang SQ, Yang W, Kontaridis MI, et al. Shp2 regulates SRC family kinase activity and Ras/Erk activation by controlling Csk recruitment. Mol Cell 2004;13:341-355.
13. Frame MC. Newest findings on the oldest oncogene; how activated src does it. J Cell Sci 2004;117:989-998.
14. Gonzalez L, Agullo-Ortuno MT, Garcia-Martinez JM, et al. Role of c-Src in human MCF7 breast cancer cell tumorigenesis. J Biol Chem 2006;281:20851-20864.
15. Alvarez RH, Kantarjian HM, Cortes JE. The role of Src in solid and hematologic malignancies: development of new-generation Src inhibitors. Cancer 2006;107:1918-1929.
16. Qin B, Ariyama H, Baba E, et al. Activated Src and Ras induce gefitinib resistance by activation of signaling pathways downstream of epidermal growth factor receptor in human gallbladder adenocarcinoma cells. Cancer Chemother Pharmacol 2006;58:577-584.
17. Hiscox S, Morgan L, Green TP, Barrow D, Gee J, Nicholson RI. Elevated Src activity promotes cellular invasion and motility in tamoxifen resistant breast cancer cells. Breast Cancer Res Treat 2006;97:263-274.
18. Coopman PJ, Mueller SC. The Syk tyrosine kinase: a new negative regulator in tumor growth and progression. Cancer Lett 2006;241:159-173.
19. Ruschel A, Ullrich A. Protein tyrosine kinase Syk modulates EGFR signalling in human mammary epithelial cells. Cell Signal 2004;16:1249-1261.
20. Moroni M, Soldatenkov V, Zhang L, et al. Progressive loss of Syk and abnormal proliferation in breast cancer cells. Cancer Res 2004;64:7346-7354.

21. Rodriguez-Viciana P, Sabatier C, McCormick F. Signaling specificity by Ras family GTPases is determined by the full spectrum of effectors they regulate. Mol Cell Biol 2004;24:4943-4954.
22. Daly RJ, Binder MD, Sutherland RL. Overexpression of the Grb2 gene in human breast cancer cell lines. Oncogene 1994;9:2723-2727.
23. Verbeek BS, Adriaansen-Slot SS, Rijksen G, Vroom TM. Grb2 overexpression in nuclei and cytoplasm of human breast cells: a histochemical and biochemical study of normal and neoplastic mammary tissue specimens. J Pathol 1997;183:195-203.
24. Yip SS, Crew AJ, Gee JM, et al. Up-regulation of the protein tyrosine phosphatase SHP-1 in human breast cancer and correlation with GRB2 expression. Int J Cancer 2000;88:363-368.
25. Lee MS, Igawa T, Chen SJ, et al. p66Shc protein is upregulated by steroid hormones in hormone-sensitive cancer cells and in primary prostate carcinomas. Int J Cancer 2004;108:672-678.
26. Rauh MJ, Blackmore V, Andrechek ER, et al. Accelerated mammary tumor development in mutant polyomavirus middle T transgenic mice expressing elevated levels of either the Shc or Grb2 adapter protein. Mol Cell Biol 1999;19:8169-8179.
27. Pelicci G, Lanfrancone L, Salcini AE, et al. Constitutive phosphorylation of Shc proteins in human tumors. Oncogene 1995;11:899-907.
28. Davol PA, Bagdasaryan R, Elfenbein GJ, Maizel AL, Frackelton AR, Jr. Shc proteins are strong, independent prognostic markers for both node-negative and node-positive primary breast cancer. Cancer Res 2003;63:6772-6783.
29. Jackson JG, Yoneda T, Clark GM, Yee D. Elevated levels of p66 Shc are found in breast cancer cell lines and primary tumors with high metastatic potential. Clin Cancer Res 2000;6:1135-1139.
30. Gu H, Neel BG. The "Gab" in signal transduction. Trends Cell Biol 2003;13:122-130.
31. Brummer T, Schramek D, Hayes VM, et al. Increased proliferation and altered growth factor dependence of human mammary epithelial cells overexpressing the Gab2 docking protein. J Biol Chem 2006;281:626-637.
32. Daly RJ, Gu H, Parmar J, et al. The docking protein Gab2 is overexpressed and estrogen regulated in human breast cancer. Oncogene 2002;21:5175-5181.
33. Bentires-Alj M, Gil SG, Chan R, et al. A role for the scaffolding adapter GAB2 in breast cancer. Nat Med 2006;12:114-121.
34. Schuuring E. The involvement of the chromosome 11q13 region in human malignancies: cyclin D1 and EMS1 are two new candidate oncogenes--a review. Gene 1995;159:83-96.
35. Sjoblom T, Jones S, Wood LD, et al. The consensus coding sequences of human breast and colorectal cancers. Science 2006;314:268-274.
36. Bentires-Alj M, Paez JG, David FS, et al. Activating mutations of the noonan syndrome-associated SHP2/PTPN11 gene in human solid tumors and adult acute myelogenous leukemia. Cancer Res 2004;64:8816-8820.
37. Bos JL. ras oncogenes in human cancer: a review. Cancer Res 1989;49:4682-4689.
38. Malaney S, Daly RJ. The ras signaling pathway in mammary tumorigenesis and metastasis. J Mammary Gland Biol Neoplasia 2001;6:101-113.
39. Han SW, Kim TY, Jeon YK, et al. Optimization of patient selection for gefitinib in non-small cell lung cancer by combined analysis of epidermal growth factor receptor mutation, K-ras mutation, and Akt phosphorylation. Clin Cancer Res 2006;12:2538-2544.
40. Shigematsu H, Lin L, Takahashi T, et al. Clinical and biological features associated with epidermal growth factor receptor gene mutations in lung cancers. J Natl Cancer Inst 2005;97:339-346.
41. Pao W, Wang TY, Riely GJ, et al. KRAS mutations and primary resistance of lung adenocarcinomas to gefitinib or erlotinib. PLoS Med 2005;2:e17.
42. Giaccone G, Gallegos Ruiz M, Le Chevalier T, et al. Erlotinib for frontline treatment of advanced non-small cell lung cancer: a phase II study. Clin Cancer Res 2006;12:6049-6055.
43. Lievre A, Bachet JB, Le Corre D, et al. KRAS mutation status is predictive of response to cetuximab therapy in colorectal cancer. Cancer Res 2006;66:3992-3995.
44. Yoon S, Seger R. The extracellular signal-regulated kinase: multiple substrates regulate diverse cellular functions. Growth Factors 2006;24:21-44.
45. Wellbrock C, Karasarides M, Marais R. The RAF proteins take centre stage. Nat Rev Mol Cell Biol 2004;5:875-885.

46. Davies H, Bignell GR, Cox C, et al. Mutations of the BRAF gene in human cancer. Nature 2002;417:949-954.
47. Sivaraman VS, Wang H, Nuovo GJ, Malbon CC. Hyperexpression of mitogen-activated protein kinase in human breast cancer. J Clin Invest 1997;99:1478-1483.
48. Schmidt CM, McKillop IH, Cahill PA, Sitzmann JV. Increased MAPK expression and activity in primary human hepatocellular carcinoma. Biochem Biophys Res Commun 1997;236:54-58.
49. Normanno N, De Luca A, Maiello MR, et al. The MEK/MAPK pathway is involved in the resistance of breast cancer cells to the EGFR tyrosine kinase inhibitor gefitinib. J Cell Physiol 2006;207:420-427.
50. Gonzalez-Garcia A, Pritchard CA, Paterson HF, Mavria G, Stamp G, Marshall CJ. RalGDS is required for tumor formation in a model of skin carcinogenesis. Cancer Cell 2005;7:219-226.
51. Malliri A, van der Kammen RA, Clark K, van der Valk M, Michiels F, Collard JG. Mice deficient in the Rac activator Tiam1 are resistant to Ras-induced skin tumours. Nature 2002;417:867-871.
52. Bai Y, Edamatsu H, Maeda S, et al. Crucial role of phospholipase Cepsilon in chemical carcinogen-induced skin tumor development. Cancer Res 2004;64:8808-8810.
53. Camonis JH, White MA. Ral GTPases: corrupting the exocyst in cancer cells. Trends Cell Biol 2005;15:327-332.
54. Chien Y, Kim S, Bumeister R, et al. RalB GTPase-mediated activation of the IkappaB family kinase TBK1 couples innate immune signaling to tumor cell survival. Cell 2006;127:157-170.
55. Sriuranpong V, Mutirangura A, Gillespie JW, et al. Global gene expression profile of nasopharyngeal carcinoma by laser capture microdissection and complementary DNA microarrays. Clin Cancer Res 2004;10:4944-4958.
56. Engers R, Mueller M, Walter A, Collard JG, Willers R, Gabbert HE. Prognostic relevance of Tiam1 protein expression in prostate carcinomas. Br J Cancer 2006;95:1081-1086.
57. Engers R, Zwaka TP, Gohr L, Weber A, Gerharz CD, Gabbert HE. Tiam1 mutations in human renal-cell carcinomas. Int J Cancer 2000;88:369-376.
58. Wells A, Grandis JR. Phospholipase C-gamma1 in tumor progression. Clin Exp Metastasis 2003;20:285-290.
59. Chen P, Xie H, Sekar MC, Gupta K, Wells A. Epidermal growth factor receptor-mediated cell motility: phospholipase C activity is required, but mitogen-activated protein kinase activity is not sufficient for induced cell movement. J Cell Biol 1994;127:847-857.
60. Thomas SM, Coppelli FM, Wells A, et al. Epidermal growth factor receptor-stimulated activation of phospholipase Cgamma-1 promotes invasion of head and neck squamous cell carcinoma. Cancer Res 2003;63:5629-5635.
61. Arteaga CL, Johnson MD, Todderud G, Coffey RJ, Carpenter G, Page DL. Elevated content of the tyrosine kinase substrate phospholipase C-gamma 1 in primary human breast carcinomas. Proc Natl Acad Sci U S A 1991;88:10435-10439.
62. Bader AG, Kang S, Zhao L, Vogt PK. Oncogenic PI3K deregulates transcription and translation. Nat Rev Cancer 2005;5:921-929.
63. Cully M, You H, Levine AJ, Mak TW. Beyond PTEN mutations: the PI3K pathway as an integrator of multiple inputs during tumorigenesis. Nat Rev Cancer 2006;6:184-192.
64. Stambolic V, Woodgett JR. Functional distinctions of protein kinase B/Akt isoforms defined by their influence on cell migration. Trends Cell Biol 2006;16:461-466.
65. Samuels Y, Ericson K. Oncogenic PI3K and its role in cancer. Curr Opin Oncol 2006;18:77-82.
66. Samuels Y, Velculescu VE. Oncogenic mutations of PIK3CA in human cancers. Cell Cycle 2004;3:1221-1224.
67. Bachman KE, Argani P, Samuels Y, et al. The PIK3CA gene is mutated with high frequency in human breast cancers. Cancer Biol Ther 2004;3:772-775.
68. Levine DA, Bogomolniy F, Yee CJ, et al. Frequent mutation of the PIK3CA gene in ovarian and breast cancers. Clin Cancer Res 2005;11:2875-2878.
69. Ikenoue T, Kanai F, Hikiba Y, et al. Functional analysis of PIK3CA gene mutations in human colorectal cancer. Cancer Res 2005;65:4562-4567.
70. Isakoff SJ, Engelman JA, Irie HY, et al. Breast cancer-associated PIK3CA mutations are oncogenic in mammary epithelial cells. Cancer Res 2005;65:10992-11000.
71. Zhao JJ, Liu Z, Wang L, Shin E, Loda MF, Roberts TM. The oncogenic properties of mutant p110alpha and p110beta phosphatidylinositol 3-kinases in human mammary epithelial cells. Proc Natl Acad Sci U S A 2005;102:18443-18448.

72. Philp AJ, Campbell IG, Leet C, et al. The phosphatidylinositol 3Î-kinase p85alpha gene is an oncogene in human ovarian and colon tumors. Cancer Res 2001;61:7426-7429.
73. Shayesteh L, Lu Y, Kuo WL, et al. PIK3CA is implicated as an oncogene in ovarian cancer. Nat Genet 1999;21:99-102.
74. Yen CC, Chen YJ, Lu KH, et al. Genotypic analysis of esophageal squamous cell carcinoma by molecular cytogenetics and real-time quantitative polymerase chain reaction. Int J Oncol 2003;23:871-881.
75. Redon R, Muller D, Caulee K, Wanherdrick K, Abecassis J, du Manoir S. A simple specific pattern of chromosomal aberrations at early stages of head and neck squamous cell carcinomas: PIK3CA but not p63 gene as a likely target of 3q26-qter gains. Cancer Res 2001;61:4122-4129.
76. Altomare DA, Testa JR. Perturbations of the AKT signaling pathway in human cancer. Oncogene 2005;24:7455-7464.
77. Cheng JQ, Altomare DA, Klein MA, et al. Transforming activity and mitosis-related expression of the AKT2 oncogene: evidence suggesting a link between cell cycle regulation and oncogenesis. Oncogene 1997;14:2793-2801.
78. Arboleda MJ, Lyons JF, Kabbinavar FF, et al. Overexpression of AKT2/protein kinase Bbeta leads to up-regulation of beta1 integrins, increased invasion, and metastasis of human breast and ovarian cancer cells. Cancer Res 2003;63:196-206.
79. Irie HY, Pearline RV, Grueneberg D, et al. Distinct roles of Akt1 and Akt2 in regulating cell migration and epithelial-mesenchymal transition. J Cell Biol 2005;171:1023-1034.
80. Bellacosa A, de Feo D, Godwin AK, et al. Molecular alterations of the AKT2 oncogene in ovarian and breast carcinomas. Int J Cancer 1995;64:280-285.
81. Bacus SS, Altomare DA, Lyass L, et al. AKT2 is frequently upregulated in HER-2/neu-positive breast cancers and may contribute to tumor aggressiveness by enhancing cell survival. Oncogene 2002;21:3532-3540.
82. Cheng JQ, Ruggeri B, Klein WM, et al. Amplification of AKT2 in human pancreatic cells and inhibition of AKT2 expression and tumorigenicity by antisense RNA. Proc Natl Acad Sci U S A 1996;93:3636-3641.
83. Roy HK, Olusola BF, Clemens DL, et al. AKT proto-oncogene overexpression is an early event during sporadic colon carcinogenesis. Carcinogenesis 2002;23:201-205.
84. Xu X, Sakon M, Nagano H, et al. Akt2 expression correlates with prognosis of human hepatocellular carcinoma. Oncol Rep 2004;11:25-32.
85. Stal O, Perez-Tenorio G, Akerberg L, et al. Akt kinases in breast cancer and the results of adjuvant therapy. Breast Cancer Res 2003;5:R37-44.
86. Nakatani K, Thompson DA, Barthel A, et al. Up-regulation of Akt3 in estrogen receptor-deficient breast cancers and androgen-independent prostate cancer lines. J Biol Chem 1999;274:21528-21532.
87. Soung YH, Lee JW, Nam SW, Lee JY, Yoo NJ, Lee SH. Mutational Analysis of AKT1, AKT2 and AKT3 Genes in Common Human Carcinomas. Oncology 2006;70:285-289.
88. Chow LM, Baker SJ. PTEN function in normal and neoplastic growth. Cancer Lett 2006;241:184-196.
89. Leslie NR, Downes CP. PTEN function: how normal cells control it and tumour cells lose it. Biochem J 2004;382:1-11.
90. Sansal I, Sellers WR. The biology and clinical relevance of the PTEN tumor suppressor pathway. J Clin Oncol 2004;22:2954-2963.
91. Saal LH, Holm K, Maurer M, et al. PIK3CA mutations correlate with hormone receptors, node metastasis, and ERBB2, and are mutually exclusive with PTEN loss in human breast carcinoma. Cancer Res 2005;65:2554-2559.
92. Knowles MA, Habuchi T, Kennedy W, Cuthbert-Heavens D. Mutation spectrum of the 9q34 tuberous sclerosis gene TSC1 in transitional cell carcinoma of the bladder. Cancer Res 2003;63:7652-7656.
93. Hay N. The Akt-mTOR tango and its relevance to cancer. Cancer Cell 2005;8:179-183.
94. Jiang WG, Sampson J, Martin TA, et al. Tuberin and hamartin are aberrantly expressed and linked to clinical outcome in human breast cancer: the role of promoter methylation of TSC genes. Eur J Cancer 2005;41:1628-1636.
95. Kataoka K, Fujimoto K, Ito D, et al. Expression and prognostic value of tuberous sclerosis complex 2 gene product tuberin in human pancreatic cancer. Surgery 2005;138:450-455.
96. Engelman JA, Janne PA, Mermel C, et al. ErbB-3 mediates phosphoinositide 3-kinase activity in gefitinib-sensitive non-small cell lung cancer cell lines. Proc Natl Acad Sci U S A 2005;102:3788-3793.

97. Engelman JA, Mukohara T, Zejnullahu K, et al. Allelic dilution obscures detection of a biologically significant resistance mutation in EGFR-amplified lung cancer. J Clin Invest 2006;116:2695-2706.
98. Mellinghoff IK, Wang MY, Vivanco I, et al. Molecular determinants of the response of glioblastomas to EGFR kinase inhibitors. N Engl J Med 2005;353:2012-2024.
99. She QB, Solit D, Basso A, Moasser MM. Resistance to gefitinib in PTEN-null HER-overexpressing tumor cells can be overcome through restoration of PTEN function or pharmacologic modulation of constitutive phosphatidylinositol 3'-kinase/Akt pathway signaling. Clin Cancer Res 2003;9: 4340-4346.
100. Bianco R, Shin I, Ritter CA, et al. Loss of PTEN/MMAC1/TEP in EGF receptor-expressing tumor cells counteracts the antitumor action of EGFR tyrosine kinase inhibitors. Oncogene 2003;22:2812-2822.
101. Festuccia C, Muzi P, Millimaggi D, et al. Molecular aspects of gefitinib antiproliferative and pro-apoptotic effects in PTEN-positive and PTEN-negative prostate cancer cell lines. Endocr Relat Cancer 2005;12:983-998.
102. Wang MY, Lu KV, Zhu S, et al. Mammalian Target of Rapamycin Inhibition Promotes Response to Epidermal Growth Factor Receptor Kinase Inhibitors in PTEN-Deficient and PTEN-Intact Glioblastoma Cells. Cancer Res 2006;66:7864-7869.
103. Ferrell JE, Jr. Self-perpetuating states in signal transduction: positive feedback, double-negative feedback and bistability. Curr Opin Cell Biol 2002;14:140-148.
104. Courtois-Cox S, Genther Williams S, Reczek E, et al. A negative feedback signalling network underlies oncogene-induced senescence. Cancer Cell 2006;10:459-472.
105. O'Reilly KE, Rojo F, She QB, et al. mTOR inhibition induces upstream receptor tyrosine kinase signaling and activates Akt. Cancer Res 2006;66:1500-1508.
106. Northwood IC, Gonzalez FA, Wartmann M, Raden DL, Davis RJ. Isolation and characterization of two growth factor-stimulated protein kinases that phosphorylate the epidermal growth factor receptor at threonine 669. J Biol Chem 1991;266:15266-15276.
107. Theroux SJ, Taglienti-Sian C, Nair N, Countaway JL, Robinson HL, Davis RJ. Increased oncogenic potential of ErbB is associated with the loss of a COOH-terminal domain serine phosphorylation site. J Biol Chem 1992;267:7967-7970.
108. Huang L, Watanabe M, Chikamori M, et al. Unique role of SNT-2/FRS2beta/FRS3 docking/adaptor protein for negative regulation in EGF receptor tyrosine kinase signaling pathways. Oncogene 2006;25:6457-6466.
109. Dougherty MK, Muller J, Ritt DA, et al. Regulation of Raf-1 by direct feedback phosphorylation. Mol Cell 2005;17:215-224.
110. Lynch DK, Daly RJ. PKB-mediated negative feedback tightly regulates mitogenic signalling via Gab2. Embo J 2002;21:72-82.
111. Bao L, Kimzey A, Sauter G, Sowadski JM, Lu KP, Wang DG. Prevalent overexpression of prolyl isomerase Pin1 in human cancers. Am J Pathol 2004;164:1727-1737.
112. Mason JM, Morrison DJ, Basson MA, Licht JD. Sprouty proteins: multifaceted negative-feedback regulators of receptor tyrosine kinase signaling. Trends Cell Biol 2006;16:45-54.
113. Lo TL, Fong CW, Yusoff P, et al. Sprouty and cancer: The first terms report. Cancer Lett 2006;242:141-150.
114. Mason JM, Morrison DJ, Bassit B, et al. Tyrosine phosphorylation of Sprouty proteins regulates their ability to inhibit growth factor signaling: a dual feedback loop. Mol Biol Cell 2004;15:2176-2188.
115. Gur G, Rubin C, Katz M, et al. LRIG1 restricts growth factor signaling by enhancing receptor ubiquitylation and degradation. Embo J 2004;23:3270-3281.
116. Suzuki Y, Miura H, Tanemura A, et al. Targeted disruption of LIG-1 gene results in psoriasiform epidermal hyperplasia. FEBS Lett 2002;521:67-71.
117. Nilsson J, Vallbo C, Guo D, et al. Cloning, characterization, and expression of human LIG1. Biochem Biophys Res Commun 2001;284:1155-1161.
118. Holmlund C, Nilsson J, Guo D, et al. Characterization and tissue-specific expression of human LRIG2. Gene 2004;332:35-43.
119. Fiorini M, Ballaro C, Sala G, Falcone G, Alema S, Segatto O. Expression of RALT, a feedback inhibitor of ErbB receptors, is subjected to an integrated transcriptional and post-translational control. Oncogene 2002;21:6530-6539.

120. Anastasi S, Fiorentino L, Fiorini M, et al. Feedback inhibition by RALT controls signal output by the ErbB network. Oncogene 2003;22:4221-4234.
121. Xu D, Makkinje A, Kyriakis JM. Gene 33 is an endogenous inhibitor of epidermal growth factor (EGF) receptor signaling and mediates dexamethasone-induced suppression of EGF function. J Biol Chem 2005;280:2924-2933.
122. Ferby I, Reschke M, Kudlacek O, et al. Mig6 is a negative regulator of EGF receptor-mediated skin morphogenesis and tumor formation. Nat Med 2006;12:568-573.
123. Zhang YW, Staal B, Su Y, et al. Evidence that MIG-6 is a tumor-suppressor gene. Oncogene In press.
124. Anastasi S, Sala G, Huiping C, et al. Loss of RALT/MIG-6 expression in ERBB2-amplified breast carcinomas enhances ErbB-2 oncogenic potency and favors resistance to Herceptin. Oncogene 2005;24:4540-4548.
125. Dickinson RJ, Keyse SM. Diverse physiological functions for dual-specificity MAP kinase phosphatases. J Cell Sci 2006;119:4607-4615.
126. Ryser S, Massiha A, Piuz I, Schlegel W. Stimulated initiation of mitogen-activated protein kinase phosphatase-1 (MKP-1) gene transcription involves the synergistic action of multiple cis-acting elements in the proximal promoter. Biochem J 2004;378:473-484.
127. Sato M, Vaughan MB, Girard L, et al. Multiple oncogenic changes (K-RAS(V12), p53 knockdown, mutant EGFRs, p16 bypass, telomerase) are not sufficient to confer a full malignant phenotype on human bronchial epithelial cells. Cancer Res 2006;66:2116-2128.
128. Tsujita E, Taketomi A, Gion T, et al. Suppressed MKP-1 is an independent predictor of outcome in patients with hepatocellular carcinoma. Oncology 2005;69:342-347.
129. Furukawa T, Sunamura M, Motoi F, Matsuno S, Horii A. Potential tumor suppressive pathway involving DUSP6/MKP-3 in pancreatic cancer. Am J Pathol 2003;162:1807-1815.
130. Vicent S, Garayoa M, Lopez-Picazo JM, et al. Mitogen-activated protein kinase phosphatase-1 is overexpressed in non-small cell lung cancer and is an independent predictor of outcome in patients. Clin Cancer Res 2004;10:3639-3649.
131. Loda M, Capodieci P, Mishra R, et al. Expression of mitogen-activated protein kinase phosphatase-1 in the early phases of human epithelial carcinogenesis. Am J Pathol 1996;149:1553-1564.
132. Liao Q, Guo J, Kleeff J, et al. Down-regulation of the dual-specificity phosphatase MKP-1 suppresses tumorigenicity of pancreatic cancer cells. Gastroenterology 2003;124:1830-1845.
133. Manzano RG, Montuenga LM, Dayton M, et al. CL100 expression is down-regulated in advanced epithelial ovarian cancer and its re-expression decreases its malignant potential. Oncogene 2002;21:4435-4447.
134. Denkert C, Schmitt WD, Berger S, et al. Expression of mitogen-activated protein kinase phosphatase-1 (MKP-1) in primary human ovarian carcinoma. Int J Cancer 2002;102:507-513.
135. Givant-Horwitz V, Davidson B, Goderstad JM, Nesland JM, Trope CG, Reich R. The PAC-1 dual specificity phosphatase predicts poor outcome in serous ovarian carcinoma. Gynecol Oncol 2004;93:517-523.
136. Sanchez-Perez I, Martinez-Gomariz M, Williams D, Keyse SM, Perona R. CL100/MKP-1 modulates JNK activation and apoptosis in response to cisplatin. Oncogene 2000;19:5142-5152.
137. Small GW, Shi YY, Edmund NA, Somasundaram S, Moore DT, Orlowski RZ. Evidence that mitogen-activated protein kinase phosphatase-1 induction by proteasome inhibitors plays an antiapoptotic role. Mol Pharmacol 2004;66:1478-1490.
138. Schulze A, Lehmann K, Jefferies HB, McMahon M, Downward J. Analysis of the transcriptional program induced by Raf in epithelial cells. Genes Dev 2001;15:981-994.
139. Berset TA, Hoier EF, Hajnal A. The C. elegans homolog of the mammalian tumor suppressor Dep-1/Scc1 inhibits EGFR signaling to regulate binary cell fate decisions. Genes Dev 2005;19:1328-1340.
140. Ruivenkamp CA, van Wezel T, Zanon C, et al. Ptprj is a candidate for the mouse colon-cancer susceptibility locus Scc1 and is frequently deleted in human cancers. Nat Genet 2002;31:295-300.
141. Soubeyran P, Kowanetz K, Szymkiewicz I, Langdon WY, Dikic I. Cbl-CIN85-endophilin complex mediates ligand-induced downregulation of EGF receptors. Nature 2002;416:183-187.
142. Petrelli A, Gilestro GF, Lanzardo S, Comoglio PM, Migone N, Giordano S. The endophilin-CIN85-Cbl complex mediates ligand-dependent downregulation of c-Met. Nature 2002;416:187-190.
143. Lynch DK, Winata SC, Lyons RJ, et al. A Cortactin-CD2-associated Protein (CD2AP) Complex Provides a Novel Link between Epidermal Growth Factor Receptor Endocytosis and the Actin Cytoskeleton. J Biol Chem 2003;278:21805-21813.

144. Marmor MD, Yarden Y. Role of protein ubiquitylation in regulating endocytosis of receptor tyrosine kinases. Oncogene 2004;23:2057-2070.
145. Thien CB, Langdon WY. Cbl: many adaptations to regulate protein tyrosine kinases. Nat Rev Mol Cell Biol 2001;2:294-307.
146. Thien CB, Walker F, Langdon WY. RING finger mutations that abolish c-Cbl-directed polyubiquitination and downregulation of the EGF receptor are insufficient for cell transformation. Mol Cell 2001;7:355-365.
147. Waterman H, Katz M, Rubin C, et al. A mutant EGF-receptor defective in ubiquitylation and endocytosis unveils a role for Grb2 in negative signaling. Embo J 2002;21:303-313.
148. Moscatello DK, Holgado-Madruga M, Godwin AK, et al. Frequent expression of a mutant epidermal growth factor receptor in multiple human tumors. Cancer Res 1995;55:5536-5539.
149. Frederick L, Wang XY, Eley G, James CD. Diversity and frequency of epidermal growth factor receptor mutations in human glioblastomas. Cancer Res 2000;60:1383-1387.
150. Schmidt MH, Furnari FB, Cavenee WK, Bogler O. Epidermal growth factor receptor signaling intensity determines intracellular protein interactions, ubiquitination, and internalization. Proc Natl Acad Sci U S A 2003;100:6505-6510.
151. Lenferink AE, Pinkas-Kramarski R, van de Poll ML, et al. Differential endocytic routing of homo- and hetero-dimeric ErbB tyrosine kinases confers signaling superiority to receptor heterodimers. Embo J 1998;17:3385-3397.
152. Worthylake R, Opresko LK, Wiley HS. ErbB-2 amplification inhibits down-regulation and induces constitutive activation of both ErbB-2 and epidermal growth factor receptors. J Biol Chem 1999;274:8865-8874.
153. Muthuswamy SK, Gilman M, Brugge JS. Controlled dimerization of ErbB receptors provides evidence for differential signaling by homo- and heterodimers. Mol Cell Biol 1999;19:6845-6857.
154. Bao J, Gur G, Yarden Y. Src promotes destruction of c-Cbl: implications for oncogenic synergy between Src and growth factor receptors. Proc Natl Acad Sci U S A 2003;100:2438-2443.
155. Tanos B, Pendergast AM. Abl tyrosine kinase regulates endocytosis of the epidermal growth factor receptor. J Biol Chem 2006;281:32714-32723.
156. Chen WS, Kung HJ, Yang WK, Lin W. Comparative tyrosine-kinase profiles in colorectal cancers: enhanced arg expression in carcinoma as compared with adenoma and normal mucosa. Int J Cancer 1999;83:579-584.
157. Srinivasan D, Plattner R. Activation of Abl tyrosine kinases promotes invasion of aggressive breast cancer cells. Cancer Res 2006;66:5648-5655.
158. Feng Q, Baird D, Peng X, et al. Cool-1 functions as an essential regulatory node for EGF receptor- and Src-mediated cell growth. Nat Cell Biol 2006;8:945-956.
159. Fritz G, Just I, Kaina B. Rho GTPases are over-expressed in human tumors. Int J Cancer 1999;81:682-687.
160. Qiu RG, Abo A, McCormick F, Symons M. Cdc42 regulates anchorage-independent growth and is necessary for Ras transformation. Mol Cell Biol 1997;17:3449-3458.
161. Wu WJ, Tu S, Cerione RA. Activated Cdc42 sequesters c-Cbl and prevents EGF receptor degradation. Cell 2003;114:715-725.
162. Hirsch DS, Shen Y, Wu WJ. Growth and motility inhibition of breast cancer cells by epidermal growth factor receptor degradation is correlated with inactivation of Cdc42. Cancer Res 2006;66:3523-3530.
163. Zhang B, Srirangam A, Potter DA, Roman A. HPV16 E5 protein disrupts the c-Cbl-EGFR interaction and EGFR ubiquitination in human foreskin keratinocytes. Oncogene 2005;24:2585-2588.
164. Daly RJ. Cortactin signalling and dynamic actin networks. Biochem J 2004;382:13-25.
165. Timpson P, Lynch DK, Schramek D, Walker F, Daly RJ. Cortactin overexpression inhibits ligand-induced down-regulation of the epidermal growth factor receptor. Cancer Res 2005;65:3273-3280.
166. Hyun TS, Rao DS, Saint-Dic D, et al. HIP1 and HIP1r stabilize receptor tyrosine kinases and bind 3-phosphoinositides via epsin N-terminal homology domains. J Biol Chem 2004;279:14294-14306.
167. Rao DS, Bradley SV, Kumar PD, et al. Altered receptor trafficking in Huntingtin Interacting Protein 1-transformed cells. Cancer Cell 2003;3:471-482.
168. Rao DS, Hyun TS, Kumar PD, et al. Huntingtin-interacting protein 1 is overexpressed in prostate and colon cancer and is critical for cellular survival. J Clin Invest 2002;110:351-360.

169. Lee MP, Feinberg AP. Aberrant splicing but not mutations of TSG101 in human breast cancer. Cancer Res 1997;57:3131-3134.
170. Xu Z, Liang L, Wang H, Li T, Zhao M. HCRP1, a novel gene that is downregulated in hepatocellular carcinoma, encodes a growth-inhibitory protein. Biochem Biophys Res Commun 2003;311:1057-1066.
171. Bache KG, Slagsvold T, Cabezas A, Rosendal KR, Raiborg C, Stenmark H. The growth-regulatory protein HCRP1/hVps37A is a subunit of mammalian ESCRT-I and mediates receptor down-regulation. Mol Biol Cell 2004;15:4337-4346.
172. Kwak EL, Sordella R, Bell DW, et al. Irreversible inhibitors of the EGF receptor may circumvent acquired resistance to gefitinib. Proc Natl Acad Sci U S A 2005;102:7665-7670.
173. Ono M, Hirata A, Kometani T, et al. Sensitivity to gefitinib (Iressa, ZD1839) in non-small cell lung cancer cell lines correlates with dependence on the epidermal growth factor (EGF) receptor/extracellular signal-regulated kinase 1/2 and EGF receptor/Akt pathway for proliferation. Mol Cancer Ther 2004;3:465-472.
174. Adjei AA. Novel combinations based on epidermal growth factor receptor inhibition. Clin Cancer Res 2006;12:4446s-4450s.

18 EGFR Signaling in Invasion, Angiogenesis and Metastasis

Carol Box, Joanna Peak, Susanne Rogers, and Suzanne Eccles

CONTENTS

INTRODUCTION
TUMOR INVASION
ANGIOGENESIS AND LYMPHANGIOGENESIS
METASTASIS
CLINICAL OBSERVATIONS
THERAPEUTIC OPPORTUNITIES
REFERENCES

Abstract

Tumor invasion and metastasis are the hallmarks of advanced stage cancer and are associated with poor patient prognosis. EGFR is overexpressed in a variety of tumor types and this frequently correlates with a more aggressive tumor phenotype. In this chapter, we discuss the cellular and molecular mechanisms by which EGFR contributes to tumor progression and present evidence from experimental and clinical observations that reinforce the notion that EGFR actively contributes to the onset of metastatic disease. EGFR plays a key role in the regulation of processes central to tumor invasion including cell adhesion and motility through its interactions with molecules such as integrins, cadherins, phospholipase Cγ1 and phosphoinositide 3-kinase. In addition, EGFR signaling can contribute to both proteolysis and angiogenesis through up-regulated expression of matrix metalloproteinases (MMPs) and angiogenic cytokines *e.g.* VEGF-A and IL-8. The significance of these contributions to tumor invasion and metastasis is highlighted by the fact that a mutant, constitutively active receptor (EGFRvIII) associated with human cancers can induce these behaviors when transfected into fibroblasts. Finally, we discuss the use of EGFR antagonists to stem metastatic disease and their potential, in combination with additional novel agents, to improve treatment for cancer patients.

Key Words: invasion, adhesion, motility, proteolysis, angiogenesis, lymphangiogenesis, metastasis.

1. INTRODUCTION

For most solid tumors, patient prognosis is largely determined by the extent of tumor cell invasion and metastasis at the time of diagnosis, which reflects the fact that conventional therapies are relatively ineffective against advanced stage cancer. A greater understanding of the biology of tumor cell invasion, metastasis, and angiogenesis will hopefully contribute

From: *Cancer Drug Discovery and Development: EGFR Signaling Networks in Cancer Therapy*
Edited by: J. D. Haley and W. J. Gullick, DOI: 10.1007/978-1-59745-356-1_18
© 2008 Humana Press, a part of Springer Science+Business Media, LLC

to the development of combined modality and adjuvant therapy regimens that better control local and distant disease.

EGFR has been established as an important oncogene in many solid tumor types (*1*). Despite the lack of standardization in methodology, overexpression of EGFR is widely reported to correlate with poor prognosis in patients with head and neck cancer (SCCHN) (*2*), oesophageal, bladder, cervical, and ovarian cancers (*3*) and may adversely affect outcome in breast, gastric, colorectal, and endometrial cancers (*3*). Although increased cell proliferation (*4*) and survival (*5*) may be the dominant events resulting from EGFR overexpression, enhanced tumor cell migration (*6*), invasion (*7*), metastasis (*8*) and angiogenesis (*9*) may be of greater significance in determining patient prognosis and are the focus of this chapter.

2. TUMOR INVASION

Tumor cell invasion represents a complex process requiring coordination of a multitude of cell behaviors including dynamic adhesive interactions between cells and their underlying matrix, cell motility (in particular chemotaxis) and proteolysis.

Several studies have demonstrated a key role for EGFR in promoting tumor cell invasion in vitro (*10–12*). More recently, the development of multiphoton-based intravital imaging has enabled visualization of individual cells within experimental tumors, which has reinforced the notion that EGF, through EGFR, is an important factor regulating the invasion and intravasation of metastatic tumor cells (*13–15*). In a rat orthotopic breast carcinoma model, metastatic cells within the primary tumor were found to migrate rapidly towards endogenous and exogenous sources of EGF (*16, 17*). Macrophages play a central role in this invasive process through the establishment of a paracrine signaling loop involving EGF: colony stimulating factor-1 (CSF-1) cross-talk (*14, 18*). The central role played by the EGFR in tumor cell invasion is described below and summarized in Fig. 18.1.

2.1. Adhesion

Tumor invasion into the surrounding stroma involves complex alterations in both cell-cell and cell-matrix adhesion. Adhesion of cells to the extracellular matrix (ECM) is largely regulated by integrins, transmembrane glycoproteins that convey bi-directional signals between cells and their surroundings. Intercellular adhesion is regulated by cadherin-catenin complexes whose status can determine whether epithelial cells remain as a cohesive cluster or disaggregate to allow tumor dissemination.

2.1.1. INTEGRINS AND CELL-MATRIX INTERACTIONS

Integrin heterodimers function as receptors for matrix proteins such as collagen, laminin and fibronectin (*19*). Integrins lack intrinsic catalytic activity but interact directly with receptor tyrosine kinases (RTKs) such as EGFR, ERB-B2, VEGFR and MET to transduce cell adhesion and migration signals (*20*). Integrin activation, clustering and subsequent actin polymerisation results in phosphorylation and activation of focal adhesion kinase (FAK), a requirement of cell adhesion, spreading and migration. FAK autophosphorylation at tyrosine 397 generates a docking site for phosphoinositide 3-kinase (PI3K), SRC, FYN or phospholipase Cγ (PLCγ) (*21*). SRC subsequently phosphorylates FAK on additional residues mediating the docking of a cohort of other SH2 domain proteins.

FAK associates with activated EGFR to promote EGF-driven cell migration; this may be facilitated by co-association of FAK with integrins (*21*). Following EGF stimulation, FAK becomes dephosphorylated and inactivated resulting in detachment of tumor cells from the extracellular matrix, increased tumor cell motility, invasion and metastasis (*22*). This mechanism has been illustrated in a cervical carcinoma cell line where EGF induced cell motility

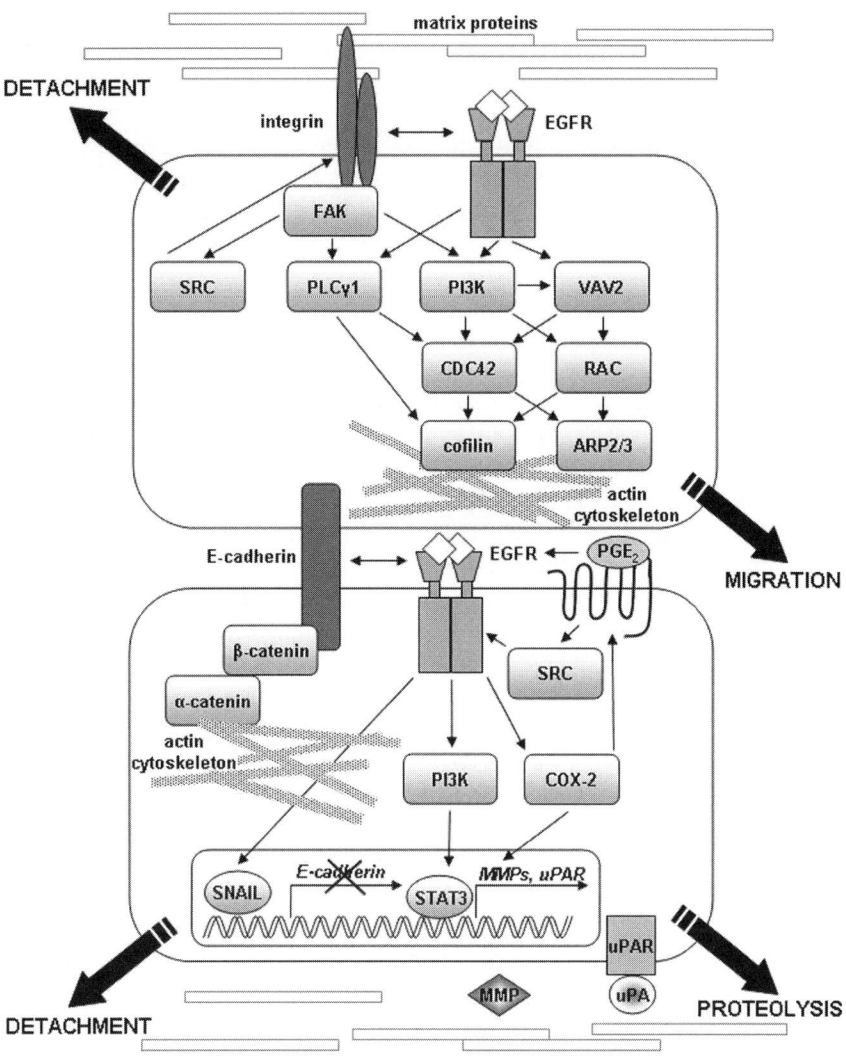

Fig. 18.1. The coordination of EGFR and integrin signaling through FAK and SRC or EGFR and cadherin-catenin signaling mediates changes in cellular adhesion required for migration. Reorganization of the actin cytoskeleton occurs in motile cells and this is regulated by the EGFR through the activation of PLCγ1, PI3K, and RHO family GTPases. Up-regulation of MMPs and uPAR through EGFR-stimulated activation of PI3K and/or COX-2 drives the proteolytic degradation of matrix proteins required for tumor cell invasion.

via the dephosphorylation of FAK and this was blocked by either an α2β1 integrin antibody or by gefitinib, a small molecule tyrosine kinase inhibitor of EGFR (23).

Growth factor-induced cell migration is distinct from migration induced by the ECM as the engagement of integrins activates FAK, SRC and PI3K and cells move as a coherent sheet with the integrity of cell-cell attachments maintained. In contrast, the ability to move individually appears to be a property of carcinoma cells in which cell-ECM and cell-cell contacts are disrupted following EGF-induced inactivation of FAK. These studies suggest that dynamic regulation of FAK leads to a fine balance with respect to the regulation of cell migration. EGF-mediated down-regulation of FAK is important for early dissemination phases, e.g., cell detachment from the primary tumor. At secondary sites, interaction with the extracellular matrix via integrins activates FAK and mediates the cell attachment required for establishment of a metastatic tumor.

Integrins can interact directly with EGFR to allow its phosphorylation by kinases such as SRC and thus its ligand-independent activation (24, 25). β1 integrin, in particular, is frequently complexed with EGFR (21, 26, 27) and links EGFR to the actin cytoskeleton. Expression is closely coordinated and reducing levels of either EGFR or β1 integrin in 3-D cultures of mammary epithelial cells modulates expression of the other. This effect was not reproducible in 2-D cultures showing that the consequences of EGFR-integrin communication are entirely context-dependent (28).

Similarly, alterations in ECM composition can change EGF-induced signaling. Mattila et al. (29) found that collagen but not fibronectin reduced EGF-induced EGFR phosphorylation through the recruitment of TCPTP (T-cell protein tyrosine phosphatase) to the cytoplasmic tail of α1β1 integrin in tumor cells. In cells lacking α1 integrin, ligand-induced EGFR phosphorylation was not attenuated, due to the absence of TCPTP in the protein complex, providing an elegant mechanism for adhesion-mediated regulation of EGF-driven signaling.

A mutant, truncated protein (EGFRvIII) is constitutively active and although it signals independently of soluble ligands such as EGF, recent work by Ning et al. (30) suggests that, in common with the full-length receptor, it interacts with integrins to regulate metastatic signaling pathways. Transfection of EGFRvIII into an ovarian cancer cell line impaired cell spreading and focal adhesions leading to a fibroblastic morphology via the reduction of α2 integrin expression. The authors suggest that this at least partially explains the more aggressive nature of ovarian cancers expressing EGFRvIII.

While β1 integrins link the EGFR to the actin cytoskeleton, α6β4 binds laminin 5 and links extracellular signals to the keratin cytoskeleton (19, 31). β4 has a uniquely large cytoplasmic domain allowing it to recruit multiple cytoplasmic signal transducers. α6β4 integrin is localized in the hemidesmosome junctions, which maintain stable adhesion between epithelial cells. The loss of hemidesmosomes (32) and overexpression of both EGFR and integrin α6β4 (31) have independently been linked with the invasive propensity of squamous cell carcinomas (SCC). EGFR associates with α6β4 in tumor cells and induces tyrosine phosphorylation of the β4 cytoplasmic domain via the SRC family kinase FYN, resulting in the disassembly of hemidesmosomes, an essential precursor for SCC invasion. Mariotti and colleagues also exogenously expressed a dominant-negative form of FYN to suppress in vitro and in vivo invasion, demonstrating the essential role of FYN in mediating EGFR-α6β4 integrin-mediated tumor progression.

A novel mechanism for the coordinated function of EGFR and integrins in tumor metastasis has recently been proposed by Yan and Shao (33). Periostin, a secretory protein normally found in osteoblasts, binds to αVβ5 and is required for the interaction of this integrin with EGFR to promote tumor cell migration and invasion. The authors demonstrated that the periostin-induced association of αVβ5 and EGFR results in increased expression of matrix metalloproteinase (MMP)-9, vimentin and fibronectin and that this is responsible for the invasive phenotype in EGFR and periostin co-overexpressing tumor cells.

2.1.2. E-cadherin and Cell-cell Interactions

EGFR activation results not only in the break-up of tumor cell-extracellular matrix interactions but also in the disruption of cell-cell junctions, facilitating epithelial-to-mesenchymal transition and tumor cell migration. The rapid dissolution of intercellular adhesions is an early step in metastasis involving loss of cadherin function. Cadherins mediate homophilic adhesion interactions between cells (34). Loss of E-cadherin has been observed in highly invasive human tumor cells (*35–38*) and its re-expression can reverse the invasive phenotype (*39, 40*) and restore epithelial morphology (*41, 42*).

The down-regulation of E-cadherin in invasive tumors is regulated by the phosphorylation and dephosphorylation of catenins. β-catenin, γ-catenin (plakoglobin) and p120^{CAS} each associate with the cytoplasmic tail of E-cadherin and are regulated by RTK-mediated phosphorylation. β- and γ-catenin also link cadherins to the actin cytoskeleton via α-catenin thus furnishing a role for cadherins in both adhesive and migratory aspects of tumor cell invasion. Stimulation with EGF or overexpression of EGFR in cancer cells causes down-regulation of E-cadherin-mediated adhesion correlating with the increased phosphorylation of β-catenin (*43*). This impairment of E-cadherin-dependent adhesion can occur via alternative mechanisms depending on the duration of the EGF signal. First, caveolin-mediates the endocytosis of E-cadherin and β-catenin resulting in the redistribution rather than degradation of E-cadherin following transient exposure (hours) to EGF. Secondly, there is a down-regulation of E-cadherin expression at the transcriptional level possibly through the induction of the transcriptional repressor SNAIL following chronic exposure (days) to EGF (*44*). For further discussion on the cross-talk between E-cadherin and EGFR refer to Chapter 10.

2.2. Motility

It has been proposed that tumor invasion reflects a dysregulation of cell motility (*45, 46*). A role for EGFR in driving motogenic pathways in normal cells and cancer cells has been well defined (*47–51*). Indeed, transfection of the constitutively active mutant, EGFRvIII, into fibroblasts increased their motility. This observation reinforces the importance of EGFR-driven motility in tumor progression (*52*). It was initially suggested that the motility and mitogenic signaling pathways downstream of EGFR were separable (*49*). There is clearly overlap and cross-talk between the various pathways (*52, 53*), however. Some of the key players acting downstream of EGFR to regulate migration and thus invasion of cancer cells are described below.

2.2.1. PHOSPHOLIPASE C GAMMA1 (PLCγ1)

Autophosphorylation of EGFR is essential for the generation of a motile phenotype as it allows for recruitment of PLCγ1 (*54*). Both pharmacological and genetic approaches have demonstrated that PLCγ1 activity is essential for EGFR-mediated cell motility (*49*) and tumor invasion in vitro and in vivo (*55–58*).

PLCγ1 has been implicated in regulation of the early stages of cell motility (*59*). Direct visualization of events following EGF stimulation revealed that phosphoinositol 4,5-bisphosphate (PIP$_2$) hydrolysis occurs predominantly at the leading edge of cells, which results in the redistribution of the PIP$_2$-binding, actin regulatory proteins, cofilin and gelsolin to the submembranous cytoskeleton where initial actin polymerization gives rise to lamellipod extension (*60, 61*). Other actin-modifying proteins that may become activated following PIP$_2$ hydrolysis include vinculin, talin and α-actinin (*62, 63*). Proteins activated further down the PLCγ1 signaling cascade, for example protein kinase C (PKC) enzymes, may also contribute to the motility response (*64*).

2.2.2. MITOGEN-ACTIVATED PROTEIN KINASE (MAPK)

Early work indicated that MAPK activity alone was insufficient for EGF-stimulated cell migration (*49*). Subsequent studies, however, demonstrated that MAPK contributes to growth factor-induced motility of tumor cells (*65, 66*). The magnitude and duration of MAPK activation, partially influenced by the level of EGFR expression, is thought to determine the involvement of MAPK (ERK1/2) in early and late stages of cell migration (*53*). MAPK can interact with the cytoskeletal machinery by phosphorylating myosin light chain kinase that, in turn, phosphorylates myosin light chains to generate the tractional force required to move the cell forward (*67*).

2.2.3. PHOSPHOINOSITIDE 3-KINASE (PI3K)

PI3Ks have a long-established role in the regulation of cell motility based on extensive studies monitoring leukocyte and *Dictyostelium* chemotaxis (*68*). PI3Ks also regulate EGF-driven motility and invasion of glioma, breast, and bladder cancer cell lines in vitro (*69–73*).

Rapid localized accumulation of phosphoinositol 3,4,5-trisphosphate (PIP_3), a product of class I PI3Ks, at the leading edge of motile cells forms part of the asymmetry required for directional movement (*74*). This is consistent with the role of the p85-p110α PI3K isoform in orchestrating the localized actin polymerization and lamellipod extension in response to EGF (*75*). The phosphatase PTEN antagonizes the action of PI3K by locally depleting levels of PIP_3 (*74*). PTEN is a major tumor suppressor whose loss frequently correlates with more aggressive phenotypes, indicating that it contributes to tumor cell invasion (*76, 77*). Consistent with this, restoration of wild-type PTEN expression in thyroid carcinoma and glioma cells was found to inhibit EGFR driven migration and invasion (*78, 79*).

2.2.4. RHO FAMILY GTPASES

RHO family GTPases provide one link between PI3K activity and the cytoskeleton as RHO family GEFs (guanine nucleotide exchange factors) can bind to PI3K lipid products via their PH domains (*80*). VAV2, a ubiquitously expressed GEF, is activated downstream of EGFR leading to the activation of RHO GTPases: RAC, CDC42 and RHO-A (*81–83*). RAC and CDC42 act at the front of migrating cells to coordinate actin polymerization necessary for lamellipodia and filopodia extension respectively (*84, 85*). A positive feedback loop exists between RAC and PI3K to reinforce the production of further PIP_3 (*86*). In addition, the EGF-mediated association between CDC42 and PLCγ1 is thought to facilitate PLCγ1's role in establishing cell polarity and directional movement (*87*). RHO promotes contractile actin:myosin filament assembly within the cell body necessary to translocate the cell forward (*85*).

Aberrant regulation of RHO family proteins is found in several cancers supporting the notion that they contribute to tumor cell motility and invasion (*88*). In addition, activation of RHO and CDC42 can feed back at the level of the EGFR to regulate cell motility responses as demonstrated in breast cancer cells (*89, 90*).

2.2.5. CYTOSKELETAL REGULATORS

Active RHO GTPases couple to downstream effectors, including p160 ROCK, p65 PAK, LIM kinase, and the WASP/SCAR/WAVE family of proteins that ultimately converge on the machinery that orchestrates cell movement. Two key actin regulators, cofilin and the ARP2/3 complex, function synergistically at the cytoskeleton to coordinate the remodeling activity necessary for cell locomotion (*91, 92*). Both are recruited to the cell's leading edge in response to EGF stimulation where they cause localized actin polymerization through their actin-severing and nucleating activities, respectively (*93–95*).

Cofilin, ARP2/3 and their upstream regulators LIM kinase and the WASP family are overexpressed in a variety of cancers and in an invasive subpopulation of breast cancer cells, highlighting their role in the regulation of cancer cell migration and invasion (*96, 97*). In addition, inhibition of N-WASP, ARP2/3 or cofilin prevents the EGF-driven formation of functional invadopodia (specialized membrane protrusions with extracellular protease activity) and invasion of metastatic cancer cells in vitro (*98*).

2.2.6. TRANSCRIPTIONAL REGULATORS

In addition to direct cytoskeletal regulation, signals from EGFR may act at the level of gene expression to effect tumor invasion responses, since inhibition of transcriptional regulators such as c-JUN and STAT3 downstream of EGFR blocks migration and invasion of cancer cells in vitro (*65, 99, 100*). In particular, EGFR regulation of proteases required for ECM degradation occurs at the transcriptional level (*101, 102*).

2.3. Proteolysis

Proteolysis forms an integral part of tumor cell invasion at several levels. It is required for destruction of physical ECM components that act as barriers to invasion including collagens, laminins, and fibronectin. It also leads to remodeling of intercellular or cell-ECM adhesive interactions, for example through cleavage of E-cadherin and CD44 (*103, 104*). Two major systems orchestrate tumor-associated proteolysis: the MMP/ADAMALYSIN family and the urokinase plasminogen activator (uPA) system. Two-way regulation occurs between EGFR and both these types of protease activity in the context of tumor invasion.

2.3.1. MATRIX METALLO PROTEINASES (MMPs)

Robust experimental and clinical data support a role for MMPs in the promotion of tumor invasion and metastasis (*105*). Consistent with a role for EGFR in regulating MMPs, strong correlations exist between EGFR overexpression, MMP levels/activity and enhanced tumor invasion in vitro and in vivo (*106, 107*). In addition, MMP inhibitors block EGF-driven invasion of carcinoma cell lines (*108*).

EGFR signaling up-regulates transcription of several members of the MMP family (MMP-1, MMP-7, MMP-9, MMP-10, MMP-13, and MMP-14) in a variety of tumor types, including glioma, SCCHN, pancreatic, and bladder cancers (*101, 106, 109–111*). EGFR inhibition strategies that block MMP expression also reduce cell invasion in vitro indicating that MMP production is an active mechanism by which EGFR drives tumor invasion (*106, 111*). EGFR ligands, including EGF, TGF α, amphiregulin and betacellulin regulate MMP expression differently by utilizing signaling intermediates such as PI3K, described above in the context of tumor cell migration (*106, 112, 113*). EGFR regulation of MMP activity can also occur through enzyme localization to the plasma membrane; for example, enhanced association of MMP-9 with the cell surface in response to EGF stimulation is associated with ovarian cancer cell invasion (*114*).

EGFR-mediated release of interleukins, interferons and growth factors from tumor cells may enhance tumor associated MMP activity in a more indirect way through the recruitment of inflammatory cells, a major source of MMPs (*14*). MMPs can also feed back at the level of EGFR signaling as their proteolytic activity can release and activate matrix- or membrane-bound precursor forms of EGF-like ligands (*115*).

2.3.2. UROKINASE PLASMINOGEN ACTIVATOR (uPA)

uPA is a well-characterized tumor-associated protease that displays enhanced proteolytic activity when bound to its cell surface receptor uPAR. Overexpression of uPA and uPAR correlates positively with invasive potential in a variety of cancers (*116*).

Microarray analyses have revealed that EGFR signaling induces uPAR transcription (*102, 117*). Consistent with this finding, increased levels of cell-associated uPAR and release of uPA into conditioned medium have been reported in EGF-treated tumor cells (*118, 119*). A role for uPAR:uPA in driving EGFR-mediated invasion is supported by the fact that expression of a uPAR antisense construct significantly inhibited in vitro invasion of prostate cancer cells and reduced the aggressiveness of tumor xenografts (*102*). As for MMPs, regulation can also occur at the level of cell surface expression and increased expression of uPAR in response to EGF stimulation is enhanced through decreased internalization and degradation of the uPA:uPAR complex (*119*).

Further cross-talk exists between EGFR and uPAR as intracellular signaling downstream of uPAR ligation occurs, in part, via EGFR transactivation (*120*). In support of this, EGFR inhibition blocks uPAR-associated migration, invasion and growth of tumors in mice (*121–123*). It has recently been suggested that uPAR and EGFR are engaged in the same multi-protein assembly on the cell surface thought to include integrins, such as α5β1, involved in EGFR activation by uPAR stimulation (*119, 122*).

2.4. COX-2 and Prostaglandins

The interaction of cyclooxygenase-2 (COX-2) with the EGFR is discussed in detail in Chapter 21 and we therefore include only a brief description of this relationship in the context of invasion here.

COX-2 catalyses the synthesis of prostaglandins, such as prostaglandin E_2 (PGE_2), mediators of inflammation which can also affect several aspects of tumorigenesis, including apoptosis/cell survival, angiogenesis, and invasion. The overexpression of COX-2 has been found to increase the metastatic potential of colorectal carcinoma cells through the increased activation of MMP-2 and the increased expression of membrane-type MMP-1 (*124*). The invasive phenotype of non-small cell lung cancer (NSCLC) cell lines was found to be due to COX-2-mediated up-regulation of CD44, an adhesive receptor for the extracellular matrix component hyaluronate (*125*).

Activation of EGFR up-regulates COX-2 expression in certain human tumor cells, most notably in SCCHN where overexpression of the EGFR is associated with a highly invasive phenotype. A reciprocal relationship exists as COX-2 can induce the expression and/or activation of EGFR via the production of PGE_2 (*126*). Treatment of colon cancer cells with a small molecule inhibitor of SRC blocked PGE_2-induced phosphorylation of EGFR and attenuated migration and invasion, implicating SRC as a key mediator of EGFR-COX-2 crosstalk.

One mechanism that might explain the synergistic effect of EGFR and COX-2 on tumor invasion has been proposed by Mann and colleagues (*127*). Once synthesized by COX-2, PGE_2 is inactivated by the enzyme PGDH (prostaglandin dehydrogenase). The authors demonstrate that EGF induces the transcriptional repressor SNAIL via activation of the RAS/MAPK pathway. SNAIL then binds to the promoter of PGDH and represses its expression so promoting PGE_2 activity and tumor progression. In concordance with this, treatment of tumor cell lines with the EGFR inhibitor erlotinib reversed this effect of EGF. Additional evidence arises from APC^{min} mice, which spontaneously develop preinvasive adenomas similar to the human familial adenomatous polyposis coli syndrome. The tumors lack PGDH expression and have elevated levels of EGFR. Treatment of mice with erlotinib induced PGDH production and reduced SNAIL, PGE_2, and COX-2 levels. It remains to be shown if this mechanism exists in human tumors, although PGDH and SNAIL expression analyzed by immunohistochemistry correlated inversely in matched pairs of normal tissue and colorectal carcinoma (*127*).

3. ANGIOGENESIS AND LYMPHANGIOGENESIS

The development of a blood supply is essential to sustain growing tumors and also acts as a conduit for hematogenous dissemination and metastasis. What is more, there is increasing evidence that a parallel process, lymphangiogenesis, may in some cancers contribute to spread via the lymphatics (*128*). However, clear evidence for intratumoral lymphatics is limited to certain tumor types (e.g., SCCHN, gastric cancer, and melanoma (*129–131*)) and it may be that tumor-derived lymphangiogenic cytokines serve rather to stimulate expansion of peritumoral vessels and thus facilitate access of motile tumor cells.

3.1. EGFR-mediated Regulation of Angiogenic Cytokines

In experimental systems, overexpression or activation of EGFR (and other ERB-B receptors) has been shown to regulate the transcription of genes encoding key angiogenic (VEGF-A, bFGF, IL-8) and lymphangiogenic (VEGF-C or, less frequently, VEGF-D) cytokines in many tumor cell types. For example, stimulation of SCCHN cells in vitro with EGF, heregulin or betacellulin up-regulated VEGF-C and VEGF-A secretion and this was blocked by treatment with anti-EGFR antibody (ICR62) (*132*). Similar observations have been made in glioma (*133*), prostate (*134*), gastric (*135*) and breast carcinoma cells (*136*). These studies have used a variety of stimulatory ligands (EGF, TGFα, HB-EGF) and EGFR antagonists. The latter included antibodies such as C225 (the forerunner of cetuximab) (*136*), small molecule inhibitors gefitinib (*137*) or erlotinib (*138*) and ERRP, a naturally occurring negative regulator of EGFR, which also prevented HCT116 colon carcinoma cell invasion via inhibition of FAK, MEK, and RAC activation (*139*).

The signaling pathways by which activated EGFR induces angiogenic cytokine expression (see Fig. 18.2 for summary) have been explored in several tumor cell systems.

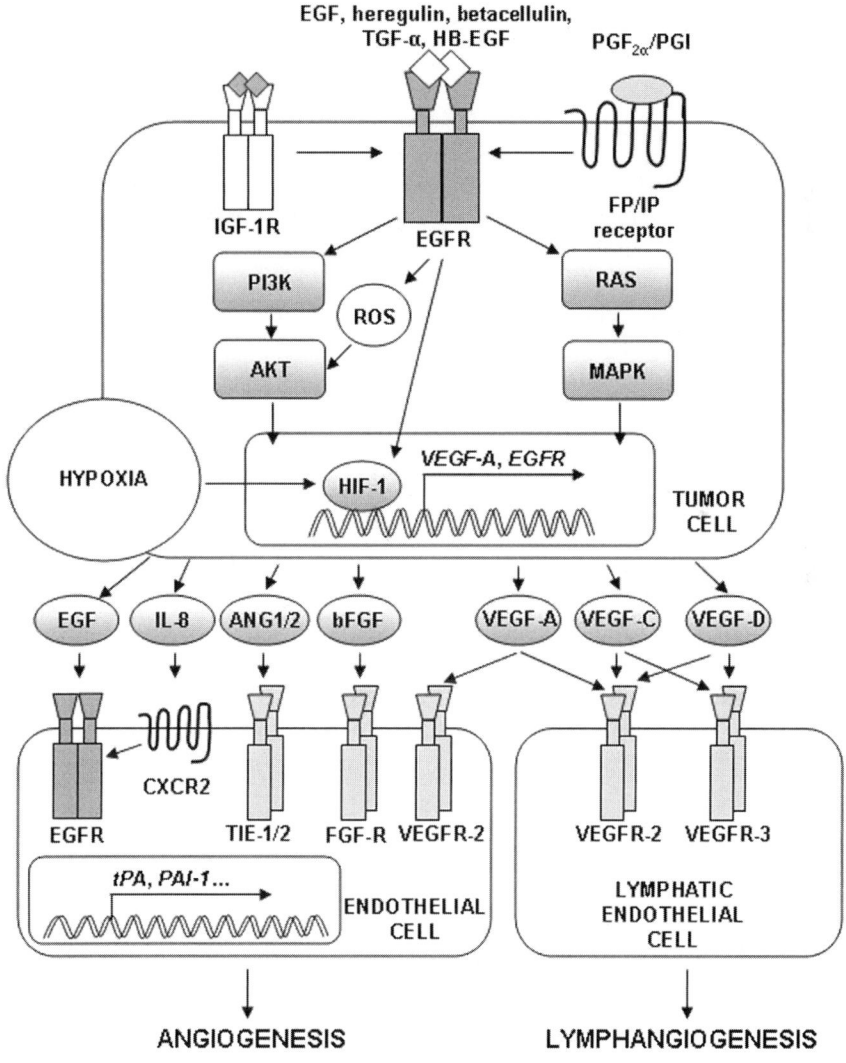

Fig. 18.2. EGFR signaling in tumor cells promotes tumor–associated angiogenesis and lymphangiogenesis by increasing the expression of a variety of angiogenic and lymphangiogenic cytokines. In addition, EGFR signaling can up-regulate HIF-1 and potentiate the effects of hypoxia on production of angiogenic factors. EGF is itself an angiogenic growth factor that can bind directly to EGFR on endothelial cells and promote angiogenesis.

It is generally accepted that the RAS-MAPK and/or PI3K-AKT pathways are central to EGFR-mediated VEGF-A up-regulation in most cell types, but only the former has been consistently linked with VEGF-C induction. P38 MAPK seems to participate in VEGF-A or VEGF-C regulation in some cell types (*135*). In glioma cells (and others in which the tumor suppressor PTEN is inactivated), the resulting hyperactivation of the PI3K pathway can cooperate with EGFR activation by transcriptionally up-regulating the proximal VEGF-A promoter; introduction of functional PTEN, or dominant negative AKT reduced VEGF-A transcription (*140*).

EGFR also cooperates with other RTKs (such as IGF-1R) and also receptors for prostanoids to up-regulate angiogenic cytokines. For example, both prostaglandin $F_2\alpha$ via the FP receptor and prostacyclin via the IP receptor transphosphorylate EGFR and thus induce VEGF-A, bFGF and angiopoietins via ERK/MEK activation in endometrial carcinoma cells (*141, 142*) and gastric carcinoma cells (*143*). PGE_2 has also been shown to stimulate VEGF expression in endothelial cells (EC) via ERK2/JNK1 signaling pathways (*144*).

Hypoxia is also a key regulator of VEGF-A via the transcription factor hypoxia inducible factor (HIF), which binds to hypoxia response elements (HRE) in the VEGF-A promoter. EGFR can up-regulate VEGF-A via both HIF-dependent and independent mechanisms and may well cooperate with hypoxia to induce angiogenesis in vivo. Inhibition of EGFR or PI3K did not completely abolish VEGF-A induction by hypoxia in glioma cells and EGF was still able to activate VEGF-A transcription in constructs lacking HREs (*145*). Both pathways were partially dependent on PI3K activity, but other signaling mechanisms were also implicated. A reciprocal relationship between tumor hypoxia and EGFR has been suggested in NSCLC, since hypoxia may induce expression of EGFR and its ligands, whereas EGFR activation up-regulates HIF-1 which acts as a survival factor for hypoxic cells (*146*). These relationships may also be important in UVB irradiated skin carcinogenesis, since EGFR activation, HIF-1α /VEGF expression and the PI3K pathway are again tightly linked (*147*). Interestingly, in transfected 3T3 fibroblasts, mutant EGFRvIII, while inducing the same levels of secreted VEGF-A as wild-type EGFR under normoxic conditions, generated much higher levels of VEGF-A in hypoxia. This hypoxic enhancement was PI3K-dependent (*148*).

EGFR activation in ovarian carcinoma cells has been shown to increase reactive oxygen species (ROS; e.g., H_2O_2), leading to activation of the AKT/p70S6K pathway and thus VEGF-A transcription. In this system, EGF-induced VEGF expression was prevented by catalase (an H_2O_2 scavenger) and rapamycin (an mTOR inhibitor) and involved HIF-1α induction (*11*).

3.2. EGFR Signaling in Endothelial Cells (EC)

EGFR is also expressed on endothelial cells and can be directly influenced by ligands produced in the tumor environment and by inhibitors designed primarily to target tumor cells (Fig. 18.2). EC in xenograft tumors producing high levels of EGF or TGFα expressed activated EGFR and were particularly sensitive to apoptosis induced by EGFR inhibitors (*149*). In hepatocellular carcinoma, betacellulin was predominantly expressed by the tumor cells, but EGFR was localized to sinusoidal EC, again offering opportunities for paracrine stimulation (*150*). HB-EGF and EGF activated EGFR and thus the plasminogen activator system and tubulogenesis in human microvascular EC in vitro (*151*). Both glioma cells and cerebral microvascular endothelial cells responded chemotactically to several tumor-derived ligands, including EGF and TGFα (*152*). Also, IL-8 mediated EC migration was shown to depend on transactivation of EGFR by the IL-8 receptor, CXCR2 (*153*).

4. METASTASIS

EGFR may contribute to metastasis, as indicated in the above sections, by up-regulation of tumor cell motility and expression of several families of proteases, thus potentiating invasion of surrounding tissues and access to vascular channels. EGFR-induced angiogenic and lymphangiogenic cytokines may also increase the number of vessels in and around tumors and enhance their permeability. All of these mechanisms combine to increase the probability of dissemination to lymph nodes and distant organs. There is also the possibility that EGFR may contribute to patterns of metastasis by tumor cells responding to high local ligand concentrations by chemomigration or enhanced survival in specific sites. For example, it has been suggested that tumor cells overexpressing EGFR have a predilection for metastasis to liver, where there are high concentrations of TGFα (*154*). Similarly, EGFR overexpression is associated with increased risk of breast cancer metastasis to brain (*155*), and high grade gliomas also express high levels of EGFR and one or more ligands (*156*). Thus, in the brain there may be opportunities for autocrine, juxtacrine, and paracrine EGFR activation, which could become ligand-independent in the case of expression of the EGFRvIII mutant. A further example is advanced ovarian carcinoma, where high HB-EGF expression is correlated with ADAM-17 (the protease which releases it from sequestration) and this may be linked to LPA-mediated EGFR transactivation in this disease (*157*).

5. CLINICAL OBSERVATIONS

EGFR expression is reportedly strongly associated with tumor cell invasion, lymph node metastasis and hence more advanced tumor stage in multiple tumor types.

An inverse relationship between EGFR expression and intercellular adhesion has been found to correlate with metastasis in clinical samples. The loss of membrane-bound E-cadherin was found to coincide with increased EGFR immunohistochemical staining and the presence of lymph node metastasis in breast cancer (*158*). Similarly, a reduction in membrane expression of the E-cadherin regulator β-catenin was found to associate with EGFR expression and a more invasive phenotype in oral cancer (*159*).

Up-regulation of EGFR and/or other ERB-B family members is associated with higher levels of MMPs, which are fundamental to tumor progression and invasion (*160–163*). Also, EGFR levels correlate with VEGF-A and/or VEGF-C expression (*164*) and in some cases with intratumoral microvessel density (MVD) (*9, 165*). HIF-1 was positively associated with EGFR levels, MVD and levels of angiogenic cytokines bFGF and PDGF-BB in invasive breast cancer (*166*). Correlative studies have clearly illustrated the clinical significance of these observations. For example, in colorectal carcinoma, increased expression of VEGF-A was associated with lymphatic metastases (*167*) and in NSCLC with early tumor relapse and shorter patient survival (*168, 169*). Higher levels of other EGFR-regulated angiogenic growth factors (e.g., bFGF and IL-8) correlated significantly with a shorter time to local relapse in SCCHN (*170*), and poor patient survival in breast (*171*) and ovarian cancers (*172*), respectively.

6. THERAPEUTIC OPPORTUNITIES

Clear evidence of anti-angiogenic effects of EGFR antagonists has been observed in preclinical xenograft models (*173*) and reviewed in (*174*). Gefitinib has been shown to exert both indirect anti-angiogenic effects (by down-regulation of angiogenic cytokines such as VEGF, IL-8, bFGF and COX-2) and direct effects by targeting EGFR expressing EC (*137*).

With the relatively recent development of small molecule inhibitors of both COX-2 and the EGFR, this close relationship in regulating carcinoma invasion is beginning to be exploited for therapeutic purposes. Based upon the functions of COX-2 and EGFR in regulating tumor cell invasion, clinical trials are planned with combined drugs as chemopreventative agents to stem the malignant progression of early stage lesions (*126*).

In several experimental models acquired resistance to anti-EGFR antibodies was related to up-regulated VEGF (and in one case also COX-2 and activated MAPK) resulting in enhanced angiogenesis (*175, 176*). It has thus been suggested that simultaneous inhibition of EGFR and VEGFR signaling pathways may offer therapeutic advantages (*177–179*). This has been achieved by a combination of blocking antibodies, pharmacological agents (erlotinib, gefitinib, sorafenib) or, more recently, by dual specificity kinase inhibitors such as ZD6474 (AstraZeneca) and AEE788 (Novartis). ZD6474 prevented (and reversed) the resistance seen in erbitux or gefitinib treated colon carcinoma xenografts (*175*). Early clinical trials have also combined erlotinib with an anti-VEGF antibody, bevacizumab (*180*).

Other potentially interesting combinations include gefitinib plus camptothecin (a topoisomerase 1 inhibitor) in gastric carcinomas. SN38 (the active metabolite of camptothecin) activates EGFR and induces expression of HB-EGF, amphiregulin, TGFα and IL-8 via ROS and PKC, followed by MMP activation and release of ligands, which potentially stimulate tumor cells and EC via autocrine and paracrine mechanisms. It has been suggested that gefitinib could overcome all of these undesirable potential resistance mechanisms induced by camptothecin (*181*) or similar EGFR-dependent MAPK activation induced in tumor cells and EC by irradiation (*182*).

In summary, this chapter focuses on the central role played by the EGFR in promoting tumor invasion and metastasis. EGFR regulation of processes including cell adhesion, motility, proteolysis, and angiogenesis relies on its interaction with a plethora of key molecular players detailed above. Our understanding of EGFR biology in cancer progression raises the possibility that EGFR antagonists will be effective against advanced stage disease and highlights the potential for exploiting key molecular interactions in the development of more effective combinatorial therapeutic strategies.

REFERENCES

1. Salomon DS, Brandt R, Ciardiello F, Normanno N. Epidermal growth factor-related peptides and their receptors in human malignancies. Crit Rev Oncol Hematol 1995;19:183-232.
2. Dassonville O, Formento JL, Francoual M, et al. Expression of epidermal growth factor receptor and survival in upper aerodigestive tract cancer. J Clin Oncol 1993;11:1873-8.
3. Nicholson RI, Gee JM, Harper ME. EGFR and cancer prognosis. Eur J Cancer 2001;37 Suppl 4:S9-15.
4. Imai Y, Leung CK, Friesen HG, Shiu RP. Epidermal growth factor receptors and effect of epidermal growth factor on growth of human breast cancer cells in long-term tissue culture. Cancer Res 1982;42:4394-8.
5. Lin J, Adam RM, Santiestevan E, Freeman MR. The phosphatidylinositol 3′-kinase pathway is a dominant growth factor-activated cell survival pathway in LNCaP human prostate carcinoma cells. Cancer Res 1999;59:2891-7.
6. Westermark B, Magnusson A, Heldin CH. Effect of epidermal growth factor on membrane motility and cell locomotion in cultures of human clonal glioma cells. J Neurosci Res 1982;8:491-507.
7. Lund-Johansen M, Bjerkvig R, Humphrey PA, Bigner SH, Bigner DD, Laerum OD. Effect of epidermal growth factor on glioma cell growth, migration, and invasion in vitro. Cancer Res 1990;50:6039-44.
8. Sainsbury JR, Farndon JR, Needham GK, Malcolm AJ, Harris AL. Epidermal-growth-factor receptor status as predictor of early recurrence of and death from breast cancer. Lancet 1987;1:1398-402.
9. de Jong JS, van Diest PJ, van der Valk P, Baak JP. Expression of growth factors, growth-inhibiting factors, and their receptors in invasive breast cancer. II: Correlations with proliferation and angiogenesis. J Pathol 1998;184:53-7.
10. Price J, Wilson HM, Haites, NE. Epidermal growth factor (EGF) increases the in vitro invasion, motility and adhesion interactions of the primary renal cell carcinoma cell line, A704. Eur J Cancer 1996;32A:1977-82.

11. Liu LZ, Hu XW, Xia C, et al. Reactive oxygen species regulate epidermal growth factor-induced vascular endothelial growth factor and hypoxia-inducible factor-1alpha expression through activation of AKT and P70S6K1 in human ovarian cancer cells. Free Radic Biol Med 2006;41:1521-33.
12. Damstrup L, Rude Voldborg B, Spang-Thomsen M, Brunner N, Skovgaard Poulsen H. In vitro invasion of small-cell lung cancer cell lines correlates with expression of epidermal growth factor receptor. Br J Cancer 1998;78:631-40.
13. Condeelis J SJ. Intravital imaging of cell movement in tumours. Nat Rev Cancer 2003;3:921-30.
14. Wyckoff J, Wang W, Lin EY, et al. A paracrine loop between tumor cells and macrophages is required for tumor cell migration in mammary tumors. Cancer Res 2004;64:7022-9.
15. Xue C, Wyckoff J, Liang F, et al. Epidermal growth factor receptor overexpression results in increased tumor cell motility in vivo coordinately with enhanced intravasation and metastasis. Cancer Res 2006;66:192-7.
16. Wyckoff J. The collection of the motile population of cells from a living tumour. Cancer Res 2000;60:5401-4.
17. Wyckoff J. A critical step in metastasis: in vivo analysis of intravasation at the primary tumor. Cancer Res 2000;60:2504-11.
18. Goswami S, Sahai E, Wyckoff JB, et al. Macrophages promote the invasion of breast carcinoma cells via a colony-stimulating factor-1/epidermal growth factor paracrine loop. Cancer Res 2005;65:5278-83.
19. Hynes RO, Lively JC, McCarty JH, et al. The diverse roles of integrins and their ligands in angiogenesis. Cold Spring Harb Symp Quant Biol 2002;67:143-53.
20. Guo W, Giancotti FG. Integrin signalling during tumour progression. Nat Rev Mol Cell Biol 2004;5:816-26.
21. Sieg DJ, Hauck CR, Ilic D, et al. FAK integrates growth-factor and integrin signals to promote cell migration. Nat Cell Biol 2000;2:249-56.
22. Lu Z, Jiang G, Blume-Jensen P, Hunter T. Epidermal growth factor-induced tumor cell invasion and metastasis initiated by dephosphorylation and downregulation of focal adhesion kinase. Mol Cell Biol 2001;21:4016-31.
23. Yamanaka I, Koizumi M, Baba T, Yamashita S, Suzuki T, Kudo R. Epidermal growth factor increased the expression of alpha2beta1-integrin and modulated integrin-mediated signaling in human cervical adenocarcinoma cells. Exp Cell Res 2003;286:165-74.
24. Moro L, Venturino M, Bozzo C, et al. Integrins induce activation of EGF receptor: role in MAP kinase induction and adhesion-dependent cell survival. Embo J 1998;17:6622-32.
25. Cabodi S, Moro L, Bergatto E, et al. Integrin regulation of epidermal growth factor (EGF) receptor and of EGF-dependent responses. Biochem Soc Trans 2004;32:438-42.
26. Miyamoto S, Teramoto H, Gutkind JS, Yamada KM. Integrins can collaborate with growth factors for phosphorylation of receptor tyrosine kinases and MAP kinase activation: roles of integrin aggregation and occupancy of receptors. J Cell Biol 1996;135:1633-42.
27. Yu X, Miyamoto S, Mekada E. Integrin alpha 2 beta 1-dependent EGF receptor activation at cell-cell contact sites. J Cell Sci 2000;113 (Pt 12):2139-47.
28. Wang F, Weaver VM, Petersen OW, et al. Reciprocal interactions between beta1-integrin and epidermal growth factor receptor in three-dimensional basement membrane breast cultures: a different perspective in epithelial biology. Proc Natl Acad Sci USA 1998;95:14821-6.
29. Mattila E, Pellinen T, Nevo J, Vuoriluoto K, Arjonen A, Ivaska J. Negative regulation of EGFR signalling through integrin-alpha1beta1-mediated activation of protein tyrosine phosphatase TCPTP. Nat Cell Biol 2005;7:78-85.
30. Ning Y, Zeineldin R, Liu Y, Rosenberg M, Stack MS, Hudson LG. Down-regulation of integrin alpha2 surface expression by mutant epidermal growth factor receptor (EGFRvIII) induces aberrant cell spreading and focal adhesion formation. Cancer Res 2005;65:9280-6.
31. Mariotti A, Kedeshian PA, Dans M, Curatola AM, Gagnoux-Palacios L, Giancotti FG. EGF-R signaling through Fyn kinase disrupts the function of integrin alpha6beta4 at hemidesmosomes: role in epithelial cell migration and carcinoma invasion. J Cell Biol 2001;155:447-58.
32. Schenk P. The fate of hemidesmosomes in laryngeal carcinoma. Arch Otorhinolaryngol 1979;222:187-98.
33. Yan W, Shao R. Transduction of a mesenchyme-specific gene periostin into 293T cells induces cell invasive activity through epithelial-mesenchymal transformation. J Biol Chem 2006;281:19700-8.

34. Lilien J, Balsamo J. The regulation of cadherin-mediated adhesion by tyrosine phosphorylation/dephosphorylation of beta-catenin. Curr Opin Cell Biol 2005;17:459-65.
35. Behrens J, Mareel MM, Van Roy FM, Birchmeier W. Dissecting tumor cell invasion: epithelial cells acquire invasive properties after the loss of uvomorulin-mediated cell-cell adhesion. J Cell Biol 1989;108:2435-47.
36. Birchmeier W, Behrens J. Cadherin expression in carcinomas: role in the formation of cell junctions and the prevention of invasiveness. Biochim Biophys Acta 1994;1198:11-26.
37. Pignatelli M, Ansari TW, Gunter P, et al. Loss of membranous E-cadherin expression in pancreatic cancer: correlation with lymph node metastasis, high grade, and advanced stage. J Pathol 1994;174:243-8.
38. Sommers CL, Thompson EW, Torri JA, Kemler R, Gelmann EP, Byers SW. Cell adhesion molecule uvomorulin expression in human breast cancer cell lines: relationship to morphology and invasive capacities. Cell Growth Differ 1991;2:365-72.
39. Frixen UH, Behrens J, Sachs M, et al. E-cadherin-mediated cell-cell adhesion prevents invasiveness of human carcinoma cells. J Cell Biol 1991;113:173-85.
40. Vleminckx K, Vakaet L, Jr., Mareel M, Fiers W, van Roy F. Genetic manipulation of E-cadherin expression by epithelial tumor cells reveals an invasion suppressor role. Cell 1991;66:107-19.
41. Hajra KM, Fearon ER. Cadherin and catenin alterations in human cancer. Genes Chromosomes Cancer 2002;34:255-68.
42. Perl AK, Wilgenbus P, Dahl U, Semb H, Christofori G. A causal role for E-cadherin in the transition from adenoma to carcinoma. Nature 1998;392:190-3.
43. Lilien J, Balsamo J, Arregui C, Xu G. Turn-off, drop-out: functional state switching of cadherins. Dev Dyn 2002;224:18-29.
44. Lu Z, Ghosh S, Wang Z, Hunter T. Downregulation of caveolin-1 function by EGF leads to the loss of E-cadherin, increased transcriptional activity of beta-catenin, and enhanced tumor cell invasion. Cancer Cell 2003;4:499-515.
45. Wells A. Tumor invasion: role of growth factor-induced cell motility. Adv Cancer Res 2000;78:31-101.
46. Wells A, Kassis J, Solava J, Turner T, Lauffenburger DA. Growth factor-induced cell motility in tumor invasion. Acta Oncol 2002;41:124-30.
47. Blay J, Brown KD. Epidermal growth factor promotes the chemotactic migration of cultured rat intestinal epithelial cells. J Cell Physiol 1985;124:107-12.
48. Brandt BH, Roetger A, Dittmar T, et al. c-erbB-2/EGFR as dominant heterodimerization partners determine a motogenic phenotype in human breast cancer cells. Faseb J 1999;13:1939-49.
49. Chen P, Gupta K, Wells A. Cell movement elicited by epidermal growth factor receptor requires kinase and autophosphorylation but is separable from mitogenesis. J Cell Biol 1994;124:547-55.
50. Dittmar T, Husemann A, Schewe Y, et al. Induction of cancer cell migration by epidermal growth factor is initiated by specific phosphorylation of tyrosine 1248 of c-erbB-2 receptor via EGFR. Faseb J 2002;16:1823-5.
51. Hudson LG, McCawley LJ. Contributions of the epidermal growth factor receptor to keratinocyte motility. Microsc Res Tech 1998;43:444-55.
52. Pedersen MW, Tkach V, Pedersen N, Berezin V, Poulsen HS. Expression of a naturally occurring constitutively active variant of the epidermal growth factor receptor in mouse fibroblasts increases motility. Int J Cancer 2004;108:643-53.
53. Kruger JS, Reddy KB. Distinct mechanisms mediate the initial and sustained phases of cell migration in epidermal growth factor receptor-overexpressing cells. Mol Cancer Res 2003;1:801-9.
54. Chen P, Xie H, Sekar MC, Gupta K, Wells A. Epidermal growth factor receptor-mediated cell motility: phospholipase C activity is required, but mitogen-activated protein kinase activity is not sufficient for induced cell movement. J Cell Biol 1994;127:847-57.
55. Xie H, Turner T, Wang MH, Singh RK, Siegal GP, Wells A. In vitro invasiveness of DU-145 human prostate carcinoma cells is modulated by EGF receptor-mediated signals. Clin Exp Metastasis 1995;13:407-19.
56. Kassis J, Moellinger J, Lo H, Greenberg NM, Kim HG, Wells A. A role for phospholipase C-gamma-mediated signaling in tumor cell invasion. Clin Cancer Res 1999;5:2251-60.
57. Khoshyomn S, Penar PL, Rossi J, Wells A, Abramson DL, Bhushan A. Inhibition of phospholipase C-gamma1 activation blocks glioma cell motility and invasion of fetal rat brain aggregates. Neurosurgery 1999;44:568-77; discussion 77-8.

58. Turner T, Epps-Fung MV, Kassis J, Wells A. Molecular inhibition of phospholipase cgamma signaling abrogates DU-145 prostate tumor cell invasion. Clin Cancer Res 1997;3:2275-82.
59. Wells A, Ware MF, Allen FD, Lauffenburger DA. Shaping up for shipping out: PLCgamma signaling of morphology changes in EGF-stimulated fibroblast migration. Cell Motil Cytoskeleton 1999;44:227-33.
60. Chou J, Stolz DB, Burke NA, Watkins SC, Wells A. Distribution of gelsolin and phosphoinositol 4,5-bisphosphate in lamellipodia during EGF-induced motility. Int J Biochem Cell Biol 2002;34:776-90.
61. Mouneimne G, Soon L, DesMarais V, et al. Phospholipase C and cofilin are required for carcinoma cell directionality in response to EGF stimulation. J Cell Biol 2004;166:697-708.
62. Fukami K, Furuhashi K, Inagaki M, Endo T, Hatano S, Takenawa T. Requirement of phosphatidylinositol 4,5-bisphosphate for alpha-actinin function. Nature 1992;359:150-2.
63. Gilmore AP, Burridge K. Regulation of vinculin binding to talin and actin by phosphatidyl-inositol-4-5-bisphosphate. Nature 1996;381:531-5.
64. Iwabu A, Smith K, Allen FD, Lauffenburger DA, Wells A. Epidermal growth factor induces fibroblast contractility and motility via a protein kinase C delta-dependent pathway. J Biol Chem 2004;279:14551-60.
65. Hauck CR, Sieg DJ, Hsia DA, et al. Inhibition of focal adhesion kinase expression or activity disrupts epidermal growth factor-stimulated signaling promoting the migration of invasive human carcinoma cells. Cancer Res 2001;61:7079-90.
66. Rigot V, Lehmann M, Andre F, Daemi N, Marvaldi J, Luis J. Integrin ligation and PKC activation are required for migration of colon carcinoma cells. J Cell Sci 1998;111 (Pt 20):3119-27.
67. Klemke RL, Cai S, Giannini AL, Gallagher PJ, de Lanerolle P, Cheresh DA. Regulation of cell motility by mitogen-activated protein kinase. J Cell Biol 1997;137:481-92.
68. Merlot S, Firtel RA. Leading the way: Directional sensing through phosphatidylinositol 3-kinase and other signaling pathways. J Cell Sci 2003;116:3471-8.
69. Park CM, Park MJ, Kwak HJ, et al. Ionizing Radiation Enhances Matrix Metalloproteinase-2 Secretion and Invasion of Glioma Cells through Src/Epidermal Growth Factor Receptor-Mediated p38/Akt and Phosphatidylinositol 3-Kinase/Akt Signaling Pathways. Cancer Res 2006;66:8511-9.
70. Price JT, Tiganis T, Agarwal A, Djakiew D, Thompson EW. Epidermal growth factor promotes MDA-MB-231 breast cancer cell migration through a phosphatidylinositol 3′-kinase and phospholipase C-dependent mechanism. Cancer Res 1999;59:5475-8.
71. Sawyer C, Sturge J, Bennett DC, et al. Regulation of breast cancer cell chemotaxis by the phosphoinositide 3-kinase p110delta. Cancer Res 2003;63:1667-75.
72. Shien T, Doihara H, Hara H, et al. PLC and PI3K pathways are important in the inhibition of EGF-induced cell migration by gefitinib ('Iressa', ZD1839). Breast Cancer 2004;11:367-73.
73. Theodorescu D, Laderoute KR, Gulding KM. Epidermal growth factor receptor-regulated human bladder cancer motility is in part a phosphatidylinositol 3-kinase-mediated process. Cell Growth Differ 1998;9:919-28.
74. Funamoto S, Meili R, Lee S, Parry L, Firtel RA. Spatial and temporal regulation of 3-phosphoinositides by PI 3-kinase and PTEN mediates chemotaxis. Cell 2002;109:611-23.
75. Hill K, Welti S, Yu J, et al. Specific requirement for the p85-p110alpha phosphatidylinositol 3-kinase during epidermal growth factor-stimulated actin nucleation in breast cancer cells. J Biol Chem 2000;275:3741-4.
76. Tang JM, He QY, Guo RX, Chang XJ. Phosphorylated Akt overexpression and loss of PTEN expression in non-small cell lung cancer confers poor prognosis. Lung Cancer 2006;51:181-91.
77. Tsuruta H, Kishimoto H, Sasaki T, et al. Hyperplasia and Carcinomas in Pten-Deficient Mice and Reduced PTEN Protein in Human Bladder Cancer Patients. Cancer Res 2006;66:8389-96.
78. Furukawa K, Kumon Y, Harada H, et al. PTEN gene transfer suppresses the invasive potential of human malignant gliomas by regulating cell invasion-related molecules. Int J Oncol 2006;29:73-81.
79. Soula-Rothhut M, Coissard C, Sartelet H, et al. The tumor suppressor PTEN inhibits EGF-induced TSP-1 and TIMP-1 expression in FTC-133 thyroid carcinoma cells. Exp Cell Res 2005;304:187-201.
80. Rossman KL, Der CJ, Sondek J. GEF means go: turning on RHO GTPases with guanine nucleotide-exchange factors. Nat Rev Mol Cell Biol 2005;6:167-80.
81. Marcoux N, Vuori K. EGF receptor mediates adhesion-dependent activation of the Rac GTPase: a role for phosphatidylinositol 3-kinase and Vav2. Oncogene 2003;22:6100-6.

82. Tamas P, Solti Z, Bauer P, et al. Mechanism of epidermal growth factor regulation of Vav2, a guanine nucleotide exchange factor for Rac. J Biol Chem 2003;278:5163-71.
83. Tu S, Wu WJ, Wang J, Cerione RA. Epidermal growth factor-dependent regulation of Cdc42 is mediated by the Src tyrosine kinase. J Biol Chem 2003;278:49293-300.
84. Nobes CD, Hall A. Rho GTPases control polarity, protrusion, and adhesion during cell movement. J Cell Biol 1999;144:1235-44.
85. Raftopoulou M, Hall A. Cell migration: Rho GTPases lead the way. Dev Biol 2004;265:23-32.
86. Bokoch GM, Vlahos CJ, Wang Y, Knaus UG, Traynor-Kaplan AE. Rac GTPase interacts specifically with phosphatidylinositol 3-kinase. Biochem J 1996;315 (Pt 3):775-9.
87. Chou J, Burke NA, Iwabu A, Watkins SC, Wells A. Directional motility induced by epidermal growth factor requires Cdc42. Exp Cell Res 2003;287:47-56.
88. Sahai E, Marshall CJ. RHO-GTPases and cancer. Nat Rev Cancer 2002;2:133-42.
89. Caceres M, Guerrero J, Martinez J. Overexpression of RhoA-GTP induces activation of the Epidermal Growth Factor Receptor, dephosphorylation of focal adhesion kinase and increased motility in breast cancer cells. Exp Cell Res 2005;309:229-38.
90. Hirsch DS, Shen Y, Wu WJ. Growth and motility inhibition of breast cancer cells by epidermal growth factor receptor degradation is correlated with inactivation of Cdc42. Cancer Res 2006;66:3523-30.
91. Condeelis JS, Wyckoff JB, Bailly M, et al. Lamellipodia in invasion. Semin Cancer Biol 2001;11:119-28.
92. DesMarais V, Ghosh M, Eddy R, Condeelis J. Cofilin takes the lead. J Cell Sci 2005;118:19-26.
93. Bailly M, Macaluso F, Cammer M, Chan A, Segall JE, Condeelis JS. Relationship between Arp2/3 complex and the barbed ends of actin filaments at the leading edge of carcinoma cells after epidermal growth factor stimulation. J Cell Biol 1999;145:331-45.
94. Chan AY, Bailly M, Zebda N, Segall JE, Condeelis JS. Role of cofilin in epidermal growth factor-stimulated actin polymerization and lamellipod protrusion. J Cell Biol 2000;148:531-42.
95. Kempiak SJ, Yip SC, Backer JM, Segall JE. Local signaling by the EGF receptor. J Cell Biol 2003;162:781-7.
96. Condeelis J, Singer RH, Segall JE. The great escape: when cancer cells hijack the genes for chemotaxis and motility. Annu Rev Cell Dev Biol 2005;21:695-718.
97. Yamaguchi H, Condeelis J. Regulation of the actin cytoskeleton in cancer cell migration and invasion. Biochim Biophys Acta 2006.
98. Yamaguchi H, Lorenz M, Kempiak S, et al. Molecular mechanisms of invadopodium formation: the role of the N-WASP-Arp2/3 complex pathway and cofilin. J Cell Biol 2005;168:441-52.
99. Malliri A, Symons M, Hennigan RF, et al. The transcription factor AP-1 is required for EGF-induced activation of rho-like GTPases, cytoskeletal rearrangements, motility, and in vitro invasion of A431 cells. J Cell Biol 1998;143:1087-99.
100. Zhou W, Grandis JR, Wells A. STAT3 is required but not sufficient for EGF receptor-mediated migration and invasion of human prostate carcinoma cell lines. Br J Cancer 2006;95:164-71.
101. Itoh M, Murata T, Suzuki T, et al. Requirement of STAT3 activation for maximal collagenase-1 (MMP-1) induction by epidermal growth factor and malignant characteristics in T24 bladder cancer cells. Oncogene 2006;25:1195-204.
102. Mamoune A, Kassis J, Kharait S, et al. DU145 human prostate carcinoma invasiveness is modulated by urokinase receptor (uPAR) downstream of epidermal growth factor receptor (EGFR) signaling. Exp Cell Res 2004;299:91-100.
103. Kajita M, Itoh Y, Chiba T, et al. Membrane-type 1 matrix metalloproteinase cleaves CD44 and promotes cell migration. J Cell Biol 2001;153:893-904.
104. Noe V, Fingleton B, Jacobs K, et al. Release of an invasion promoter E-cadherin fragment by matrilysin and stromelysin-1. J Cell Sci 2001;114:111-8.
105. Deryugina EI, Quigley JP. Matrix metalloproteinases and tumor metastasis. Cancer Metastasis Rev 2006;25:9-34.
106. O-charoenrat P, Rhys-Evans P, Modjtahedi H, Court W, Box G, Eccles S. Overexpression of epidermal growth factor receptor in human head and neck squamous carcinoma cell lines correlates with matrix metalloproteinase-9 expression and in vitro invasion. Int J Cancer 2000;86:307-17.
107. O-charoenrat P, Rhys-Evans PH, Archer DJ, Eccles SA. C-erbB receptors in squamous cell carcinomas of the head and neck: clinical significance and correlation with matrix metalloproteinases and vascular endothelial growth factors. Oral Oncol 2002;38:73-80.

108. Rosenthal EL, Johnson TM, Allen ED, Apel IJ, Punturieri A, Weiss SJ. Role of the plasminogen activator and matrix metalloproteinase systems in epidermal growth factor- and scatter factor-stimulated invasion of carcinoma cells. Cancer Res 1998;58:5221-30.
109. Lal A, Glazer CA, Martinson HM, et al. Mutant epidermal growth factor receptor up-regulates molecular effectors of tumor invasion. Cancer Res 2002;62:3335-9.
110. Tan X, Egami H, Abe M, Nozawa F, Hirota M, Ogawa M. Involvement of MMP-7 in invasion of pancreatic cancer cells through activation of the EGFR mediated MEK-ERK signal transduction pathway. J Clin Pathol 2005;58:1242-8.
111. Van Meter TE, Broaddus WC, Rooprai HK, Pilkington GJ, Fillmore HL. Induction of membrane-type-1 matrix metalloproteinase by epidermal growth factor-mediated signaling in gliomas. Neuro-oncol 2004;6:188-99.
112. Kondapaka SB, Fridman R, Reddy KB. Epidermal growth factor and amphiregulin up-regulate matrix metalloproteinase-9 (MMP-9) in human breast cancer cells. Int J Cancer 1997;70:722-6.
113. O-charoenrat P, Wongkajornsilp A, Rhys-Evans PH, Eccles SA. Signaling pathways required for matrix metalloproteinase-9 induction by betacellulin in head-and-neck squamous carcinoma cells. Int J Cancer 2004;111:174-83.
114. Ellerbroek SM, Halbleib JM, Benavidez M, et al. Phosphatidylinositol 3-kinase activity in epidermal growth factor-stimulated matrix metalloproteinase-9 production and cell surface association. Cancer Res 2001;61:1855-61.
115. Prenzel N, Zwick E, Daub H, et al. EGF receptor transactivation by G-protein-coupled receptors requires metalloproteinase cleavage of proHB-EGF. Nature 1999;402:884-8.
116. Laufs S, Schumacher J, Allgayer H. Urokinase-receptor (u-PAR): an essential player in multiple games of cancer: a review on its role in tumor progression, invasion, metastasis, proliferation/dormancy, clinical outcome and minimal residual disease. Cell Cycle 2006;5:1760-71.
117. Li Y, Sarkar FH. Down-regulation of invasion and angiogenesis-related genes identified by cDNA microarray analysis of PC3 prostate cancer cells treated with genistein. Cancer Lett 2002;186:157-64.
118. Festuccia C, Angelucci A, Gravina GL, et al. Epidermal growth factor modulates prostate cancer cell invasiveness regulating urokinase-type plasminogen activator activity. EGF-receptor inhibition may prevent tumor cell dissemination. Thromb Haemost 2005;93:964-75.
119. Henic E, Sixt M, Hansson S, Hoyer-Hansen G, Casslen B. EGF-stimulated migration in ovarian cancer cells is associated with decreased internalization, increased surface expression, and increased shedding of the urokinase plasminogen activator receptor. Gynecol Oncol 2006;101:28-39.
120. Guerrero J, Santibanez JF, Gonzalez A, Martinez J. EGF receptor transactivation by urokinase receptor stimulus through a mechanism involving Src and matrix metalloproteinases. Exp Cell Res 2004;292:201-8.
121. Jo M, Thomas KS, O'Donnell DM, Gonias SL. Epidermal growth factor receptor-dependent and -independent cell-signaling pathways originating from the urokinase receptor. J Biol Chem 2003;278:1642-6.
122. Liu D, Aguirre Ghiso J, Estrada Y, Ossowski L. EGFR is a transducer of the urokinase receptor initiated signal that is required for in vivo growth of a human carcinoma. Cancer Cell 2002;1:445-57.
123. Unlu A, Leake RE. The effect of EGFR-related tyrosine kinase activity inhibition on the growth and invasion mechanisms of prostate carcinoma cell lines. Int J Biol Markers 2003;18:139-46.
124. Tsujii M, Kawano S, DuBois RN. Cyclooxygenase-2 expression in human colon cancer cells increases metastatic potential. Proc Natl Acad Sci USA 1997;94:3336-40.
125. Dohadwala M, Luo J, Zhu L, et al. Non-small cell lung cancer cyclooxygenase-2-dependent invasion is mediated by CD44. J Biol Chem 2001;276:20809-12.
126. Choe MS, Zhang X, Shin HJ, Shin DM, Chen ZG. Interaction between epidermal growth factor receptor- and cyclooxygenase 2-mediated pathways and its implications for the chemoprevention of head and neck cancer. Mol Cancer Ther 2005;4:1448-55.
127. Mann JR, Backlund MG, Buchanan FG, et al. Repression of prostaglandin dehydrogenase by epidermal growth factor and snail increases prostaglandin E2 and promotes cancer progression. Cancer Res 2006;66:6649-56.
128. Cao Y. Opinion: emerging mechanisms of tumour lymphangiogenesis and lymphatic metastasis. Nat Rev Cancer 2005;5:735-43.
129. Beasley NJ, Prevo R, Banerji S, et al. Intratumoral lymphangiogenesis and lymph node metastasis in head and neck cancer. Cancer Res 2002;62:1315-20.

130. Shields JD, Borsetti M, Rigby H, et al. Lymphatic density and metastatic spread in human malignant melanoma. Br J Cancer 2004;90:693-700.
131. Shimizu K, Kubo H, Yamaguchi K, et al. Suppression of VEGFR-3 signaling inhibits lymph node metastasis in gastric cancer. Cancer Sci 2004;95:328-33.
132. O-charoenrat P, Rhys-Evans P, Modjtahedi H, Eccles SA. Vascular endothelial growth factor family members are differentially regulated by c-erbB signaling in head and neck squamous carcinoma cells. Clin Exp Metastasis 2000;18:155-61.
133. Goldman CK, Kim J, Wong WL, King V, Brock T, Gillespie GY. Epidermal growth factor stimulates vascular endothelial growth factor production by human malignant glioma cells: a model of glioblastoma multiforme pathophysiology. Mol Biol Cell 1993;4:121-33.
134. Ravindranath N, Wion D, Brachet P, Djakiew D. Epidermal growth factor modulates the expression of vascular endothelial growth factor in the human prostate. J Androl 2001;22:432-43.
135. Akagi M, Kawaguchi M, Liu W, et al. Induction of neuropilin-1 and vascular endothelial growth factor by epidermal growth factor in human gastric cancer cells. Br J Cancer 2003;88:796-802.
136. Petit AM, Rak J, Hung MC, et al. Neutralizing antibodies against epidermal growth factor and ErbB-2/neu receptor tyrosine kinases down-regulate vascular endothelial growth factor production by tumor cells in vitro and in vivo: angiogenic implications for signal transduction therapy of solid tumors. Am J Pathol 1997;151:1523-30.
137. Hirata A, Ogawa S, Kometani T, et al. ZD1839 (Iressa) induces antiangiogenic effects through inhibition of epidermal growth factor receptor tyrosine kinase. Cancer Res 2002;62:2554-60.
138. Pore N, Jiang Z, Gupta A, Cerniglia G, Kao GD, Maity A. EGFR tyrosine kinase inhibitors decrease VEGF expression by both hypoxia-inducible factor (HIF)-1-independent and HIF-1-dependent mechanisms. Cancer Res 2006;66:3197-204.
139. Rishi AK, Parikh R, Wali A, et al. EGF receptor-related protein (ERRP) inhibits invasion of colon cancer cells and tubule formation by endothelial cells in vitro. Anticancer Res 2006;26:1029-37.
140. Pore N, Liu S, Haas-Kogan DA, O'Rourke DM, Maity A. PTEN mutation and epidermal growth factor receptor activation regulate vascular endothelial growth factor (VEGF) mRNA expression in human glioblastoma cells by transactivating the proximal VEGF promoter. Cancer Res 2003;63:236-41.
141. Sales KJ, List T, Boddy SC, et al. A novel angiogenic role for prostaglandin F2alpha-FP receptor interaction in human endometrial adenocarcinomas. Cancer Res 2005;65:7707-16.
142. Smith OP, Battersby S, Sales KJ, Critchley HO, Jabbour HN. Prostacyclin receptor up-regulates the expression of angiogenic genes in human endometrium via cross talk with epidermal growth factor Receptor and the extracellular signaling receptor kinase 1/2 pathway. Endocrinology 2006;147:1697-705.
143. Ding YB, Shi RH, Tong JD, et al. PGE2 up-regulates vascular endothelial growth factor expression in MKN28 gastric cancer cells via epidermal growth factor receptor signaling system. Exp Oncol 2005;27:108-13.
144. Pai R, Szabo IL, Soreghan BA, Atay S, Kawanaka H, Tarnawski AS. PGE(2) stimulates VEGF expression in endothelial cells via ERK2/JNK1 signaling pathways. Biochem Biophys Res Commun 2001;286:923-8.
145. Maity A, Pore N, Lee J, Solomon D, O'Rourke DM. Epidermal growth factor receptor transcriptionally up-regulates vascular endothelial growth factor expression in human glioblastoma cells via a pathway involving phosphatidylinositol 3Î-kinase and distinct from that induced by hypoxia. Cancer Res 2000;60:5879-86.
146. Swinson DE, O'Byrne KJ. Interactions between hypoxia and epidermal growth factor receptor in non-small-cell lung cancer. Clin Lung Cancer 2006;7:250-6.
147. Li Y, Bi Z, Yan B, Wan Y. UVB radiation induces expression of HIF-1alpha and VEGF through the EGFR/PI3K/DEC1 pathway. Int J Mol Med 2006;18:713-9.
148. Clarke K, Smith K, Gullick WJ, Harris AL. Mutant epidermal growth factor receptor enhances induction of vascular endothelial growth factor by hypoxia and insulin-like growth factor-1 via a PI3 kinase dependent pathway. Br J Cancer 2001;84:1322-9.
149. Baker CH, Kedar D, McCarty MF, et al. Blockade of epidermal growth factor receptor signaling on tumor cells and tumor-associated endothelial cells for therapy of human carcinomas. Am J Pathol 2002;161:929-38.
150. Moon W, Park, HS, Yu, KH, Park, MY, Kim, KR, Jang KY, Kim, JS, Cho, BH. Expression of betacellulin and epidermal growth factor in hepatocellular carcinoma: implications for angiogenesis. Human Pathol 2006;37:1324-32.

151. Ushiro S, Ono M, Izumi H, et al. Heparin-binding epidermal growth factor-like growth factor: p91 activation induction of plasminogen activator/inhibitor, and tubular morphogenesis in human microvascular endothelial cells. Jpn J Cancer Res 1996;87:68-77.
152. Brockmann MA, Ulbricht U, Gruner K, Fillbrandt R, Westphal M, Lamszus K. Glioblastoma and cerebral microvascular endothelial cell migration in response to tumor-associated growth factors. Neurosurgery 2003;52:1391-9.
153. Schraufstatter IU, Trieu K, Zhao M, Rose DM, Terkeltaub RA, Burger M. IL-8-mediated cell migration in endothelial cells depends on cathepsin B activity and transactivation of the epidermal growth factor receptor. J Immunol 2003;171:6714-22.
154. Parker C, Roseman BJ, Bucana CD, Tsan R, Radinsky R. Preferential activation of the epidermal growth factor receptor in human colon carcinoma liver metastases in nude mice. J Histochem Cytochem 1998;46:595-602.
155. Tham YL, Sexton K, Kramer R, Hilsenbeck S, Elledge R. Primary breast cancer phenotypes associated with propensity for central nervous system metastases. Cancer 2006;107:696-704.
156. Ekstrand AJ, James CD, Cavenee WK, Seliger B, Pettersson RF, Collins VP. Genes for epidermal growth factor receptor, transforming growth factor alpha, and epidermal growth factor and their expression in human gliomas in vivo. Cancer Res 1991;51:2164-72.
157. Tanaka Y, Miyamoto S, Suzuki SO, et al. Clinical significance of heparin-binding epidermal growth factor-like growth factor and a disintegrin and metalloprotease 17 expression in human ovarian cancer. Clin Cancer Res 2005;11:4783-92.
158. Jones JL, Royall JE, Walker RA. E-cadherin relates to EGFR expression and lymph node metastasis in primary breast carcinoma. Br J Cancer 1996;74:1237-41.
159. Odajima T, Sasaki Y, Tanaka N, et al. Abnormal beta-catenin expression in oral cancer with no gene mutation: correlation with expression of cyclin D1 and epidermal growth factor receptor, Ki-67 labeling index, and clinicopathological features. Hum Pathol 2005;36:234-41.
160. Curran S, Murray GI. Matrix metalloproteinases in tumour invasion and metastasis. J Pathol 1999;189:300-8.
161. Dalberg K, Eriksson E, Enberg U, Kjellman M, Backdahl M. Gelatinase A, membrane type 1 matrix metalloproteinase, and extracellular matrix metalloproteinase inducer mRNA expression: correlation with invasive growth of breast cancer. World J Surg 2000;24:334-40.
162. Koshiba T, Hosotani R, Wada M, et al. Involvement of matrix metalloproteinase-2 activity in invasion and metastasis of pancreatic carcinoma. Cancer 1998;82:642-50.
163. O-charoenrat P, Modjtahedi H, Rhys-Evans P, Court WJ, Box GM, Eccles SA. Epidermal growth factor-like ligands differentially up-regulate matrix metalloproteinase 9 in head and neck squamous carcinoma cells. Cancer Res 2000;60:1121-8.
164. O-charoenrat P, Rhys-Evans P, Eccles SA. Expression of vascular endothelial growth factor family members in head and neck squamous cell carcinoma correlates with lymph node metastasis. Cancer 2001;92:556-68.
165. Raspollini MR, Castiglione F, Garbini F, et al. Correlation of epidermal growth factor receptor expression with tumor microdensity vessels and with vascular endothelial growth factor expression in ovarian carcinoma. Int J Surg Pathol 2005;13:135-42.
166. Bos R, van Diest PJ, de Jong JS, van der Groep P, van der Valk P, van der Wall E. Hypoxia-inducble factor-1alpha is associated with angiogenesis, and expression of bFGF, PDGF-BB, and EGFR in invasive breast cancer. Histopathology 2005;46:31-6.
167. George ML, Tutton MG, Janssen F, et al. VEGF-A, VEGF-C, and VEGF-D in colorectal cancer progression. Neoplasia 2001;3:420-7.
168. Han H, Silverman JF, Santucci TS, et al. Vascular endothelial growth factor expression in stage I non-small cell lung cancer correlates with neoangiogenesis and a poor prognosis. Ann Surg Oncol 2001;8:72-9.
169. Yuan A, Yu CJ, Chen WJ, et al. Correlation of total VEGF mRNA and protein expression with histologic type, tumor angiogenesis, patient survival and timing of relapse in non-small-cell lung cancer. Int J Cancer 2000;89:475-83.
170. Dietz A, Rudat V, Conradt C, Weidauer H, Ho A, Moehler T. Prognostic relevance of serum levels of the angiogenic peptide bFGF in advanced carcinoma of the head and neck treated by primary radiochemotherapy. Head Neck 2000;22:666-73.

171. Benoy IH, Salgado R, Van Dam P, et al. Increased serum interleukin-8 in patients with early and metastatic breast cancer correlates with early dissemination and survival. Clin Cancer Res 2004;10:7157-62.
172. Kassim SK, El-Salahy EM, Fayed ST, et al. Vascular endothelial growth factor and interleukin-8 are associated with poor prognosis in epithelial ovarian cancer patients. Clin Biochem 2004;37:363-9.
173. Ciardiello F, Caputo R, Bianco R, et al. Inhibition of growth factor production and angiogenesis in human cancer cells by ZD1839 (Iressa), a selective epidermal growth factor receptor tyrosine kinase inhibitor. Clin Cancer Res 2001;7:1459-65.
174. Ellis LM. Epidermal growth factor receptor in tumor angiogenesis. Hematol Oncol Clin North Am 2004;18:1007-21, viii.
175. Ciardiello F, Bianco R, Caputo R, et al. Antitumor activity of ZD6474, a vascular endothelial growth factor receptor tyrosine kinase inhibitor, in human cancer cells with acquired resistance to antiepidermal growth factor receptor therapy. Clin Cancer Res 2004;10:784-93.
176. Viloria-Petit A, Crombet T, Jothy S, et al. Acquired resistance to the antitumor effect of epidermal growth factor receptor-blocking antibodies in vivo: a role for altered tumor angiogenesis. Cancer Res 2001;61:5090-101.
177. Bozec A, Fischel JL, Milano G. Epidermal growth factor receptor/angiogenesis dual targeting: preclinical experience. Curr Opin Oncol 2006;18:330-4.
178. Ciardiello F, Troiani T, Bianco R, et al. Interaction between the epidermal growth factor receptor (EGFR) and the vascular endothelial growth factor (VEGF) pathways: a rational approach for multitarget anticancer therapy. Ann Oncol 2006;17:vii109-vii14.
179. van Cruijsen H, Giaccone G, Hoekman, K. Epidermal growth factor receptor and angiogenesis: opportunities for combined anticancer strategies. Int J Cancer 2006;118:883-8.
180. Herbst RS, Johnson DH, Mininberg E, et al. Phase I/II trial evaluating the anti-vascular endothelial growth factor monoclonal antibody bevacizumab in combination with the HER-1/epidermal growth factor receptor tyrosine kinase inhibitor erlotinib for patients with recurrent non-small-cell lung cancer. J Clin Oncol 2005;23:2544-55.
181. Kishida O, Miyazaki Y, Murayama Y, et al. Gefitinib ("Iressa", ZD1839) inhibits SN38-triggered EGF signals and IL-8 production in gastric cancer cells. Cancer Chemother Pharmacol 2005;55:393-403.
182. Bozec A, Formento P, Ciccolini J, et al. Response of endothelial cells to a dual tyrosine kinase receptor inhibition combined with irradiation. Mol Cancer Ther 2005;4:1962-71.

19 Constitutive Activation of Truncated EGF Receptors in Glioblastoma

Carol J. Wikstrand and Darell D. Bigner

CONTENTS

    INTRODUCTION
    SIGNAL TRANSDUCTION VIA EGFRWT: SYNOPSIS
    SIGNAL TRANSDUCTION BY EGFRvIII
    CONSEQUENCES OF GLIOMA-ASSOCIATED EGFRvIII SIGNALING
        FOR THERAPEUTIC TARGETING
    CONCLUSION

Abstract

The pathways of signal transduction utilized by EGFRwt are briefly reviewed, and those used by EGFRvIII compared and contrasted to them, in an effort to elucidate the correlation between expression of EGFRwt and/or EGFRvIII and tumor growth. We expect that effective targeting of the EGFR-mediated growth advantage in gliomas will require inhibition of both EGFRwt and EGFRvIII signaling pathways, as the majority of glioblastomas will express both. Successful targeting of this signaling cascade will be a valuable adjunct to the other specific receptor targeting mechanisms (Mab constructs, ligand bullets) available and demonstrably effective against EGFRwt- and EGFRvIII-expressing tumor cells.

Key Words: gene amplification, immunotherapy, mutation, nervous system neoplasms, signal transduction.

1. INTRODUCTION

The involvement of increased and/or aberrant EGFR activity in human cancers, including breast (*1*) and ovarian (*2*) cancers, non-small cell lung carcinomas (*3*), and head and neck tumors (*4–6*), has been well documented (*7, 8*), and the observation that tumors express "elevated," as opposed to normal, levels of EGFRwt (*5, 8–10*) has led to attempts to correlate aberrant "overexpression" (never strictly defined) with overall or disease-free survival in patients (*6, 11*). In general, increased EGFR expression was reported to correlate with a poorer clinical outcome in several malignancies, including bladder, breast, lung, and head and neck cancers (*6, 12, 13*). It was originally postulated that EGFR expression and/or gene amplification promoted tumor development by increasing ligand-activated signaling through EGFRwt kinase activity (*12, 14*). The increased receptor expression was reported to be associated with increased production of ligands, such as TGF-α, by the same tumor cells, which raised the possibility of receptor activation by autocrine pathways (*3, 6, 10*).

From: *Cancer Drug Discovery and Development: EGFR Signaling Networks in Cancer Therapy*
Edited by: J. D. Haley and W. J. Gullick, DOI: 10.1007/978-1-59745-356-1_19
© 2008 Humana Press, a part of Springer Science+Business Media, LLC

Gliomas were one of the first tumor types to be reported to express EGFRwt (15), and it was suggested that amplification of the *EGFRwt* gene in these tumors could result in possible rearrangement and production of variant EGFR molecules (16). This effect was further supported by Wong et al. (17), who reported that the increased expression of EGFRwt in gliomas was almost invariably associated with gene amplification. With fluorescence in situ hybridization, it was demonstrated that in the majority of malignant gliomas (or xenografts derived from them) exhibiting amplification of the *EGFR* gene, the amplicon was contained within double minute (dmin) chromosomes (18, 19). Gene amplification is primarily associated with GBM and not with astrocytomas of grades II/III or pilocytic astrocytomas (20–24), as estimates of the frequency of *EGFR* gene amplification by genetic analyses in human tumors range from 36% to 60% for GBM and 10% to 22% for AA (25–31). Within primary, or *de novo* GBM, *EGFR* gene amplification or EGFRwt protein expression was quite common (>63%), but rare in secondary, or progressive GBM (<0%) (32–34)

Amplification of the *EGFRwt* gene in gliomas is frequently accompanied by rearrangement (35, 36) and mutations (summarized in Kuan et al. [*37*]), leading to co-expression of wild-type and variant EGFR on the glioma cell surface (*16, 22, 28, 38*). Several genomic variants have been described (*36*), the most frequently detected variant being EGFRvIII (or de2-7, Δ2-7), which has been found in 41–54% of GBM cases exhibiting *EGFRwt* gene amplification (*25, 27, 32*). The EGFRvIII rearrangement and protein expression, however, can be found in both GBM (4–8%) and AA (1–12%) that do not exhibit amplification (*23, 25*, Wikstrand et al., unpublished data). The EGFRvIII receptor contains an in-frame deletion of exons 2–7 from the extracellular region, does not bind ligand, and is constitutively activated (*9, 13, 35, 37*) (Fig. 19.1). While EGFRvIII has also been described in head and neck squamous cell carcinoma (*4*), non-small cell lung cancer (*39*), and breast cancer (*8, 40*), gene amplification is far less common (10% in head and neck cancers [*4*]) and appears to be primarily characteristic of astrocytic lineage tumors (*12*). Another significant difference between gliomas and EGFR-expressing lung adenocarcinomas is the occurrence of mutations in the kinase domain of EGFRwt; in a comprehensive study of over 566 human tumors, Sihto et al. (*41*) reported that almost 90% of all EGFR kinase domain deletions in lung cancer were either deletions in exon 19 or missense mutations in exon 21. Analysis for the presence for such mutations in 95 gliomas revealed none, suggesting that the biology of EGFR expression in gliomas is quite different from that in lung cancer (*42*).

The correlation between expression of EGFRwt and/or EGFRvIII and tumor growth has been investigated extensively in both retrospective analyses of human tumors and model systems involving transfected human tumor cell-derived xenografts. The presence of EGFRwt has been reported to be associated with a poorer clinical outcome in a number of malignancies, including bladder, breast, lung, and head and neck cancers (*6, 12, 13*). Within gliomas, however, attempts to correlate *EGFR* amplification alone with outcome in GBM or AA patients have to date provided inconclusive or contradictory results (reviewed in Liu et al. [*23*]). The most recent analyses with large patient cohorts have shown no evidence of *EGFRwt* gene amplification as an independent prognosticator of survival (*23, 43*). Several groups have noted, however, that in multivariate analyses there is a trend for *EGFRwt* gene amplification to be associated with better prognosis in older patients and worse prognosis in younger patients (*26, 44*). As younger patients more often develop secondary GBMs and older patients primary GBMs (*29, 32, 45, 46*), this association between EGFR and age could also be associated with other mechanisms of tumor progression. Although signaling via the EGFR pathway has been demonstrated to contribute to radiation resistance in many tumor types, including glioma (*32, 47*), more recent studies found no association between EGFR amplification and response to radiation treatment, progression-free survival, or overall

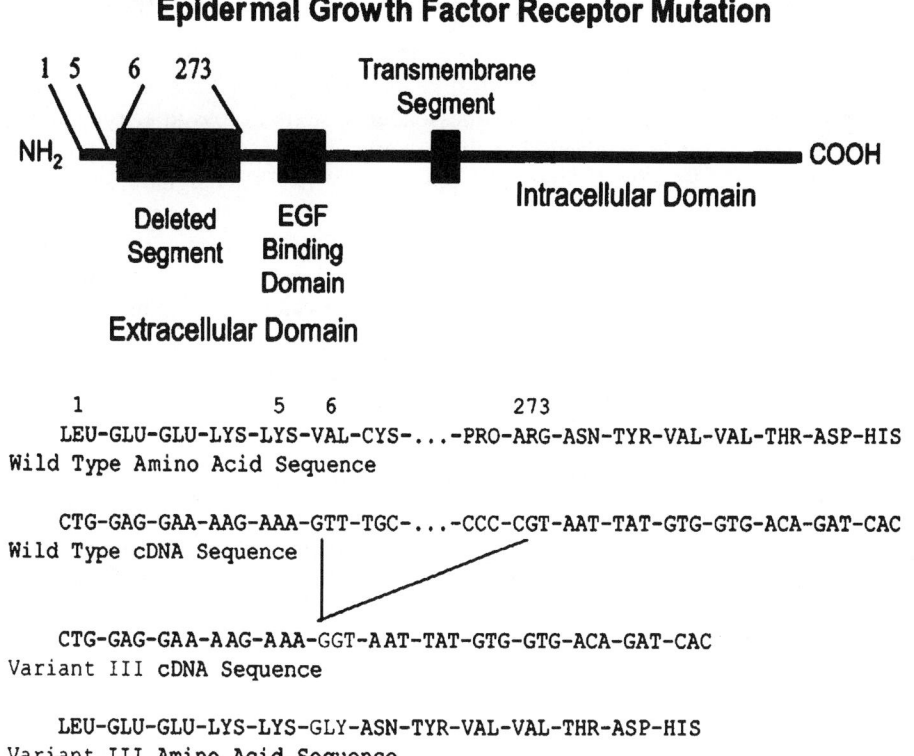

Fig. 19.1. Depiction of the EGFRvIII Protein.

survival in gliomas (*30, 48*). Finally, the association between responsiveness to tyrosine kinase inhibitor (TKI) therapy (gefitinib and erlotinib) and EGFRwt expression has been shown in turn to be associated with somatic mutations within exons 19 and 21 (*41, 42, 49*); however, as these mutations are not present in gliomas or head and neck squamous adenocarcinomas, this genetic variation is not a factor contributing to progression in these tumors.

Far fewer studies of EGFRvIII expression as it relates to various parameters of tumor behavior have been performed. Liu et al. (*23*) have observed a trend toward decreased survival among AA patients with any EGFR abnormality, while Aldape et al. (*25*) reported that EGFRvIII expression was strongly associated with reduced survival in AA patients ($P < 0.002$), although there was no association with survival within the GBM cohort ($P = 0.84$). As the AA patients with the worst prognosis also were the eldest, with tumors exhibiting a clinical behavior similar to that of GBM, the presence of EGFRvIII in this group might identify those AA patients with the worst prognosis. Similarly, Heimberger et al. (*50, 51*) found no correlation between EGFRvIII and overall survival, although a slight trend toward negative outcome was noted for patients <40 years of age with EGFRvIII+ tumors. Although EGFRvIII has been associated with enhanced invasiveness and infiltration in both in vitro and in vivo assays (*52, 53*), presumably by increasing proliferation and reducing apoptosis, there has been no significant observed increase in EGFRvIII in patients presenting with multifocal disease or gliomatosis cerebri, but a trend toward higher levels of EGFRvIII expression has been seen in tumors with ependymal dissemination (*51*).

2. SIGNAL TRANSDUCTION VIA EGFRwt: SYNOPSIS

Chapters 1–15 of this volume provide a comprehensive summary of the established mechanisms of EGFRwt ligand binding, receptor dimerization and mobilization, internalization, signaling through various second messenger systems, cross-talk, regulation, and inhibition. For the purpose of discussing these components of signaling as mediated by glioma cell-associated EGFRvIII, the major pathways of EGFRwt signal transduction are presented in Fig. 19.2.

As summarized by Mendelsohn and Baselga (*12*) the EGFRwt receptor system is a "rich multilayered network…which allows for horizontal interactions and permits multiple combinatorial responses". This network, which can be activated by a number of stimuli that do not interact directly with the EGFR itself (*54*), and by homodimeric and heterodimeric complexes formed between ErbB family receptors (*55, 56*), generates a high degree of cross-talk and activation of diverse second messenger systems (*55, 57*).

2.1. Cell Membrane Localization

A variety of cell surface receptors, including EGFRwt, are naturally associated with lipid rafts and specialized plasma membrane vesicular organelles known as caveolae (*58*). By immunocytochemistry and measurement of in vitro binding to caveolin scaffolding domain peptides, Abulrob et al. (*58*) have demonstrated association of EGFRwt with caveolin-1 or -3 via the caveolin-binding motif within the kinase domain of EGFR.

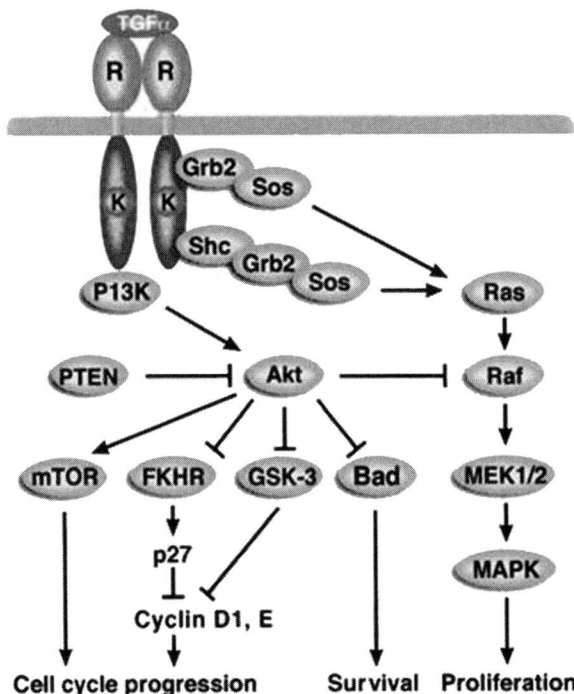

Fig. 19.2. Epidermal Growth Factor Receptor Signaling. The process of ligand-receptor and receptor-receptor interaction leads to activation of key intracellular-signaling pathways that regulate gene transcription, cell cycle progression, and a variety of cellular responses that promote malignant behaviors (Mendelsohn J, Baselga J, J Clin Oncol., 21 *14*, 2003: 2787–2799; reprinted with permission from the American Society of Clinical Oncology).

2.2. Ligand Binding, Dimerization, and Autophosphorylation

Following binding of EGF or TNF-α to EGFRwt, the monomeric receptor undergoes dimerization, resulting in kinase activation, and autophosphorylation primarily of tyrosine residues Tyr^{845}, Tyr^{992}, Tyr^{1045}, Tyr^{1068}, Tyr^{1086}, Tyr^{1148}, and Tyr^{1173} (*54, 59*).

2.3. Endosomal Localization

While it is the consensus that most mitogenic signaling is generated by activated receptors at the plasma membrane (*60*), it has been demonstrated that once formed, the receptor-ligand complex is released from caveolae, as EGFRwt is no longer associated with caveolin-1, and the receptor complex is found in the cytosol (*58*). Specifically, following EGF or TNF-α stimulation, the former sequestration of non-phosphorylated EGFRwt within caveolae is rapidly reversed; phosphorylated EGF-EGFR complexes are internalized in Rab5-positive endosomes via coated pit- and coated vesicle-mediated endocytosis. Signaling by the complex can occur from within the endosome (*61*), although this is probably not the major source of signaling. It is not until the complex progresses to lysosomes that degradation and attenuation of receptor signaling occurs via the phosphorylation of c-Cbl, an E3 ubiquitin ligase, which directs its degradation (*56, 62*).

2.4. Signaling Pathways

Whether from the membrane or endosomes, ligand-EGFRwt complexes utilize a variety of pathways, as depicted in Fig. 19.2. The major pathway that activated ErbB family receptors, including EGFRwt, use is the recruitment of either Grb2-Sos or Shc-Grb2-Sos complexes that activate Ras, which in turn ultimately stimulates phosphorylation of the MAPKs Erk 1 and 2 through sequential activation of c-Raf and MEK 1/2 [*12*]). The ERKs are considered components of "proliferation pathways" and are primarily involved in the activation of transcription factors involved in mitogenic signaling and cell proliferation, and they may promote cell-cycle progression by inducing cyclin D1 (*60, 62*). EGFRwt also activates "anti-apoptosis" pathways primarily through the phosphatidylinositol 3-kinase (PI3K) and the downstream protein-serine/threonine kinase Akt (*12, 57, 62*). The probable mechanism is by tyrosine phosphorylation of Gab1 (a Grb2-associated binder) by the EGFR kinase; phosphorylated Gab1 then recruits SHP-2 (a tyrosine phosphatase with Src homology domain) and PI3-kinase, which results in the activation of Akt, which in turn activates NF-κB, and this results in inhibition of factors inducing apoptosis (*57*). A third, but minor pathway used by EGFRwt is the stress-activated protein kinase pathway involving protein kinase C and Jak/Stat transcription factors; this is primarily mediated through the recruitment of adapter proteins with SH2 domains, which serve to dock the Src kinases, and this results in the triggering of STATs and NF-κB, among others (*57, 12, 60*). The EGFRwt signaling system then uses multiple pathways, with cross-talk at all levels: homodimerization of EGFRwt and heterodimerization with other ErbB family receptors, recruitment of adapter molecules, and activation of Ras, PI3K, and PKC pathways, resulting in induction of the transcription of genes that regulate cell transcription and prevent apoptosis.

3. SIGNAL TRANSDUCTION BY EGFRvIII

The majority of in vitro studies defining the signaling by EGFRvIII have been performed with cell lines engineered to express either EGFRwt, or EGFRvIII, or both. The most widely used model is the U87MG cell line, expressing low levels of endogenous EGFRwt (*63*), and its transfected derivatives U87MG$_{wtEGFR}$, expressing enhanced levels of EGFRwt, and U87MG$_{\Delta EGFR}$, expressing enhanced levels of EGFRvIII and low levels of endogenous EGFRwt (*9, 64, 65*).

Multiple groups have examined this system with consistent results; it is proposed that the U87MG$_{\Delta EGFR}$ cell line, co-expressing EGFRvIII and endogenous EGFRwt, represents a close approximation of a particularly aggressive subset of human glioblastomas—"those tumors in which p16 deletion, allelic loss on chromosome 10q, and EGFR activation occur, while p53 is nonmutated" (65).

3.1. Cell Membrane Localization

EGFRvIII, like EGFRwt, is expressed on the cell surface, frequently at densities >10^6 molecules per cell, as detected by specific monoclonal antibody (Mab L8A4) in FACs analysis under conditions preventing internalization (38, 59) (Fig. 19.3). While EGFRwt colocalizes with caveolin-1 and lipid rafts, and binding of ligand results in the release of EGFRwt from caveolae (58), EGFRvIII does not colocalize with caveolin-1 or rafts (58). Indeed, the prevention of constitutive autophosphorylation of EGFRvIII by kinase inhibitor AG1478 results in an increased association of EGFRvIII with caveolin-1, suggesting that phosphorylation regulates the degree of ligand-induced or constitutive signaling by regulating release from caveolae.

3.2 Ligand Binding, Dimerization and Autophosphorylation

There is no evidence for regulation of EGFRvIII by EGF or TGF-α; EGFRvIII is constitutively activated (37). Although earlier studies reported that EGFRvIII homodimerization or heterodimerization with EGFRwt or other ErbB family members was undetectable or insignificant (66–68), it has since been established that not only does homodimerization of EGFRvIII occur (69, 70), but it is highly dependent upon a conformation induced by N-linked core glycosylation (62, 71). The degree of autophosphorylation of EGFRvIII had been described as significantly less than that induced by ligand binding to EGFRwt (59, 67, 69). Recent studies, however, have established that the degree of autophosphorylation and kinase activity per molecule of dimeric EGFRvIII is comparable to that of the EGF-stimulated EGFRwt (58, 62, 71). Furthermore, the phosphorylation pattern of EGFRvIII is identical to that obtained following EGF-EGFRwt interaction as determined by phosphopeptide analysis (71). In addition, these authors have demonstrated that the conformation-specific anti-

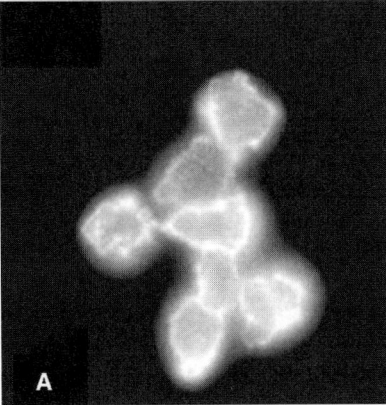 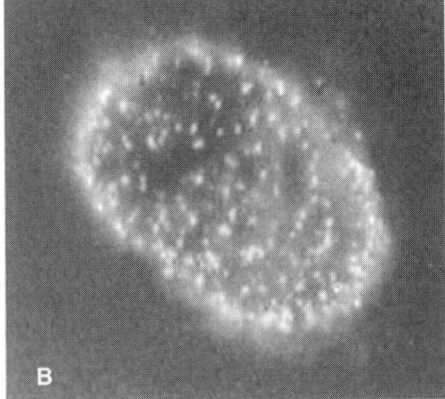

Fig. 19.3. EGFRvIII Mab L8A4, noninternalizing conditions. Cell surface expression of EGFRvIII on U87MG-EGFRvIII cells. The extensive display shown in panel A is demonstrated at higher magnification (panel B) to be due to multiple discrete patches of labeling.

body P2, which recognizes an epitope in the EGFRwt intracellular domain that is unmasked only upon phosphorylation of tyrosines 992, 1068, and 1086, also recognizes constitutively phosphorylated EGFRvIII, which suggests that there is a similar phosphorylation-induced conformational change in both receptors (71). Thus, it would appear that the ligand-induced and EGFRvIII constitutive phosphorylation patterns are highly similar, if not identical. The crucial observation is that constitutively activated EGFRvIII receptor trafficking is different from that of EGFRwt; it has been reported to be slower than that of ligand-activated EGFRwt, and to resemble the random entrapment kinetics of non-activated EGFRwt (59). Mab L8A4-EGFRvIII complexes formed at the cell surface are readily and rapidly internalized, however, resulting in detectable cytoplasmic, perinuclear vesicular localization corresponding to endosomes and lysosomes within five minutes (72). More definitively, Abulrob et al. (58) have demonstrated that EGFRvIII, unassociated with caveolae, is endocytosed and remains in the endosomal compartment, where the truncated receptor sustains its phosphorylated, activated state; Liu et al. (62) have demonstrated that EGFRvIII is quite proficient at signaling from within endosomes. Thus, despite the differences between EGFRwt and EGFRvIII in caveolar localization, speed of endocytosis, and lysosomal sorting, ultimately, activated EGFRvIII ends up in the endosomal compartment, quite capable of sustained signaling.

3.3. Signaling Pathways

The signaling pathways used by EGFRvIII are, not surprisingly, those primarily used by EGFRwt. Early studies readily identified the association between EGFRvIII and Grb2, with or without involvement of the adapter protein Shc, culminating in the recruitment of Ras-GTP (66–68, 73). Prigent et al. (67), using derivatives of EGFRvIII containing single or multiple mutations at critical autophosphorylation sites in the U87MG transfectant system, demonstrated that EGFRvIII constitutively associates with the adapter protein Shc and Grb2 via specific phosphorylation sites, Shc recruiting Ras through phosphorylated Tyr-1148, and Grb2 primarily through Tyr-1068. The centrality of the Shc-Grb2- or Grb2-Ras pathway to EGFRvIII signaling has been demonstrated by many groups. Klingler-Hoffman et al. (69, 70) demonstrated that the activation of ERK1/2 via EGFRvIII-to-Ras-to-MAPK was essential for the proliferation of U87MG-EGFRvIII expressing cells both in vitro and in tumor xenografts, a general observation supported by other studies (66, 74–76). Recently, Zhan and O'Rourke (76) reported that the tyrosine phosphatase SHP-2 modulates the MAPK kinase MEK-mediated signaling pathway via recruitment of SHP-2 to Gab-1; dephosphorylation of components of the MAPK pathway by SHP-2 thereby modulates EGFRvIII tyrosine phosphorylation, decreasing proliferation. This is in contrast to the observation of the action of SHP-2 in regulation of EGFRwt-mediated pathways; there the primary effect of SHP-2 was reported to be downregulation of the Gab1/PI3 kinase/Akt pathway (55, 76). These observed effects on the two major pathways involved in EGFR stimulation provide the first clue to differential regulation of maintained signaling and downstream activation effects of EGFRwt and EGFRvIII.

The use of the PI3K-Akt pathway by EGFRvIII was similarly established quite early and subsequently verified by many groups (47, 77–81). Klingler-Hoffman et al. (70) established that EGFRvIII autophosphorylation allows for recruitment of the PI3K p85 regulatory subunit, consequently activating the catalytic subunit of PI3K, and contributing to the growth advantage in vitro mediated by the MAPK-pathway seen in the U87MG transfectant system. In addition, the EGFRvIII-mediated activation of PI3K results in the activation of c-Jun N-terminal kinase (JNK; 82), an interaction not seen in EGFRwt-expressing cells.

However, the clearest dissection of the contributions of the various pathways in EGFRvIII-mediated signaling is obtained only with specific inhibition of one pathway versus another, or suppression/inactivation of one receptor versus the other in the U87MG cell system, where EGFRvIII expression is coincident with low levels of endogenous EGFRwt. Several studies have been performed to isolate the effects of each pathway.

3.3.1. MAPK Pathway Inhibition

The tyrosine kinase AG1478 competes with adenosine triphosphate and effects greater inhibition of EGFRvIII than EGFRwt by reducing ERK1/2 activation (*78*). By decreasing EGFRvIII autophosphorylation, it causes a downregulation of Bcl-X_L expression, although this is not sufficient to induce apoptosis in vitro or inhibit growth of EGFRvIII-expressing tumors in vivo (*64*). Similarly, treatment of U87MG-EGFRvIII cells with the MEK inhibitor PD98059 also results in no ERK1/2 activation and decreased cell proliferation (*69*). Treatment with either AG1478 or PD98059 renders U87MG-EGFRvIII cells, but not U87MGwt cells, susceptible to apoptosis following exposure to cisplatin (CDDP), which indicates that for EGFRvIII, the MAPK pathway is involved in regulating cell survival through inhibition of EGFRvIII tyrosine phosphorylation (p Tyr). As EGFRvIII p Tyr is modulated by SHP-2-dependent MAPK pathway activation and EGFRwt p Tyr is modulated by PI3K signaling events (*76*), this provides a targetable separation of pathways.

3.3.2. PI3K Pathway Inhibition

In a similar fashion, two inhibitors of the PI3K pathway, LY294002 and wortmannin, have been studied for their effects on EGFRvIII signaling. Klingler-Hoffman et al. (*70*) demonstrated that while PI3K signaling (as demonstrated by inhibition with wortmannin) was necessary to maintain the growth advantage conferred by EGFRvIII, suppression of PI3K signaling was not sufficient to inhibit anchorage independence in U87MG-EGFRvIII cells. Treatment of EGFRvIII-positive cell lines with LY294002 or wortmannin, as reported by Kuan et al. (*37*), "decreased JNK activity and induced the loss of transformed cell properties (anchorage independent growth, growth in low-serum medium), which suggests that the transforming activity of EGFRvIII involves the constitutive activation of both PI3K and JNK activity" (*37, 66, 70, 82*). Klingler-Hoffmann et al. (*68*) were able to elucidate the different downstream effects of the PI3K versus MAPK pathways by using variants of the TCPTP tyrosine phosphatase. TC45, which inhibits MAPK ERK2 and PI3K signaling, inhibited both the proliferation and anchorage-independent growth of U87MG-EGFRvIII. However, the variant TC45-D182A, which suppresses activation of only ERK2, but not PI3K, only inhibited cell proliferation, which suggests that one of the cardinal diagnostic features of neoplastic progression, anchorage-independent growth in vitro, is attributable to the PI3K pathway, as earlier suggested by Moscatello et al. (*66*) for glioblastoma cells, and by Li et al. (*80*) for EGFRvIII-transfected NIH3T3 cells. In addition, Narita et al. (*77*) have shown that treatment of U87MG-EGFRvIII cells with LY294002 not only reduced levels of P-Akt, as expected, but concomitantly up-regulated p27 (the cyclin-dependent kinase inhibitor). As U87MG-EGFRvIII normally exhibits low levels of p27 and high levels of P-Akt, the effects of the PI3K inhibitor were to increase p27 levels and to downregulate tumorigenicity in vivo. Therefore, it is apparent that the constitutively active EGFRvIII acts to increase cell proliferation by decreasing the expression of p27 via activation of the PI3K-Akt pathway.

Finally, the effects of "natural" inhibitors of EGFRvIII signaling have revealed some further information. As noted in the introduction, the presence of EGFRvIII and PTEN in the same tumor appears to be antagonistic; the mechanism for this antagonism has been proposed to be via the PI3K pathway. The normal PTEN gene product inhibits PI3K signaling by dephosphorylation of the lipid products of PI3K signaling (PIP3), thus impeding the phosphorylation of Akt (*77*). Inactivation of PTEN, however, results in the prolongation of the lifespan of EGFRvIII-induced PI3K lipid products, resulting in high levels of PI3K signaling and therefore growth advantage (*70*); thus the presence of EGFRvIII in the absence of normal PTEN expression will lead to cell proliferation. Herstatin, a naturally occurring product of the *HER-2* gene, which inhibits EGFRwt by binding to its extracellular domain and blocking dimerization (*83*), is capable of preventing tumor formation by U87MG cells in vivo. Staverosky et al. (*84*) found that although herstatin bound to EGFRvIII, the variant receptor still dimerized and was capable of signaling through both MAPK and PI3K pathways, while EGFRwt exposed to herstatin could use only the MAPK pathway. Thus, a powerful inhibitor of EGFRwt-driven growth in vitro and in vivo is ineffective versus EGFRvIII at the level of receptor dimerization.

4. CONSEQUENCES OF GLIOMA-ASSOCIATED EGFRvIII SIGNALING FOR THERAPEUTIC TARGETING

In a review of EGFRvIII as an immunotherapeutic target, in 2000, we stated: "In addition to the capacity to localize putative effectors, a tumor-cell distinctive molecule which mediates biologic function central to cell growth advantage, metabolism, adhesiveness/motility, or drug resistance, would have a great therapeutic targeting potential" (35). This introductory statement is still applicable. Currently, a number of strategies for targeting EGFRwt or EGFRvIII—either as localizing targets for the delivery of cytocidal Mab-isotope, Mab-drug, Mab-toxin agents, or tumor vaccines, or as inhibition mediators of cell proliferation by TKIs, antisense oligonucleotides or constructs—are being explored.

4.1. EGFRvIII as Localizing Target

As has been extensively summarized elsewhere (37) EGFRwt has been targeted on tumor cells, notably by the chimerized/human Mabs IMC-C225 (cetuximab) and E7.6.3, both of which presumably block the binding of ligand to EGFR, but cause receptor-mediated internalization, preventing downstream signaling and abolishing cell proliferation, EGFR tyrosine phosphorylation, and ultimately resulting in apoptosis. While this approach, especially in combination with chemotherapy or radiation, has resulted in impressive responses in some tumor systems, the widespread normal tissue distribution of EGFRwt limits approaches by this route. Conversely, EGFRvIII is an excellent target for specific Mab delivery of a variety of payloads, as to date its expression appears confined to tumor cells, and immunoreagents specific for its extracellular domain have been extensively characterized (37, 85, 86). As was shown for the fully human anti-EGFRwt Mab E7.6.3 (87), unarmed anti-EGFRvIII-specific Mab Y10 is capable of inhibiting DNA synthesis and cellular proliferation of EGFRvIII-expressing cells in vitro, presumably by receptor internalization and inhibition of downstream signaling, and of producing an average 286% increase in survival, with 25% cures, in animals bearing EGFRvIII-expressing intracranial xenografts (88). Mab Y10 (murine IgG2a) was demonstrated to mediate cell death of EGFRvIII-positive tumor cells by both complement-mediated and Fc-receptor-bearing effector cells in a murine homologue model system, which suggests that its cytocidal effects in vivo could be the result of both inhibitory induction of apoptosis and direct, cytotoxic killing pathways.

Of more interest therapeutically, however, is the exploitation of the demonstrable rapid internalization of specific Mab-EGFRvIII complexes (72, 89). As previously summarized, Zalutsky (91) has developed labeling strategies designed to maximize stability and minimize lysosomal degradation and dehalogenation of labeled Mabs, scFv, F(ab')$_2$, or other constructs for delivering isotope (either α- or γ-emitters) by receptor-mediated internalization to the cytoplasm of EGFRvIII-expressing cells (72, 89–92). Similarly, delivery of toxin, rather than isotope, can be achieved by the same targeting Mabs, and this has been an active area of research, with *Pseudomonas* exotoxin A–antibody constructs exhibiting significant long-term survival in rodent intracranial models of EGFRvIII-expressing gliomas (37, 93). These approaches are predicated upon the tumor-specific localizing attribute of the EGFRvIII extracellular domain, however, and exploit the rapid internalization capacity of this noncaveolin bound receptor, not the downstream signaling activities of the molecule.

4.2. EGFRvIII Peptide as a Tumor Vaccine

Both animal and human clinical studies have shown promise in vaccination trials with malignant gliomas utilizing the EGFRvIII 14 amino acid peptide (PEP3) shown in Fig. 19.1, which contains the new glycine inserted at the fusion junction of the EGFRvIII receptor protein. Because the glycine at the mutant protein fusion junction is not present in the wild-type EGFR protein, PEP3 contains true tumor-specific epitopes. Both cell-mediated and antibody mechanisms are thought to have played a role in the successful vaccine trials in animals and humans. The first trial conducted at Duke by Sampson and Bigner utilized pulsing of autologous dendritic cells with KLH-PEP3. The pulsed dendritic cells were then readministered to the patients. No significant toxicities were observed, and promising survival increases relative to historical controls were seen. The second clinical vaccine trials were done in multi-institutional studies conducted at Duke and at M.D. Anderson. They also showed promising increases in survival in malignant glioma patients compared to historical controls. In the latter trials, KLH-PEP3 was simply administered systematically, simultaneously with GMCSF. The EGFRvIII PEP-3 peptide vaccine approach has now been licensed by a biotechnology company, and multi-institutional, randomized, pivotal trials are being planned. This vaccine approach should be promising also in head and neck squamous cell carcinoma, as well as in malignant gliomas (*94–97*).

4.3. EGFRvIII as Signaling Target

The consensus of investigators of normal EGFRwt and variant EGFRvIII signaling mechanisms is that given the usual coincident expression of both receptors (>90% of EGFRvIII+ gliomas express EGFRwt [*23, 35*]) efforts that target both the wild-type and vIII receptors would be optimal (*12, 23, 27*). The excessive cross-talk between these receptors and other family receptors, primarily through the PI3K/Akt and MAPK (p44/p42) pathways, however, creates some conundrums: (a) While it has been conventionally accepted that the RAS/RAF/MAPK cascade can be activated by EGFR family receptors, it is now evident that RAS may well activate the PI3K-AKT pathway as well, and in this guise, be a more potent suppressor of radiation-induced apoptosis (*47*); and (b) both of these pathways are also essential survival pathways for normal astrocytes and neurons, as well as for glioma cells (summarized in Chakravarti et al. [*47*]). Therefore, the general blockade of such pathways must be considered with caution to avoid bystander death of normal cells. Targeting of potential upstream tumor-specific activators or mediators associated with these pathways, such as RTKs and RAS, would therefore be optimal. In addition, for particularly aggressive or resistant cell populations such as those emerging in therapy-refractory GBM, inhibition of a single pathway is not likely to be successful; experimental evidence has indeed indicated that a two-point blockade (for example, HER1/EGFR and PI3K) in animal models of glioma was synergistic using sub-optimal doses of the single agents (*98*). Currently, with the exception of the use of radiolabeled or toxin-conjugated ligands (EGFRwt) or Mabs (EGFRwt and EGFRvIII) to block downstream signaling, the major approaches include specific kinase inhibitors of various steps of the signal transduction pathways, antisense oligonucleotides and or ribozymes to reduce or impede receptor function.

4.4. TKIs

Although in many tumor types the observed clinical response to TKIs has failed to correlate with the promising effects demonstrated in preclinical studies (summarized in Sok et al. [*4*]), approaches using various TKIs are being actively investigated. Many investigators, assuming that EGFRwt and EGFRvIII "selectively" or "preferentially" activate the PI3K-Akt pathway, have concentrated on inhibition of this pathway (*56, 77, 99*). The Thomas and Narita groups both used the PI3K inhibitor LY294002 to investigate the effects of reduced levels of phosphorylated Akt in EGFRwt- and EGFRvIII-expressing cells, respectively. It was rapidly apparent that the loss of PTEN, a tumor-suppressor protein that inhibits the PI3K signaling pathway, was associated with resistance to EGFR kinase inhibitors targeting PI3K in gliomas (56, 77, 99). These data corroborated those of Klingler-Hoffmann et al. (70), who demonstrated that EGFRvIII expression and signaling and PTEN inactivation cooperated to produce high levels of PI3K signaling in GBM cells, but that inhibition of EGFRvIII-mediated PI3K activation alone did not appreciably suppress tumorigenicity in vivo (69). As PTEN losses/mutations have been variably reported to occur in 30%-50% of GBM (summarized in Narita et al. (77), the effects of this targeting could be expected to be mixed, depending upon the PTEN status of a targeted tumor. In addition, Chakravarti et al. (100) have demonstrated for EGFRwt, and presumably for EGFRvIII, that the targeting of this growth factor by the TKI AG1478 could result in the up-regulation of insulin-like growth factor receptor 1 (IGF-1), resulting in sustained signaling through the PI3K pathway, effectively negating the suppression of EGFR-mediated PI3K pathways and thus providing a mechanism of resistance to anti-EGFR therapeutic approaches.

In addition to cross-talk mediated by Ras between the PI3K/Akt and MAPK pathways (47), the MAPK pathway has recently been stressed as a major route for EGFRwt and EGFRvIII signaling (67, 69, 72, 76). Therefore, as suggested by Biernat et al. (27), and in accord with the caution of Chakravarti et al. (47) concerning inhibition of pathways used by normal cells, a very feasible approach would be to simultaneously target the EGFRwt and EGFRvIII pathways in glioma cells by inhibiting SHP-2, which mediates the phosphorylation of Akt and EGFRwt via PI3K (55, 57, 76), and of EGFRvIII via MAPK. Similarly, the small molecule irreversible EGFR/ERB2 inhibitor HKI-272, which has been shown to have a greater inhibitory effect than gefitinib or erlotinib on the growth of EGFRvIII+ tumors in in vivo model systems, has been demonstrated to reduce levels of phospho-EGFR, phospho-Akt, and phospho-ERK1/2 (101), thereby providing a dual pathway-targeting reagent.

Exploiting the fact that the genetic deletion and resultant fusion event generating EGFRvIII is directly upstream of a GTA triplet, which is subsequently transcribed into a ribozyme target codon (GUA), Halatsch et al. (102) have attempted to curtail EGFRvIII gene expression at the mRNA level by creating an anti-EGFRvIII hairpin ribozyme. Administration of the construct via retrovirus to EGFRvIII-expressing target cells in vitro resulted in a >90% reduction in EGFRvIII mRNA levels, 69% inhibition of proliferation, and >95% decrease in colony formation in agar, suggesting that this approach could selectively and significantly inhibit EGFRvIII-mediated growth advantages. Inhibition of EGFRvIII at the protein level has been investigated by O'Rourke et al. (65); they have shown that the p185*neu* ectodomain-derived mutant (carboxyl terminal deletion mutant) forms heterodimers with EGFRvIII proteins, reducing the phosphotyrosine content and kinase activity of assayed EGFRvIII monomers. Creation of pharmaceutical agents mimicking the p185 ectodomain could then be used to create receptor assemblies that are defective in signaling, effectively silencing the growth advantage conferred by EGFRvIII.

5. CONCLUSION

The effective targeting of EGFR-mediated growth advantage in gliomas will require inhibition of both EGFRwt and EGFRvIII signaling pathways, as the majority of GBMs either express both or will eventually express both. In addition to ligand (EGFRwt) or specific Mab approaches (both) which abrogate the original induction, or compromise the endogenous signaling (EGFRvIII), further targeting of upstream or downstream events used by these receptors must recognize that they use the same basic pathways. They may stress different pathways, and be differentially inhibited by small molecule TKIs, but they use mechanisms crucial to bystander normal cells. Thus the approaches outlined above that do not inactivate all RAS, or all PI3K pathways, but target upstream (Shc, Grb2) steps would be optimal. The prospects of specific targeting via mRNA transcription or protein-dimerization of these family proteins are significant in providing the specific blockade required. Successful implementation of signaling cascade targeting will be a valuable adjunct to the other specific receptor targeting mechanisms (Mab constructs, ligand bullets) available and demonstrably effective against EGFRwt- and EGFRvIII-expressing tumor cells.

REFERENCES

1. Arteaga CL, Hurd SD, Dugger TC, Winnier AR, Robertson JB. Epidermal growth factor receptors in human breast carcinoma cells: a potential selective target for transforming growth factor α-*Pseudomonas* exotoxin 40 fusion protein. Cancer Res 1994;54:4703–9.
2. Owens OJ, Steward C, Leake RE, McNicol AM. A comparison of biochemical and immunohistochemical assessment of EGFR expression in ovarian cancer. Anticancer Res 1992;12:1455–8.
3. Rusch V, Baselga J, Cordon-Cardo C, et al. Differential expression of the epidermal growth factor receptor and its ligands in primary non-small cell lung cancers and adjacent benign lung. Cancer Res 1993;53:2379–85.
4. Sok JC, Coppelli FM, Thomas SM, et al. Mutant epidermal growth factor receptor (EGFRvIII) contributes to head and neck cancer growth and resistance to EGFR targeting. Clin Cancer Res 2006;12:5064–73.
5. Grandis JR, Tweardy DJ. Elevated levels of transforming growth factor alpha and epidermal growth factor receptor messenger RNA are early markers of carcinogenesis in head and neck cancer. Cancer Res 1993;53:3579–84.
6. Grandis JR, Melhem, MF, Gooding WE, et al. Levels of TGF-α and EGFR protein in head and neck squamous cell carcinoma and patient survival. J Natl Cancer Inst 1998;90:824–32.
7. Nicholson RI, Gee JM, Harper ME. EGFR and cancer prognosis. Eur J Cancer 2001;37(Suppl 4):S9-S15.
8. Wikstrand CJ, Hale LP, Batra SK, et al. Monoclonal antibodies against EGFRvIII are tumor specific and react with breast and lung carcinomas and malignant gliomas. Cancer Res 1995;55:3140–8.
9. Nishikawa R, Ji X-D, Harmon RC, et al. A mutant epidermal growth factor receptor common in human glioma confers enhanced tumorigenicity. Proc Natl Acad Sci USA 1994;91:7727–31.
10. Salomon D, Brandt R, Ciardiello F, Normanno N. Epidermal growth factor-related peptides and their receptors in human malignancies. Crit Rev Oncol Hematol 1995;19:182–232.
11. Ang KK, Berkey BA, Tu X, et al. Impact of epidermal growth factor receptor expression on survival and pattern of relapse in patients with advanced head and neck carcinoma. Cancer Res 2002;62:7350–6.
12. Mendelsohn J, Baselga J. Status of epidermal growth factor receptor antagonists in the biology and treatment of cancer. J. Clin Oncol 2003;21:2787–99.
13. Moscatello DK, Holgado-Madruga M, Godwin AK, et al. Frequent expression of a mutant epidermal growth factor receptor in multiple human tumors. Cancer Res 1995;55:5536–9.
14. Wong AJ, Croce CM. Oncogenes and signal transduction. Hosp Pract 1993;28:128–41.
15. Libermann TA, Razon N, Bartal AD, Yarden Y, Schlessinger J, Soreq H. Expression of epidermal growth factor receptors in human brain tumors. Cancer Res 1984;44:753–60.
16. Libermann TA, Nusbaum HR, Razon N, et al. Amplification, enhanced expression and possible rearrangement of EGF receptor gene in primary human brain tumours of glial origin. Nature 1985;313:144–7.
17. Wong AJ, Bigner SH, Bigner DD, Kinzler KW, Hamilton SR, Vogelstein B. Increased expression of the epidermal growth factor receptor gene in malignant gliomas is invariably associated with gene amplification. Proc Natl Acad Sci USA 1987;84:6899–903.
18. Sauter G, Maeda T, Waldman F, Davis RL, Feuerstein BG. Patterns of epidermal growth factor receptor amplification in malignant gliomas. Am J Pathol 1996;148:1047–53.
19. Goike HM, Asplund AC, Pettersson EH, Liu L, Sanoudou D, Collins VP. Acquired rearrangement of an amplified epidermal growth factor receptor (EGFR) gene in a human glioblastoma xenograft. J Neuropathol Exp Neurol 1999;58:697–701.

20. Agosti RM, Leuthold M, Gullick WJ, Yasargil MG, Wiestler OD. Expression of the epidermal growth factor receptor in astrocytic tumours is specifically associated with glioblastoma multiforme. Virchows Archiv A Pathol Anat Histopathol 1992;420:321–5.
21. Torp SH, Helseth E, Dalen A, Unsgaard G. Epidermal growth factor receptor expression in human gliomas. Cancer Immunol Immunother 1991;33:61–4.
22. Wong AJ, Ruppert JM, Bigner SH, et al. Structural alterations of the epidermal growth factor receptor gene in human gliomas. Proc Natl Acad Sci USA 1992;89:2965–9.
23. Liu L, Bäcklund LM, Nilsson BR, et al. Clinical significance of *EGFR* amplification and the aberrant EGFRvIII transcript in conventionally treated astrocytic gliomas. J Mol Med 2005;83:917–26.
24. Shinojima N, Tada K, Shiraishi S, et al. Prognostic value of epidermal growth factor receptor in patients with glioblastoma multiforme. Cancer Res 2003;63:6962–70.
25. Aldape KD, Ballman K, Furth A, et al. Immunohistochemical detection of EGFRvIII in high malignancy grade astrocytomas and evaluation of prognostic significance. J Neuropathol Exp Neurol 2004;63:700–7.
26. Batchelor TT, Betensky RA, Esposito JM, et al. Age-dependent prognostic effects of genetic alterations in glioblastoma. Clin Cancer Res 2004;10:228–33.
27. Biernat W, Huang H, Yokoo H, Kleihues P, Ohgaki H. Predominant expression of mutant EGFR (EGFRvIII) is rare in primary glioblastomas. Brain Pathol 2004;14:131–6.
28. McLendon RE, Wikstrand CJ, Matthews MR, Al-Baradei R, Bigner SH, Bigner DD. Glioma-associated antigen expression in oligodendroglial neoplasms: Tenascin and epidermal growth factor receptor. J Histochem Cytochem 2000;48:1103–10.
29. Rich JN, Hans C, Jones B, et al. Gene expression profiling and genetic markers in glioblastoma survival. Cancer Res 2005;65:4051–8.
30. Shih HA, Betensky RA, Dorfman MV, Louis DN, Loeffler JS, Batchelor TT. Genetic analyses for predictors of radiation response in glioblastoma. Int J Rad Oncol Biol Phys 2005;63:704–10.
31. Smith JS, Tachibana I, Passe SM, et al. PTEN mutation, EGFR amplification, and outcome in patients with anaplastic astrocytoma and glioblastoma multiforme. J Natl Cancer Inst 2001;93:1246–56.
32. Barker FG, Simmons ML, Chang SM, et al. EGFR overexpression and radiation response in glioblastoma multiforme. Int J Radiat Oncol Biol Phys 2001;51:410–8.
33. von Deimling A, Louis DN, Wiestler OD. Molecular pathways in the formation of gliomas. Glia 1995;15:328–38.
34. Watanabe K, Trachibana O, Sato K, Yonekawa Y, Kleihues P, Ohgaki H. Overexpression of the EGF receptor and p53 mutations are mutually exclusive in the evolution of primary and secondary glioblastomas. Brain Pathol 1996;6:217–24.
35. Wikstrand CJ, Reist CJ, Archer GE, Zalutsky MR, Bigner DD. The class III variant of the epidermal growth factor receptor (EGFRvIII): characterization and utilization as an immunotherapeutic target. J Neurovirol 1998;4:148–58.
36. Frederick L, Wang XY, Eley G, James CD. Diversity and frequency of epidermal growth factor receptor mutations in human gliomas. Cancer Res 2000;60:1383–7.
37. Kuan C-T, Wikstrand CJ, Bigner DD. EGF mutant receptor vIII as a molecular target in cancer therapy. Endocr Rel Cancer 2001;8:83–96.
38. Wikstrand CJ, McLendon RE, Friedman AH, Bigner DD. Cell surface localization and density of the tumor-associated variant of the epidermal growth factor receptor, EGFRvIII. Cancer Res 1997;57:4130–40.
39. Okamoto I, Kenyon LC, Emlet DR, et al. Expression of constitutively activated EGFRvIII in non-small cell lung cancer. Cancer Sci 2003;94:50–6.
40. Ge H, Gong X, Tang CK. Evidence of high incidence of EGFRvIII expression and coexpression with EGFR in human invasive breast cancer by laser capture microdissection and immunohistochemical analysis. Int J Cancer 2002;98:357–61.
41. Sihto H, Puputti M, Pulli L, et al. Epidermal growth factor receptor domain II, IV, and kinase domain mutations in human solid tumors. J Mol Med 2005;83:976–83.
42. Marie Y, Carpentier AF, Omuro AMP, et al. EGFR tyrosine kinase domain mutations in human gliomas. Neurology 2005;64:1444–5.
43. Ohgaki H, Dessen P, Jourde B, et al. Genetic pathways to glioblastoma: a population-based study. Cancer Res 2004;64: 6892–9.

44. Simmons ML, Lamborn KR, Takahashi M, et al. Analysis of complex relationships between age, p53, epidermal growth factor receptor, and survival in glioblastoma patients. Cancer Res 2001;61:1122–8.
45. Kleihues P, Cavenee WK. World Health Organization Classification of Tumours. Pathology and Genetics of Tumours of the Nervous System. Lyon: IARC Press, 2000.
46. Dropcho EJ, Soong SJ. The prognostic impact of prior low grade histology in patients with anaplastic gliomas: A case-control study. Neurology 1996;47:684–90.
47. Chakravarti A, Chakladar A, Delaney MA, Latham DE, Loeffler JS. The epidermal growth factor receptor pathway mediates resistance to sequential administration of radiation and chemotherapy in primary human glioblastoma cells in a RAS-dependent manner. Cancer Res 2002;62: 4307–15.
48. Sarkaria JN, Carlson BL, Schroeder MA, et al. Use of an orthotopic xenograft model for assessing the effect of epidermal growth factor receptor amplification on glioblastoma radiation response. Clin Cancer Res 2006;12:2264–71.
49. Lynch TJ, Bell DW, Sordella R, et al. Activating mutations in the epidermal growth factor receptor underlying responsiveness of non-small-cell lung cancer to gefitinib. N Engl J Med 2004;350:2129–39.
50. Heimberger AB, Hlatky R, Suki D, et al. Prognostic effect of epidermal growth factor receptor and EGFRvIII in glioblastoma multiforme patients. Clin Cancer Res 2005;11:1462–6.
51. Heimberger AB, Suki D, Yang D, Shi W, Aldape K. The natural history of EGFR and EGFRvIII in glioblastoma patients. J Transl Med 2005;3:38–43.
52. Nagane M, Coufal F, Lin H, Bogler O, Cavenee WK, Huang HJ. A common mutant epidermal growth factor receptor confers enhanced tumorigenicity on human glioblastoma cells by increasing proliferation and reducing apoptosis. Cancer Res 1996;56:5079–86.
53. Tysnes BB, Haugland HK, Bjerkvig R. Epidermal growth factor and laminin receptors contribute to migratory and invasive properties of gliomas. Invasion Metastasis 1997;17:270–80.
54. Amos S, Martin PM, Polar GA, Parsons SJ, Hussaini IM. Phorbol 12-myristate 13-acetate induces epidermal growth factor receptor transactivation via protein kinase Cδ/c-Src pathways in glioblastoma cells. J Biol Chem 2005;280:7729–38.
55. Kapoor GS, Kapitonov D, O'Rourke DM. Transcriptional regulation of signal regulatory protein α1 inhibitory receptors by epidermal growth factor receptor signaling. Cancer Res 2004;64:6444–52.
56. Thomas CY, Chouinard M, Cox M, Parsons S, Stallings-Mann M, Garcia R, Jove R, Wharen R. Spontaneous activation and signaling by overexpressed epidermal growth factor receptors in glioblastoma cells. Int J Cancer 104:19–27, 2003.
57. Kapoor GS, Zhan Y, Johnson GR, O'Rourke DM. Distinct domains in the SHP-2 phosphatase differentially regulate epidermal growth factor receptor/NF-κB activation through Gab1 in glioblastoma cells. Mol Cell Biol 2004;24:823–36.
58. Abulrob A, Giuseppin S, Andrade MF, McDermid A, Moreno M, Stanimirovic D. Interactions of EGFR and caveolin-1 in human glioblastoma cells: evidence that tyrosine phosphorylation regulates EGFR association with caveolae. Oncogene 2004;23:6967–79.
59. Huang H-JS, Nagane M, Klingbeil CK, et al. The enhanced tumorigenic activity of a mutant epidermal growth factor receptor common in human cancers is mediated by threshold levels of constitutive tyrosine phosphorylation and unattenuated signaling. J Biol Chem 1997;272:2927–35.
60. Habib AA, Chun SJ, Neel BG, Vartanian T. Increased expression of epidermal growth factor receptor induces sequestration of extracellular signal-related kinases and selective attenuation of specific epidermal growth factor-mediated signal transduction pathways. Mol Cancer Res 2003;1:219–33.
61. Wang Y, Pennock S, Chen X, Wang Z. Endosomal signaling of epidermal growth factor receptor stimulates signal transduction pathways leading to cell survival. Mol Cell Biol 2002;22:7279–90.
62. Liu K-J, Chen C-T, Hu WS, et al. Expression of cytoplasmic-domain substituted epidermal growth factor receptor inhibits tumorigenicity of EGFR-overexpressed human glioblastoma multiforme. Int J Oncol 2004;24:581–90.
63. Ponten J, MacIntyre EH. Long term culture of normal and neoplastic human glia. Acta Pathol Microbiol Scand 1968;74:465–86.
64. Nagane M, Narita Y, Mishima K, et al. Human glioblastoma xenografts overexpressing a tumor-specific mutant epidermal growth factor receptor sensitized to cisplatin by the AG1478 tyrosine kinase inhibitor. J Neurosurg 2001;95:472–479.
65. O'Rourke DM, Nute EJL, Davis JG, et al. Inhibition of a naturally occurring EGFR oncoprotein by the p185*neu* ectodomain: implications for subdomain contributions to receptor assembly. Oncogene 1998;16:1197–207.

66. Moscatello DK, Montgomery RB, Sundareshan P, McDanel H, Wong MY, Wong AJ. Transformation and altered signal transduction by a naturally occurring mutant EGF receptor. Oncogene 1996;13:85–96.
67. Prigent SA, Nagane M, Lin H, et al. Enhanced tumorigenic behavior of glioblastoma cells expressing a truncated epidermal growth factor receptor is mediated through the Ras-Shc-Grb2 pathway. J Biol Chem 1996;271:25639–45.
68. Chu CT, Everiss KD, Wikstrand CJ, Batra SK, Kung HJ, Bigner DD. Receptor dimerization is not a factor in the signaling activity of a transforming variant epidermal growth factor receptor (EGFRvIII). Biochem J 1997;324:855–61.
69. Klingler-Hoffman M, Fodero-Tavoletti MT, Mishima K, et al. The protein tyrosine phosphatase TCPTP suppresses the tumorigenicity of glioblastoma cells expressing a mutant epidermal growth factor receptor. J Biol Chem 2001;276:46313–8.
70. Klingler-Hoffmann M, Bukczynska P, Tiganis T. Inhibition of phosphatidylinositol 3-kinase signaling negates the growth advantage imparted by a mutant epidermal growth factor receptor on human glioblastoma cells. Int J Cancer 2003;105:331–9.
71. Fernandes H, Cohen S Bishayee S. Glycosylation-induced conformational modification positively regulates receptor-receptor association. A study with an aberrant epidermal growth factor receptor (EGFRvIII/ΔEGFR) expressed in cancer cells. J Biol Chem 2001;276:5375–83.
72. Reist CJ, Archer GE, Kurpad SN, et al. Tumor-specific anti-epidermal growth factor receptor variant III monoclonal antibodies: use of the tyramine-cellobiose radioiodination method enhances cellular retention and uptake in tumor xenografts. Cancer Res 1995;55:4375–82.
73. Feldkamp MM, Lau N, Rak J, Kerbel RS, Guha A. Normoxic and hypoxic regulation of vascular endothelial growth factor (VEGF) by astrocytoma cells is mediated by Ras. Int J Cancer 1999;81:118–24.
74. Lorimer IA, Lavictoire SJ. Activation of extracellular-regulated kinases by normal and mutant EGF receptors. Biochim Biophys Acta 2001;1538:1–9.
75. Montgomery RB, Moscatello DK, Wong AJ, Cooper JA, Stahl WL. Differential modulation of mitogen-activated protein (MAP) kinase/extracellular signal-related kinase kinase and MAP kinase activities by a mutant epidermal growth factor receptor. J Biol Chem 1995;270:30562–6.
76. Zhan Y, O'Rourke DM. SHP-2-dependent mitogen-activated protein kinase activation regulates EGFRvIII but not wild-type epidermal growth factor receptor phosphorylation and glioblastoma cell survival. Cancer Res 2004;64:8292–8298.
77. Narita Y, Nagane M, Mishima K, Huang H-JS, Furnari FB, Cavenee WK. Mutant epidermal growth factor receptor signaling down-regulates p27 through activation of the phosphatidylinositol 3-kinase/Akt pathway in glioblastomas. Cancer Res 2002;62:6764–9.
78. Sordella R, Bell DW, Haber DA, Settleman J. Gefitinib-sensitizing EGFR mutations in lung cancer activate anti-apoptotic pathways. Science 2004;305:1163–7.
79. Choe G, Horvath S, Cloughesy TF, et al. Analysis of the phosphatidylinositol 3′-kinase signaling pathway in glioblastoma patients in vivo. Cancer Res 2003;63:2742–6.
80. Li B, Yuan M, Kim IA, Chang CM, Bernhard EJ, Shu HK. Mutant epidermal growth factor receptor displays increased signaling through the phosphatidylinositol-3 kinase/AKT pathway and promotes radioresistance in cells of astrocytic origin. Oncogene 2004;23:4594–602.
81. Batra SK, Castelino-Prabhu S, Wikstrand CJ, et al. Epidermal growth factor ligand-independent, unregulated, cell-transforming potential of a naturally occurring human mutant *EGFRvIII* gene. Cell Growth Differ. 1995;6:1251–9.
82. Antonyak MA, Moscatello DK, Wong AJ. Constitutive activation of c-Jun N-terminal kinase by a mutant epidermal growth factor receptor. J Biol Chem 1998;273:2817–22.
83. Justman AQ, Clinton GM. Herstatin, an autoinhibitor of the human epidermal growth factor receptor 2 tyrosine kinase, modulates epidermal growth factor signaling pathways resulting in growth arrest. J Biol Chem 2002;277:20618–24.
84. Staverosky JA, Muldoon LL, Guo S, Evans AJ, Neuwelt EA, Clinton GM. Herstatin, an autoinhibitor of the epidermal growth factor receptor family, blocks the intracranial growth of glioblastoma. Clin Cancer Res 2005;11:335–40.
85. Wikstrand CJ, Sampson JH, Bigner DD. EGFRvIII: an oncogene deletion mutant cell surface receptor target expressed by multiple tumour types. Emerg Ther Targets 2000;4:497–514.
86. Hills D, Rowlinson-Busza G, Gullick WJ. Specific targeting of a mutant, activated EGF receptor found in glioblastoma using a monoclonal antibody. Int J Cancer 1995;63:537–43.

87. Yang X-D, Jia X-C, Corvalan JRF, Wang P, Davis CG, Jakobovits A. Eradication of established tumors by a fully human monoclonal antibody to the epidermal growth factor receptor without concomitant chemotherapy. Cancer Res 1999;59:1236–43.
88. Sampson, JH, Crotty LE, Lee S, et al. Unarmed, tumor-specific monoclonal antibody effectively treats brain tumors. Proc Natl Acad Sci USA 2000;97:7503–8.
89. Reist CJ, Archer GE, Wikstrand CJ, Bigner DD, Zalutsky MR. Improved targeting of an anti-epidermal growth factor receptor variant III monoclonal antibody in tumor xenografts after labeling using *N*-succinimidyl 5-iodo-3-pyridinecarboxylate. Cancer Res 1997;57:1510–5.
90. Wikstrand CJ, Cokgor I, Sampson JH, Bigner DD. Monoclonal antibody therapy of human gliomas: current status and future approaches. Cancer Metastasis Rev 1999;18:451–64.
91. Zalutsky MR. Growth factor receptors as molecular targets for cancer diagnosis and therapy. Q J Nucl Med 1997;41:71–7.
92. Foulon CF, Reist CJ, Bigner DD, Zalutsky MR. Radioiodination via D-amino acid peptide enhances cellular retention and tumor xenograft targeting of an internalizing anti-epidermal growth factor receptor variant III monoclonal antibody. Cancer Res 2000;60:4453–60.
93. Archer GE, Sampson JH, Lorimer IAJ, et al. Regional treatment of epidermal growth factor receptor vIII-expressing neoplastic meningitis with a single-chain immunotoxin MR1. Clin Cancer Res 1999;5:2646–52.
94. Heimberger AB, Hussain SF, Aldape K, et al. Tumor-specific peptide vaccination in newly-diagnosed patients with GBM. Abstract 2529. Presentation for the 2006 ASCO Annual Meeting Proceedings. J Clin Oncol 2006;24(18S):107s.
95. Erdal S, Bigner DD, Davis FG. Theoretical estimation of dermal exposure to known and suspected animal neurocarcinogens. Abstract EP-08. Presented at Society for Neuro-Oncology Ninth Annual Meeting, Toronto, Ontario, Canada, November 18–21, 2004. Neuro-Oncology 2004;6:341.
96. Sok JC, Coppelli FM, Thomas SM, et al. Mutant epidermal growth factor receptor (EGFRvIII) contributes to head and neck cancer growth and resistance to EGFR targeting. Clin Cancer Res 2006;12(17):5064–73.
97. Heimberger AB, Crotty LE, Archer GE, et al. Epidermal growth factor receptor VIII peptide vaccination is efficacious against established intracerebral tumors. Clin Cancer Res 2003;9:4247–54.
98. Fan QW, Specht KM, Zhang C, Goldenberg DD, Shokat KM, Weiss WA. Combinatorial efficacy achieved through two-point blockade within a signaling pathway—a chemical genetic approach. Cancer Res 2003;63:8930–8.
99. Mellinghoff IK, Wang MY, Vivanco I, et al. Molecular determinants of the response of glioblastomas to EGFR kinase inhibitors. N Engl J Med 2005;353:2012–24.
100. Chakravarti A, Loeffler JS, Dyson NJ. Insulin-like growth factor receptor I mediates resistance to anti-epidermal growth factor receptor therapy in primary human glioblastoma cells through continued activation of phosphoinositide 3-kinase signaling. Cancer Res 2002;62:200–7.
101. Ji H, Zhao X, Yuza Y, et al. Epidermal growth factor receptor variant III mutations in lung tumorigenesis and sensitivity to tyrosine kinase inhibitors. Proc Natl Acad Sci USA 2006;103:7817–22.
102. Halatsch ME, Schmidt U, Botefur IC, Holland JF, Ohnuma T. Marked inhibition of glioblastoma target cell tumorigenicity in vitro by retrovirus-mediated transfer of a hairpin ribozyme against deletion-mutant epidermal growth factor receptor messenger RNA. J Neurosurg 2000;92:297–305.

20 EGFR Mutations, Other Molecular Alterations Related to Sensitivity to EGFR Inhibitors, and Molecular Testing for EGFR-Targeted Therapies in Non-Small Cell Lung Cancer

David A. Eberhard

Contents

Introduction
EGFR Tyrosine Kinase Domain (TKD) Mutations in NSCLC
EGFR Tyrosine Kinase Domain Mutations in Tumor Types Other than NSCLC
Relationship of EGFR TKD Mutations to EGFR TKI Sensitivity And Clinical Outcomes In NSCLC Patients
EGFR Expression and Gene Copy Number in NSCLC
Kras Mutation in NSCLC and Primary Resistance to EGFR TKIS
Other Molecular Characteristics Related to NSCLC Sensitivity to EGFR Inhibitors
Molecular Testing in Clinical Trials and Clinical Practice
Pathology Sample and Assay Considerations for the Molecular Testing of NSCLC in Clinical Tumor Samples
Conclusion
References

Abstract

Clinical response to EGFR inhibitors has varied considerably from patient to patient. In this chapter, the molecular, pathological and clinical correlates of therapeutic response and survival outcome are examined.

From: *Cancer Drug Discovery and Development: EGFR Signaling Networks in Cancer Therapy*
Edited by: J. D. Haley and W. J. Gullick, DOI: 10.1007/978-1-59745-356-1_20
© 2008 Humana Press, a part of Springer Science+Business Media, LLC

Key Words: Epidermal Growth Factor Receptor, Tyrosine Kinase Inhibitors, Molecular Diagnostics, Mutations, Fluorescence In Situ Hybridization, Immunohistochemistry, Lung Cancer.

1. INTRODUCTION

"From bench to bedside": the vision of rational molecular mechanism-based drug development and patient management has progressed into a new era of reality in oncology therapeutics. Scientific discovery does not end at the bedside, however, as the clinical testing and use of molecularly targeted therapeutics continues to reveal new insights into the mechanisms of cancer and human biology, which were not anticipated from experimental systems and disease models. Clinical observations with targeted therapies can point toward new directions for basic research, which greatly deepen our understanding of the mechanisms of human diseases and facilitate the development of more relevant disease models, closing the loop of bench to bedside, then back again.

Clinical experience with targeted therapeutics in oncology has provided several examples where tumor types or subsets having molecular genetic alterations of a proto-oncogene which activate its function are remarkably responsive to inhibitors of that molecule, revealing a strong dependence of the tumor on the genetically altered molecule and its signaling pathways. Examples of this include KIT mutations in gastrointestinal stromal tumors, BCR-ABL fusion in chronic myelogenous leukemia, and PDFGR mutations in dermatofibrosarcoma protuberans which are related to imatinib sensitivity, as well as HER2 amplification and response to trastazumab in breast cancer. The concept that tumors may be "addicted" to a particular oncogene is strengthened by observations that activating mutations may be accompanied by gene amplification and protein overexpression, strengthening signaling through the oncogenic pathway. Remarkably, when tumors with oncogene mutations become resistant to inhibitors of the oncogene, they may not lose their dependence on the original oncogenic signaling pathway. Imatinib resistance results from mutations in c-kit or bcr-abl, which prevent the drug from binding to its target region in their tyrosine kinase domains. HER2-positive breast cancers which become resistant to trastuzumab can still be responsive to other HER2-directed therapies such as the tyrosine kinase inhibitor (TKI), lapatinib, or the HER2 heterodimerization inhibitor, pertuzumab. Thus, oncogene addiction can represent an "Achilles' heel" for some tumor types on which to focus further drug development. We must be careful, however, not to assume that if tumors that have oncogene mutations or activation are very sensitive to oncogene inhibitors, then tumors that do not display the same genetic alterations will not be sensitive to inhibitors. Ultimately, activation of signaling through the oncogenic pathway, rather than any one specific molecular alteration in a signaling molecule, may be the most important indicator of tumor dependence on the pathway and the potential degree of clinical benefit derived from inhibition of the pathway. This concept has been supported by investigations of HER2 activation in ovarian cancers treated with pertuzumab (1).

The epidermal growth factor receptor (EGFR; HER1; ErbB1) family of receptor tyrosine kinases (HER1-4; ErbB1-4) is one of the longest-known and best-studied groups of molecules in the field of tumor biology. Nonclinical evidence for their role in oncogenesis includes a viral oncogene homolog (v-ErbB), the induction of transformation and tumor formation in cell and animal models, and the inhibition of tumor initiation and growth when their activities are neutralized experimentally. Prior to 2004, the genetic evidence implicating the EGFR in human cancers was limited to the frequent amplification and rearrangement of EGFR in a subset of glioblastomas. The activity of trastuzumab in the treatment of a subset of breast cancers which exhibit gene amplification of EGFR's sister molecule, HER2, added to the optimism that targeting the EGFR would yield further clinical successes.

However, the extensive efforts behind the development of EGFR tyrosine kinase inhibitors (TKIs) and anti-EGFR antibodies were fueled by beliefs that these drugs would be active in a wide range of tumors beyond glioblastomas, including the most common and most lethal tumor types, such as lung cancer, colorectal cancer, and pancreatic cancer.

The initial clinical evidence suggesting a prominent role of the EGFR in non-small cell lung cancer (NSCLC) and several other epithelial tumor types were demonstrations that the EGFR and/or its activating ligands were "overexpressed" in tumor samples from a significant number of patients (*2*, *3*). Many reports have justified the significance of "overexpression" of these molecules by implicit analogy with the pathological levels of HER2 overexpression which result from gene amplification in breast cancer. However, in the clinical experience of EGFR TKIs in NSCLC and the anti-EGFR monoclonal antibody cetuximab in colorectal cancer, the concept of EGFR "overexpression" has shown limited usefulness in terms of identifying patients who are most likely to respond to and benefit from these therapies, and it has become apparent that the molecular pathology of EGFR in various tumor types is substantially different from that of HER2 in breast cancer. This experience has given us many lessons regarding the complexity and interrelations between tumor and patient genetics, phenotypes and molecular therapies, and the challenges in applying molecular testing of clinical solid tumor samples to patient selection and decision making in these diseases.

During phase II trials of the EGFR TKIs, gefitinib, and erlotinib, in NSCLC it was recognized that there were a number of patient and tumor characteristics that were associated with a higher likelihood of tumor responses to EGFR TKI monotherapy, including a history of minimal or never smoking, Asian ethnicity, female gender, and adenocarcinoma pathologic diagnosis, particularly tumors with histologic features of bronchioloalveolar carcinoma (BAC)(*4–7*). Prospectively defined subgroup analyses in controlled phase III studies confirmed the relationship between some of these features, particularly never-smoking, with increased survival benefit from EGFR TKI treatment (*8–11*). The clinicopathologic features of never-smoking status, female gender and adenocarcinoma tumor type are known to be co-associated in NSCLC (reviewed by (*12*)), and are also favorable prognostic variables in the absence of EGFR TKI therapy, although the prognostic significance of histologic type differs between studies and may be related to stage or treatment (*13–18*). Therefore, it appears that some lung adenocarcinomas that tend to arise in non-smoking females may exemplify a biologically distinct entity that especially benefits from EGFR TKI treatment. Some NSCLC patients treated with gefitinib or erlotinib exhibited dramatic radiographic responses and clinical improvements so profound as to be called a "Lazarus effect," with patients going from deathbed to tennis court in a few weeks. Groups at the Dana-Farber Cancer Institute, Massachusetts General Hospital and Memorial Sloan-Kettering Cancer Center correctly suspected that such responses to EGFR TKIs might be associated with somatic activating mutations in the tyrosine kinase domain (TKD) of the EGFR and confirmed this hunch by retrospectively sequencing the EGFR in tumor samples from patients who had responded to gefitinib or erlotinib treatment (*19–21*). The discovery of EGFR TKD mutations and their relationship to response and clinical benefit from TKIs has had a major impact in our understanding of the etiology, biology, and classification of NSCLC, and it has raised important issues regarding patient selection in the treatment of this disease. However, EGFR mutations are not the whole story of molecular relationships to response and survival with EGFR TKIs in NSCLC. Evidence that EGFR gene copy number may be predictive of EGFR TKI treatment effects in NSCLC was first provided by groups at the University of Colorado and Bologna, Italy, and at the University of Toronto. Additional studies examining the relationship of EGFR molecular genetics, EGFR signaling pathways, and other aspects of NSCLC pathobiology, such as epithelial-mesenchymal differentiation, to the effects of EGFR TKIs have been provided by several groups around the world and these continue to be areas of intense investigation. In addition to being a rich scientific field, the work raises important and controversial questions regarding the role and conduct of molecular testing in guiding therapeutic decisions for lung cancer patients.

Various aspects of the evolving knowledge and experience regarding the molecular and cellular biology of EGFR mutations, their clinicopathologic associations, and their relationship to EGFR TKI treatment in NSCLC have been addressed in several reviews and updates over the past three years (22–31) and a collection of review articles (32). The purpose of this chapter is to provide a comprehensive and up-to-date review of the primary literature and current knowledge regarding EGFR TKD mutations, their role in NSCLC biology and treatment, other molecular characteristics that affect NSCLC responses to EGFR TKIs, and considerations regarding the application of molecular tests to clinical samples of NSCLC.

2. EGFR TYROSINE KINASE DOMAIN (TKD) MUTATIONS IN NSCLC

2.1. Molecular and Mechanistic Aspects of EGFR TKD Mutations

2.1.1. SPECTRUM AND PREVALENCE OF EGFR TKD MUTATIONS

The prevalence of somatic mutations in the tyrosine kinase domain region, encoded by exons 18-21, of the EGFR in NSCLC ranges from about 10-15% in the United States and Europe to 20-60% in East Asian populations (22, 33). The clinical associations of EGFR mutations are addressed in more detail in Section 2.2.1. The majority (85-90%) of mutations are exon 19 deletions (e19del) involving ELREA residues 746-750 and the substitution (point or missense) exon 21 mutation L858R, with the reported frequencies of e19del vs. L858R generally being about 1:1 to 2:1. Substitutions at G719X, D761Y, T790M and L861X, and exon 20 insertions, occur much less frequently than the "classical" e19del and L858R mutations, but have been reported by multiple groups. A few dozen other mutations, nearly all single-base substitutions, have been reported only once or very rarely. The significance of these novel or very rare mutations is open to debate. PCR-based sequencing artifacts can result from formalin fixation of tumor tissues or the use of very small tumor samples, and different mutation detection techniques vary in their sensitivities and their abilities to detect mutations that are present in only a small fraction of tumor cells or amplified alleles (see Sections 9.1.3 and 9.2). The methods used in studies of EGFR mutations in clinical NSCLC samples should be carefully considered, especially when the data seem unusual in terms of mutation frequencies or the numbers of novel substitution mutations (34, 35). Gu et al. (36) have created a public database of reported somatic EGFR mutations or sequence variations in NSCLC which can be accessed at http://www.cityofhope.org/cmdl/egfr_db, and authors are encouraged to submit new data to that database. The Sanger Institute Cancer Genome Project COSMIC website (http://www.sanger.ac.uk/genetics/CGP/cosmic/) has a very useful compendium of reported mutations and sequence variations in many genes including the EGFR in a variety of cancer types.

2.1.2. EGFRvIII in NSCLC

The groups who discovered the EGFR TKD mutations in NSCLC began their investigations by direct sequencing the coding sequence of the entire gene and focused further investigations on the TKD exons after finding mutations in this region. The EGFR variant III extracellular domain deletion of exons 2-7, which is well known in glioblastomas, has also been investigated recently in NSCLC by several groups using RT-PCR to analyze mRNA transcript sequences. Sasaki et al. (37) detected EGFRvIII in eight of 252 (3%) NSCLC cases; seven of the eight were in squamous cell carcinomas. These authors showed that EGFR gene copy number was higher in EGFRvIII-positive cases than in non-vIII cases, and that the EGFRvIII was exclusive of EGFR TKD mutations found in 60 cases. Ji et al. (38) detected EGFRvIII in none of 123 lung adenocarcinomas and in three of 56 squamous cell carcinomas. Ohtsuka et al. (39) found

EGFRvIII in zero of 31 squamous cell, zero of four adenosquamous, and in one of seven large cell carcinomas. These authors did not find any cases having EGFRvIII in a previous report (*40*). EGFRvIII immunohistochemistry using variant-specific antibodies in earlier studies gave somewhat variable results, with reports of EGFRvIII being present in NSCLC and absent in normal lung (Sonnweber et al: 42% in NSCLC overall (*41*); Garcia de Palazzo et al: two of 13 squamous cell carcinoma, zero of ten adenocarcinomas, three of nine other; 16% overall (*42*)) and present in both NSCLC (42% of squamous cell and 41% of adenocarcinomas) and in normal lung (*43*). In contrast to glioblastomas, which can show the type III *EGFR* gene rearrangements, it is very likely that EGFRvIII expression in NSCLC results from alternative splicing rather than from actual genetic alterations (*43*).

2.1.3. Cytogenetics of EGFR TKD Mutations in NSCLC

The tumor cytogenetic status associated with EGFR TKD mutations in NSCLC has been inferred largely from the analysis of relative peak heights of the wild-type and mutant alleles in sequencing chromatograms. These analyses suggest that most EGFR mutations are heterozygous. The accuracy of this interpretation, however, depends on the tumor cell content of the tumor tissue sample, since non-tumor stromal, vacular, and inflammatory cells will contribute wild-type sequence. Furthermore, fluorescence in situ hybridization (FISH) cytogenetic studies have demonstrated that about 30-50% of NSCLC cases acquire EGFR gene copy number gains, and several reports indicate that there is some degree of association between NSCLC cases showing EGFR mutation and increased copy number by FISH (see Section 5.4). Sequencing chromatograms showed only the mutant allele in 33% of cases (*44*), and a comparison of peak heights in sequencing chromatograms was interpreted as showing amplification of the mutant allele in about 40% of cases (*33*). The original reports describing EGFR mutations included one case with homozygous in-frame deletion at exon 19 (*19*) and two cases with homozygous exon 19 deletions (*21*). The absence of wild-type sequence in sequencing chromatograms could be due to homozygous mutations, loss of a wild-type allele or selective amplification of a mutant allele. In order to more precisely define the cytogenetic alterations associated with EGFR mutations, a combination of different techniques is necessary. Conde et al. (*45*) described a case that was EGFR-amplified by FISH and showed only mutated EGFR in the sequence analysis, indicating selective amplification of the mutant allele. Ma et al. (*46*) provided a detailed examination of a NSCLC case in which homozygous EGFR mutation in primary tumor and metastasis occurred through a combination of LOH, with deletion of a normal allele resulting in a hemizygous state, together with amplification of the mutant allele. These types of changes may not be unusual since NSCLC frequently show complex cytogenetic alterations with extensive chromosomal gains, losses, and rearrangements (*47, 48*).

2.1.4. Oncogenic Signaling by Mutant EGFRs

The effects of the most common EGFR TKD mutations, e19del and L858R, on EGFR kinase activity, signaling pathway activation and transforming activity have been studied in detail in a variety of experimental systems. The findings from various laboratories are not always in agreement. This may reflect, at least in part, differences in experimental models such as endogenous receptors vs. transfected receptors in cells vs. purified kinases, or differences in the molecular mileu between different cell types such as expression of EGFR co-receptors and ligands, endogenous EGFR copy number, and the genetic and activation status of other signaling molecules.

2.1.4.1 Receptor Activation and Turnover
The elegant structural studies of Yun et al. (*49*) revealed that mutations activate the kinase by disrupting autoinhibitory interactions. Some studies have found that the mutant receptors

are constitutively activated in the absence of added ligand (50–55) although the mutant receptors retain ligand dependence for receptor activation (20, 56–58). The e19del and L858R mutants exhibited enhanced enzymatic properties relative to wild-type EGFR (57, 59), increased levels of autophosphorylation (20, 51, 59, 60) and prolonged signaling activation (20, 56), although the study of Pao et al. (21) gave somewhat different findings. At least some EGFR mutations may lead to altered kinetics of receptor turnover, which could contribute to prolonged receptor signaling. Unlike wild-type EGFR, the L858R and e19del mutants are stabilized by interacting with HSP90 and are sensitive to degradation following HSP90 inhibition with geldanamycin (61). Furukawa et al. (58) found that the e19 del-EGFR lacked EGF-induced phosphorylation at the Cbl binding site Tyr 1045, and cells exhibited impaired EGF-induced endocytosis, ubiquitination, and downregulation of the e19del-mutant EGFR, whereas the L858R mutant exhibited phosphorylation at Tyr 1045, and its downstream signaling was not prolonged. Chen et al. (62) found that the S768I, L861Q, E709G, and G719S mutants did not undergo ligand-induced ubiquitination and had more sustained tyrosine phosphorylation. E709G and G719S also lacked EGF-induced receptor down-regulation. The several autophosphorylation sites in the activated EGFR exhibit differential patterns of phosphorylation in the mutant receptors as compared with the wild-type receptor (50, 57, 60, 62), which may result in the differential activation of downstream signaling pathways upon which tumor cells are dependent. However, Choi et al. (52) did not observe differences in autophosphorylation patterns in the mutant receptors.

2.1.4.2. Receptor Signaling Pathways

The mutant EGFRs preferentially activate Akt and STAT signaling pathways which promote cell survival, whereas the mutant receptors appear to be unlinked to MAP kinase pathway signaling, which controls proliferation (50, 53, 55). Tumor cells expressing mutant EGFR undergo apoptosis when receptor signaling is inhibited (50, 63–65), demonstrating their dependence on survival pathways. The association of EGFR receptor mutations and Akt pathway activation has been confirmed in some immunohistochemical studies of human NSCLC tumor samples using phospho-specific antibodies (45, 66, 67), although other studies did not find significant associations between EGFR mutations and phospho-Akt IHC (68, 69).

Since the EGFR does not contain tyrosine phosphorylation sites which directly engage the p85 regulatory subunit of PI-3-kinase, the coupling of EGFR activation to Akt pathway signaling must occur indirectly. One way in which this could occur is through heterodimerization of the activated EGFR with Her3, which does contain multiple p85 binding sites and can strongly activate Akt pathway signaling (70), and may be a key link between EGFR and Akt signaling (71). Another mechanism could involve K-ras activation, which may couple to Akt either via direct binding to the p110 subunit of PI-3-kinase resulting in its activation, or through regulating the activity of PDK2, the Rictor-mTOR complex (72).

2.1.4.3. Receptor Tumorigenicity

The tumorigenicity of the19del and L858R mutations has been demonstrated in transfected cell lines and in animal models. Fibroblasts and lung epithelial cells expressing the mutant receptors acquire anchorage-independent growth and the ability to form tumors in immunocompromised mice (57, 73) and Ba/F3 cells transform to interleukin 3-independent growth (52, 74). Transgenic mice with inducible expression of L858R and e19del in type II pneumocytes developed lung adenocarcinomas, which regressed when treated with EGFR inhibitors (75, 76).

2.1.5. EGFR TKD Mutations and Sensitivity or Resistance to Inhibitors In Vitro

2.1.5.1. "Classical" EGFR TKD Mutations (Exon 19 deletion or L858R) and Increased Sensitivity to Gefitinib and Erlotinib

In addition to their effects in promoting EGFR oncogenicity through enhanced receptor signaling and activation of AKT and STAT survival pathways, the e19del and L858R mutations confer an enhanced sensitivity of the receptor to inhibition by the reversible 4-anilinoquinazoline EGFR TKIs. Receptor phosphorylation and phosphorylation of downstream signaling molecules are inhibited at several-fold lower concentrations of gefitinib and erlotinib in cell lines expressing the mutant receptors compared to those with wild-type receptors (19–21, 55, 62). In vitro kinase assays showed that e19del and L858R mutant kinases are more sensitive to enzymatic inhibition by gefitinib and erlotinib, reflecting their increased drug affinity (57, 59). Higher affinity was confirmed by direct binding measurements demonstrating that gefitinib bound 20-fold more tightly to the L858R mutant than to the wild-type enzyme (49). Liu et al. (77) used a computational structural and energetic modeling approach to show that L858R caused gefitinib move closer to the hinge region in the TK domain. However, different EGFR TKD mutants may differ in their relative sensitivies to TKIs. Carey et al. (57) performed enzyme kinetic analyses of the purified kinases, which indicated that EGFR exon 19 del(746–752) was more sensitive to erlotinib inhibition than the EGFR L858R mutant, and confirmed this differential sensitivity between mutants in growth inhibition studies of transfected cell lines (although both mutants were more sensitive than the wild-type EGFR). The higher sensitivities of the common mutant vs. wild-type receptors to inhibition by EGFR TKIs may result in different pharmacokinetic profiles related to drug efficacy and toxicity in treating tumors in vivo. In mouse allografts of NR6 cells transfected with mutant and wild-type EGFRs, Carey et al. (57) found that significant growth inhibition of tumors with wild-type EGFR receptors was only observed at doses of erlotinib approaching the maximum tolerated dose for the mouse, whereas the growth of e19del and L858R mutant tumors was inhibited by erlotinib treatment at approximately one-third the maximum tolerated dose. These preclinical observations raise an important question as to whether the doses of EGFR TKIs used clinically are sufficient to inhibit both wild-type receptors and mutant receptors in patients. Pharmacodynamic biomarker studies in humans have shown that clinical doses of gefitinib or erlotinib indeed can inhibit wild-type EGFR activation and signaling in normal cells and tumor cells (78–82).

2.1.5.2. EGFR TKD Mutations Causing Resistance to Gefitinib and Erlotinib

The e19del and L858R mutations were initially discovered by their association with gefitinib and erlotinib sensitivity in NSCLC patients, which was subsequently confirmed by in vitro experiments. Another mutation, T790M, was subsequently discovered as an acquired secondary resistance mutation occurring in NSCLC patients with tumors which had primary sensitivity mutations (L858R or e19del) but which subsequently progressed after initiation of EGFR TKI therapy. The ability of the secondary T790M mutation to convert drug-sensitive EGFR mutants (e19del and L858R) into drug-resistant receptors was then directly demonstrated by expressing the various EGFR mutant constructs in transfected cells (83, 84). Notably, an established NSCLC cell line, H1975, was then also found to have the T790M mutation, in addition to the L858R mutation which had been previously reported in this cell line (83). Engelman et al. (85) modeled acquired resistance in vitro by passaging H3255 NSCLC cells, which carry the EGFR L858R mutation and are EGFR gene-amplified, in the presence of gefitinib. Drug-resistant cells acquired T790M in a small fraction of amplified alleles, and this second mutation conferred resistance when it occurred in *cis* to the activating mutation. Structural analyses indicate that the T790M mutation impairs the interaction of the inhibitor with the binding pocket in the kinase domain (*84, 86*). The EGFR resistance mutation is analogous to imatinib resistance mutations that evolve in ABL kinase (*87*) and KIT (*88, 89*) during treatment of CML and GIST, respectively, with imatinib. This common mutation site in all three kinases is a highly conserved "gatekeeper" threonine residue near the kinase active site. In addition to its role in conferring secondary resistance to anilinoquinazoline EGFR TKIs, the T790M mutation also contributes to enhanced receptor kinase activity in concert with primary drug-sensitive activating mutations such as L858R and may, therefore, be pro-oncogenic (*55, 59, 90*).

Another rare mutation, D761Y, has been found clinically as a secondary mutation associated with acquired resistance (*91*). In cell transfection experiments, adding the D761Y mutation did not noticeably change the apparent kinase activity of L858R EGFR. The D761Y mutation decreased the gefitinib sensitivity of the L858R receptor in phosphorylation and cell survival assays, although the degree of resistance conferred by D761Y was considerably less than that of T790M (*91*).

Exon 20 insertions have been found as uncommon primary mutations in NSCLC series. Greulich et al. (*73*) found that while transformation of fibroblasts and lung epithelial cells by the "classical" EGFR TKD mutants conferred sensitivity to erlotinib and gefitinib, transformation by an exon 20 insertion made cells resistant to these inhibitors. Patients with tumors bearing exon 20 do not appear to respond to gefitinib (*92*).

2.1.5.3. In Vitro Sensitivity of Uncommon EGFR TKD Mutations to Erlotinib or Gefitinib

Comparing the effect of gefitinib on the common e19del and L858R mutants to some of the more rare primary TKD mutations, Chen et al. (*62*) reported that while gefitinib suppressed the tyrosine phosphorylation of most EGFR mutants better than the wild-type receptor, the drug had more variable effects on growth suppression in 32D cells transfected with different EGFR mutants (relative inhibition: L858R, E746-A750 del, G719S > L861Q > wt > S768I, E709G). However, Jiang et al. (*74*) found that Ba/F3 cells expressing the L858R mutant were much more sensitive to gefitinib than were cells expressing the less common G719S mutant. Examining the kinetic properties of purified enzymes, Carey et al. (*57*) determined that L861Q was much less sensitive to inhibition by erlotinib than del746-750 or L858R. Using computational modeling approaches based on structures and molecular dynamics, Liu et al. (*77*) developed an algorithm to predict the functional effect of EGFR TKD mutations, which was successfully applied to several clinically relevant mutations (T790M, L858R, G719C, L861Q, T790M + L858R double mutant, and exon 19 delL747-P753insS). Such modeling approaches might be used to rationally design optimal inhibitors for the various mutations as well as to predict their oncogenicities.

2.1.5.4. Differential Sensitivity or Resistance of EGFR TKD Mutations to Various Classes of EGFR Inhibitors

Several laboratories have examined the relative efficacies of different classes of EGFR inhibitors against EGFR receptors bearing the variety of mutations discovered in clinical samples. Importantly, the drug sensitivity or resistance associated with various mutations is drug class-specific, so that mutations that confer resistance to the anilinoquinazolines (erlotinib and gefitinib) may not be resistant to irreversible inhibitors of the EGFR kinase. Carter et al. (*93*) showed EKB-569 and CI-1033, but not GW-572016 and ZD-6474, potently inhibited the gefitinib- and erlotinib-resistant EGFR (L858R/T790M) kinase. Kwak et al. (*94*) demonstrated that HK-272, HK-356 and EKB-569 effectively signaling of the EGFR (L8585R/T790M). Kobayashi et al. (*84*) noted that the T790M mutation in the context of e19 del747-S752 could be inhibited by CL-387,785. By contrast, L858R EGFR with the D761Y "resistance" mutation was less sensitive to HKI-272 than to gefitinib (*91*). Greulich et al. (*73*) found that fibroblasts and lung epithelial cells transformed by an exon 20 insertion were resistant to erlotinib or gefitinib but were more sensitive to the irreversible inhibitor CL-387,785. Yuza et al. (*95*) compared erlotinib and HKI-272 across a series of EGFR mutants expressed in Ba/F3 cells. Erlotinib was a more potent inhibitor of the common e19 deletion mutants than was HKI-272, whereas HKI-272 more potently inhibited the L858R, other erlotinib-sensitive mutants, and erlotinib-resistant mutants including T790M and e20ins mutants. Kwak et al. (*94*) generated gefitinib-resistant NSCLC cells which did not have a second resistance mutation in the EGFR but which maintained their dependence on EGFR signaling. These cells, which acquired gefitinib resistance through a mechanism other than secondary mutations, were still sensitive to irreversible inhibitors, such as HK-272. Newer drugs in development with various kinase specificities, such as EXEL-7647, also have activity against the T790M mutation (*96*).

The EGFR mutations that confer particular sensitivity (e.g., e19del, L858R) and resistance (e.g., T790M) to erlotinib and gefitinib do not change the sensitivity of the EGFR to inhibition by the ECD-directed monoclonal antibody cetuximab (*64, 76, 97, 98*). A small clinical study of cetuximab in NSCLC showed no evidence of improved response in tumors with EGFR TKD mutations (*99, 100*).

2.2. Clinical—Pathological Relationships of EGFR TKD Mutations
2.2.1. DEMOGRAPHIC ASSOCIATIONS

After EGFR mutations in EGFR TKI responders were first identified by the Boston and New York groups, other investigators in North America, Europe, Japan, South Korea, mainland China and Taiwan have reported the incidence and clinical-pathological relationships of EGFR mutations in NSCLC. EGFR mutations in NSCLC are found more frequently in East Asian populations (20-60%) than in Western, primarily Caucasion, populations (10-17%). In both Asians and non-Asians, EGFR mutations occur more frequently in women than in men, are associated with adenocarcinoma histology, and are very often present in NSCLC arising in patients with a minimal or never-smoking history whereas current or formerly smoking patients have a much lower frequency of EGFR mutations (*26, 29, 33, 40, 44, 45, 101–122*). The statistical significance in univariate and multivariate analyses of the associations of EGFR mutations with these various clinical and pathologic features (*33, 44, 110, 114–117, 120*) may depend upon the sample sizes of the patient subgroups being compared, the demographic background of the population under study, and the accuracy of the mutation detection methodology. For example, Marchetti et al (*116*) found never smoking, female sex and adenocarcinoma (bronchioloalveolar subtype) were all independently associated with EGFR mutations status in multivariate analyses, whereas Chou et al (*35*) found no significant association of EGFR mutations with gender, smoking status or tumor histology. However, the latter study also reported an unusually high number of novel point mutations, which raises the possibility that some of the reported sequence alterations might represent technical artifacts rather than true tumor mutations ((*123*); see Section 9.1.3). Analysis of the multinational phase III study of erlotinib in advanced NSCLC, BR.21, found a significant significant association of EGFR TKD mutations with adenocarcinoma histology and Asian ethnicity, but not with gender or smoking history (*34*). This analysis also reported an unusually high number of novel point mutations, with the possibility that some of these might not represent true tumor mutations.

2.2.2. ASSOCIATIONS OF EGFR, KRAS AND p53 MUTATIONS WITH SMOKING HISTORY AND WITH EACH OTHER

A history of never or minimal smoking is the strongest clinical predictor of harboring an EGFR mutation in NSCLC *(108, 110, 114)*. Sequist et al. *(108)* found that each pack-year of smoking corresponded to a 5% decreased likelihood of having an EGFR mutation. The groups of Kosaka et al., Tokumo et al. and Mounawar et al. *(44, 120, 122)* also observed that increasing smoke exposure was inversely related to EGFR mutation rate. Pham et al. *(124)* found that mutations were less common in people who smoked for more than 15 pack-years or who stopped smoking cigarettes less than 25 years ago, and Sugio et al. *(114)* observed EGFR mutations more frequently in patients who smoked <or=20 pack-year, and in patients who quit at least 20 years before the date of diagnosis for lung cancer. It is important to recognize that this does not mean that EGFR mutations do not occur in patients who have smoked; for example, in the NSCLC case series examined by Yang et al. *(125)*, 50% of EGFR mutations occurred in current or past smokers, and in the phase III TRIBUTE clinical trial of erlotinib and chemotherapy in NSCLC, 83% of the cases with EGFR mutations had a history of smoking *(126)*. Rather, in NSCLC tumors arising in patients with a never- or minimal-smoking history, EGFR mutations are present much more commonly than in the tumors arising in patients who smoked. EGFR mutations in smokers do not carry the characteristic signatures of mutagens in cigarette smoke *(36)* suggesting that these mutations arise from a causative mechanism independent of smoking. By contrast, mutations in KRAS and p53 which are associated with clinical smoking history typically reflect alterations, such as G:C to T:A transversions and A:T-to G:C transitions, induced by the formation of DNA adducts with various reactive mutagens in tobacco smoke *(12, 44, 127, 128)*. In direct comparisons of smoking history to the occurrence of EGFR and KRAS mutations, EGFR mutations were more frequent in patients with little or distant smoking history whereas KRAS mutations were more often found in smokers than in never smokers *(33, 106, 114)*, and more often in high-dose smokers than in low-dose smokers *(114)*. Likewise, in the phase III TRIBUTE clinical trial, EGFR mutations occurred in patients who had never smoked, as well as in those with a history of smoking, whereas KRAS mutations were found only in smokers *(126)*. EGFR and KRAS mutations are nearly always mutually exclusive, that is, NSCLC tumors may contain mutations in either gene but not in both *(33, 45, 102, 105, 106, 110, 112, 114, 116, 129, 130)* although rare cases of EGFR and KRAS co-mutation have been reported *(92, 126)*. The remarkable separation of NSCLC cases with EGFR and KRAS mutations probably cannot be explained solely by their different association, or lack thereof, with exposure to mutagens in smoke, as EGFR mutations do occur with some frequency in patients who have smoked and yet KRAS mutations are very rarely seen in EGFR-mutated tumors in smokers. An attractive hypothesis is that there is functional redundancy between the two genes so that when the tumor cells already carry one of the mutations, the acquisition of the second mutation confers little additional biological advantage and does not undergo selection during tumor evolution.

A wide spectrum of p53 mutations occur in NSCLC. Some of these result from the G:C-to-T:A transversions and A:T-to-G:C transitions caused by mutagens produced by tobacco smoking, whereas others appear to be unrelated to smoking *(12, 44, 122, 127)*. In contrast to the situation of KRAS and EGFR mutations, p53 mutations are not mutually exclusive of EGFR mutations *(44, 106, 122)*. However, the spectrum of p53 mutations seen together with EGFR mutations is different from that which occurs in the absence of EGFR mutations, with the smoking-associated p53 mutations tending to be excluded from cases having EGFR mutations *(44)*. A case of EGFR-mutated NSCLC arising in a patient with Li-Fraumeni syndrome, which is caused by germline p53 mutation, has been reported *(131)*.

Although EGFR mutations in NSCLC are somatic, occurring in the tumor cells but not in normal cells from other tissues such as blood, EGFR mutations are detected in histologically normal respiratory epithelium from lung cancer patients, suggesting a localized field effect phenomenon consistent with exposure to an environmental agent (*132*). Environmental or occupational agents other than smoking, which have been implicated in lung cancer include radon, cooking fumes, asbestos, heavy metals, polyvinyl chloride, human papillomavirus infection (*12*). A study of 19 NSCLC cases associated with radon exposure found that p53 mutations were present in 9 (50%) tumors but none of these were G:C-to-T:A transversions, and KRAS mutations were absent (*133*). Thus, the genotoxic effects of radon exposure appear to be different from those of tobacco smoke.

2.2.3. Ethnicity

The association of higher EGFR mutation rates with East Asian ethnicity compared to Western populations was introduced in Section 2.2.1 above. Several studies in East Asian, U.S. and European centers analyzed both EGFR and KRAS mutations in their patient cohorts. EGFR mutation rates are consistently higher, and KRAS mutation rates are lower, in NSCLC studied in East Asian populations compared to Western, largely Caucasian, series of patients. NSCLC series comparing EGFR and KRAS mutation in series from the United States, Europe, and Australia have found mutation rates of 10-15% in EGFR and 12-30% for KRAS whereas series from Japan, China and Korea show mutation rates of 17-42% in EGFR and 3-13% in KRAS (*33, 44, 45, 102, 105, 110, 112, 114, 116, 126, 129, 130, 134, 135*). Since EGFR and KRAS mutations have different associations with smoking history (section 2.2.2), these data suggest that a higher proportion of NSCLC arising in East Asians may have a causative mechanism other than smoking, compared to Western NSCLC patients. It is possible that there could be an inherited predisposition to developing EGFR mutations in Asian peoples, or that in Asian countries or cultures there are particular exposures to environmental factors that promote EGFR mutations in the lung. Notably, within a North American patient cohort, Riely et al. (*28*) found that EGFR mutations were significantly more frequent in patients of Asian background. Whether this association persists in ethnic Asians living in the West beyond the first generation is presently unknown. Comparing African American and Caucasion patients in North America, Yang et al. (*125*) found EGFR mutations in 14% of Caucasions but in only one of 41 (2.4%) of African Americans, whereas Riely et al. (*29*) concluded there was no difference in EGFR mutation rate in African Americans compared to Caucasians. A study of Saudi Arabian patients found one EGFR mutation in 34 (3%) of NSCLC cases (*136*), suggesting that the mutations might occur less frequently in Middle Eastern than in Western and East Asian populations. EGFR mutation rates reported from various European centers have been fairly consistent, including Spain, 12-13% (*45, 115*); Italy, 10% (*116, 134*); Finland, 10% (*137*). A study of Greek and Czech patients reported an EGFR mutation frequency of 15% (*113*) but was rather unusual in that several novel EGFR mutations were reported, and the KRAS mutation frequency was only 8%.

2.2.4. Histopathologic Types of NSCLC

In NSCLC, EGFR mutations are limited largely to adenocarcinomas and are relatively rare in squamous cell and large cell carcinomas. Several studies have found that EGFR mutations in adenocarcinomas are associated with more differentiated features (*102*), including bronchioloalveolar carcinomas (BAC) or adenocarcinoma with BAC features (*40, 44, 108, 114, 116*) and papillary subtype adenocarcinomas (*40, 138*), although the large series of Shigematsu et al. (*33*) did not find an association with BAC subtype. KRAS mutations are also strongly associated with adenocarcinoma histology and occur in BAC. However, EGFR mutations in

BAC are associated with the non-mucinous subtype, whereas KRAS mutations are associated with mucinous BAC subtype (*116, 139, 140*). EGFR mutation analysis has contributed to the molecular pathologic classification of histologically heterogeneous adenosquamous carcinomas. EGFR mutations in these tumors, when present, are detected in both squamous and adenocarcinoma components (*39, 141, 142*). These tumors therefore appear to be clonal and to genetically resemble adenocarcinomas rather than pure squamous cell carcinomas.

3. EGFR TYROSINE KINASE DOMAIN MUTATIONS IN TUMOR TYPES OTHER THAN NSCLC

After the initial discovery of EGFR TKD mutations in NSCLC and their relationship to EGFR TKI response, Lynch et al. (*20*) also screened a series of 95 primary tumors and 108 cancer cell lines representing a variety of other tumor types and did not identify the mutations in their sample set. Sihto et al. (*137*) screened a larger set of 566 tumor samples representing a variety of histologic types and found EGFR TKD mutations in 11% of NSCLC but not in other tumor types. Likewise, Lee et al. (*143*) did not find EGFR TKD mutations in common cancer types other than NSCLC. Most recently, Thomas et al. (*144*) described high-throughput genotyping of oncogene mutations in 1,000 tumor samples of various types and reported EGFR TKD mutations only in NSCLC and in a case of leukemia. Additional studies have focused more deeply on specific tumor types.

3.1. Head and Neck

Several investigators have found EGFR TKD mutations in squamous cell carcinomas of the head and neck (SCCHN): Lee et al. (*145*), three of 41 (7.3%; all were exon 19 E746_A750del); Willmore-Payne et al. (*146*), two of 24 (8%; exon 20 N771YinsG and G729E); Loeffler-Ragg et al. (*147*), one of 100 (1%; K745R); and Na et al. (*148*), 17 of 108 (16%). However, other studies failed to detect activating EGFR TKD mutations in large series of SCCHN (*149, 150*). Cohen et al. (*151*) examined SCCHN, which clinically responded to gefitinib and did not detect EGFR TKD mutations in these responsive tumors.

3.2. Colorectal

In a series of 293 colorectal adenocarcinomas (CRC), Barber et al. (*152*) found only one case (0.34%) with a mutation in the EGFR TKI, whereas Nagahara et al. (*153*) reported EGFR TKD mutations in four of 33 (12%) tumor cases (but in none of 11 CRC cell lines). Moroni et al. and Ogino et al. (*154, 155*) examined two different clinical series of CRC, each including 31 patients, and both studies found one of 31 cases having missense TKD mutations (G857R, G724S). Endo et al. (*156*) found no EGFR mutations in 70 cases of CRC and Kimura et al. (*157*) found no mutations in 12 CRC cell lines.

3.3. Biliary Tract

EGFR TKD mutations in cholangicarcinomas (bile duct or gallbladder adenocarcinoma) were investigated in two studies. Gwak et al. (*158*) found the "classical" TKI-sensitive e19del mutation in three of 22 (13.6%) cholangiocarcinomas, while Leone et al. (*159*) found missense point mutations in the EGFR TKD in six of 40 (15%) cholangiocarcinomas; two of these mutations had been previously described in NSCLC including the T790M "resistance" mutation.

3.4. Esophagus

Kwak et al. (*160*) found classical e19delE746-A750 and L858R mutations in two of 17 (12%) esophageal adenocarcinomas and three of 21 (14.2%) cases of Barrett's esophagus, as well as one case of adenocarcinoma and matched Barrett's esophagus, which had a T790M mutation in both samples. Guo et al. (*161*) found novel missense or nonsense point mutations in the EGFR TKD in four of 87 specimens of primary esophageal carcinoma or dysplasia and in one esophageal cancer cell line, and Sudo et al. (*162*) found a G719D mutation in one of 50 primary esophageal cancers. However, several other studies did not detect amino acid-altering EGFR TKD mutations in series of esophageal carcinomas and cancer cell lines (*156, 157, 163–166*).

3.5. Pancreas

In pancreatic adenocarcinomas, Kwak et al. (*160*) also identified "classical" TKD mutations in two of 55 cases (3.6%), and Lee et al. (*167*) found an exon 20 substitution mutation in one of 66 cases (1.5%), while other investigators did not find amino acid-altering mutations in their series (*168–170*).

3.6. Stomach

EGFR TKD mutations have not been found in primary gastric adenocarcinomas (*156, 166, 171–173*) although a missense mutation was reported in one gastric carcinoma cell line (*157*).

3.7. Prostate

In prostate adenocarcinomas, Douglas et al. (*174*) found novel missense mutations in the EGFR TKD in four of 89 (4.4%) of localized tumors, while Curigliano et al. (*175*) found no EGFR mutations in eight hormone-refractory cases.

3.9. Breast

Most series have not found EGFR TKD mutations in breast cancers (*20, 144, 176*) although one study reported the presence of missense EGFR TKD mutations in seven of 48 (14.6%) of sporadic breast cancers and in 11 of 24 (45.8%) of cancers in BRCA1/2 mutation carriers (*177*). Unexpectedly, laser-capture microdissection of the tumors in that study showed that the majority of the EGFR mutations were detected in the stromal cells but not in tumor cells. This unusual finding remains to be verified.

3.10. Renal

Franco-Hernandez et al. (*178*) described an EGFR e19del mutation in a brain metastasis of renal cell carcinoma, while Sakaeda et al. (*179*) found no EGFR TKD mutations in 19 cases of renal cell carcinoma.

3.11. Ovarian

Schilder et al. (*180*) discovered EGFR TKD mutations in two of 57 (3.5%) of ovarian cancers. One of the mutated cases was from a clinical trial of gefitinib in ovarian cancer, and was the only patient to exhibit an objective response in that trial. Lassus et al. (*181*) (198 cases), Stadlmann et al. (*182*) (80 cases) and Lacroix et al. (*183*) (20 cases exhibiting response or stable disease on treatment with gefitinib in combination with carboplatin and paclitaxel) did not detect any amino-acid sequence altering EGFR mutations in ovarian cancers.

3.12. Glioblastoma

In addition to the well-known EGFR ECD deletions such as variant III, novel missense mutations in the EGFR ECD have been recently described in GBMs (*137, 184*). Mutations in the EGFR TKD were reported in two of 69 (3%) glioblastomas in Japan and in four of 81 (5%) glioblastomas in Switzerland (*185*) and in one of 151 (0.7%) of GBMs and gliomas (*184*) while other studies did not find TKD mutations in series of GBMs (*137, 152, 186–189*).

3.13. Sarcoma

Bode et al. (*190*) detected missense mutations (P733S and A840T) in one of 13 cases of synovial sarcoma.

3.14. Other

Amino acid sequence-altering EGFR TKD mutations were not found in hepatocellular carcinomas (*191*), nasopharyngeal carcinomas (*192*), thymomas and thymic carcinomas (*193, 194*), gastroenteropancreatic neuroendocrine tumors (*195*) or testicular germ-cell tumors (*196*).

In summary, EGFR TKD mutations occur infrequently in tumor types other than NSCLC, although continued examination of the less-common tumor types and of pathological and genetic tumor subtypes might identify occasional associations in the future. Studies that report unusual numbers of novel or rare substitution mutations should be critically evaluated for methodology, since FFPE tissue processing can introduce artifactual nucleotide changes which may not reproducibly detected (*123, 197*).

4. RELATIONSHIP OF EGFR TKD MUTATIONS TO EGFR TKI SENSITIVITY AND CLINICAL OUTCOMES IN NSCLC PATIENTS

The initial discovery of EGFR TKD mutations in NSCLC tumors that responded to EGFR TKI treatment (*19–21*) created intense interest in the possibility that mutation analysis could be used to select patients for therapy. However, a number of issues have complicated the picture, and the role for EGFR mutation testing for therapeutic decision-making is still unsettled. These issues include the predictive strength of the relationship of EGFR mutations to clinical benefit in terms of overall and progression-free survival as well as response; whether EGFR mutations are predictive of specific treatment effects of TKIs or of nonspecific responsiveness to any therapy, or are prognostic indicators irrespective of therapy; whether other clinical and molecular characteristics associated with response, survival or EGFR mutation status are superior to EGFR mutation testing, or should be used in concert with mutation testing to guide treatment decisions; and whether existing methods of mutation testing are sufficiently sensitive and accurate to be relied upon for therapeutic decision-making.

4.1. Results from Analyses of Non-Randomized Patient Cohorts

4.1.1. RETROSPECTIVE STUDIES OF TUMOR RESPONSE AND CLINICAL BENEFIT IN PATIENTS TREATED WITH EGFR TKIs

Presently, the great majority of information regarding the relationship of EGFR mutation status to therapeutic effect comes from retrospective analyses of mutations in NSCLC patients who received received erlotinib or gefitinib as second or third-line monotherapy. Rates of objective radiographic responses, i.e., tumor shrinkage, in such studies are consistently significantly higher in EGFR mutant tumors than EGFR wild-type (*35, 68, 69, 92, 101, 102, 104, 109, 110, 115, 117, 120, 121, 135, 198–204*). In these studies, the objective response rates to EGFR TKIs were 9-17% in EGFR wild type tumors and 46-94% in those having EGFR mutations. Potential factors that could underlie the differences in response rates reported for EGFR mutant tumors include the numbers of the "classical" sensitivity mutations vs. other mutations (or sequencing artifacts); case selection biases and response evaluation criteria; and perhaps demographic, pharmacogenetic/kinetic or other patient characteristics that might influence response and could differ between study cohorts. Also, these studies were generally limited to patient cohorts treated with a single EGFR TKI. Interestingly, a small retrospective comparison of patients with EGFR-mutated tumors treated with gefitinib or erlotinib noted that gefitinib had significantly higher response rate than erlotinib (78% vs 33%, p=0.0354) (*205*). While EGFR TKD mutations are often found in tumors that respond to EGFR TKIs by decreasing in size, mutations are less frequent in tumors that exhibit disease stabilization on EGFR TKI treatment (*203, 206–208*) although Chou et al. (*35*) did find that EGFR mutation status was an independent predictor for disease control (response + stable disease). In terms of clinical outcomes, several-fold increases in time to progression (TTP) or progression-free survival (PFS) have been reported for EGFR TKD mutants compared to wild-type (*35, 69, 92, 110, 115, 198–203*). Overall survival (OS) for EGFR mutants treated with EGFR TKIs was significantly prolonged vs. wild-type in some studies (*35, 68, 92, 107, 109, 110, 115, 117, 135, 198, 200–203*), while others found no relationship of mutation status to survival or an insignificant trend for better survival in mutants (*69, 104, 120, 121, 134, 199*). The small study by Jackman et al. (*205*), which found higher RR in patients with EGFR mutations treated with gefitinib compared to those treated with erlotinib, did not find a difference in time to progression or overall survival between gefitinib- treated vs. erlotinib-treated patients. Recent retrospective analyses of phase II trials of EGFR TKIs as 1st line monotherapy in chemonaive NSCLC patients have also found a strong association of EGFR mutations with tumor objective responses (*209–211*) and with prolonged TTP and survival (*210*).

4.1.2. CLINICAL TRIALS OF EGFR TKIS IN NSCLC PATIENTS PROSPECTIVELY SELECTED FOR EGFR TKD MUTATIONS

The results from several phase II trials in which patients were prospectively screened for EGFR TKD mutations in order to be selected for gefitinib or erlotinib therapy have been recently presented at meetings and are being published as full reports (*212–215*). Reily et al. and Costa et al. (*28, 216*) have summarized the data from prospective studies reported as abstracts or full papers to date. The overall objective response rate across the studies was approximately 80%, validating the association between EGFR mutations and high response rate indicated from retrospective studies. Median progression-free survivals ranged from 7.7 to 12.9 months. Median overall survival was 15.4 months in one study and had not yet been reached in the rest.

4.1.3. DIFFERENCES IN EGFR TKI TREATMENT EFFECT IN PATIENTS WITH EXON 19 DELETION VS. L858R VS. OTHER MUTATIONS IN TUMORS

Although both e19del and L858R are "classical" TKI-sensitive mutations, they may not be equivalent in terms of treatment effects of TKIs or prognosis. Retrospective studies of EGFR TKI-treated patients found those having tumors with e19del had higher response rates than L858R (*69, 117, 205, 217*). Another small study, which prospectively selected patients based on clinical characteristics but had retrospective mutation analysis, reported that tumors having exon 19 deletions responded well to EGFR TKIs, whereas tumors with point mutations exhibited only less-durable response or stable disease (*207*). However, Costa et al. (*216*) examined the combined data from 5 phase II studies which prospectively selected patients for gefitinib therapy based on the presence of EGFR mutations. The response rate was 80.3% (53 of 66 patients) for exon 19 deletion and 81.8% (27 of 33 patients) for L858R, indicating no difference between the two mutation types.

Improved OS and TTP in e19del mutants vs. L858R were reported by Jackman et al., Riely et al. and Hirsch et al. (*69, 205, 217*), although Mitsudomi et al. (*117*) did not find that that mutation class affected survival. In surgical resection patients who were not treated with

EGFR TKIs, those with deletions in exon 19 had worse survival and those with the L858R mutation had better survival compared to patients wild-type patients but this was not statistically significant (*33*).

Comparing the classical drug-sensitive mutations to other uncommon mutations, Ichihara et al. 2007 found that the presence of e19del or L858R mutation was a more powerful predictor of TKI response than other EGFR mutations.

4.1.4. EGFR TKD Mutations and Response to Cetuximab in NSCLC

In a phase II trial of cetuximab as single agent in recurrent NSCLC, EGFR mutation status was analyzed in 39 patients. Of three responders in the trial, two had tissue available and neither had a mutation. Of 3 patients with EGFR mutations, two had stable disease as best response and one progressed on treatment. This small clinical trial did not suggest any association of EGFR mutation status with response to cetuximab (*99, 100*).

4.1.5. Prediction and Prognosis in Patient Cohorts Not Treated with EGFR Inhibitors

Since control groups for treatment are not included in these retrospective studies of erlotinib- or gefitinib-treated patients, they leave open the question of whether EGFR TKD mutation status is predictive for deriving greater clinical benefit with EFGR TKIs, or is a prognostic factor irrespective of specific treatment.

In studies of NSCLC patients who underwent surgical tumor resections and did not receive specific anticancer therapies, several groups (*33, 44, 103, 218*) found no significant differences in survival related to overall EGFR mutation status, although Tsao et al. (*103*) noted a trend for shorter median OS in EGFR mutants. By contrast, Ohtsuka et al. (*40*) found that patients with tumor EGFR mutations had a significantly better prognosis than those with wild-type tumors. Notably, when EGFR mutation subtypes were compared, patients with exon 19 deletions had poorer survival and those with L858R had better survivals, than those without EGFR mutations (*33*). Takeuchi et al. (*219*) used gene expression profiling to classify tumors into "terminal respiratory unit (TRU)" and "non-TRU" types, and found that the presence of EGFR mutations was a significant predictor of shorter postoperative survival for TRU-type tumors. In another profiling approach, Shibata et al. (*220*) used array chromosomal genomic hybridization (CGH) to identify chromosomal numerical changes associated with EGFR mutational status, and categorized tumors into CGH "EGFR-MUT" and "EGFR-WT" groups. The CGH "EGFR-MUT" group had a significantly poorer disease-free survival than the "EGFR-WT" group even though EGFR mutation status alone was not significantly related to DFS.

Regarding advanced or metastatic disease treated with chemotherapy, Sequist et al. (*108*) recently described a retrospective clinical study of NSCLC patients who were routinely referred for EGFR mutation testing as part of clinical care. In patients with metastatic tumors, the RR to EGFR TKI was 54% in EGFR mutants vs. 0% in wild-type ($p < 0.0001$), while the RR to chemotherapy was 25% in EGFR mutants vs. 34% in wild-type ($p = 0.41$). After adjusting for other independent clinical predictors of survival, median predicted survival was 3.1 years for EGFR mutants vs. 1.6 years for wild-type across all treatment modalities, suggesting that EGFR mutation is a favorable prognostic factor regardless of treatment in the metastatic setting. In other retrospective studies of chemotherapy-treated patients, Hotta et al. (*221*) found that EGFR mutations were significantly associated with a better PFS in first-line cytotoxic chemotherapy regimens, whereas Lee et al. (*222*) concluded that RR and TTP were not affected by EGFR or KRAS mutation status.

In summary, in advanced or metastatic disease, EGFR mutations may be a favorable prognostic factor for survival with chemotherapy or other treatment, although EGFR mutations do not appear to be predictive of higher response rates with chemotherapy treatment. The data regarding the prognostic implications of EGFR mutations for survival in early-stage patients who underwent surgical resection as initial therapy are somewhat conflicting.

4.2. Retrospective Analyses of Randomized Phase III Clinical Trials of EGFR TKIs in Advanced or Metastatic NSCLC

4.2.1. EGFR TKD Mutations as Predictive vs. Prognostic Factors

Several large phase III randomized placebo-controlled studies of erlotinib and gefitinb in advanced or metastatic NSCLC were completed or in progress at the time of the discovery of EGFR mutations in NSCLC. These included 2nd/3rd line EGFR TKI monotherapy after chemotherapy failure (erlotinib: BR.21 (8); gefitinib: ISEL (9)) and first-line combinations of EGFR TKI with chemotherapy (erlotinib: TRIBUTE (10) and TALENT (296); gefitinib: INTACT 1 (223) and INTACT 2 (224)). In the overall patient populations under study, erlotinib monotherapy provided a significant survival benefit in 2nd/3rd line in the BR.21 study, which allowed for the successful approval of erlotinib in this setting in the United States, whereas ISEL showed a nonsignificant trend for improved survival benefit with gefitinib. By contrast, the TRIBUTE, TALENT and INTACT 1 and 2 studies showed that no clinical benefit was conferred by combining an EGFR TKI with first-line chemotherapy in nonselected patients. When interest in molecular predictors of EGFR TKI efficacy developed, attempts were made to collect archived FFPE tumor samples from as many patients in these trials as possible in order to assess clinical outcomes in molecular subgroups. There were high hopes that these large controlled studies would provide more definitive answers to some of the questions raised above regarding the relationship of EGFR mutations to predictive vs. prognostic outcomes.

In the molecular analysis of the BR.21 trial (34), the RR of EGFR mutants was 16%, vs. 7% for wild-type tumors (p=0.37). There was no significant difference in survival benefit from erlotinib treatment in patients with classical e19del and L858R mutations (hazard ratio, HR: 0.65) compared to wild-type (HR: 0.73) (34). In the placebo arm of BR.21, patients with e19del and L858R mutations had a median OS of 9.1 months compared to 3.5 months for wild-type patients (34, 225). Thus, this study suggests that EGFR mutations might have positive prognostic impact, but have no predictive value for erlotinib survival benefit. In the molecular analysis of ISEL (226), tumors with EGFR mutations had a higher RR to gefitinib than tumors without EGFR mutations (37.5% vs. 2.6%), but there were insufficient data for survival analysis.

In the molecular analysis of TRIBUTE (126), EGFR mutations were associated with longer survival, irrespective of treatment (P < .001). EGFR mutations were associated with improved response rate in patients treated with erlotinib + chemotherapy (P<.05), but not in patients treated with chemotherapy alone. In patients treated with erlotinib + chemotherapy, EGFR mutations were associated with a trend toward an erlotinib benefit on TTP (P=.092), but not with improved survival (P=.96). In a combined molecular analysis of the two INTACT trials (199), the RR was higher for EGFR mutants vs. wild-type in the gefitinib + chemotherapy arm but not in the chemotherapy alone arm (not statistically significant). EGFR mutations were associated with a significantly prolonged OS and a trend for prolonged TTP irrespective of gefitinib treatment. In TALENT, the RR was higher in EGFR mutants vs. wild-type in the chemotherapy + erlotinib arm vs. chemo alone arm (not significant), and survival and PFS showed trends which were consistent with the results of TRIBUTE and INTACT (227). Overall, the analyses of the phase III first-line trials produced results that, while not statistically significant in all studies, were fairly consistent across the trials and which indicate that in first-line NSCLC, the presence of EGFR mutations is predictive of improved RR over wild-type when EGR TKI is added to chemotherapy, but is prognostic for improved survival vs. wild-type in chemotherapy-treated patients irrespective of whether they also receive a EGFR TKI.

These studies, together with the uncontrolled studies described in the previous sections, indicate that in advanced or metastatic NSCLC: 1) EGFR mutations are a positive prognostic factor for survival in patients who are presently or have previously been treated with chemotherapy, irrespective of EGFR TKI treatment; 2) EGFR mutations are predictive of increased tumor response rates to EGFR TKIs in patients regardless of previous or concurrent chemotherapy; 3) EGFR mutations are not predictive of increased tumor response to chemotherapy.

4.2.2. CHALLENGES ENCOUNTERED IN MOLECULAR ANALYSES OF PHASE III CLINICAL TRIALS

The operational and technical challenges encountered in performing these analyses in multicenter (and often multinational) phase III clinical trials will be very useful as lessons in helping to plan and implement molecular testing in future drug development efforts. The archival tumor specimens available in NSCLC patients are obtained and prepared in a variety ways: larger surgical resections and excisional biopsies; small biopsies obtained via bronchial endoscopy or by using a cutting needle to obtain a thin core of tissue; cytology specimens such as fine-needle aspirates or sputum samples, where tumor cells suspended in fluids can be prepared in cell blocks or smeared directly on microscope slides prior to fixation. The amount of tumor available in these samples, and the method by which the tumor cells were preserved, may not be technically compatible with the requirements of the molecular assay procedure. Sometimes the tumor samples obtained for diagnosis are entirely consumed by prior diagnostic testing, so there is no remaining archival tumor sample available for testing. Patients were not required to have an adequate tumor sample available for molecular analyses in order to be enrolled in these trials. Thus, the number of patients with successful EGFR mutation testing out of the total number of patients enrolled in the phase III trials were: BR.21: 177 of 731 (24%); ISEL: 215 of 1692 (13%) *(226)*; TRIBUTE: 228 of 1079 (21%) *(126)*; INTACT: 312 of 2130 (15%) *(199)*; TALENT: 191 of 1172 (16%) *(227)*. The relatively small number of patients with analyzable tumor samples, together with the performance of retrospective subgroup analyses in each arm of a clinical trial that was randomized for treatment but not for mutational status, resulted in severe statistical limitations. The subgroup sample numbers were often too small to achieve statistical significance in subgroups comparisons even when trends appeared obvious, and it was difficult to avoid imbalances in patient demographic and other characteristics that may influence outcome such as performance status, tumor stage, age, ethnicity, etc. Furthermore, the small amount of tumor present in many NSCLC samples results in a limited reliability of mutational analysis results. Some studies required that each tumor be tested more than once and that only those with consistent results were included in the analysis (e.g., *(126)*) while other studies included the results from samples that were too small to allow confirmatory testing *(103)*. Confirmatory testing is advisable when possible to avoid artifactual or spurious results *(123)*.

4.3. EGFR Mutations Associated with Acquired or Primary Resistance to EGFR TKIs in NSCLC

NSCLC tumors with classical drug-sensitive EGFR TKD mutations frequently show an initial response to erlotinib or gefitinib, but the duration of response can be quite variable and ultimately most patients will develop disease progression despite TKI therapy. Such tumors can be thought of as having developed acquired resistance to therapy while on treatment. When the recurrent tumors could be biopsied for re-analysis, a second substitution mutation associated with resistance to gefitinib and erlotinib, T790M, was found in about 50% of cases *(83, 91)*. The secondary resistance mutations were easily detected in the tumor recurrences after treatment but were rarely detected in primary tumors. Kosaka et al. (*228*) noted that NSCLC patients with acquired gefitinib resistance and secondary T790M mutations tended to be women, never smokers, and carrying deletion mutations, but the T790M was not associated with the duration of gefitinib administration. Another mutation, D761Y, occurs much more rarely as a second mutation associated with acquired resistance (*91*). Exon 20 insertions have been found as uncommon primary mutations in NSCLC series and are associated with TKI resistance in experimental systems (*73*) and in patients (*92*), but these do not seem to occur as secondary mutations in the context of recurrent tumors that have a primary sensitivity mutation and that develop acquired resistance on therapy.

Although the T790M mutation seems to develop secondarily after EGFR TKI treatment of NSCLC tumors that have a primary sensitivity EGFR TKD mutation, it is likely that in many cases the T790M mutation is already present in a subpopulation of tumor cells prior to therapy. During treatment, the growth of cells without T790M is inhibited, whereas the cells bearing the resistance mutation are not inhibited, so the T790M-containing cell population expands and ultimately gives rise to clinically evident recurrent tumor. Evidence that EGFR TKI treatment is not necessary for the resistance mutation to occur comes from occasional cases of primary tumors and atypical adenomatous hyperplasia (*44, 229*) and an NSCLC cell line (NCI-H1975) in which T790M mutations in conjunction with another TKD mutation were detected by direct sequencing. Inukai M et al. 2006 also found one case of T790M+L858R, as well as one of D761Y+L858R and one of e20ins+L858R, out of 280 primary NSCLC tumors prior to or without TKI treatment which were examined by direct sequencing. These authors then examined the same series of tumors using a highly sensitive mutant-enriched assay and discovered nine additional cases containing the T790M mutation. The T790M mutation occurred with an EGFR e19del or L858R mutation in four cases, with a KRAS mutation in two cases, and in the absence of additional EGFR or KRAS mutations in four cases. In these cases, T790M mutations showed no association with sex, smoking status, or histology but were significantly more frequent in advanced tumors than in early-stage tumors. Notably, that study also found that primary T790M mutation was present in three of seven patients whose tumors also had sensitivity mutations but did not respond to gefitinib, whereas T790M was absent in 19 tumors with sensitivity mutations that responded to gefitinib. Likewise, Giaccone G et al. 2006 found a T790M mutation in a primary EGFR-mutated tumor that did not respond to erlotinib. These observations suggest that NSCLC tumors may harbor variable numbers of tumor cells having the T790M mutation. If the initial proportion of tumor cells with T790M is rather large, the tumor might be non- or poorly-responsive to erlotinib or gefitinib. If the proportion of T790M-containing cells is small, the tumor may initially respond but later re-grow as the resistant cells proliferate.

Bell et al. (*111*) added a fascinating twist to the T790M story by describing a family with multiple cases of NSCLC associated with germline transmission of this mutation, suggesting a basis for inherited susceptibility to lung cancer. Four of six tumors analyzed in that study showed a secondary somatic activating EGFR mutation, arising in *cis* with the germline EGFR mutation T790M. However, Vikis et al. (*90*) screened 237 lung cancer family probands and did not find any with T790M mutations, so may be an uncommon association.

5. EGFR EXPRESSION AND GENE COPY NUMBER IN NSCLC

The development programs of EGFR-targeted therapies began well before the discovery of EGFR TKD mutations in NSCLC, and it was anticipated that EGFR protein overexpression or gene amplification might be related to efficacy of EGFR inhibitors, similar to the paradigm established for anti-HER2 (trastuzumab) therapy in breast cancers. The relationship of EGFR expression and gene copy number in NSCLC to clinical outcome with gefitib or erlotinib therapy has been investigated in several studies. The varied results of these studies indicate that EGFR expression, gene copy number and TKD mutation may be partially, but not completely, related to one another and may each contribute to some extent to sensitivity to EGFR TKI treatment. However, the results of the studies may be dependent on the particular assays used, which emphasizes the importance of developing robust assays for a clearly defined molecular endpoint that are suitable for clinical specimens.

5.1. EGFR Expression

EGFR expression in clinical tumor samples may be assessed by IHC for protein or quantitative reverse-transcriptase PCR (qRT-PCR) for mRNA. The interpretation of IHC assays is highly subjective, and different scoring systems have been employed by different laboratories. Two scoring systems have been used that have clinical validation. Tsao et al. (*34*) used a threshold of 10% or more cells showing staining, regardless of staining intensity, to define "IHC positive". This was clinically validated by correlation with NSCLC patient survival with erlotinib treatment. The Colorado group (*69*) developed a system that uses staining intensity levels and the percentage of stained cells as multipliers to produce a final product score that is a continuous variable. A cutoff can be applied to this score to define "low" vs. "high", or "positive" vs. "negative". This system was clinically validated by correlation with NSCLC patient survival with gefitinib treatment.

Although some retrospective studies found no relationship between the level of tumor EGFR protein expression assessed by IHC and tumor response or survival in patients treated with single-agent gefitinib (*68, 230*) or erlotinib (*231*), others found significantly higher objective response rate, longer time to progression, and longer survival in EGFR IHC-positive vs. IHC-negative patients treated with gefitinib (*69, 232*) or at least noted a possible association between response and high EGFR expression (*233*). Analyses of the placebo-controlled phase III studies demonstrated that EGFR expression status by IHC does impact patient outcomes in $2^{nd}/3^{rd}$ line monotherapy setting. In BR.21, survival was significantly longer in the erlotinib-treated group vs. placebo in patients with positive EGFR expression in univariate analyses, while in multivariate analyses EGFR expression was significantly associated with higher ORR but survival after erlotinib treatment was not influenced by EGFR status (*34*). Further analysis of the BR.21 data found that patients with EGFR IHC-positive tumors who never smoked had the greatest survival benefit from erlotinib relative to placebo (*234*). In the ISEL study, EGFR IHC-positive patients had significantly better survival with gefitinib vs. placebo than patients with IHC-negative tumors, and IHC-positive patients had a higher response rate than IHC-negative patients (*226*). EGFR IHC status was not associated with outcome in patients treated with chemotherapy alone (*235*).

Most pathology laboratories have experience in performing immunohistochemistry but this technique has limitations and is subject to variables that can negatively impact its reproduceability and reliability. There is considerable heterogeneity of EGFR expression levels within NSCLC tumors, such that small diagnostic biopsies are poorly representative of EGFR expression in the whole tumor (*236, 237*). Different antibodies and detection techniques can give different results when analyzing the same specimens, and even the results obtained using a standardized EGFR assay kit can be changed if the assay performance protocol is altered (*238*). Finally, IHC interpretation (scoring) criteria differ between various laboratories that may affect the classification of tumors as positive or negative. However, Clark et al. (*239*) examined the effect of varying the cutoff for classifying patients in BR.21 as being either IHC-positive or negative, and found no significant differences in survival benefit between different cutoff points. Consistent with this, Helfrich et al. (*240*) examined

EGFR expression and sensitivity to gefitinib in 23 NSCLC cell lines, and concluded that the presence of EGFR protein was necessary for drug effect but that expression levels were not sufficient for predicting sensitivity.

Dziadziuszko et al. (*241*) examined EGFR mRNA expression by real-time quantitative reverse-transcriptase PCR (qRT-PCR) in the same cohort of gefitinib-treated NSCLC patients previously reported by Cappuzzo et al. (*69*). EGFR mRNA was significantly higher in responders to gefitinib as compared with nonresponders. Patients with high expression had a significantly greater response rate and PFS than patients with low expression, and a modest trend toward longer survival. EGFR mRNA expression was significantly correlated with protein expression assessed by IHC.

5.2. EGFR Gene Copy Number

Assessment of EGFR gene copy number by fluorescence in situ hybridization (FISH) affords a more quantitative, objective assay interpretation than does IHC and so could be expected to be give more reproducible results between laboratories. Furthermore, two-color FISH using a chromosomal centromeric control probe allows the distinction of true gene amplification vs. aneusomy on an individual cell basis. Across studies, series of NSCLC show EGFR gene amplification in about 10-15% of cases, and increased EGFR gene copy number associated with chromosome 7 polysomy occurs in a larger proportion of cases, about 20-40% (Varella-Garcia M 2006; and see references below). Quantitative PCR (qPCR) is another method of assessing gene copy number or "gene dosage." For both FISH and qPCR methods, there may be differences in published studies about the definitions of increased copy number/gene dosage versus gene amplification, and whether "positive" assays include both increased copy number and amplification, or only amplification. These technical and interpretive differences must be kept in mind when comparing study results.

Several retrospective studies of uncontrolled NSCLC cohorts have shown significantly increased response rates and prolonged survival in tumors showing EGFR amplification or high copy number (FISH-positive) compared to FISH-negative patients treated with gefitinib (*69, 232, 242, 243*). In the study of Cappuzzo et al. (*69*), FISH appeared to be a stronger predictor of survival benefit than IHC. However, other studies did not find a relationship between EGFR FISH status and response, TTP/PFS or survival in NSCLC patients on gefitinib therapy (*110, 134, 201*). Han et al. (*92*) did find an association of high EGFR FISH gene copy number with better objective response to gefitinib in univariate analysis, but copy number was not significantly associated with prolonged survival. EGFR FISH status was not associated with outcome in chemotherapy-treated patients (*235*).

Retrospective analyses of controlled phase III studies support the predictive value of EGFR FISH for predicting response and benefit from EGFR TKI treatment of advanced or metastatic NSCLC that failed chemotherapy. In BR.21, EGFR FISH-positive patients showed a higher response rate to erlotinib than FISH-negative patients and had significantly prolonged survival in the erlotinib-treated group than in the placebo arm, although survival was not influenced by EGFR gene copy number in multivariate analysis (*34*). In ISEL, high EGFR copy number was associated with significantly improved survival on gefitinib treatment and with increased response rate to gefitinib (*226*).

Very recently, results were reported for a clinical study, ONCOBELL, in which NSCLC patients treated with gefitinib were prospectively evaluated for EGFR FISH status (*244*). EGFR FISH-positive patients, compared with negative patients, had significantly higher RR and longer TTP, and showed a trend for longer survival. Consistent with the observed associations between EGFR gene copy number and EGFR TKI sensitivity in NSCLC patients, Helfrich et al. (*240*) found a significant correlation between EGFR gene copy number assessed by FISH and gefitinib sensitivity in 23 NSCLC lines. EGFR copy number by FISH and EGFR mutations do not appear to share the same ethnic associations. Unlike EGFR mutations, the frequency of EGFR amplification and high polysomy by FISH appears to be similar in East Asian and Western populations (*245*). NSCLC patients in the Middle East appear to have a high EGFR amplification rate assessed by FISH and a low rate of EGFR mutations (*136*). Because EGFR gene copy number increases are more often associated with chromosome 7 polysomy than with selective EGFR gene amplification as assessed by FISH in NSCLC, Buckingham et al. (*204*) investigated the relationship of chromosome 7 polysomy to gefitinib efficacy in advanced NSCLC patients. Polysomy was significantly associated with increased objective response and overall survival.

The relationship between gefitinib sensitivity and EGFR gene dosage has also been investigated using quantitative PCR (qPCR) methods. Takano et al. (*202*) found that high gene dosage by qPCR was significantly associated with response rate and TTP but not with OS in gefitinib-treated NSCLC patients. Bell et al. (*199*) analyzed samples from the phase II IDEAL trials of gefitinib. EGFR gene amplification by qPCR was associated with increased response rate, but because there were a limited number of samples analyzed and some of the amplified cases also had EGFR TKD mutations, the relationship of amplified wild-type EGFR to response could not be assessed. The number of samples was too low to allow meaningful assessment of the relationship of amplification to TTP and OS. Dziadziuszko et al. (*241*) analyzed the same cohort previously studied by Cappuzzo et al. (*69*) and found that EGFR gene dosage did not predict response, PFS, or overall survival. Quite importantly, EGFR gene dosage was not related to FISH positivity in that study. The reasons for discordance between copy number assessment by FISH versus qPCR are not clear and should be investigated further.

5.3. Relationship of EGFR Gene Copy Number and EGFR Expression in NSCLC

Significant correlations in NSCLC between EGFR gene copy number by FISH and protein expression by IHC have been reported by several groups (*69, 235, 245–247*). However, Dacic S et al. 2006 observed that EGFR protein expression appeared to be uncoupled from FISH gene amplification in most cases (although good correlation did occur in a subset of squamous cell carcinomas) and Willmore-Payne et al. (*169*) concluded that polysomy for chromosome 7 was not related to EGFR protein overexpression. Likewise, Argiris et al. (*206*) reported that EGFR gene amplification by FISH was not correlated with EGFR IHC, and Bell et al. (*199*) found that *EGFR* amplification by qPCR accounted for only a small subset of cases with high levels of protein expression by IHC. Dziadziuszko et al. (*241*) reported that EGFR mRNA expression was significantly higher in FISH-positive (high copy number or amplified) patients.

5.4. Relationship of EGFR Mutations to Gene Copy Number and Expression in NSCLC

Associations between high EGFR gene copy number and the presence of EGFR TKD mutations have been noted in several studies of primary NSCLC tumors (*45, 69, 92, 109, 110, 137, 206, 242, 244, 248*), sometimes reaching statistical significance (*92, 110, 206, 244*), and in series of NSCLC cell lines (*56, 60, 240*). Investigating gene dosage and amplification by qPCR, Takano et al. (*202*) determined that high EGFR copy numbers were caused by selective amplification of mutant alleles, while Dziadziuszko et al. (*241*) concluded that EGFR gene dosage was not associated with EGFR mutation status and Bell et al. (*199*) found that of 10 of 14 (80%) cases with EGFR amplification had amplification of wild-type alleles.

EGFR mutations and EGFR protein expression by IHC have been reported to be both associated with one another (*40, 249*) and not associated (*103*). Two studies investigating EGFR mutation and EGFR mRNA expression found no significant association (*109, 241*).

6. KRAS MUTATION IN NSCLC AND PRIMARY RESISTANCE TO EGFR TKIS

Since the EGFR signals through the K-ras to activate signaling through the the MAP kinase/Erk and Akt pathways, KRAS mutations might be predicted to subvert tumor cell dependence on EGFR activation and thus cause a lack of sensitivity to EGFR inhibitors. Several groups investigating this question in clinical series have reported consistently that KRAS mutations are associated with non-response, i.e., primary resistance, to gefitinib or erlotinib treatment in NSCLC patients (*92, 110, 126, 130, 134, 209, 250*).

As discussed previously in sections 2.2.2 and 2.2.3, EGFR mutation rates are higher and KRAS mutation rates are lower in East Asian populations or in non-smokers, compared to Western Caucasian populations or smokers, respectively. Therefore, the associations of East Asian ethnicity or non-smoking status with higher NSCLC response rates to EGFR TKIs might reflect a summation of two separate molecular factors: a higher frequency of a molecular alteration that makes tumors very sensitive to the drugs (EGFR mutation), together with a lower frequency of an alteration which causes tumors to be drug-resistant (KRAS mutation).

The reported associations of KRAS mutations with time to progression and survival in patients treated with EGFR TKI monotherapy are less consistent than the association with non-response: Han et al. (*92*) found that TTP and OS were not significantly different by KRAS status; Massarelli et al. (*134*) reported that KRAS mutations were associated with significantly shorter median time to progression but not with survival, compared to KRAS wild-type; while Endoh et al. (*130*) found that survival was significantly shorter in patients with KRAS mutations. In the phase III TRIBUTE study, patients with KRAS mutation who received erlotinib together with chemotherapy fared considerably worse than did patients with KRAS mutations who received chemotherapy alone, or patients with wild-type KRAS who received either treatment (*126*). The possible mechanistic basis for this apparent interaction between KRAS mutation, EGFR TKI, and chemotherapy on survival in NSCLC presently is not clear. KRAS mutations have also been associated with poor response rates and TTP to the EGFR-targeted antibody cetuximab in colorectal cancer patients (*251–253*).

In experimental cell systems, the ability to demonstrate a relationship of KRAS mutation and resistance to EGFR inhibitors may depend on the type of model employed and the examined endpoints. For example, Uchida et al. (*254*) could induce gefitinib resistance by transfecting cells with activated KRAS expression constructs, whereas Suzuki et al. (*255*) and Yauch et al. (*65*) did not note a relationship between the mutation status of endogenous KRAS and gefitinib or erlotinib sensitivity in panels of NSCLC cell lines.

7. OTHER MOLECULAR CHARACTERISTICS RELATED TO NSCLC SENSITIVITY TO EGFR INHIBITORS

A variety of other parameters related to EGFR expression, activation and signaling have been investigated for their relationship to EGFR-targeted drug sensitivity or resistance in NSCLC. The aims of the studies have been to provide a better understanding of the various factors that influence drug sensitivity, to gauge the relative importance of these factors, and to determine which molecular endpoints or combinations of endpoints might be best used to guide clinical decision-making.

7.1. EGFR Intron 1 Simple Sequence Repeats and Promoter Single-nucleotide Polymorphisms

Germline genetic variants may influence EGFR expression levels. Lower numbers of intron 1 CA repeats (associated with higher gene expression levels) and -216G/T SNPs may be associated with increased tumor sensitivity to EGFR TKI treatment, as well as an increased tendency for patients to develop mechanism-related toxicities such as skin rash (86, 110, 256–258). Nomura et al. (259) recently described a broad investigation of the prevalence and associations of EGFR polymorphisms, mutations and amplification across a multi-ethnic patient cohort. Polymorphisms associated with increased EGFR expression (lower numbers of intron 1 CA repeats and SNPs at -216 and -191) were rare in East Asians as compared to other ethnicities. EGFR mutations were more often associated with shorter intron 1 CA repeats, and amplification of the shorter allele of CA repeats often occurred in tumors having EGFR mutations, particularly in East Asian patients.

7.2. AKT Phosphorylation

Consistent with the hypothesis that AKT phosphorylation may be indicative of tumors in which EGFR downstream signaling is activated, Cappuzzo et al. (260) first reported that gefitinib-treated NSCLC patients whose tumors expressed phospho-Akt by IHC had a better response rate, disease control rate, and time to progression than patients with phospho-Akt-negative tumors. Subsequent studies, however, have suggested that phospho-Akt status alone is not strongly associated with clinical benefit from EGFR TKI treatment (226, 244). Other studies suggested that phospho-Akt status may be related to improved response or outcome when combined with EGFR mutation status (68, 69), EGFR FISH or IHC (69, 261), chromosome 7 polysomy (204) or KRAS mutation status (92). However, the phase II ONCOBELL trial of gefitinib, which enrolled patients prospectively based on never-smoking status, EGFR FISH positivity or phospho-Akt positivity by IHC, failed to show any predictive value of phospho-Akt status alone or in combination with EGFR FISH status (244).

7.3. PTEN Loss, PIK3CA Mutation, IGFR-1 Expression

PTEN loss, mutational activation of PI-3-kinase, or activation of RTKs such as IGFR-1 might be expected to result in EGFR-independent activation of AKT signaling, making this cell survival pathway resistant to EGFR inhibitors. Buckingham et al. (204) found a significant association of PTEN expression with longer overall survival in gefitinib-treated patients. However, PTEN expression alone was not related to NSCLC outcome with gefitinib treatment in other studies (135, 262) although Endoh et al. (130) found that in tumors with EGFR mutations, survival was longer in those with high PIK3CA or PTEN expression than in those with low expression of these molecules. In the latter study, the two patients who had PIK3CA mutations had partial responses to gefitinib. Surprisingly, high IGFR-1 expression was found to be significantly associated with longer survival in gefitinib-treated NSCLC although not with greater RR or TTP (262).

7.4. Co-expression of HER2, HER3 and EGFR Ligands; MET Amplification

Experiments with panels of NSCLC lines and with transgenic mice indicated that an EGFR TKI-sensitive phenotype maybe related to the expression of the EGFR together with its co-receptors, HER2 and HER3, and ligands that activate the EGFR signaling complex; HER3 expression in particular was related to EGFR TKI sensitivity (65, 263, 264). Importantly, HER3 appears to provide a key link between EGFR activation and PI-3-kinase/AKT signaling (71). In 2005, Hirata A et al. found that overexpression of HER2 by transfection of NSCLC cells produced an increased sensitivity to gefitinib, which appeared to be mediated by heterodimerization with HER3. Therefore, HER3 may play an important role in the formation of heteromeric complexes with EGFR and HER2, which drive NSCLC tumor cell growth and survival. Examination of tumor samples from gefitinib-treated patients confirmed the association with sensitivity of high HER3 expression (*263*) and co-expression of EGFR, HER2, and HER3 or HER4 (*265*). Other studies of primary tumor samples from treated patients indicated that increased HER2 gene copy number was related to responses to gefitinib (*69, 244*) but HER2 protein alone (*266*) or HER3 gene copy numbers (*261*) were not related to response. NSCLC tumors with HER2 mutations appear to be poorly responsive to gefitinib (*92*). Recently, Engelman et al. (*267*) described a HER3-mediated association between MET amplification and acquired resistance to gefitinib, raising the possibility that high levels of MET expression might in some way compete with EGFR for its critical signaling partner, HER3. This could represent a second mechanism for developing acquired resistance in NSCLC, which recur after an initial response to EGFR TKI but do not develop resistance mutations (e.g., T790M) in the EGFR.

7.5. Epithelial vs. Mesenchymal Differentiation

NSCLC show a wide range of cellular differentiation in tumors from different patients, and often even within the tumor in a single patient. Well-differentiated tumors are associated with the expression of epithelial differentiation markers such as E-cadherin, whereas more poorly-differentiated tumors show loss of epithelial differentiation markers and can begin to show differentiation markers generally associated with a mesenchymal phenotype, such as vimentin. The relationship of the range of differentiation observed in human NSCLC tumors to the experimental phenomenon of "epithelial-mesenchymal transition" (EMT) remains controversial (*268*). In NSCLC cell lines, epithelial differentiation is associated with sensivity to erlotinib or gefitinib, while a more mesenchymal phenotype is associated with EGFR TKI resistance (*65, 269, 270*). In the phase III TRIBUTE trial, patients whose tumors were E-cadherin-positive by IHC exhibited a significantly longer time to progression and a non-significant trend toward longer survival with erlotinib + chemotherapy treatment versus chemotherapy alone (*65*). E-cadherin expression appears to play a key role in determining EGFR TKI sensitivity since restoring E-cadherin expression increases sensitivity to EGFR inhibitors in NSCLC cell lines (*271*).

7.6. EMP-1 Expression

Jain et al. (*272*) developed an experimental model of acquired gefitinib resistance and used differential gene expression profiling to identify epithelial membrane protein-1 (*272*) as a marker of resistance. The association of EMP-1 expression with gefitinib resistance was confirmed in a series of tumor samples from gefitinib-treated NSCLC patients.

7.7. Transcript Expression and Proteomic Profiling Signatures

Microarray analyses of mRNA expression in training sets of NSCLC cell lines with varying degrees of EGFR sensitivity were used to develop gene expression signatures that differentiated sensitive vs. resistant cell lines. The signatures were validated against a second test of NSCLC lines of unknown sensitivity (*273*) or against primary NSCLC tumors where the expression signature identified tumors with high levels of EGFR activation or EGFR mutations (*274*). Proteomic approaches have included analysis of tumor tissues from gefitinib-responsive and non-responsive patients by 2-D gel electrophoresis to identify a panel of discriminator proteins whose predictive power was validated in a second tumor test set using a specific immunoassay (*275*); and mass spectrometric analysis of serum from NSCLC patients patients treated with gefitinib or erlotinib, which generated spectrographic signatures whose predictive power was validated in additional test sets of sera from erlotinib- or gefitinib-treated patients (*276*).

7.8. Utility of Various Molecular Data Related to EGFR TKI Efficacy

The different tumor molecular characteristics related to EGFR TKI efficacy described in the previous section suggest potential avenues for predictive molecular diagnostics. Whether these can be developed into clinically useful tests for patient selection will depend on the further demonstrations of the robustness of the tests and their predictive power.

Regardless of whether assays for these various molecular characteristics are suitable as tests for patient selection for therapy, the research data are valuable in suggesting strategies for combining targeted therapeutics. For example, PI-3-kinase inhibition potentiated gefitinib in EGFR TKI-resistant A549 cells which do not express HER3 (*277*); inhibition of AKT-mTOR signaling with rapamycin enhanced the effect of HK-272 in lung tumors of EGFR L858R+T790M transgenic mice (*278*); histone deacetylase (HDAC) inhibition restored E-cadherin expression and EGFR TKI responsiveness in gefitinib-resistant, E-cadherin-deficient NSCLC cells (*271*); and the HER2 heterodimerization inhibitor, pertuzumab, in combination with erlotinib was superior to monotherapy in xenograft models (*279*).

8. MOLECULAR TESTING IN CLINICAL TRIALS AND CLINICAL PRACTICE

The studies above indicate that a number of different molecular characteristics may be related to the efficacy of EGFR inhibitors in NSCLC, and that some of these characteristics may be mechanistically related in various ways, and some may be independent of others. The data suggest that there are several possible approaches to molecular testing for patient selection and therapeutic decision-making in the clinical setting. Careful and critical evaluation and testing will be needed to determine the preferable assays for clinical use. It may well be that combinations of assays will be needed to achieve the desired results (*68, 69, 92, 135, 198, 232, 244*). Ultimately, prospective clinical data will be needed to establish the power of molecular testing. Some phase II trials of EGFR TKI have been completed in patients prospectively selected for EGFR mutations (*212–215*) and for EGFR FISH or phospho-AKT positivity (*244*). Furthermore, the Dana-Farber/MGH laboratories have instituted routine EGFR mutation testing in their NSCLC patients as part of their clinical/pathological evaluation protocol and are prospectively following patient outcomes (*108*). These studies support the ability of molecular testing to enrich clinical trial and clinical practice populations for enhanced therapeutic efficacy. More clinical trials of EGFR TKIs in NSCLC which incorporate molecular testing for EGFR mutations, FISH, IHC and other endpoints in order to select patients or for secondary analyses are underway and are being planned (for current information regarding federally and privately supported clinical trials, see http://www.clinicaltrials.gov/), and will be reported as they are completed over the next few years. In the end, the strength of the combined data from multiple studies in various settings that test the efficacy and safety of the drug, as well as the value and reliability of the molecular tests, will determine whether testing becomes an accepted part of therapeutic decision-making.

9. PATHOLOGY SAMPLE AND ASSAY CONSIDERATIONS FOR THE MOLECULAR TESTING OF NSCLC IN CLINICAL TUMOR SAMPLES

The acceptable level of rigor required of a molecular assay may be different for an experimental or clinical trial situation where the main goal is to create subject cohorts that are enriched for a molecular characteristic, compared to clinical practice where the assay is used to make individual treatment decisions. The accuracy and reproducibility (both technical and clinical) of molecular assessment is highly dependent on every step of the testing process: the quality of the sample and the degree to which the sample is representative of the whole disease burden within the patient, the performance characteristics of the assay reagents and procedure, and the approach used to interpret the results of the assay.

9.1. Pathology Samples

9.1.1. Sample Type

Because gaining wide access to intrathoracic lesions requires major surgery, approaches to sample acquisition for pathological diagnosis and staging attempt to be minimally invasive: biopsies obtained by bronchoscopy, mediastinoscopy, or core needle biopsy; or cytology samples obtained by fine-needle aspiration or sputum sampling. The tumor sample obtained by these techniques is quite small in size. Larger excisional biopsies may be performed if the lesion is easily accessible. Surgical excision of the entire tumor with curative intent is only attempted for limited-stage lesions. Molecular analyses of EGFR can be successfully performed on small biopsy and aspiration samples (*200, 242*). The limitations of these sample types, however, must be recognized, with tumor heterogeneity being a major issue.

9.1.2. Tumor Heterogeneity

NSCLC tumors are notoriously heterogeneous in several aspects: between different regions or cell subpopulations within a single tumor mass, between multiple synchronous tumor masses in the same patient, between primary tumors and metachronous metastases, and over the course of tumor evolution and progression during treatment (as in the acquisition of EGFR T790M mutations). The sample size, sampling location and timing of sample acquisition can all influence the degree to which a tumor sample is representative of the disease burden within the patient at any particular time during the course of disease.

9.1.2.1. Intra-tumor Regional Heterogeneity of EGFR IHC and FISH
Ferrigan L et al. examined EGFR IHC in 36 resected cases of NSCLC compared to their matched preoperative diagnostic biopsies in order to determine whether the IHC status of the resected tumor could reliably be predicted from the small diagnostic biopsy (*237*). There was considerable intratumor regional heterogeneity of EGFR expression in the resected tumors and a poor predictive value of the results obtained with the diagnostic biopsies, indicating that EGFR IHC of small diagnostic biopsies would have limited usefulness in accurately assessing patient tumor status for making treatment decisions. Likewise, Taillade et al. (*236*) compared the expression of several biomarkers including EGFR in patients having both a bronchial biopsy and a surgical resection sample. For EGFR IHC there was no significant correlation between the numbers of positive cells in the two sample types, and there was a discordance rate of 18% in the assessment of the samples as being "EGFR-positive" or "EGFR negative." The guidelines published by the Colorado group for the performance and interpretation of EGFR FISH in NSCLC include a caution regarding intratumor heterogeneity of EGFR gene copy number, where EGFR amplification may be present in specific foci of tumor cells or diffusely interspaced among non-amplified tumor nuclei (*280*). Therefore, the Colorado guidelines recommend examining several different areas within a tumor for EGFR FISH analysis.

9.1.2.2. Cellular or Molecular Subpopulations of EGFR Mutations within a Tumor
Mutational analyses of EGFR in tumor samples using sensitive detection techniques demonstrated the presence of relatively small numbers of mutated genes that were not evident using less sensitive direct sequencing techniques. The presence of primary EGFR mutations

in a background of wild-type sequence can reflect a mixture of tumor cells and non-tumor stromal cells in a primary tumor sample (*281*). Analyses of the T790M second mutation in tumors with primary EGFR sensitivity mutations demonstrated the presence of double mutant subpopulations that could reflect minor clones of cells or subpopulations of mutant alleles in a background of gene amplification (*282*). NSCLC lines that presumably represent "pure" tumor cell populations also show heterogeneity in EGFR mutation status (*283*). In an EGFR TKI-resistant cell line model having both EGFR sensitivity mutation and gene amplification, a sensitive detection assay demonstrated a T790M-containing subpopulation (*85*). Those authors proposed that "allelic dilution" of biologically significant gene mutations may go undetected by direct sequencing in cancers with amplified oncogenes.

9.1.2.3. EGFR Mutation Heterogeneity between Multiple Tumors in the Same Patient

Gallegos Ruiz et al. (*284*) examined mutations and chromosomal abnormalities in 3 patients with multiple NSCLC tumors and found that the tumors were clonal in one patient and genetically different in two patients. Kozuki et al. (*229*) described a variety of differences in the EGFR mutational status between lesions in patients who had synchronous or metachronous multiple adenocarcinomas and/or atypical adenomatous hyperplasia and concluded that EGFR mutations may occur randomly even in multiple lesions in a single patient.

9.1.2.4. EGFR FISH and IHC in NSCLC Primary Tumors and Metastases

Italiano et al. (*285*) found a 27% discordance in EGFR FISH status, and 33% discordance in EGFR IHC status, of primary NSCLC tumors compared to their metastases. Their series included cases in which the primary tumors were FISH- or IHC-positive and the metastases were negative, and cases having FISH- or IHC-negative primaries and test-positive metastases.

9.1.2.5. EGFR FISH and Mutations in Tumors Sampled over Time During Therapy

In the ONCOBELL trial, Cappuzzo et al. (*244*) collected nine pairs of tumor samples taken at the time of original diagnosis and after chemotherapy, and 14 pairs of samples taken at the time of original diagnosis and after initiating gefitinib therapy, with or without prior chemotherapy. In the samples taken before and after chemotherapy, there was 89% concordance for both EGFR FISH and mutations. In samples taken before and during gefitinib therapy, there was 64% concordance for EGFR FISH and 50% for mutations.

9.1.3. Sample Fixation and Storage

The molecular integrity of tumor tissues is optimally preserved by flash freezing of fresh tissue samples or by fixation in alcohol. However, since routinely processed archival pathology samples are fixed in formalin (or other fixative such as Bouin's solution) and embedded in paraffin blocks, clinically useful assays must be applicable to such specimen preparations. Some EGFR mutation analyses using formalin-fixed paraffin-embedded (FFPE) NSCLC samples have reported unusually high numbers of novel substitution mutations including C → T/G → A or A → G/T → C transitions (*34, 35*). Marchetti et al. (*123*) analyzed 70 FFPE NSCLC samples and identified 45 unusual "mutations" were identified, including the 22 transitions reported by Tsao et al. (*34*). However, these unusual sequence alterations were also found in FFPE samples of normal tissues. The sequence changes were shown to be artifacts related to formalin fixation resulting from postmortem deamination of cytosine or adenine resulting in uracil or hypoxanthine residues, respectively. The occurrence of C → T/G → A transitions could be prevented by the addition of uracil-N-glycosylase to the DNA template prior to PCR amplification. Gallegos Ruiz et al. (*197*) compared EGFR and KRAS sequence analyses in 47 matched frozen and FFPE tumor samples and detected 10 nucleotide changes in FFPE samples that were not found in the frozen specimens. Upon re-analysis, these nucleotide changes could not be confirmed and were most likely the result of paraffin embedding and fixation procedures.

In regard to FISH analysis, pathologist consensus recommendations for HER2 FISH testing are to avoid the use of Bouin's fixative because it can cause the loss of FISH signals (*286*) and it is probable that EGFR FISH testing is similarly affected by fixation. In general, any fixative containing heavy metal ions will likely interfere with DNA analytical procedures, including FISH as well as PCR used for sequence analysis.

Fixation conditions and storage conditions can greatly affect IHC results in NSCLC tissues. A study of EGFR IHC (Dako pharmDx kit) performance on NSCLC and other tumor samples prepared with 8 commonly used fixatives showed that unbuffered formalin (4% or 10%), acetic formalin alcohol and Pen-Fix all resulted in acceptable levels of EGFR signal, while Bouin's fixative or 4% neutral buffered formalin resulted in a lower percentage of positively stained tumor cells, and Prefer fixative resulted in poor preservation of tissue morphology and poor EGFR staining (*287*). When NSCLC tissue sections are cut from paraffin blocks and then stored for various periods of time as unstained sections mounted on glass microscope slides prior to performing EGFR IHC assays, a time-dependent loss of immunoreactivity is observed (*287–289*). DNA is less susceptible to degradation in cut-sections over time, but long-term storage of cut sections may result in decreased quality of FISH and DNA mutational assay results. The molecular degradation that occurs over time in slide-mounted cut sections stored in ambient atmospheric conditions probably is due to oxidation and humidity. One approach that has been attempted to prevent this is to dip the slides in paraffin after sectioning in order to create a protective coating during storage of the sections. If this approach is used, extreme care must be taken to ensure that the de-paraffinization process is absolutely complete prior to peforming the assay, with particular attention paid to frequent refreshment of the xylenes or other solvent solutions used for deparaffinization. Any traces of residual paraffin remaining in the sections will inhibit antibody or probe penetration into the tissue section and cause loss of signal in IHC or FISH assays, and reduce the efficiency of PCR reactions for sequencing.

9.2. Assay Sensitivity

Direct sequencing is the gold standard for determining amplicon sequences and establishing the identity of mutations and sequence variations. However, direct sequencing is laborious, has a rather low sensitivity, and requires relatively pure samples without contaminating nontumor cells for reliable mutation analysis. Therefore, a variety of alternative techniques have been devised to allow efficient mutation screening and for the high-sensitivity detection of specific EGFR mutations in a high background of contaminating wild-type sequence. Such techniques include dHPLC/SURVEYOR for mutation screening and high-sensivity detection (*281*), s-RT-MELT (*290*), Scorpion Amplified Refractory Mutation System technology (*203, 291*); mutant-enriched PCR (*292, 293*); peptide nucleic acid-locked nucleic acid (PNA-LNA) PCR clamp assay (*292, 294*); Cycleave PCR technique (*214*); and high-resolution melting analysis (*295*). Such high-sensitivity techniques can increase the probability of successful mutation determination from small samples and also obviate the need for laborious tumor macrodissection or laser-capture microdissection to isolate tumor cells. The development of ultra high-sensitivity assays raises the very exciting possibility that mutation analysis could be performed on DNA in pleural fluid (*208, 292*) or tumor DNA circulating in the blood, which would allow repeated sequence analysis at any time during a patient's clinical course without the need to obtain tumor tissue samples. Kimura et al. (*203*) used Scorpion-ARMS assay to detect EGFR mutations in serum DNA obtained from Japanese patients with NSCLC before first-line gefitinib monotherapy. EGFR mutations (E746_A750del and L858R) were detected in 13 of 27 (48.1%) patients. EGFR mutations were seen significantly more frequently in patients with a partial response than in patients with stable disease or progressive disease and median progression-free survival and overall survival were significantly longer in patients with EGFR mutations than in patients without EGFR mutations. In pairs of tumor and serum samples obtained from 11 patients, the EGFR mutation status in the tumors was consistent with those in the serum of eight of 11 (72.7%) of the paired samples.

The sensitivity of FISH is influenced by probe size and fluorophore labeling, hybridization conditions, and the completeness of proteinase digestion of the tissue prior to hybridization (*280*). Importantly, interpreting the FISH assay depends on quantitating the numbers of hybridization signals within cell nuclei. Suboptimal assay conditions or poor tissue quality may decrease hybridization signal intensity or increase background signal, but the numbers of hybridization signals will not change. This would result in an increased number of assay failures but not in an increased number of false-negative test results.

In contrast to FISH, interpretation of IHC assays depends on qualitative signal intensity. Poor quality tissues, inappropriate fixation or suboptimal assay conditions may reduce signal intensity and thus lead to an increased number of false-negative assay results. For commercially available assay kits, altering the manufacturer's recommended protocol may reduce assay performance, or can even result in increased assay sensitivity. Derecskei et al. (*238*) altered the protocol provided for the Dako pharmDx EGFR IHC kit and converted four out of eight EGFR-negative tumors into EGFR-positive in a study of 50 lung adenocarcinoma cases. Thus, the reproducibility of IHC assays is critically dependent on close adherence to standardized methodologies that may be problematic if the test is widely used in many testing laboratories.

10. CONCLUSION

The discovery of EGFR mutations in NSCLC, and their relationships to tumor responses to EGFR TKIs, has been an important and exciting advance in our understanding of molecular subtypes related to the pathogenesis, biology and treatment of this disease. However, the molecular characteristics that may influence the sensitivity of NSCLC tumors to EGFR TKIs are multifactorial and may be interrelated to, or independent from, one another in varying degrees. As usually occurs in a rapidly moving area of scientific inquiry, the available data at times appear to be somewhat conflicting, and there are continuing challenges to better understand the various data and to reconcile the apparent conflicts. At the time of this writing, it remains to be seen which molecular endpoints or clinical characteristics will ultimately gain clinical acceptance and use in guiding clinical decision–making.

Activating mutations in the EGFR, together with EGFR gene amplification, may indicate genetic oncogene addiction for some NSCLC, representing their "Achilles' heel." Many tumors recur after an initial response to TKIs because they develop secondary EGFR mutations that block the effect of the drug. Strategies for treating mutated tumors may include irreversible or second generation EGFR TKIs that can circumvent the secondary mutations or other mechanisms that develop in tumors addicted to the EGFR signal. However, mutations and gene amplifications are not the whole story underlying NSCLC responsiveness to EGFR TKIs, as some wild-type and non-amplified tumors also respond. Other tumors may not be genetically addicted to EGFR activation, but could still be driven to a more aggressive phenotype by EGFR signaling. Inhibiting the EGFR in such tumors could cause a shift toward biological quiescence or more benign behavior, resulting in delayed tumor progression and prolonged survival: "taming the beast." These tumors may have increased EGFR, co-receptor and ligand expression or other molecular phenotypic characteristics that are linked to activation of EGFR signaling. By contrast, other tumors may have molecular genetic or phenotypic alterations, such as KRAS mutation or loss of epithelial differentiation in primary tumors, or MET amplification in some cases of acquired resistance, which subvert the influence of EGFR signaling and make them non- responsive to EGFR inhibition. The variety of molecular alterations linked to sensitivity or resistance to TKIs suggest two basic strategies for patient selection: testing to identify tumors which have a high likelihood of tumor response or clinical benefit, and therefore should be treated; or testing for those which have a low chance of responding and therefore should be excluded from treatment.

Regardless of the strategy – whether to find Achilles' heel, or to name the beasts that can or cannot be tamed – the success depends on having a dependable test that can be used to accomplish the task. A molecular test result is dependent upon three components: 1) the sample and preanalytical variables (how the sample for assay is obtained from the patient's tumor; how the sample is processed including fixation, storage and preparation for assay; sample size and composition of tumor vs. non-tumor cells); 2) the assay technique (reagents and procedure); 3) assay result interpretation (scoring). All three of these components influence the robustness of the test, and the parameters of all three components must be defined - in the environment in which they are intended to be used - before an assay can be used as a test to investigate clinical correlations with any confidence in the result. No matter how well a molecular assay performs technically using non-clinical samples in the research laboratory, it is not yet acceptable as a clinically useful test until the application to clinical samples has been technically validated, and reproduceable and reliable methods of interpreting assay results have been established.

REFERENCES

1. Gordon MS, Matei D, Aghajanian C, et al. Clinical activity of pertuzumab (rhuMAb 2C4), a HER dimerization inhibitor, in advanced ovarian cancer: potential predictive relationship with tumor HER2 activation status. J Clin Oncol 2006;24:4324–32.
2. Rusch V, Baselga J, Cordon-Cardo C, et al. Differential expression of the epidermal growth factor receptor and its ligands in primary non-small cell lung cancers and adjacent benign lung. Cancer Res 1993;53:2379–85.
3. Ciardiello F, De Vita F, Orditura M, Tortora G. The role of EGFR inhibitors in nonsmall cell lung cancer. Curr Opin Oncol 2004;16:130–5.
4. Fukuoka M, Yano S, Giaccone G, et al. Multi-institutional randomized phase II trial of gefitinib for previously treated patients with advanced non-small-cell lung cancer (The IDEAL 1 Trial) [corrected]. J Clin Oncol 2003;21:2237–46.
5. Kris MG, Natale RB, Herbst RS, et al. Efficacy of gefitinib, an inhibitor of the epidermal growth factor receptor tyrosine kinase, in symptomatic patients with non-small cell lung cancer: a randomized trial. Jama 2003;290:2149–58.
6. Ho C, Murray N, Laskin J, Melosky B, Anderson H, Bebb G. Asian ethnicity and adenocarcinoma histology continues to predict response to gefitinib in patients treated for advanced non-small cell carcinoma of the lung in North America. Lung Cancer 2005;49:225–31.
7. Miller VA, Kris MG, Shah N, et al. Bronchioloalveolar pathologic subtype and smoking history predict sensitivity to gefitinib in advanced non-small-cell lung cancer. J Clin Oncol 2004;22:1103–9.
8. Shepherd FA, Rodrigues Pereira J, Ciuleanu T, et al. Erlotinib in previously treated non-small-cell lung cancer. N Engl J Med 2005;353:123–32.
9. Thatcher N, Chang A, Parikh P, et al. Gefitinib plus best supportive care in previously treated patients with refractory advanced non-small-cell lung cancer: results from a randomised, placebo-controlled, multicentre study (Iressa Survival Evaluation in Lung Cancer). Lancet 2005;366:1527–37.
10. Herbst RS, Prager D, Hermann R, et al. TRIBUTE: a phase III trial of erlotinib hydrochloride (OSI-774) combined with carboplatin and paclitaxel chemotherapy in advanced non-small-cell lung cancer. J Clin Oncol 2005;23:5892–9.

11. Chang A, Parikh P, Thongprasert S, et al. Gefitinib (IRESSA) in patients of Asian origin with refractory advanced non-small cell lung cancer: subset analysis from the ISEL study. J Thorac Oncol 2006;1:847–55.
12. Subramanian J, Govindan R. Lung cancer in never smokers: a review. J Clin Oncol 2007;25:561–70.
13. Bryant A, Cerfolio RJ. Differences in epidemiology, histology, and survival between cigarette smokers and never-smokers who develop non-small cell lung cancer. Chest 2007;132:185–92.
14. Zhou W, Heist RS, Liu G, et al. Smoking cessation before diagnosis and survival in early stage non-small cell lung cancer patients. Lung Cancer 2006;53:375–80.
15. Batevik R, Grong K, Segadal L, Stangeland L. The female gender has a positive effect on survival independent of background life expectancy following surgical resection of primary non-small cell lung cancer: a study of absolute and relative survival over 15 years. Lung Cancer 2005;47:173–81.
16. Itaya T, Yamaoto N, Ando M, et al. Influence of histological type, smoking history and chemotherapy on survival after first-line therapy in patients with advanced non-small cell lung cancer. Cancer Sci 2007;98:226–30.
17. Tsuchiya T, Akamine S, Muraoka M, et al. Stage IA non-small cell lung cancer: vessel invasion is a poor prognostic factor and a new target of adjuvant chemotherapy. Lung Cancer 2007;56:341–8.
18. Ramnath N, Demmy TL, Antun A, et al. Pneumonectomy for bronchogenic carcinoma: analysis of factors predicting survival. Ann Thorac Surg 2007;83:1831–6.
19. Paez JG, Janne PA, Lee JC, et al. EGFR mutations in lung cancer: correlation with clinical response to gefitinib therapy. Science 2004;304:1497–500.
20. Lynch TJ, Bell DW, Sordella R, et al. Activating mutations in the epidermal growth factor receptor underlying responsiveness of non-small-cell lung cancer to gefitinib. N Engl J Med 2004;350:2129–39.
21. Pao W, Miller V, Zakowski M, et al. EGF receptor gene mutations are common in lung cancers from "never smokers" and are associated with sensitivity of tumors to gefitinib and erlotinib. Proc Natl Acad Sci USA 2004;101:13306–11.
22. Pao W, Miller VA. Epidermal growth factor receptor mutations, small-molecule kinase inhibitors, and non-small-cell lung cancer: current knowledge and future directions. J Clin Oncol 2005;23:2556–68.
23. Johnson BE, Janne PA. Epidermal growth factor receptor mutations in patients with non-small cell lung cancer. Cancer Res 2005;65:7525–9.
24. Hirsch FR, Witta S. Biomarkers for prediction of sensitivity to EGFR inhibitors in non-small cell lung cancer. Curr Opin Oncol 2005;17:118–22.
25. Janne PA, Engelman JA, Johnson BE. Epidermal growth factor receptor mutations in non-small-cell lung cancer: implications for treatment and tumor biology. J Clin Oncol 2005;23:3227–34.
26. Shigematsu H, Gazdar AF. Somatic mutations of epidermal growth factor receptor signaling pathway in lung cancers. Int J Cancer 2006;118:257–62.
27. Bunn PA, Jr., Dziadziuszko R, Varella-Garcia M, et al. Biological markers for non-small cell lung cancer patient selection for epidermal growth factor receptor tyrosine kinase inhibitor therapy. Clin Cancer Res 2006;12:3652–6.
28. Riely GJ, Pao W, Pham D, et al. Clinical course of patients with non-small cell lung cancer and epidermal growth factor receptor exon 19 and exon 21 mutations treated with gefitinib or erlotinib. Clin Cancer Res 2006;12:839–44.
29. Riely GJ, Politi KA, Miller VA, Pao W. Update on epidermal growth factor receptor mutations in non-small cell lung cancer. Clin Cancer Res 2006;12:7232–41.
30. Rosell R, Taron M, Reguart N, Isla D, Moran T. Epidermal growth factor receptor activation: how exon 19 and 21 mutations changed our understanding of the pathway. Clin Cancer Res 2006;12:7222–31.
31. Ono M, Kuwano M. Molecular mechanisms of epidermal growth factor receptor (EGFR) activation and response to gefitinib and other EGFR-targeting drugs. Clin Cancer Res 2006;12:7242–51.
32. CCR Focus. Clin Cancer Res 2006;12:7222–70.
33. Shigematsu H, Lin L, Takahashi T, et al. Clinical and biological features associated with epidermal growth factor receptor gene mutations in lung cancers. J Natl Cancer Inst 2005;97:339–46.
34. Tsao MS, Sakurada A, Cutz JC, et al. Erlotinib in lung cancer - molecular and clinical predictors of outcome. N Engl J Med 2005;353:133–44.
35. Chou TY, Chiu CH, Li LH, et al. Mutation in the tyrosine kinase domain of epidermal growth factor receptor is a predictive and prognostic factor for gefitinib treatment in patients with non-small cell lung cancer. Clin Cancer Res 2005;11:3750–7.

36. Gu D, Scaringe WA, Li K, et al. Database of somatic mutations in EGFR with analyses revealing indel hotspots but no smoking-associated signature. Hum Mutat 2007;28:760–70.
37. Sasaki H, Kawano O, Endo K, Yukiue H, Yano M, Fujii Y. EGFRvIII mutation in lung cancer correlates with increased EGFR copy number. Oncol Rep 2007;17:319–23.
38. Ji H, Zhao X, Yuza Y, et al. Epidermal growth factor receptor variant III mutations in lung tumorigenesis and sensitivity to tyrosine kinase inhibitors. Proc Natl Acad Sci USA 2006;103:7817–22.
39. Ohtsuka K, Ohnishi H, Fujiwara M, et al. Abnormalities of epidermal growth factor receptor in lung squamous-cell carcinomas, adenosquamous carcinomas, and large-cell carcinomas: tyrosine kinase domain mutations are not rare in tumors with an adenocarcinoma component. Cancer 2007;109:741–50.
40. Ohtsuka K, Ohnishi H, Furuyashiki G, et al. Clinico-pathological and biological significance of tyrosine kinase domain gene mutations and overexpression of epidermal growth factor receptor for lung adenocarcinoma. J Thorac Oncol 2006;1:787–95.
41. Sonnweber B, Dlaska M, Skvortsov S, Dirnhofer S, Schmid T, Hilbe W. High predictive value of epidermal growth factor receptor phosphorylation but not of EGFRvIII mutation in resected stage I non-small cell lung cancer (NSCLC). J Clin Pathol 2006;59:255–9.
42. Garcia de Palazzo IE, Adams GP, Sundareshan P, et al. Expression of mutated epidermal growth factor receptor by non-small cell lung carcinomas. Cancer Res 1993;53:3217–20.
43. Okamoto I, Kenyon LC, Emlet DR, et al. Expression of constitutively activated EGFRvIII in non-small cell lung cancer. Cancer Sci 2003;94:50–6.
44. Kosaka T, Yatabe Y, Endoh H, Kuwano H, Takahashi T, Mitsudomi T. Mutations of the epidermal growth factor receptor gene in lung cancer: biological and clinical implications. Cancer Res 2004;64:8919–23.
45. Conde E, Angulo B, Tang M, et al. Molecular context of the EGFR mutations: evidence for the activation of mTOR/S6K signaling. Clin Cancer Res 2006;12:710–7.
46. Ma ES, Wong CL, Siu D, Chan WK. Amplification, mutation and loss of heterozygosity of the EGFR gene in metastatic lung cancer. Int J Cancer 2007;120:1828–31; author reply 32–3.
47. Balsara BR, Testa JR. Chromosomal imbalances in human lung cancer. Oncogene 2002;21:6877–83.
48. Sy SM, Wong N, Lee TW, et al. Distinct patterns of genetic alterations in adenocarcinoma and squamous cell carcinoma of the lung. Eur J Cancer 2004;40:1082–94.
49. Yun CH, Boggon TJ, Li Y, et al. Structures of lung cancer-derived EGFR mutants and inhibitor complexes: mechanism of activation and insights into differential inhibitor sensitivity. Cancer Cell 2007;11:217–27.
50. Sordella R, Bell DW, Haber DA, Settleman J. Gefitinib-sensitizing EGFR mutations in lung cancer activate anti-apoptotic pathways. Science 2004;305:1163–7.
51. Arao T, Fukumoto H, Takeda M, Tamura T, Saijo N, Nishio K. Small in-frame deletion in the epidermal growth factor receptor as a target for ZD6474. Cancer Res 2004;64:9101–4.
52. Choi SH, Mendrola JM, Lemmon MA. EGF-independent activation of cell-surface EGF receptors harboring mutations found in gefitinib-sensitive lung cancer. Oncogene 2007;26:1567–76.
53. Sakai K, Arao T, Shimoyama T, et al. Dimerization and the signal transduction pathway of a small in-frame deletion in the epidermal growth factor receptor. Faseb J 2006;20:311–3.
54. Sakai K, Yokote H, Murakami-Murofushi K, Tamura T, Saijo N, Nishio K. In-frame deletion in the EGF receptor alters kinase inhibition by gefitinib. Biochem J 2006;397:537–43.
55. Schiffer HH, Reding EC, Fuhs SR, et al. Pharmacology and signaling properties of epidermal growth factor receptor isoforms studied by bioluminescence resonance energy transfer. Mol Pharmacol 2007;71:508–18.
56. Amann J, Kalyankrishna S, Massion PP, et al. Aberrant epidermal growth factor receptor signaling and enhanced sensitivity to EGFR inhibitors in lung cancer. Cancer Res 2005;65:226–35.
57. Carey KD, Garton AJ, Romero MS, et al. Kinetic analysis of epidermal growth factor receptor somatic mutant proteins shows increased sensitivity to the epidermal growth factor receptor tyrosine kinase inhibitor, erlotinib. Cancer Res 2006;66:8163–71.
58. Furukawa M, Nagatomo I, Kumagai T, et al. Gefitinib-sensitive EGFR lacking residues 746–750 exhibits hypophosphorylation at tyrosine residue 1045, hypoubiquitination, and impaired endocytosis. DNA Cell Biol 2007;26:178–85.
59. Mulloy R, Ferrand A, Kim Y, et al. Epidermal growth factor receptor mutants from human lung cancers exhibit enhanced catalytic activity and increased sensitivity to gefitinib. Cancer Res 2007;67:2325–30.

60. Okabe T, Okamoto I, Tamura K, et al. Differential constitutive activation of the epidermal growth factor receptor in non-small cell lung cancer cells bearing EGFR gene mutation and amplification. Cancer Res 2007;67:2046–53.
61. Shimamura T, Lowell AM, Engelman JA, Shapiro GI. Epidermal growth factor receptors harboring kinase domain mutations associate with the heat shock protein 90 chaperone and are destabilized following exposure to geldanamycins. Cancer Res 2005;65:6401–8.
62. Chen YR, Fu YN, Lin CH, et al. Distinctive activation patterns in constitutively active and gefitinib-sensitive EGFR mutants. Oncogene 2006;25:1205–15.
63. Tracy S, Mukohara T, Hansen M, Meyerson M, Johnson BE, Janne PA. Gefitinib induces apoptosis in the EGFRL858R non-small-cell lung cancer cell line H3255. Cancer Res 2004;64:7241–4.
64. Mukohara T, Engelman JA, Hanna NH, et al. Differential effects of gefitinib and cetuximab on non-small-cell lung cancers bearing epidermal growth factor receptor mutations. J Natl Cancer Inst 2005;97:1185–94.
65. Yauch RL, Januario T, Eberhard DA, et al. Epithelial versus mesenchymal phenotype determines in vitro sensitivity and predicts clinical activity of erlotinib in lung cancer patients. Clin Cancer Res 2005;11:8686–98.
66. Suzuki S, Igarashi S, Hanawa M, Matsubara H, Ooi A, Dobashi Y. Diversity of epidermal growth factor receptor-mediated activation of downstream molecules in human lung carcinomas. Mod Pathol 2006;19:986–98.
67. Ikeda S, Takabe K, Inagaki M, Funakoshi N, Suzuki K, Shibata T. Correlation between EGFR gene mutation pattern and Akt phosphorylation in pulmonary adenocarcinomas. Pathol Int 2007;57:268–75.
68. Han SW, Hwang PG, Chung DH, et al. Epidermal growth factor receptor (EGFR) downstream molecules as response predictive markers for gefitinib (Iressa, ZD1839) in chemotherapy-resistant non-small cell lung cancer. Int J Cancer 2005;113:109–15.
69. Cappuzzo F, Hirsch FR, Rossi E, et al. Epidermal growth factor receptor gene and protein and gefitinib sensitivity in non-small-cell lung cancer. J Natl Cancer Inst 2005;97:643–55.
70. Yarden Y, Sliwkowski MX. Untangling the ErbB signalling network. Nat Rev Mol Cell Biol 2001;2:127–37.
71. Soltoff SP, Carraway KL, 3rd, Prigent SA, Gullick WG, Cantley LC. ErbB3 is involved in activation of phosphatidylinositol 3-kinase by epidermal growth factor. Mol Cell Biol 1994;14:3550–8.
72. Zhang J, Lodish HF. Identification of K-ras as the major regulator for cytokine-dependent Akt activation in erythroid progenitors in vivo. Proc Natl Acad Sci USA 2005;102:14605–10.
73. Greulich H, Chen TH, Feng W, et al. Oncogenic transformation by inhibitor-sensitive and -resistant EGFR mutants. PLoS Med 2005;2:e313.
74. Jiang J, Greulich H, Janne PA, Sellers WR, Meyerson M, Griffin JD. Epidermal growth factor-independent transformation of Ba/F3 cells with cancer-derived epidermal growth factor receptor mutants induces gefitinib-sensitive cell cycle progression. Cancer Res 2005;65:8968–74.
75. Politi K, Zakowski MF, Fan PD, Schonfeld EA, Pao W, Varmus HE. Lung adenocarcinomas induced in mice by mutant EGF receptors found in human lung cancers respond to a tyrosine kinase inhibitor or to down-regulation of the receptors. Genes Dev 2006;20:1496–510.
76. Ji H, Li D, Chen L, et al. The impact of human EGFR kinase domain mutations on lung tumorigenesis and in vivo sensitivity to EGFR-targeted therapies. Cancer Cell 2006;9:485–95.
77. Liu B, Bernard B, Wu JH. Impact of EGFR point mutations on the sensitivity to gefitinib: insights from comparative structural analyses and molecular dynamics simulations. Proteins 2006;65:331–46.
78. Malik SN, Siu LL, Rowinsky EK, et al. Pharmacodynamic evaluation of the epidermal growth factor receptor inhibitor OSI-774 in human epidermis of cancer patients. Clin Cancer Res 2003;9:2478–86.
79. Baselga J, Albanell J, Ruiz A, et al. Phase II and tumor pharmacodynamic study of gefitinib in patients with advanced breast cancer. J Clin Oncol 2005;23:5323–33.
80. Rojo F, Tabernero J, Albanell J, et al. Pharmacodynamic studies of gefitinib in tumor biopsy specimens from patients with advanced gastric carcinoma. J Clin Oncol 2006;24:4309–16.
81. Calvo E, Malik SN, Siu LL, et al. Assessment of erlotinib pharmacodynamics in tumors and skin of patients with head and neck cancer. Ann Oncol 2007;18:761–7.
82. Agulnik M, da Cunha Santos G, Hedley D, et al. Predictive and pharmacodynamic biomarker studies in tumor and skin tissue samples of patients with recurrent or metastatic squamous cell carcinoma of the head and neck treated with erlotinib. J Clin Oncol 2007;25:2184–90.

83. Pao W, Miller VA, Politi KA, et al. Acquired resistance of lung adenocarcinomas to gefitinib or erlotinib is associated with a second mutation in the EGFR kinase domain. PLoS Med 2005;2:e73.
84. Kobayashi S, Boggon TJ, Dayaram T, et al. EGFR mutation and resistance of non-small-cell lung cancer to gefitinib. N Engl J Med 2005;352:786–92.
85. Engelman JA, Mukohara T, Zejnullahu K, et al. Allelic dilution obscures detection of a biologically significant resistance mutation in EGFR-amplified lung cancer. J Clin Invest 2006;116:2695–706.
86. Liu G, Gurubhagavatula S, Zhou W, et al. Epidermal growth factor receptor polymorphisms and clinical outcomes in non-small-cell lung cancer patients treated with gefitinib. Pharmacogenomics J 2007.
87. Shah NP, Nicoll JM, Nagar B, et al. Multiple BCR-ABL kinase domain mutations confer polyclonal resistance to the tyrosine kinase inhibitor imatinib (STI571) in chronic phase and blast crisis chronic myeloid leukemia. Cancer Cell 2002;2:117–25.
88. Antonescu CR, Besmer P, Guo T, et al. Acquired resistance to imatinib in gastrointestinal stromal tumor occurs through secondary gene mutation. Clin Cancer Res 2005;11:4182–90.
89. Wardelmann E, Merkelbach-Bruse S, Pauls K, et al. Polyclonal evolution of multiple secondary KIT mutations in gastrointestinal stromal tumors under treatment with imatinib mesylate. Clin Cancer Res 2006;12:1743–9.
90. Vikis H, Sato M, James M, et al. EGFR-T790M is a rare lung cancer susceptibility allele with enhanced kinase activity. Cancer Res 2007;67:4665–70.
91. Balak MN, Gong Y, Riely GJ, et al. Novel D761Y and common secondary T790M mutations in epidermal growth factor receptor-mutant lung adenocarcinomas with acquired resistance to kinase inhibitors. Clin Cancer Res 2006;12:6494–501.
92. Han SW, Kim TY, Jeon YK, et al. Optimization of patient selection for gefitinib in non-small cell lung cancer by combined analysis of epidermal growth factor receptor mutation, K-ras mutation, and Akt phosphorylation. Clin Cancer Res 2006;12:2538–44.
93. Carter TA, Wodicka LM, Shah NP, et al. Inhibition of drug-resistant mutants of ABL, KIT, and EGF receptor kinases. Proc Natl Acad Sci USA 2005;102:11011–6.
94. Kwak EL, Sordella R, Bell DW, et al. Irreversible inhibitors of the EGF receptor may circumvent acquired resistance to gefitinib. Proc Natl Acad Sci U S A 2005;102:7665–70.
95. Yuza Y, Glatt KA, Jiang J, et al. Allele-Dependent Variation in the Relative Cellular Potency of Distinct EGFR Inhibitors. Cancer Biol Ther 2007;6.
96. Gendreau SB, Ventura R, Keast P, et al. Inhibition of the T790M gatekeeper mutant of the epidermal growth factor receptor by EXEL-7647. Clin Cancer Res 2007;13:3713–23.
97. Perez-Torres M, Guix M, Gonzalez A, Arteaga CL. Epidermal growth factor receptor (EGFR) antibody down-regulates mutant receptors and inhibits tumors expressing EGFR mutations. J Biol Chem 2006;281:40183–92.
98. Steiner P, Joynes C, Bassi R, et al. Tumor growth inhibition with cetuximab and chemotherapy in non-small cell lung cancer xenografts expressing wild-type and mutated epidermal growth factor receptor. Clin Cancer Res 2007;13:1540–51.
99. Tsuchihashi Z, Khambata-Ford S, Hanna N, Janne PA. Responsiveness to cetuximab without mutations in EGFR. N Engl J Med 2005;353:208–9.
100. Lilenbaum RC. The evolving role of cetuximab in non-small cell lung cancer. Clin Cancer Res 2006;12:4432s-5s.
101. Huang SF, Liu HP, Li LH, et al. High frequency of epidermal growth factor receptor mutations with complex patterns in non-small cell lung cancers related to gefitinib responsiveness in Taiwan. Clin Cancer Res 2004;10:8195–203.
102. Tomizawa Y, Iijima H, Sunaga N, et al. Clinicopathologic significance of the mutations of the epidermal growth factor receptor gene in patients with non-small cell lung cancer. Clin Cancer Res 2005;11:6816–22.
103. Tsao AS, Tang XM, Sabloff B, et al. Clinicopathologic characteristics of the EGFR gene mutation in non-small cell lung cancer. J Thorac Oncol 2006;1:231–9.
104. Hsieh MH, Fang YF, Chang WC, et al. Complex mutation patterns of epidermal growth factor receptor gene associated with variable responses to gefitinib treatment in patients with non-small cell lung cancer. Lung Cancer 2006;53:311–22.
105. Bae NC, Chae MH, Lee MH, et al. EGFR, ERBB2, and KRAS mutations in Korean non-small cell lung cancer patients. Cancer Genet Cytogenet 2007;173:107–13.

106. Zhang W, Stabile LP, Keohavong P, et al. Mutation and polymorphism in the EGFR-TK domain associated with lung cancer. J Thorac Oncol 2006;1:635–47.
107. Satouchi M, Negoro S, Funada Y, et al. Predictive factors associated with prolonged survival in patients with advanced non-small-cell lung cancer (NSCLC) treated with gefitinib. Br J Cancer 2007;96:1191–6.
108. Sequist LV, Joshi VA, Janne PA, et al. Response to treatment and survival of patients with non-small cell lung cancer undergoing somatic EGFR mutation testing. Oncologist 2007;12:90–8.
109. Taron M, Ichinose Y, Rosell R, et al. Activating mutations in the tyrosine kinase domain of the epidermal growth factor receptor are associated with improved survival in gefitinib-treated chemorefractory lung adenocarcinomas. Clin Cancer Res 2005;11:5878–85.
110. Ichihara S, Toyooka S, Fujiwara Y, et al. The impact of epidermal growth factor receptor gene status on gefitinib-treated Japanese patients with non-small-cell lung cancer. Int J Cancer 2007;120:1239–47.
111. Bell DW, Gore I, Okimoto RA, et al. Inherited susceptibility to lung cancer may be associated with the T790M drug resistance mutation in EGFR. Nat Genet 2005;37:1315–6.
112. Suzuki M, Shigematsu H, Iizasa T, et al. Exclusive mutation in epidermal growth factor receptor gene, HER-2, and KRAS, and synchronous methylation of nonsmall cell lung cancer. Cancer 2006;106:2200–7.
113. Murray S, Timotheadou E, Linardou H, et al. Mutations of the epidermal growth factor receptor tyrosine kinase domain and associations with clinicopathological features in non-small cell lung cancer patients. Lung Cancer 2006;52:225–33.
114. Sugio K, Uramoto H, Ono K, et al. Mutations within the tyrosine kinase domain of EGFR gene specifically occur in lung adenocarcinoma patients with a low exposure of tobacco smoking. Br J Cancer 2006;94:896–903.
115. Cortes-Funes H, Gomez C, Rosell R, et al. Epidermal growth factor receptor activating mutations in Spanish gefitinib-treated non-small-cell lung cancer patients. Ann Oncol 2005;16:1081–6.
116. Marchetti A, Martella C, Felicioni L, et al. EGFR mutations in non-small-cell lung cancer: analysis of a large series of cases and development of a rapid and sensitive method for diagnostic screening with potential implications on pharmacologic treatment. J Clin Oncol 2005;23:857–65.
117. Mitsudomi T, Kosaka T, Endoh H, et al. Mutations of the epidermal growth factor receptor gene predict prolonged survival after gefitinib treatment in patients with non-small-cell lung cancer with postoperative recurrence. J Clin Oncol 2005;23:2513–20.
118. Mu XL, Li LY, Zhang XT, et al. Gefitinib-sensitive mutations of the epidermal growth factor receptor tyrosine kinase domain in chinese patients with non-small cell lung cancer. Clin Cancer Res 2005;11:4289–94.
119. Kim KS, Jeong JY, Kim YC, et al. Predictors of the response to gefitinib in refractory non-small cell lung cancer. Clin Cancer Res 2005;11:2244–51.
120. Tokumo M, Toyooka S, Kiura K, et al. The relationship between epidermal growth factor receptor mutations and clinicopathologic features in non-small cell lung cancers. Clin Cancer Res 2005;11:1167–73.
121. Wu YL, Zhong WZ, Li LY, et al. Epidermal growth factor receptor mutations and their correlation with gefitinib therapy in patients with non-small cell lung cancer: a meta-analysis based on updated individual patient data from six medical centers in mainland China. J Thorac Oncol 2007;2:430–9.
122. Mounawar M, Mukeria A, Le Calvez F, et al. Patterns of EGFR, HER2, TP53, and KRAS mutations of p14arf expression in non-small cell lung cancers in relation to smoking history. Cancer Res 2007;67:5667–72.
123. Marchetti A, Felicioni L, Buttitta F. Assessing EGFR mutations. N Engl J Med 2006;354:526–8; author reply -8.
124. Pham D, Kris MG, Riely GJ, et al. Use of cigarette-smoking history to estimate the likelihood of mutations in epidermal growth factor receptor gene exons 19 and 21 in lung adenocarcinomas. J Clin Oncol 2006;24:1700–4.
125. Yang SH, Mechanic LE, Yang P, et al. Mutations in the tyrosine kinase domain of the epidermal growth factor receptor in non-small cell lung cancer. Clin Cancer Res 2005;11:2106–10.
126. Eberhard DA, Johnson BE, Amler LC, et al. Mutations in the epidermal growth factor receptor and in KRAS are predictive and prognostic indicators in patients with non-small-cell lung cancer treated with chemotherapy alone and in combination with erlotinib. J Clin Oncol 2005;23:5900–9.
127. Le Calvez F, Mukeria A, Hunt JD, et al. TP53 and KRAS mutation load and types in lung cancers in relation to tobacco smoke: distinct patterns in never, former, and current smokers. Cancer Res 2005;65:5076–83.

128. DeMarini DM. Genotoxicity of tobacco smoke and tobacco smoke condensate: a review. Mutat Res 2004;567:447–74.
129. Soung YH, Lee JW, Kim SY, et al. Mutational analysis of EGFR and K-RAS genes in lung adenocarcinomas. Virchows Arch 2005;446:483–8.
130. Endoh H, Yatabe Y, Kosaka T, Kuwano H, Mitsudomi T. PTEN and PIK3CA expression is associated with prolonged survival after gefitinib treatment in EGFR-mutated lung cancer patients. J Thorac Oncol 2006;1:629–34.
131. Bemis LT, Robinson WA, McFarlane R, et al. EGFR-mutant lung adenocarcinoma in a patient with Li-Fraumeni syndrome. Lancet Oncol 2007;8:559–60.
132. Tang X, Shigematsu H, Bekele BN, et al. EGFR tyrosine kinase domain mutations are detected in histologically normal respiratory epithelium in lung cancer patients. Cancer Res 2005;65:7568–72.
133. Vahakangas KH, Samet JM, Metcalf RA, et al. Mutations of p53 and ras genes in radon-associated lung cancer from uranium miners. Lancet 1992;339:576–80.
134. Massarelli E, Varella-Garcia M, Tang X, et al. KRAS mutation is an important predictor of resistance to therapy with epidermal growth factor receptor tyrosine kinase inhibitors in non-small-cell lung cancer. Clin Cancer Res 2007;13:2890–6.
135. Han SW, Kim TY, Lee KH, et al. Clinical predictors versus epidermal growth factor receptor mutation in gefitinib-treated non-small-cell lung cancer patients. Lung Cancer 2006;54:201–7.
136. Al-Kuraya K, Siraj AK, Bavi P, et al. High epidermal growth factor receptor amplification rate but low mutation frequency in Middle East lung cancer population. Hum Pathol 2006;37:453–7.
137. Sihto H, Puputti M, Pulli L, et al. Epidermal growth factor receptor domain II, IV, and kinase domain mutations in human solid tumors. J Mol Med 2005;83:976–83.
138. Kim YH, Ishii G, Goto K, et al. Dominant papillary subtype is a significant predictor of the response to gefitinib in adenocarcinoma of the lung. Clin Cancer Res 2004;10:7311–7.
139. Sakuma Y, Matsukuma S, Yoshihara M, et al. Distinctive evaluation of nonmucinous and mucinous subtypes of bronchioloalveolar carcinomas in EGFR and K-ras gene-mutation analyses for Japanese lung adenocarcinomas: confirmation of the correlations with histologic subtypes and gene mutations. Am J Clin Pathol 2007;128:100–8.
140. Finberg KE, Sequist LV, Joshi VA, et al. Mucinous Differentiation Correlates with Absence of EGFR Mutation and Presence of KRAS Mutation in Lung Adenocarcinomas with Bronchioloalveolar Features. J Mol Diagn 2007;9:320–6.
141. Kang SM, Kang HJ, Shin JH, et al. Identical epidermal growth factor receptor mutations in adenocarcinomatous and squamous cell carcinomatous components of adenosquamous carcinoma of the lung. Cancer 2007;109:581–7.
142. Toyooka S, Kiura K, Mitsudomi T. EGFR mutation and response of lung cancer to gefitinib. N Engl J Med 2005;352:2136; author reply .
143. Lee JW, Soung YH, Kim SY, et al. Absence of EGFR mutation in the kinase domain in common human cancers besides non-small cell lung cancer. Int J Cancer 2005;113:510–1.
144. Thomas RK, Baker AC, Debiasi RM, et al. High-throughput oncogene mutation profiling in human cancer. Nat Genet 2007;39:347–51.
145. Lee JW, Soung YH, Kim SY, et al. Somatic mutations of EGFR gene in squamous cell carcinoma of the head and neck. Clin Cancer Res 2005;11:2879–82.
146. Willmore-Payne C, Holden JA, Layfield LJ. Detection of EGFR- and HER2-activating mutations in squamous cell carcinoma involving the head and neck. Mod Pathol 2006;19:634–40.
147. Loeffler-Ragg J, Witsch-Baumgartner M, Tzankov A, et al. Low incidence of mutations in EGFR kinase domain in Caucasian patients with head and neck squamous cell carcinoma. Eur J Cancer 2006;42:109–11.
148. Na, II, Kang HJ, Cho SY, et al. EGFR mutations and human papillomavirus in squamous cell carcinoma of tongue and tonsil. Eur J Cancer 2007;43:520–6.
149. Temam S, Kawaguchi H, El-Naggar AK, et al. Epidermal growth factor receptor copy number alterations correlate with poor clinical outcome in patients with head and neck squamous cancer. J Clin Oncol 2007;25:2164–70.
150. Chung CH, Ely K, McGavran L, et al. Increased epidermal growth factor receptor gene copy number is associated with poor prognosis in head and neck squamous cell carcinomas. J Clin Oncol 2006;24:4170–6.

151. Cohen EE, Lingen MW, Martin LE, et al. Response of some head and neck cancers to epidermal growth factor receptor tyrosine kinase inhibitors may be linked to mutation of ERBB2 rather than EGFR. Clin Cancer Res 2005;11:8105–8.
152. Barber TD, Vogelstein B, Kinzler KW, Velculescu VE. Somatic mutations of EGFR in colorectal cancers and glioblastomas. N Engl J Med 2004;351:2883.
153. Nagahara H, Mimori K, Ohta M, et al. Somatic mutations of epidermal growth factor receptor in colorectal carcinoma. Clin Cancer Res 2005;11:1368–71.
154. Moroni M, Veronese S, Benvenuti S, et al. Gene copy number for epidermal growth factor receptor (EGFR) and clinical response to antiEGFR treatment in colorectal cancer: a cohort study. Lancet Oncol 2005;6:279–86.
155. Ogino S, Meyerhardt JA, Cantor M, et al. Molecular alterations in tumors and response to combination chemotherapy with gefitinib for advanced colorectal cancer. Clin Cancer Res 2005;11:6650–6.
156. Endo K, Konishi A, Sasaki H, et al. Epidermal growth factor receptor gene mutation in non-small cell lung cancer using highly sensitive and fast TaqMan PCR assay. Lung Cancer 2005;50:375–84.
157. Kimura T, Maesawa C, Ikeda K, Wakabayashi G, Masuda T. Mutations of the epidermal growth factor receptor gene in gastrointestinal tract tumor cell lines. Oncol Rep 2006;15:1205–10.
158. Gwak GY, Yoon JH, Shin CM, et al. Detection of response-predicting mutations in the kinase domain of the epidermal growth factor receptor gene in cholangiocarcinomas. J Cancer Res Clin Oncol 2005;131:649–52.
159. Leone F, Cavalloni G, Pignochino Y, et al. Somatic mutations of epidermal growth factor receptor in bile duct and gallbladder carcinoma. Clin Cancer Res 2006;12:1680–5.
160. Kwak EL, Jankowski J, Thayer SP, et al. Epidermal growth factor receptor kinase domain mutations in esophageal and pancreatic adenocarcinomas. Clin Cancer Res 2006;12:4283–7.
161. Guo M, Liu S, Lu F. Gefitinib-sensitizing mutations in esophageal carcinoma. N Engl J Med 2006;354:2193–4.
162. Sudo T, Mimori K, Nagahara H, et al. Identification of EGFR mutations in esophageal cancer. Eur J Surg Oncol 2007;33:44–8.
163. Janmaat ML, Gallegos-Ruiz MI, Rodriguez JA, et al. Predictive factors for outcome in a phase II study of gefitinib in second-line treatment of advanced esophageal cancer patients. J Clin Oncol 2006;24:1612–9.
164. Puhringer-Oppermann FA, Stein HJ, Sarbia M. Lack of EGFR gene mutations in exons 19 and 21 in esophageal (Barrett's) adenocarcinomas. Dis Esophagus 2007;20:9–11.
165. Hanawa M, Suzuki S, Dobashi Y, et al. EGFR protein overexpression and gene amplification in squamous cell carcinomas of the esophagus. Int J Cancer 2006;118:1173–80.
166. Dragovich T, McCoy S, Fenoglio-Preiser CM, et al. Phase II trial of erlotinib in gastroesophageal junction and gastric adenocarcinomas: SWOG 0127. J Clin Oncol 2006;24:4922–7.
167. Lee J, Jang KT, Ki CS, et al. Impact of epidermal growth factor receptor (EGFR) kinase mutations, EGFR gene amplifications, and KRAS mutations on survival of pancreatic adenocarcinoma. Cancer 2007;109:1561–9.
168. Tzeng CW, Frolov A, Frolova N, et al. Epidermal growth factor receptor (EGFR) is highly conserved in pancreatic cancer. Surgery 2007;141:464–9.
169. Willmore-Payne C, Volmar KE, Huening MA, Holden JA, Layfield LJ. Molecular diagnostic testing as an adjunct to morphologic evaluation of pancreatic ductal system brushings: potential augmentation for diagnostic sensitivity. Diagn Cytopathol 2007;35:218–24.
170. Immervoll H, Hoem D, Kugarajh K, Steine SJ, Molven A. Molecular analysis of the EGFR-RAS-RAF pathway in pancreatic ductal adenocarcinomas: lack of mutations in the BRAF and EGFR genes. Virchows Arch 2006;448:788–96.
171. Mammano E, Belluco C, Sciro M, et al. Epidermal growth factor receptor (EGFR): mutational and protein expression analysis in gastric cancer. Anticancer Res 2006;26:3547–50.
172. Becker JC, Muller-Tidow C, Stolte M, et al. Acetylsalicylic acid enhances antiproliferative effects of the EGFR inhibitor gefitinib in the absence of activating mutations in gastric cancer. Int J Oncol 2006;29:615–23.
173. Mimori K, Nagahara H, Sudo T, et al. The epidermal growth factor receptor gene sequence is highly conserved in primary gastric cancers. J Surg Oncol 2006;93:44–6.

174. Douglas DA, Zhong H, Ro JY, et al. Novel mutations of epidermal growth factor receptor in localized prostate cancer. Front Biosci 2006;11:2518–25.
175. Curigliano G, Pelosi G, De Pas T, et al. Absence of epidermal growth factor receptor gene mutations in patients with hormone refractory prostate cancer not responding to gefitinib. Prostate 2007;67:603–4.
176. Reis-Filho JS, Pinheiro C, Lambros MB, et al. EGFR amplification and lack of activating mutations in metaplastic breast carcinomas. J Pathol 2006;209:445–53.
177. Weber F, Fukino K, Sawada T, et al. Variability in organ-specific EGFR mutational spectra in tumour epithelium and stroma may be the biological basis for differential responses to tyrosine kinase inhibitors. Br J Cancer 2005;92:1922–6.
178. Franco-Hernandez C, Martinez-Glez V, Arjona D, et al. EGFR sequence variations and real-time quantitative polymerase chain reaction analysis of gene dosage in brain metastases of solid tumors. Cancer Genet Cytogenet 2007;173:63–7.
179. Sakaeda T, Okamura N, Gotoh A, et al. EGFR mRNA is upregulated, but somatic mutations of the gene are hardly found in renal cell carcinoma in Japanese patients. Pharm Res 2005;22:1757–61.
180. Schilder RJ, Sill MW, Chen X, et al. Phase II study of gefitinib in patients with relapsed or persistent ovarian or primary peritoneal carcinoma and evaluation of epidermal growth factor receptor mutations and immunohistochemical expression: a Gynecologic Oncology Group Study. Clin Cancer Res 2005;11:5539–48.
181. Lassus H, Sihto H, Leminen A, et al. Gene amplification, mutation, and protein expression of EGFR and mutations of ERBB2 in serous ovarian carcinoma. J Mol Med 2006;84:671–81.
182. Stadlmann S, Gueth U, Reiser U, et al. Epithelial growth factor receptor status in primary and recurrent ovarian cancer. Mod Pathol 2006;19:607–10.
183. Lacroix L, Pautier P, Duvillard P, et al. Response of ovarian carcinomas to gefitinib-carboplatin-paclitaxel combination is not associated with EGFR kinase domain somatic mutations. Int J Cancer 2006;118:1068–9.
184. Lee JC, Vivanco I, Beroukhim R, et al. Epidermal Growth Factor Receptor Activation in Glioblastoma through Novel Missense Mutations in the Extracellular Domain. PLoS Med 2006;3:e485.
185. Fukushima T, Favereaux A, Huang H, et al. Genetic alterations in primary glioblastomas in Japan. J Neuropathol Exp Neurol 2006;65:12–8.
186. Marie Y, Carpentier AF, Omuro AM, et al. EGFR tyrosine kinase domain mutations in human gliomas. Neurology 2005;64:1444–5.
187. Mellinghoff IK, Wang MY, Vivanco I, et al. Molecular determinants of the response of glioblastomas to EGFR kinase inhibitors. N Engl J Med 2005;353:2012–24.
188. Lassman AB, Rossi MR, Raizer JJ, et al. Molecular study of malignant gliomas treated with epidermal growth factor receptor inhibitors: tissue analysis from North American Brain Tumor Consortium Trials 01–03 and 00–01. Clin Cancer Res 2005;11:7841–50.
189. Haas-Kogan DA, Prados MD, Tihan T, et al. Epidermal growth factor receptor, protein kinase B/Akt, and glioma response to erlotinib. J Natl Cancer Inst 2005;97:880–7.
190. Bode B, Frigerio S, Behnke S, et al. Mutations in the tyrosine kinase domain of the EGFR gene are rare in synovial sarcoma. Mod Pathol 2006;19:541–7.
191. Su MC, Lien HC, Jeng YM. Absence of epidermal growth factor receptor exon 18–21 mutation in hepatocellular carcinoma. Cancer Lett 2005;224:117–21.
192. Lee SC, Lim SG, Soo R, et al. Lack of somatic mutations in EGFR tyrosine kinase domain in hepatocellular and nasopharyngeal carcinoma. Pharmacogenet Genomics 2006;16:73–4.
193. Meister M, Schirmacher P, Dienemann H, et al. Mutational status of the epidermal growth factor receptor (EGFR) gene in thymomas and thymic carcinomas. Cancer Lett 2007;248:186–91.
194. Suzuki E, Sasaki H, Kawano O, et al. Expression and mutation statuses of epidermal growth factor receptor in thymic epithelial tumors. Jpn J Clin Oncol 2006;36:351–6.
195. Gilbert JA, Lloyd RV, Ames MM. Lack of mutations in EGFR in gastroenteropancreatic neuroendocrine tumors. N Engl J Med 2005;353:209–10.
196. Bignell G, Smith R, Hunter C, et al. Sequence analysis of the protein kinase gene family in human testicular germ-cell tumors of adolescents and adults. Genes Chromosomes Cancer 2006;45:42–6.
197. Gallegos Ruiz MI, Floor K, Rijmen F, Grunberg K, Rodriguez JA, Giaccone G. EGFR and K-ras mutation analysis in non-small cell lung cancer: Comparison of paraffin embedded versus frozen specimens. Cell Oncol 2007;29:257–64.

198. Han SW, Kim TY, Hwang PG, et al. Predictive and prognostic impact of epidermal growth factor receptor mutation in non-small-cell lung cancer patients treated with gefitinib. J Clin Oncol 2005;23:2493–501.
199. Bell DW, Lynch TJ, Haserlat SM, et al. Epidermal growth factor receptor mutations and gene amplification in non-small-cell lung cancer: molecular analysis of the IDEAL/INTACT gefitinib trials. J Clin Oncol 2005;23:8081–92.
200. Shih JY, Gow CH, Yu CJ, et al. Epidermal growth factor receptor mutations in needle biopsy/aspiration samples predict response to gefitinib therapy and survival of patients with advanced nonsmall cell lung cancer. Int J Cancer 2006;118:963–9.
201. Sone T, Kasahara K, Kimura H, et al. Comparative analysis of epidermal growth factor receptor mutations and gene amplification as predictors of gefitinib efficacy in Japanese patients with nonsmall cell lung cancer. Cancer 2007;109:1836–44.
202. Takano T, Ohe Y, Sakamoto H, et al. Epidermal growth factor receptor gene mutations and increased copy numbers predict gefitinib sensitivity in patients with recurrent non-small-cell lung cancer. J Clin Oncol 2005;23:6829–37.
203. Kimura H, Kasahara K, Kawaishi M, et al. Detection of epidermal growth factor receptor mutations in serum as a predictor of the response to gefitinib in patients with non-small-cell lung cancer. Clin Cancer Res 2006;12:3915–21.
204. Buckingham LE, Coon JS, Morrison LE, et al. The prognostic value of chromosome 7 polysomy in non-small cell lung cancer patients treated with gefitinib. J Thorac Oncol 2007;2:414–22.
205. Jackman DM, Yeap BY, Sequist LV, et al. Exon 19 deletion mutations of epidermal growth factor receptor are associated with prolonged survival in non-small cell lung cancer patients treated with gefitinib or erlotinib. Clin Cancer Res 2006;12:3908–14.
206. Argiris A, Hensing T, Yeldandi A, et al. Combined analysis of molecular and clinical predictors of gefitinib activity in advanced non-small cell lung cancer: epidermal growth factor receptor mutations do not tell the whole story. J Thorac Oncol 2006;1:52–60.
207. van Zandwijk N, Mathy A, Boerrigter L, et al. EGFR and KRAS mutations as criteria for treatment with tyrosine kinase inhibitors: retro- and prospective observations in non-small-cell lung cancer. Ann Oncol 2007;18:99–103.
208. Kimura H, Fujiwara Y, Sone T, et al. EGFR mutation status in tumour-derived DNA from pleural effusion fluid is a practical basis for predicting the response to gefitinib. Br J Cancer 2006;95:1390–5.
209. Giaccone G, Gallegos Ruiz M, Le Chevalier T, et al. Erlotinib for frontline treatment of advanced non-small cell lung cancer: a phase II study. Clin Cancer Res 2006;12:6049–55.
210. Jackman DM, Yeap BY, Lindeman NI, et al. Phase II clinical trial of chemotherapy-naive patients > or = 70 years of age treated with erlotinib for advanced non-small-cell lung cancer. J Clin Oncol 2007;25:760–6.
211. Niho S, Kubota K, Goto K, et al. First-line single agent treatment with gefitinib in patients with advanced non-small-cell lung cancer: a phase II study. J Clin Oncol 2006;24:64–9.
212. Inoue A, Suzuki T, Fukuhara T, et al. Prospective phase II study of gefitinib for chemotherapy-naive patients with advanced non-small-cell lung cancer with epidermal growth factor receptor gene mutations. J Clin Oncol 2006;24:3340–6.
213. Asahina H, Yamazaki K, Kinoshita I, et al. A phase II trial of gefitinib as first-line therapy for advanced non-small cell lung cancer with epidermal growth factor receptor mutations. Br J Cancer 2006;95:998–1004.
214. Yoshida K, Yatabe Y, Park JY, et al. Prospective validation for prediction of gefitinib sensitivity by epidermal growth factor receptor gene mutation in patients with non-small cell lung cancer. J Thorac Oncol 2007;2:22–8.
215. Sunaga N, Tomizawa Y, Yanagitani N, et al. Phase II prospective study of the efficacy of gefitinib for the treatment of stage III/IV non-small cell lung cancer with EGFR mutations, irrespective of previous chemotherapy. Lung Cancer 2007;56:383–9.
216. Costa DB, Kobayashi S, Tenen DG, Huberman MS. Pooled analysis of the prospective trials of gefitinib monotherapy for EGFR-mutant non-small cell lung cancers. Lung Cancer 2007.
217. Hirsch FR, Franklin, W.A., McCoy, J., Cappuzzo, F., Varella-Garcia, M., Witta, S.E., Gumerlock, P., West, H., Gandara, D.R., Bunn, P.A. Jr. Predicting clinical benefit from EGFR TKIs: Not all EGFR mutations are equal. J Clin Oncol 2006;24:7072.

218. Na, II, Rho JK, Choi YJ, et al. The survival outcomes of patients with resected non-small cell lung cancer differ according to EGFR mutations and the P21 expression. Lung Cancer 2007;57:96–102.
219. Takeuchi T, Tomida S, Yatabe Y, et al. Expression profile-defined classification of lung adenocarcinoma shows close relationship with underlying major genetic changes and clinicopathologic behaviors. J Clin Oncol 2006;24:1679–88.
220. Shibata T, Uryu S, Kokubu A, et al. Genetic classification of lung adenocarcinoma based on array-based comparative genomic hybridization analysis: its association with clinicopathologic features. Clin Cancer Res 2005;11:6177–85.
221. Hotta K, Kiura K, Toyooka S, et al. Clinical significance of epidermal growth factor receptor gene mutations on treatment outcome after first-line cytotoxic chemotherapy in Japanese patients with non-small cell lung cancer. J Thorac Oncol 2007;2:632–7.
222. Lee KH, Han SW, Hwang PG, et al. Epidermal growth factor receptor mutations and response to chemotherapy in patients with non-small-cell lung cancer. Jpn J Clin Oncol 2006;36:344–50.
223. Giaccone G, Herbst RS, Manegold C, et al. Gefitinib in combination with gemcitabine and cisplatin in advanced non-small-cell lung cancer: a phase III trial--INTACT 1. J Clin Oncol 2004;22:777–84.
224. Herbst RS, Giaccone G, Schiller JH, et al. Gefitinib in combination with paclitaxel and carboplatin in advanced non-small-cell lung cancer: a phase III trial--INTACT 2. J Clin Oncol 2004;22:785–94.
225. Pao W, Ladanyi M, Miller VA. Erlotinib in lung cancer. N Engl J Med 2005;353:1739–41; author reply -41.
226. Hirsch FR, Varella-Garcia M, Bunn PA, Jr., et al. Molecular predictors of outcome with gefitinib in a phase III placebo-controlled study in advanced non-small-cell lung cancer. J Clin Oncol 2006;24:5034–42.
227. Gatzemeier U, Heller, A., Foernzler, D., Moecks, J., Ward, C., de Rosa, F., Sauter, G., Brennscheidt, U. Exploratory analyses EGFR, KRAS mutations and other molecular markers in tumors of NSCLC patients (pts) treated with chemotherapy +/- erlotinib (TALENT). J Clin Oncol (Meeting Abstracts) 2005;23:7028.
228. Kosaka T, Yatabe Y, Endoh H, et al. Analysis of epidermal growth factor receptor gene mutation in patients with non-small cell lung cancer and acquired resistance to gefitinib. Clin Cancer Res 2006;12:5764–9.
229. Kozuki T, Hisamoto A, Tabata M, et al. Mutation of the epidermal growth factor receptor gene in the development of adenocarcinoma of the lung. Lung Cancer 2007.
230. Parra HS, Cavina R, Latteri F, et al. Analysis of epidermal growth factor receptor expression as a predictive factor for response to gefitinib ('Iressa', ZD1839) in non-small-cell lung cancer. Br J Cancer 2004;91:208–12.
231. Perez-Soler R, Chachoua A, Hammond LA, et al. Determinants of tumor response and survival with erlotinib in patients with non--small-cell lung cancer. J Clin Oncol 2004;22:3238–47.
232. Hirsch FR, Varella-Garcia M, Cappuzzo F, et al. Combination of EGFR gene copy number and protein expression predicts outcome for advanced non-small-cell lung cancer patients treated with gefitinib. Ann Oncol 2007;18:752–60.
233. Santoro A, Cavina R, Latteri F, et al. Activity of a specific inhibitor, gefitinib (Iressa, ZD1839), of epidermal growth factor receptor in refractory non-small-cell lung cancer. Ann Oncol 2004;15:33–7.
234. Clark GM, Zborowski DM, Santabarbara P, et al. Smoking history and epidermal growth factor receptor expression as predictors of survival benefit from erlotinib for patients with non-small-cell lung cancer in the National Cancer Institute of Canada Clinical Trials Group study BR.21. Clin Lung Cancer 2006;7:389–94.
235. Dziadziuszko R, Holm B, Skov BG, et al. Epidermal growth factor receptor gene copy number and protein level are not associated with outcome of non-small-cell lung cancer patients treated with chemotherapy. Ann Oncol 2007;18:447–52.
236. Taillade L, Penault-Llorca F, Boulet T, et al. Immunohistochemichal expression of biomarkers: a comparative study between diagnostic bronchial biopsies and surgical specimens of non-small-cell lung cancer. Ann Oncol 2007;18:1043–50.
237. Ferrigan L, Wallace WA. Predicting non-small cell lung cancer expression of epidermal growth factor receptor and matrix metalloproteinase 9 from immunohistochemical staining of diagnostic biopsy samples. Eur J Cancer 2004;40:1589–92.
238. Derecskei K, Moldvay J, Bogos K, Timar J. Protocol modifications influence the result of EGF receptor immunodetection by EGFR pharmDx in paraffin-embedded cancer tissues. Pathol Oncol Res 2006;12:243–6.

239. Clark GM, Zborowski DM, Culbertson JL, et al. Clinical utility of epidermal growth factor receptor expression for selecting patients with advanced non-small cell lung cancer for treatment with erlotinib. J Thorac Oncol 2006;1:837–46.
240. Helfrich BA, Raben D, Varella-Garcia M, et al. Antitumor activity of the epidermal growth factor receptor (EGFR) tyrosine kinase inhibitor gefitinib (ZD1839, Iressa) in non-small cell lung cancer cell lines correlates with gene copy number and EGFR mutations but not EGFR protein levels. Clin Cancer Res 2006;12:7117–25.
241. Dziadziuszko R, Witta SE, Cappuzzo F, et al. Epidermal growth factor receptor messenger RNA expression, gene dosage, and gefitinib sensitivity in non-small cell lung cancer. Clin Cancer Res 2006;12:3078–84.
242. Daniele L, Macri L, Schena M, et al. Predicting gefitinib responsiveness in lung cancer by fluorescence in situ hybridization/chromogenic in situ hybridization analysis of EGFR and HER2 in biopsy and cytology specimens. Mol Cancer Ther 2007;6:1223–9.
243. Hirsch FR, Varella-Garcia M, McCoy J, et al. Increased epidermal growth factor receptor gene copy number detected by fluorescence in situ hybridization associates with increased sensitivity to gefitinib in patients with bronchioloalveolar carcinoma subtypes: a Southwest Oncology Group Study. J Clin Oncol 2005;23:6838–45.
244. Cappuzzo F, Ligorio C, Janne PA, et al. Prospective study of gefitinib in epidermal growth factor receptor fluorescence in situ hybridization-positive/phospho-Akt-positive or never smoker patients with advanced non-small-cell lung cancer: the ONCOBELL trial. J Clin Oncol 2007;25:2248–55.
245. Jeon YK, Sung SW, Chung JH, et al. Clinicopathologic features and prognostic implications of epidermal growth factor receptor (EGFR) gene copy number and protein expression in non-small cell lung cancer. Lung Cancer 2006;54:387–98.
246. Hirsch FR, Varella-Garcia M, Bunn PA, Jr., et al. Epidermal growth factor receptor in non-small-cell lung carcinomas: correlation between gene copy number and protein expression and impact on prognosis. J Clin Oncol 2003;21:3798–807.
247. Suzuki S, Dobashi Y, Sakurai H, Nishikawa K, Hanawa M, Ooi A. Protein overexpression and gene amplification of epidermal growth factor receptor in nonsmall cell lung carcinomas. An immunohistochemical and fluorescence in situ hybridization study. Cancer 2005;103:1265–73.
248. Willmore-Payne C, Holden JA, Layfield LJ. Detection of epidermal growth factor receptor and human epidermal growth factor receptor 2 activating mutations in lung adenocarcinoma by high-resolution melting amplicon analysis: correlation with gene copy number, protein expression, and hormone receptor expression. Hum Pathol 2006;37:755–63.
249. Suzuki M, Shigematsu H, Hiroshima K, et al. Epidermal growth factor receptor expression status in lung cancer correlates with its mutation. Hum Pathol 2005;36:1127–34.
250. Pao W, Wang TY, Riely GJ, et al. KRAS mutations and primary resistance of lung adenocarcinomas to gefitinib or erlotinib. PLoS Med 2005;2:e17.
251. Lievre A, Bachet JB, Le Corre D, et al. KRAS mutation status is predictive of response to cetuximab therapy in colorectal cancer. Cancer Res 2006;66:3992–5.
252. Di Fiore F, Blanchard F, Charbonnier F, et al. Clinical relevance of KRAS mutation detection in metastatic colorectal cancer treated by Cetuximab plus chemotherapy. Br J Cancer 2007;96:1166–9.
253. Benvenuti S, Sartore-Bianchi A, Di Nicolantonio F, et al. Oncogenic activation of the RAS/RAF signaling pathway impairs the response of metastatic colorectal cancers to anti-epidermal growth factor receptor antibody therapies. Cancer Res 2007;67:2643–8.
254. Uchida A, Hirano S, Kitao H, et al. Activation of downstream epidermal growth factor receptor (EGFR) signaling provides gefitinib-resistance in cells carrying EGFR mutation. Cancer Sci 2007;98:357–63.
255. Suzuki T, Nakagawa T, Endo H, et al. The sensitivity of lung cancer cell lines to the EGFR-selective tyrosine kinase inhibitor ZD1839 ('Iressa') is not related to the expression of EGFR or HER-2 or to K-ras gene status. Lung Cancer 2003;42:35–41.
256. Nie Q, Wang Z, Zhang GC, et al. The epidermal growth factor receptor intron1 (CA) n microsatellite polymorphism is a potential predictor of treatment outcome in patients with advanced lung cancer treated with Gefitinib. Eur J Pharmacol 2007.
257. Han SW, Jeon YK, Lee KH, et al. Intron 1 CA dinucleotide repeat polymorphism and mutations of epidermal growth factor receptor and gefitinib responsiveness in non-small-cell lung cancer. Pharmacogenet Genomics 2007;17:313–9.

258. Amador ML, Oppenheimer D, Perea S, et al. An epidermal growth factor receptor intron 1 polymorphism mediates response to epidermal growth factor receptor inhibitors. Cancer Res 2004;64:9139–43.
259. Nomura M, Shigematsu H, Li L, et al. Polymorphisms, mutations, and amplification of the EGFR gene in non-small cell lung cancers. PLoS Med 2007;4:e125.
260. Cappuzzo F, Magrini E, Ceresoli GL, et al. Akt phosphorylation and gefitinib efficacy in patients with advanced non-small-cell lung cancer. J Natl Cancer Inst 2004;96:1133–41.
261. Cappuzzo F, Toschi L, Domenichini I, et al. HER3 genomic gain and sensitivity to gefitinib in advanced non-small-cell lung cancer patients. Br J Cancer 2005;93:1334–40.
262. Cappuzzo F, Toschi L, Tallini G, et al. Insulin-like growth factor receptor 1 (IGFR-1) is significantly associated with longer survival in non-small-cell lung cancer patients treated with gefitinib. Ann Oncol 2006;17:1120–7.
263. Fujimoto N, Wislez M, Zhang J, et al. High expression of ErbB family members and their ligands in lung adenocarcinomas that are sensitive to inhibition of epidermal growth factor receptor. Cancer Res 2005;65:11478–85.
264. Engelman JA, Janne PA, Mermel C, et al. ErbB-3 mediates phosphoinositide 3-kinase activity in gefitinib-sensitive non-small cell lung cancer cell lines. Proc Natl Acad Sci USA 2005;102:3788–93.
265. Nishio M, Taguchi F, Ohyanagi F, et al. Gefitinib efficacy associated with multiple expression of HER family in non-small cell lung cancer. Anticancer Res 2006;26:3761–5.
266. Cappuzzo F, Gregorc V, Rossi E, et al. Gefitinib in pretreated non-small-cell lung cancer (NSCLC): analysis of efficacy and correlation with HER2 and epidermal growth factor receptor expression in locally advanced or metastatic NSCLC. J Clin Oncol 2003;21:2658–63.
267. Engelman JA, Zejnullahu K, Mitsudomi T, et al. MET amplification leads to gefitinib resistance in lung cancer by activating ERBB3 signaling. Science 2007;316:1039–43.
268. Cardiff RD. Epithelial to Mesenchymal Transition Tumors: Fallacious or Snail's Pace? Clin Cancer Res 2005;11:8534–7.
269. Thomson S, Buck E, Petti F, et al. Epithelial to mesenchymal transition is a determinant of sensitivity of non-small-cell lung carcinoma cell lines and xenografts to epidermal growth factor receptor inhibition. Cancer Res 2005;65:9455–62.
270. Frederick BA, Helfrich BA, Coldren CD, et al. Epithelial to mesenchymal transition predicts gefitinib resistance in cell lines of head and neck squamous cell carcinoma and non-small cell lung carcinoma. Mol Cancer Ther 2007;6:1683–91.
271. Witta SE, Gemmill RM, Hirsch FR, et al. Restoring E-cadherin expression increases sensitivity to epidermal growth factor receptor inhibitors in lung cancer cell lines. Cancer Res 2006;66:944–50.
272. Jain A, Tindell CA, Laux I, et al. Epithelial membrane protein-1 is a biomarker of gefitinib resistance. Proc Natl Acad Sci USA 2005;102:11858–63.
273. Coldren CD, Helfrich BA, Witta SE, et al. Baseline gene expression predicts sensitivity to gefitinib in non-small cell lung cancer cell lines. Mol Cancer Res 2006;4:521–8.
274. Balko JM, Potti A, Saunders C, Stromberg A, Haura EB, Black EP. Gene expression patterns that predict sensitivity to epidermal growth factor receptor tyrosine kinase inhibitors in lung cancer cell lines and human lung tumors. BMC Genomics 2006;7:289.
275. Okano T, Kondo T, Fujii K, et al. Proteomic signature corresponding to the response to gefitinib (Iressa, ZD1839), an epidermal growth factor receptor tyrosine kinase inhibitor in lung adenocarcinoma. Clin Cancer Res 2007;13:799–805.
276. Taguchi F, Solomon B, Gregorc V, et al. Mass spectrometry to classify non-small-cell lung cancer patients for clinical outcome after treatment with epidermal growth factor receptor tyrosine kinase inhibitors: a multicohort cross-institutional study. J Natl Cancer Inst 2007;99:838–46.
277. Ihle NT, Paine-Murrieta G, Berggren MI, et al. The phosphatidylinositol-3-kinase inhibitor PX-866 overcomes resistance to the epidermal growth factor receptor inhibitor gefitinib in A-549 human non-small cell lung cancer xenografts. Mol Cancer Ther 2005;4:1349–57.
278. Li D, Shimamura T, Ji H, et al. Bronchial and Peripheral Murine Lung Carcinomas Induced by T790M-L858R Mutant EGFR Respond to HKI-272 and Rapamycin Combination Therapy. Cancer Cell 2007;12:81–93.
279. Friess T, Scheuer W, Hasmann M. Combination treatment with erlotinib and pertuzumab against human tumor xenografts is superior to monotherapy. Clin Cancer Res 2005;11:5300–9.

280. Varella-Garcia M. Stratification of non-small cell lung cancer patients for therapy with epidermal growth factor receptor inhibitors: the EGFR fluorescence in situ hybridization assay. Diagn Pathol 2006;1:19.
281. Janne PA, Borras AM, Kuang Y, et al. A rapid and sensitive enzymatic method for epidermal growth factor receptor mutation screening. Clin Cancer Res 2006;12:751–8.
282. Inukai M, Toyooka S, Ito S, et al. Presence of Epidermal Growth Factor Receptor Gene T790M Mutation as a Minor Clone in Non-Small Cell Lung Cancer. Cancer Res 2006;66:7854–8.
283. Nagai Y, Miyazawa H, Huqun, et al. Genetic heterogeneity of the epidermal growth factor receptor in non-small cell lung cancer cell lines revealed by a rapid and sensitive detection system, the peptide nucleic acid-locked nucleic acid PCR clamp. Cancer Res 2005;65:7276–82.
284. Gallegos Ruiz MI, van Cruijsen H, Smit EF, et al. Genetic heterogeneity in patients with multiple neoplastic lung lesions: a report of three cases. J Thorac Oncol 2007;2:12–21.
285. Italiano A, Vandenbos FB, Otto J, et al. Comparison of the epidermal growth factor receptor gene and protein in primary non-small-cell-lung cancer and metastatic sites: implications for treatment with EGFR-inhibitors. Ann Oncol 2006;17:981–5.
286. Bilous M, Dowsett M, Hanna W, et al. Current perspectives on HER2 testing: a review of national testing guidelines. Mod Pathol 2003;16:173–82.
287. Atkins D, Reiffen KA, Tegtmeier CL, Winther H, Bonato MS, Storkel S. Immunohistochemical detection of EGFR in paraffin-embedded tumor tissues: variation in staining intensity due to choice of fixative and storage time of tissue sections. J Histochem Cytochem 2004;52:893–901.
288. Olapade-Olaopa EO, MacKay EH, Habib FK. Variability of immunohistochemical reactivity on stored paraffin slides. J Clin Pathol 1998;51:943.
289. Olapade-Olaopa EO, Ogunbiyi JO, MacKay EH, et al. Further characterization of storage-related alterations in immunoreactivity of archival tissue sections and its implications for collaborative multicenter immunohistochemical studies. Appl Immunohistochem Mol Morphol 2001;9:261–6.
290. Li J, Berbeco R, Distel RJ, Janne PA, Wang L, Makrigiorgos GM. s-RT-MELT for rapid mutation scanning using enzymatic selection and real time DNA-melting: new potential for multiplex genetic analysis. Nucleic Acids Res 2007;35:e84.
291. Kimura H, Fujiwara Y, Sone T, et al. High sensitivity detection of epidermal growth factor receptor mutations in the pleural effusion of non-small cell lung cancer patients. Cancer Sci 2006;97:642–8.
292. Soh J, Toyooka S, Ichihara S, et al. EGFR mutation status in pleural fluid predicts tumor responsiveness and resistance to gefitinib. Lung Cancer 2007;56:445–8.
293. Asano H, Toyooka S, Tokumo M, et al. Detection of EGFR gene mutation in lung cancer by mutant-enriched polymerase chain reaction assay. Clin Cancer Res 2006;12:43–8.
294. Tanaka T, Nagai Y, Miyazawa H, et al. Reliability of the peptide nucleic acid-locked nucleic acid polymerase chain reaction clamp-based test for epidermal growth factor receptor mutations integrated into the clinical practice for non-small cell lung cancers. Cancer Sci 2007;98:246–52.
295. Nomoto K, Tsuta K, Takano T, et al. Detection of EGFR mutations in archived cytologic specimens of non-small cell lung cancer using high-resolution melting analysis. Am J Clin Pathol 2006;126:608–15.
296. Gatzemeier U, Pluzanska A, Szczesna A, et al. Phase III study of erlotinib in combination with cisplatin and gemcitabine in advanced non-small-cell lung cancer: the Tarceva Lung Cancer Investigation Trial. J Clin Oncol. 2007;25:1545–52.

21 Crosstalk Between COX-2 and EGFR: A Potential Therapeutic Opportunity

Andrew J. Dannenberg and Kotha Subbaramaiah

CONTENTS

INTRODUCTION
PROSTAGLANDIN BIOSYNTHESIS
EGFR SIGNALING AND CANCER
FUTURE DIRECTIONS
REFERENCES

Abstract

Cyclooxygenase-2 (COX-2), the inducible form of COX, and epidermal growth factor receptor (EGFR) are considered pharmacological targets to prevent or treat cancer. Key data implicating a causal relationship between COX-2, EGFR and carcinogenesis and possible mechanisms of action are reviewed. Evidence of crosstalk between COX-2 and EGFR is discussed. The potential of COX-2-derived prostaglandins to reduce tumor sensitivity to EGFR inhibitors is considered.

Key Words: cyclooxygenase-2, prostaglandins, epidermal growth factor receptor, crosstalk, cancer.

1. INTRODUCTION

Extensive efforts are underway to develop targeted therapies that will inhibit carcinogenesis. In this regard, both COX-2, the inducible form of COX, and the EGFR represent promising pharmacological targets. Crosstalk exists between COX-2 and EGFR (*1*). In preclinical studies, combining an inhibitor of COX-2 with an inhibitor of EGFR tyrosine kinase was more effective than either agent alone in suppressing tumor formation and growth (*1, 2*). Here we focus on evidence that COX-2-derived prostaglandins (PGs) play a role in carcinogenesis and potentially reduce the sensitivity of tumors to therapies targeting EGFR.

2. PROSTAGLANDIN BIOSYNTHESIS

COX enzymes catalyze the synthesis of PGs from arachidonic acid (Fig. 21.1). The first step in PG synthesis is hydrolysis of phospholipids to produce free arachidonic acid. This reaction is catalyzed by phospholipase A_2. Next, COX catalyzes a reaction in which molecular oxygen is inserted into arachidonic acid to form an unstable intermediate, PGG_2, which is

From: *Cancer Drug Discovery and Development: EGFR Signaling Networks in Cancer Therapy*
Edited by: J. D. Haley and W. J. Gullick, DOI: 10.1007/978-1-59745-356-1_21
© 2008 Humana Press, a part of Springer Science+Business Media, LLC

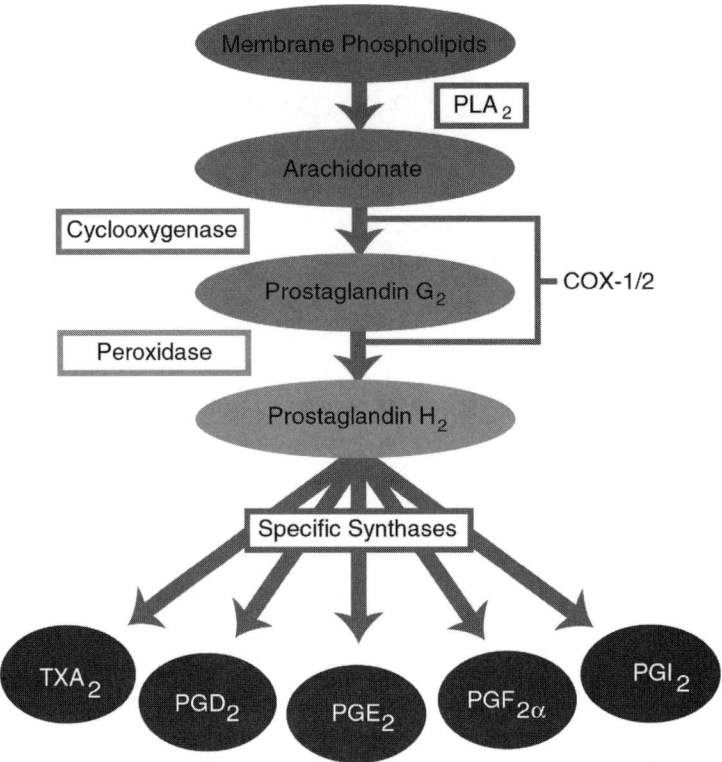

Fig. 21.1. **Arachidonic Acid Metabolism.** Arachidonic acid is released from membrane phospholipids by phopholipase A_2 (PLA_2). It is then metabolized by cyclooxygenases (COX-1, COX-2) to prostaglandin H_2 (PGH_2). PGH_2 is converted to a variety of eicosanoids by specific synthases.

converted to PGH_2. Specific isomerases then convert PGH_2 to several PGs and thromboxane A_2 (TxA_2).

There are two isoforms of COX: COX-1 and COX-2. These two enzymes differ in many respects (3, 4). COX-1 is expressed constitutively in most tissues and appears to be responsible for the production of PGs that control normal physiological functions including maintenance of the gastric mucosa, regulation of renal blood flow and platelet aggregation. In contrast, COX-2 is not detected in most normal tissues. However, it is rapidly induced by both inflammatory and mitogenic stimuli resulting in increased PG synthesis in neoplastic and inflamed tissues (4, 5). COX-2 can be selectively inhibited even though the active sites of COX-1 and COX-2 have similar structures. A substitution of isoleucine in COX-1 with valine in the NSAID binding site of COX-2 creates a void volume located to the side of the central active site channel in COX-2 (6). Compounds synthesized to bind in this additional space inhibit COX-2 but not COX-1. In contrast to conventional NSAIDs that are dual inhibitors of COX-1 and COX-2, selective COX-2 inhibitors do not suppress platelet function or increase the risk of a bleeding complication (7).

2.1. Regulation of COX-2 Expression

COX-2 is overexpressed in a variety of premalignant and malignant tissues (Table 21.1) (8–26). Up-regulation of COX-2 occurs because of deregulated transcriptional and post-transcriptional control. Oncogenes, growth factors, cytokines, and tumor promoters stimulate

Table 21.1
COX-2 is Commonly Overexpressed in Premalignant and Malignant Tissues

Organ site	Premalignancy	Malignancy
Colon	Adenoma	Adenocarcinoma
Lung	Atypical Adenomatous Hyperplasia	Adenocarcinoma, Squamous Cell Carcinoma
Head and Neck	Leukoplakia	Squamous Cell Carcinoma
Esophagus	Barrett's Esophagus, Squamous Dysplasia	Adenocarcinoma, Squamous Cell Carcinoma
Stomach	Metaplasia	Adenocarcinoma
Liver	Chronic Hepatitis	Hepatocellular Carcinoma
Pancreas	Pancreatic Intraepithelial Neoplasia	Adenocarcinoma
Breast	Ductal carcinoma *in situ*	Adenocarcinoma
Bladder	Dysplasia	Transitional Cell Carcinoma, Squamous Cell Carcinoma
Cervix	Cervical Intraepithelial Neoplasia	Adenocarcinoma, Squamous Cell Carcinoma
Penis	Penile Intraepithelial Neoplasia	Squamous Cell Carcinoma
Skin	Actinic Keratoses	Squamous Cell Carcinoma

COX-2 transcription via protein kinase C (PKC) and Ras-mediated signaling (Fig. 21.2) (*1, 4, 5, 27–30*). For example, increased amounts of COX-2 have been found in breast cancers that overexpress HER-2/neu because of enhanced Ras signaling (Fig. 21.2) (*28*). Depending on the cell type and stimulus, different transcription factors including AP-1, NF-IL6, NF-κB, NFAT and PEA3 can stimulate *COX-2* transcription (*5, 27, 28, 31, 32*). Although *COX-2* transcription can be enhanced by many factors, much less is known about negative effectors. Wild-type but not mutant p53 can inhibit *COX-2* transcription in vitro (*33*). Consistent with this finding, elevated levels of COX-2 have been found in cancers of the stomach, esophagus, lung and breast that express mutant rather than wild-type p53 (*34, 35*). Like p53, *APC* tumor suppressor gene status may also impact on COX-2 expression (*36*). Recent evidence suggests that the nuclear receptor corepressor (NCoR) may also play a role in suppressing *COX-2* transcription in normal cells (*37*). Taken together, these findings suggest that the balance between activation of oncogenes and inactivation of tumor suppressor genes modulates the expression of COX-2 in tumors.

Posttranscriptional mechanisms also appear to be important in regulating amounts of COX-2 in tumors. The 3′-untranslated region (UTR) of COX-2 mRNA contains a series of AU-rich elements (AREs) that affect both mRNA decay and protein translation (Fig. 21.2) (*38*). *Trans*-acting ARE binding factors form complexes with the COX-2 3′-UTR and regulate both COX-2 mRNA stability and translation. Enhanced binding of HuR, an RNA binding protein, to the AU-enriched region of the COX-2 3′-UTR contributes to the increase in message stability found in colon cancer (Fig. 21.2) (*39*). Other proteins, e.g., tristetraprolin, AUF1, that bind to the 3′-UTR can increase mRNA degradation (*40*). Overexpression of COX-2 may also reflect deregulated translation. For example, TIA-1, an ARE binding protein, functions as a translational silencer. Deficient TIA-1 mRNA binding was found in colon cancer cells that overexpressed COX-2 protein (*41*). Collectively, these findings suggest that changes in the relative amounts or binding activity of these functionally distinct ARE-binding proteins are likely to modulate levels of COX-2 in tumors.

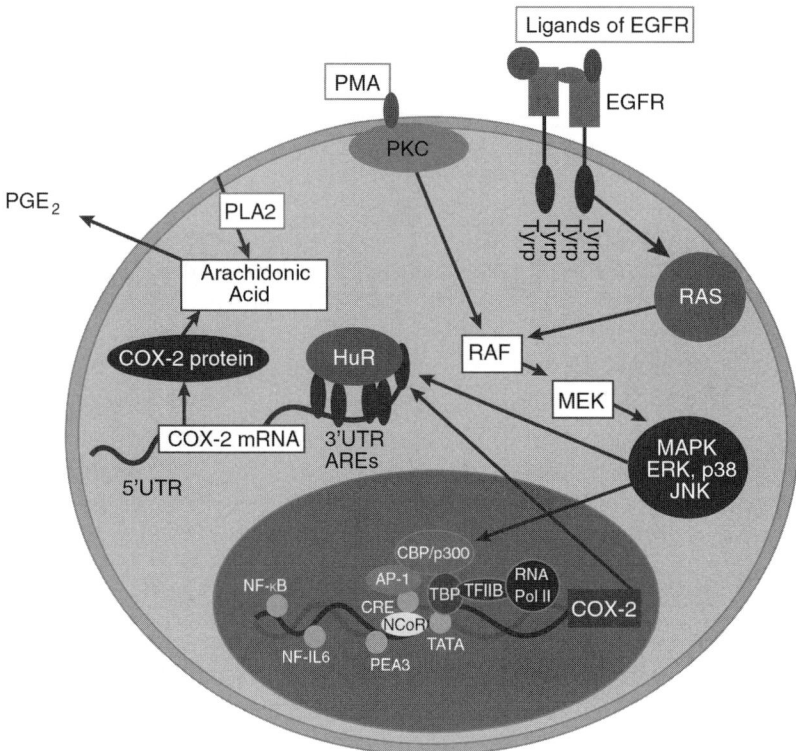

Fig. 21.2. **Regulation of COX-2 Expression in Cancers.** COX-2 is induced by a variety of stimuli including oncogenes, growth factors and tumor promoters (phorbol esters, PMA). Stimulation of Ras or PKC signaling enhances mitogen-activated protein kinase (MAPK) activity that results, in turn, in increased *COX-2* transcription. A variety of transcription factors including AP-1 and PEA3 mediate the induction of COX-2. Levels of COX-2 can also be affected by post-transcriptional mechanisms. The 3′-untranslated region (3′-UTR) of COX-2 mRNA contains a series of AU-enriched elements (ARE) that regulate message stability. Augmented binding of HuR, an RNA binding protein, to the AREs of the COX-2 3′-UTR explains, in part, the observed increase in COX-2 message stability in some tumors.

2.2. Prostaglandin Receptors, Signaling and Carcinogenesis

Overexpression of COX-2 leads to increased amounts of prostanoids in tumors. Prostanoids affect a variety of mechanisms that have been implicated in carcinogenesis. For example, PGE_2 can stimulate cell proliferation and motility while inhibiting immune surveillance and apoptosis (42–50). Importantly, PGE_2 can also induce angiogenesis, in part, by stimulating the production of proangiogenic factors including vascular endothelial growth factor (VEGF) (51,52). These important mechanisms linking COX-2-derived PGs to carcinogenesis have been the subject of several reviews (3, 53, 54). Defining the downstream signaling mechanisms by which prostanoids stimulate carcinogenesis is an active area of investigation. Prostanoids (PGE_2, $PGF_{2\alpha}$, PGD_2, TxA_2 and PGI_2) mediate their biological actions by binding to G protein coupled receptors that contain seven transmembrane domains. Multiple prostanoid receptors have been cloned and defined pharmacologically, including four subtypes of the EP (PGE) receptor (EP_1, EP_2, EP_3, EP_4), the FP receptor (PGF receptor), the DP receptor (PGD receptor), the IP receptor (PGI receptor) and the TP receptor (Tx receptor). PGE_2 is the most abundant prostanoid detected in most epithelial malignancies. Because it can stimulate tumor growth, numerous studies have attempted to define the link between PGE_2, EP receptors and carcinogenesis.

EP receptors play an important role in the development and growth of tumors. The availability of EP receptor knockout mice has facilitated studies of tumor growth, immune function and angiogenesis. PGE_2 promotes the formation of colorectal carcinogenesis through activation of EP receptors. In support of this idea, the induction of aberrant crypt foci by azoxymethane, a colon carcinogen, was reduced in $EP_1^{-/-}$ and $EP_4^{-/-}$ receptor mice (55). In $Apc^{\Delta 716}$ mice, a murine model of familial adenomatous polyposis (FAP), homozygous deletion of the gene encoding the EP_2 receptor caused a significant reduction in the number and size of intestinal polyps through inhibition of angiogenesis (56). Suppression of angiogenesis was due at least, in part, to decreased levels of VEGF. The importance of host stromal PGE_2-EP_3 signaling was highlighted in a xenograft study that found a marked decrease in tumor-associated angiogenesis in $EP_3^{-/-}$ mice (57). PGE_2 also exerts potent immunosuppressive effects by modulating dendritic cell function and causing an imbalance between type 1 and type 2 cytokines (58). An important role has been established for the EP_2 receptor in PGE_2-mediated suppression of dendritic cell differentiation and function and for reduced antitumor cellular immune responses in vivo (59).

Complementary in vitro studies have provided significant insights into procarcinogenic signaling mechanisms that are activated by PGE_2. For example, stimulation of either EP_2 or EP_4 activates TCF-β-catenin-mediated transcription that leads, in turn, to increased expression of a variety of genes, e.g., *cyclin D1* and *c-myc* that have been implicated in carcinogenesis (Fig. 21.3) (60).PGE_2 also has organ site-specific effects. Estrogen drives the growth of hormone-dependent breast cancer. The final step in the synthesis of estrogen is catalyzed by aromatase, the product of the *CYP19* gene. Binding of PGE_2 to EP receptors stimulates adenylyl cyclase activity and enhances production of cAMP, which leads, in turn, to stimulation of *CYP19*, the gene encoding aromatase (61).Consequently, estrogen biosynthesis is increased, which leads to enhanced proliferation of tumor cells. In addition to PGE_2, other prostanoids including TxA_2 and PGI_2 impact on carcinogenesis but less is known about the downstream signaling mechanisms (3, 62).

2.3. Evidence that Targeting COX-2 Inhibits Carcinogenesis

As detailed above, COX-2-derived prostanoids have a variety of procarcinogenic effects. Both animal and human studies have been carried out to investigate the potential role of COX-2 in driving the formation and progression of tumors. The most specific data supporting a cause-and-effect relationship between COX-2 and carcinogenesis come from genetic studies. Multiparous female transgenic mice engineered to overexpress human *COX-2* in mammary glands developed metastatic tumors (63). In other related studies, transgenic mice that overexpressed COX-2 developed epidermal hyperplasia and dysplasia and pancreatic neoplasia, respectively (64, 65). These results imply a causal link between expression of COX-2 and the development of premalignant lesions of the skin and pancreas. Consistent with the overexpression data, a marked reduction in the formation of skin, intestinal and mammary neoplasia was found in COX-2$^{-/-}$ mice (66–68). The importance of host COX-2 was highlighted by the finding that transplantable tumor growth was reduced in COX-2 deficient mice (69). The importance of arachidonic acid metabolism in tumorigenesis is underscored by evidence that knocking out the *COX-1* gene also protected against the formation of intestinal and skin tumors (70). In addition to genetic evidence, numerous pharmacological studies suggest that COX-2 is a therapeutic target. Treatment with selective inhibitors of COX-2 reduced the formation and growth of numerous tumor types in experimental animals (71–80). Collectively, these preclinical results provided a strong rationale for evaluating whether targeting COX-2 would be beneficial in either preventing or treating human cancer.

The first clinical trial to evaluate the anticancer properties of a selective COX-2 inhibitor was carried out in FAP patients. This patient population was chosen because of the strength of

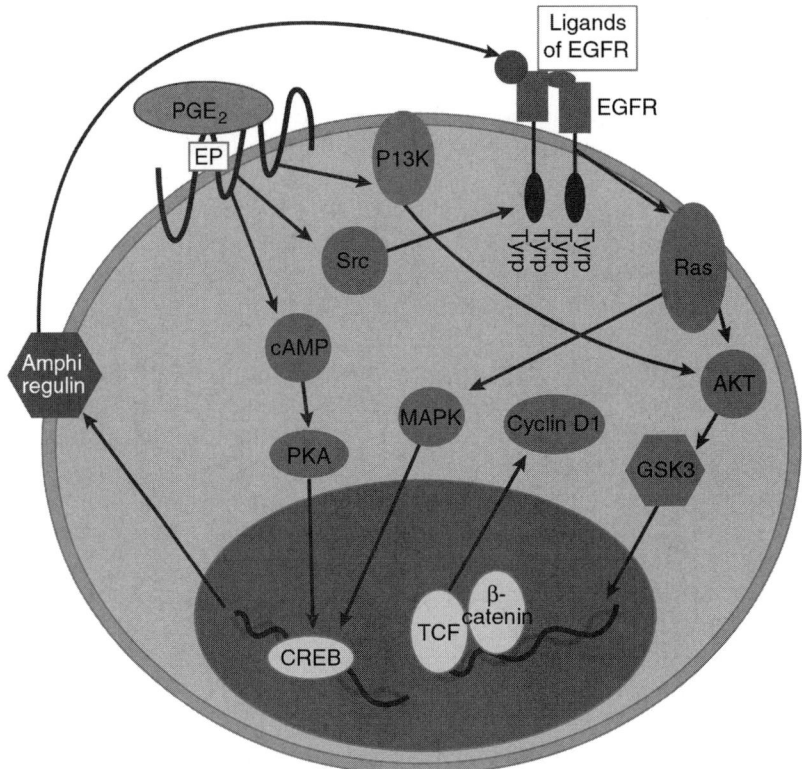

Fig. 21.3. PGE$_2$ Activates Signal Transduction Pathways that Have Been Implicated in Carcinogenesis. PGE$_2$ activates cellular signaling in an EP receptor-dependent manner. For example, PGE$_2$-mediated activation of EP$_2$ and EP$_4$ receptors leads to enhanced adenylate cyclase activity and cAMP production. cAMP, in turn, activates PKA-CREB dependent expression of genes including *amphiregulin*. Amphiregulin, a ligand of EGFR, stimulates EGFR-Ras-MAPK signaling. Additionally, activation of EP receptors stimulates TCF-β-catenin-mediated transcription of genes including *cyclin D1*.

the preclinical data and prior evidence that sulindac, a dual inhibitor of COX-1/COX-2, reduced the number of colorectal polyps in FAP patients (*81*). Treatment with celecoxib 400 mg bid for six months led to a 28% reduction in the number of colorectal polyps (p = 0.003) (*82*). Based on these results, the US FDA approved celecoxib as adjunctive therapy for the management of polyps in FAP patients. Stimulated by the FAP findings, several large placebo controlled clinical trials were carried out to evaluate whether selective COX-2 inhibitors could prevent the recurrence of sporadic colorectal adenomas (*83–85*). Treatment with either celecoxib or rofecoxib led to a significant reduction in the recurrence of sporadic colorectal adenomas (*83–85*). However, use of both celecoxib and rofecoxib was associated with an increased risk of serious cardiovascular events leading to the voluntary withdrawal of rofecoxib from the market (*86, 87*). Some investigators have postulated that cardiovascular toxicity was a consequence of an exaggerated thrombotic response due to suppression of COX-2-mediated prostacyclin production in the endothelium with unaffected generation of COX-1-derived thromboxane A$_2$ by platelets (*88*). In contrast to the beneficial antineoplastic effects observed in the colorectal polyp prevention trials, selective

COX-2 inhibitors have not been found to be active in suppressing carcinogenesis in patients with esophageal squamous dysplasia, Barrett's esophagus or gastric intestinal metaplasia (*89–91*). Although active efforts are underway to elucidate the mechanisms underlying the cardiovascular toxicity of selective COX-2 inhibitors, it seems unlikely that this class of agents will be used to treat premalignancy in the near term in any population with the possible exception of FAP patients.

In cancer patients, there is generally a greater willingness to tolerate potential side effects if an agent has demonstrable antitumor activity. Given the strength of the preclinical findings, a number of small clinical treatment trials have been carried out to evaluate the potential utility of selective COX-2 inhibitors. Promising results have been reported in some but not all cancer treatment studies (*92–97*). Currently, it is uncertain if selective COX-2 inhibitors will augment the antitumor activity of other targeted therapies, a topic that remains an active research question. In this context, we note that important interactions have been identified between COX-2 and EGFR. The link between EGFR and carcinogenesis and the rationale for simultaneously targeting COX-2 and EGFR as a potential therapeutic strategy is reviewed below.

3. EGFR SIGNALING AND CANCER

EGF was originally discovered in the early 1960s when bioassays revealed accelerated eyelid opening in animals treated with protein extracts prepared from submaxillary glands (*98*). Over the past 40 years, significant progress has been made in improving our understanding of the molecular mechanisms responsible for the biologic effects of this growth factor and the EGFR (ErbB1) (*99*). The ErbB family of receptors is comprised of the EGFR, ErbB2 (HER2), ErbB3 (HER3) and ErbB4 (HER4). Binding of ligands including EGF to the ectodomain of these receptors results in the formation of homodimeric and heterodimeric complexes, which is followed rapidly by activation of the receptors' intrinsic tyrosine kinase. Phosphorylation of specific C-terminal tyrosine residues and the recruitment of specific second messengers activate intracellular signaling pathways that play key roles in development, differentiation, migration and proliferation. Activation of ErbB receptor signaling has been linked to cancer. Mechanisms involved in activation of the ErbB receptor pathway include: (*1*) receptor overexpression (*100*), (*2*) mutation of receptors resulting in ligand-independent activation (*101, 102*), (*3*) autocrine activation by overproduction of ligand (*99*) and (*4*) transactivation through other receptor systems (*103, 104*). Overexpression of EGFR correlates with poor prognosis in several malignancies (*100, 105*). Importantly, EGFR signaling induces its cognate ligands, creating autocrine loops that can amplify EGFR activity.

Several major signaling pathways mediate the downstream effects of activated EGFR. Activation of EGFR can stimulate the Ras→Raf→MAP kinase pathway (*106*). Elevated MAP kinase activity has been reported in a number of tumors when compared with corresponding non-neoplastic tissues, and correlated with EGFR and ligand expression (*107*). A second EGFR-driven pathway involves phosphatidylinositol 3-kinase (PI3K) and Akt (*108, 109*). Activation of EGFR can also lead to enhanced signaling via Jak/Stat or PKC. These pathways regulate gene transcription and thereby modulate cell proliferation, apoptosis, angiogenesis and malignant transformation. Two strategies for blocking the action of the EGFR include antibodies directed against the ectodomain and drugs that inhibit protein-tyrosine kinase activity. Therapies that target EGFR have already been found to be beneficial in the treatment of cancers of the lung, pancreas, head and neck and colon (*110–113*). Ongoing efforts to target EGFR as a strategy for treating cancer are discussed throughout the volume, but notably in detail in Chapters 2, 3, 16, 20, 22 and 23.

3.1. Combined Targeting of the EGFR and COX-2

As detailed above, both COX-2 and the EGFR are targets for anticancer therapy. In this context, it is important to consider the rationale for combined targeting of the EGFR and COX-2. Activation of EGFR signaling leads to increased MAPK activity resulting, in turn, in activator protein-1 (AP-1)-mediated induction of *COX-2* transcription (Fig. 21.2) (*1*) and enhanced synthesis of PGs including PGE_2. Considerable evidence has accumulated indicating that COX-2-derived PGE_2 can activate EGFR signaling and thereby stimulate tumor cell proliferation (*114–116*) (Fig. 21.3). The mechanism(s) by which this occurs appear to be complex and context specific. In one study, the ability of PGE_2 to transactivate EGFR was very rapid and depended on matrix metalloproteinase activity (*114*). PGE_2 activated metalloproteinase activity resulting in shedding of active EGFR ligand from the plasma membrane. This led, in turn, to increased EGFR signaling and enhanced DNA synthesis. In another study, treatment with PGE_2 activated the cAMP/protein kinase A (PKA) pathway leading to increased expression of amphiregulin, a ligand of the EGFR (*115*). PGE_2 also has been observed to transactivate EGFR via an intracellular Src-mediated event independent of the release of an extracellular ligand of EGFR (Fig. 21.3) (*116*). In this instance, following stimulation by PGE_2, EP_4 receptors form a signaling complex with β-arrestin 1 and c-Src, resulting in the transactivation of EGFR and increased Akt signaling (*117*). Regardless of the precise mechanism, exposure to COX-2-derived PGE_2 may initiate a positive feedback loop whereby activation of EGFR results in enhanced expression of COX-2 and increased synthesis of PGs. This leads, in turn, to a further enhancement of EGFR activity. The potential importance of this positive feedback loop for driving tumor growth provides a rationale, in part, for a therapeutic regimen that combines inhibitors of EGFR and COX-2.

Crosstalk between EGFR and COX-2 may be important for tumor invasion, the epithelial-to-mesenchymal transition (EMT) and metastasis. EMT involves dedifferentiation of epithelial cells to fibroblastoid migratory cells with a markedly altered mesenchymal gene expression profile. E-cadherin plays a role in epithelial intercellular adhesion, and down-regulation of E-cadherin levels is a hallmark of EMT (*118*). Reduced expression of E-cadherin in human tumors is associated with invasion, metastasis, and decreased survival (*119*). Several findings strongly suggest that EGFR signaling and COX-2-derived PGE_2 play a role in EMT. Chronic EGF treatment disrupts cell-to-cell adhesion, suppresses expression of E-cadherin, and induces EMT in human tumor cells overexpressing EGFR (*120*). These effects are a consequence, at least in part, of EGF-mediated induction of Snail, a known repressor of E-cadherin transcription. Overexpression of COX-2 in intestinal epithelial cells can suppress the expression of E-cadherin and enhance adhesion to extracellular matrix (*121*). Recently, this work was extended to non-small cell lung cancer (*122*). In non-small cell lung cancer cells, overexpression of COX-2 or treatment with exogenous PGE_2 led to reduced expression of E-cadherin and decreased cell aggregation. These effects were attributed to up-regulation of the transcriptional repressors ZEB1 and Snail. The ability of treatment with either PGE_2 or EGF to induce Snail and suppress E-cadherin underscores the potential significance of pharmacologically targeting crosstalk between COX-2 and EGFR as an anticancer strategy. In another relevant study, non-small cell lung cancer cells that expressed E-cadherin were more sensitive to growth inhibition by erlotinib, an inhibitor of EGFR tyrosine kinase, than cells that had lost E-cadherin expression and gained the expression of mesenchymal markers (*123*). This study suggested that the EMT status of a tumor may help to determine its responsiveness to EGFR-targeted therapies. Because COX-2-derived PGE_2 can suppress the expression of E-cadherin and induce a mesenchymal phenotype, it's possible that treatment with a COX-2 inhibitor will induce E-cadherin and thereby sensitize tumor cells to agents that inhibit EGFR. Findings such as these also strengthen the rationale for a treatment regimen combining inhibitors of EGFR and COX-2.

In the discussion above, we emphasized the potential importance of crosstalk between EGFR and COX-2 as a rationale for combination therapy. It also should be stressed that EGFR and its downstream pathways can be activated independent of COX-2/PGE$_2$. Similarly, COX-2/PGE$_2$ and its effectors can act independently of EGFR. For example, COX-2-derived PGE$_2$ can induce cell proliferation by an EGFR-independent mechanism (124). These mutually independent procarcinogenic effects further support a combinatorial approach targeting both EGFR and COX-2.

Preclinical studies have been carried out to evaluate whether combining an inhibitor of EGFR tyrosine kinase with an inhibitor of COX-2 will be more effective than using either agent alone. For example, combining celecoxib, a selective COX-2 inhibitor, with gefitinib, an EGFR tyrosine kinase inhibitor, was more effective than either agent alone in suppressing the growth of experimental head and neck squamous cell carcinoma (125). Torrance et al. addressed this point by evaluating the number of intestinal adenomas that developed in Apc^{Min} mice after treatment with a dual inhibitor of COX-1/COX-2 combined with an inhibitor of EGFR tyrosine kinase (2). Apc^{Min} mice, which normally develop numerous intestinal polyps due to a mutation in the *APC* tumor suppressor gene, were almost completely protected from adenomas after treatment with the combination regimen.

The scientific rationale and experimental findings described above have stimulated interest in evaluating combined inhibition of COX-2 and EGFR in cancer patients. The combination of gefitinib and celecoxib was evaluated in a phase I study of 19 patients with unresectable recurrent locoregional and/or distant metastatic head and neck squamous cell carcinoma with progressive disease (126). The regimen was well tolerated and the response rate of 22% compared favorably with the overall response rates of 11% and 4% seen in prior gefitinib single agent phase II studies. The investigators considered the results to be promising enough to warrant further study of a regimen combining inhibitors of EGFR and COX-2. A second Phase 1 trial was carried out in 22 subjects with advanced non-small cell lung cancer (127). In this instance, celecoxib was combined with erlotinib. No dose limiting toxicities were observed. 33% of patients displayed a partial response, including patients both with and without activating EGFR mutations. Based on preclinical evidence that COX-2 overexpression can mediate resistance to EGFR tyrosine kinase inhibition (124) and the results of this Phase 1 study, the investigators are planning a phase II trial of celecoxib and erlotinib versus erlotinib and placebo in advanced non-small cell lung cancer.

4. FUTURE DIRECTIONS

Although significant progress has been made in understanding the interaction between COX-2 and EGFR, many unanswered questions remain. Under what circumstances is the interaction between these two pathways of physiological significance? For example, is crosstalk between COX-2-derived PGE$_2$ and EGFR an adaptive mechanism that is important for wound healing? If so, are there particular subsets of patients for whom combined therapy can be predicted to cause unacceptable toxicity? In chronic inflammatory states such as ulcerative colitis, will the interaction between these two pathways reduce the threshold for carcinogenesis? Will COX-2 inhibitors augment the antitumor activity of EGFR inhibitors? Although the initial Phase 1 results are encouraging, the results are by no means definitive. Will COX-2 inhibitors induce a mesenchymal to epithelial transition and thereby sensitize tumors to therapies that target EGFR? Is the interaction between these two pathways important in tumor stem cells? There is recent evidence to suggest that the increased levels of PGE$_2$ in tumors reflect reduced catabolism in addition to increased synthesis (128). Hence, it will be of interest to determine whether changes in the catabolism of PGE$_2$ have important effects on EGFR signaling, EMT and the response to EGFR inhibitors. Are there biomarkers that can be used to identify patients who are most or least likely to benefit from combined therapy? Answers to these questions and others will be critical to both understand the physiological significance of crosstalk between COX-2 and EGFR and to determine the potential benefit of combining inhibitors of COX-2 and EGFR to treat cancer.

ACKNOWLEDGMENTS

We acknowledge support from the USPH Service Grants RO1-CA111469, P01-CA77839 and P01-CA106451 and the Center for Cancer Prevention Research.

REFERENCES

1. Dannenberg AJ, Subbaramaiah K. Targeting cyclooxygenase-2 in human neoplasia: rationale and promise. Cancer Cell 2003;4:431-6.
2. Torrance CJ, Jackson PE, Montgomery E, et al. Combinatorial chemoprevention of intestinal neoplasia. Nat Med 2000; 6:1024-8.
3. Gupta RA, DuBois RN. Colorectal cancer prevention and treatment by inhibition of cyclooxygenase-2. Nat Rev Cancer 2001;1:11-21.
4. Smith WL, DeWitt DL, Garavito RM. Cyclooxygenases: structural, cellular and molecular biology. Annu Rev Biochem 2000;69:145-82.
5. Subbaramaiah K, Telang N, Ramonetti JT, et al. Transcription of cyclooxygenase 2 is enhanced in transformed mammary epithelial cells. Cancer Res 1996;56:4424 9.
6. Kurumbail RG, Stevens AM, Gierse JK, et al. Structural basis for selective inhibition of cyclooxygenase-2 by anti-inflammatory agents. Nature 1996;384:644-8.
7. Leese PT, Hubbard RC, Karim A, Isakson PC, Yu SS, Geis GS. Effects of celecoxib, a novel cyclooxygenase-2 inhibitor, on platelet function in healthy adults: a randomized, controlled trial. J Clin Pharm 2000;40:124-32.
8. Eberhart CE, Coffey RJ, Radhika A, Giardiello FM, Ferrenbach S, Dubois RN. Up-regulation of cyclooxygenase 2 gene expression in human colorectal adenomas and adenocarcinomas. Gastroenterology 1994;107:1183-8.
9. Sung JJ, Leung WK, Go MY et al. Cyclooxygenase-2 expression in Helicobacter pylori-associated premalignant and malignant gastric lesions. Am J Pathol 2000;157:729-35.
10. Ristimaki A, Honkanen N, Jankala H, Sipponen P, Harkonen M. Expression of cyclooxygenase-2 in human gastric carcinoma. Cancer Res 1997;57:1276-80.
11. Wilson KT, Fu S, Ramanujam KS, Meltzer SJ. Increased expression of inducible nitric oxide synthase and cyclooxygenase-2 in Barrett's esophagus and associated adenocarcinomas. Cancer Res 1998;58:2929-34.
12. Zimmermann KC, Sarbia M, Weber AA, Borchard F, Gabbert HE, Schror K. Cyclooxygenase-2 expression in human esophageal carcinoma. Cancer Res 1999;59:198-204.
13. Kondo M, Yamamoto H, Nagano H, et al. Increased expression of COX-2 in nontumor liver tissue is associated with shorter disease-free survival in patients with hepatocellular carcinoma. Clin Cancer Res 1999;5:4005-12.
14. Koga H, Sakisaka S, Ohishi M, et al. Expression of cyclooxygenase-2 in human hepatocellular carcinoma: relevance to tumor dedifferentiation. Hepatology 1999;29:688-96.
15. Tucker ON, Dannenberg AJ, Yang EK, et al. Cyclooxygenase-2 expression is up-regulated in human pancreatic cancer. Cancer Res 1999;59:987-90.
16. Chan G, Boyle JO, Yang EK, et al. Cyclooxygenase-2 expression is up-regulated in squamous cell carcinoma of the head and neck. Cancer Res 1999;59:991-4.
17. Wolff H, Saukkonen K, Anttila S, Karialainen A, Vainio H, Ristimaki A. Expression of cyclooxygenase-2 in human lung carcinoma. Cancer Res 1998;58:4997-5001.
18. Soslow RA, Dannenberg AJ, Rush D, et al. COX-2 is expressed in human pulmonary, colonic, and mammary tumors. Cancer 2000; 89:2637-45.
19. Parrett ML, Harris RE, Joarder FS, et al. Cyclooxygenase-2 gene expression in human breast cancer. Int J Oncol 1997;10:503-7.
20. Shirahama T. Cyclooxygenase-2 expression is up-regulated in transitional cell carcinoma and its preneoplastic lesions in the human urinary bladder. Clin Cancer Res 2000;6:2424-30.

21. Mohammed SI, Knapp DW, Bostwick DG, et al. Expression of cyclooxygenase-2 (COX-2) in human invasive transitional cell carcinoma (TCC) of the urinary bladder. Cancer Res 1999;59:5647-50.
22. Kulkarni S, Rader JS, Zhang F, et al: Cyclooxygenase-2 is overexpressed in human cervical cancer. Clin Cancer Res 2001;7:429-34.
23. Tong BJ, Tan J, Tajeda L, et al. Heightened expression of cyclooxygenase-2 and peroxisome proliferator-activated receptor-delta in human endometrial adenocarcinoma. Neoplasia 2000;2:483-90.
24. Golijanin D, Tan J.T., Kazior A, et al: Cyclooxygenase-2 and microsomal prostaglandin E synthase-1 are overexpressed in squamous cell carcinoma of the penis. Clin Cancer Res 2004;10:1024-31.
25. Muller-Decker K, Reinerth G, Krieg P, et al. Prostaglandin-H synthase isozyme expression in normal and neoplastic human skin. Int J Cancer 1999;82:648-56.
26. Buckman SY, Gresham A, Hale P, et al. COX-2 expression is induced by UVB exposure in human skin: implications for the development of skin cancer. Carcinogenesis 1998;19:723-9.
27. Inoue H, Yokoyama C, Hara S, Tone Y, Tanabe T. Transcriptional regulation of human prostaglandin endoperoxide synthase 2 gene by lipopolysaccharide and phorbol ester in vascular endothelial cells. Involvement of both nuclear factor for interleukin 6 expression site and cAMP response element. J Biol Chem 1995;270:24965 71.
28. Subbaramaiah K, Norton L, Gerald W, Dannenberg AJ. Cyclooxygenase-2 is overexpressed in HER-2/neu-positive breast cancer. J Biol Chem 2002; 277:18649-57.
29. Subbaramaiah K, Hart JC, Norton L, Dannenberg AJ. Microtubule-interfering agents stimulate the transcription of cyclooxygenase-2. Evidence for involvement of ERK1/2 and p38 mitogen-activated protein kinase pathways. J Biol Chem 2000; 275:14838-45.
30. Zhang F, Subbaramaiah K, Altorki N, Dannnberg AJ. Dihydroxy bile acids activate the transcription of cyclooxygenase-2. J Biol Chem 1998;273:2424-8.
31. Xie W, Herschman HR. v-src induces prostaglandin synthase 2 gene expression by activation of the c-Jun N-terminal kinase and the c-Jun transcription factor. J Biol Chem 1995;270:27622-8.
32. de Gregorio R, Iniguez MA, Fresno M, Alemany S. Cot kinase induces cyclooxygenase-2 expression in T cells through activation of the nuclear factor of activated T cells. J Biol Chem 2001;276:27003-09.
33. Subbaramaiah K, Altorki N, Chung WJ, Mestre J, Sampat A, Dannenberg AJ. Inhibition of cyclooxygenase-2 gene expression by p53. J Biol Chem 1999;274:10911-5.
34. Leung WK, To K-F, Ng YP, et al. Association between cyclo-oxygenase-2 overexpression and missense p53 mutations in gastric cancer. Br J Cancer 2001; 84:335-9.
35. Ristimaki A, Sivula A, Lundin J, et al. Prognostic significance of elevated cyclooxygenase-2 expression in breast cancer. Cancer Res 2002; 62:632-5.
36. Araki Y, Okamura S, Hussain SP, et al. Regulation of cyclooxygenase-2 expression by the Wnt and Ras pathways. Cancer Res 2003;63:728-34.
37. Subbaramaiah K, Dannenberg AJ. Cyclooxygenase-2 transcription is regulated by human papillomavirus 16 E6 and E7 oncoproteins: evidence of a corepressor/coactivator exchange. Cancer Res 2007;67:3976-85.
38. Dixon DA, Kaplan CD, McIntyre TM, Zimmerman GA, Prescott SM. Post-transcriptional control of cyclooxygenase-2 gene expression. The role of the 3′-unstranslated region. J Biol Chem 2000;275:11750-7.
39. Dixon DA, Tolley ND, King PH, et al. Altered expression of the mRNA stability factor HuR promotes cyclooxygenase-2 expression in colon cancer cells. J Clin Invest 2001;108:1657-65.
40. Sawaoka H, Dixon DA, Oates JA, Boutaud O. Tristetraprolin binds to the 3′-untranslated region of cyclooxygenase-2 mRNA. A polyadenylation variant in a cancer cell line lacks the binding site. J Biol Chem 2003; 278:13928-35.
41. Dixon DA, Balch GC, Kedersha N, et al. Regulation of cyclooxygenase-2 expression by the translational silencer TIA-1. J Exp Med 2003;198:475-81.
42. Sheng H, Shao J, Morrow JD, Dubois RN. Modulation of apoptosis and Bcl-2 expression by prostaglandin E_2 in human colon cancer cells. Cancer Res 1998;58:362-6.
43. Sheng H, Shao J, Washington MK, Dubois RN. Prostaglandin E2 increases growth and motility of colorectal carcinoma cells. J Biol Chem 2001;276:18075-81.
44. Cohen EG, Almahmeed T, Du B, et al. Microsomal prostaglandin E synthase-1 is overexpressed in head and neck squamous cell carcinoma. Clin Cancer Res 2003; 9:3425-30.

45. Tsujii M, DuBois RN. Alterations in cellular adhesion and apoptosis in epithelial cells overexpressing prostaglandin endoperoxide synthase-2. Cell 1995;83:493-501.
46. Goodwin JS, Bankhurst AD, Messner RP. Suppression of human T-cell mitogenesis by prostaglandin. Existence of a prostaglandin producing suppressor cell. J Exp Med 1977;146:1719-34.
47. Goodwin JS, Ceuppens J. Regulation of immune response by prostaglandins. J Clin. Immunol 1983;3:295-315.
48. Balch CM, Dougherty PA, Cloud GA, Tilden AB. Prostaglandin E_2-mediated suppression of cellular immunity in colon cancer patients. Surgery 1984;95:71-7.
49. Huang M, Stolina M, Sharma S, et al: Non-small cell lung cancer cyclooxygenase-2-dependent regulation of cytokine balance in lymphocytes and macrophages: up-regulation of interleukin 10 and down-regulation of interleukin 12 production. Cancer Res 1998;58:1208-16.
50. Stolina M, Sharma S, Lin Y, et al. Specific inhibition of cyclooxygenase-2 restores antitumor reactivity by altering the balance of IL-10 and IL-12 synthesis. J Immunol 2000;164:361-70.
51. Ben-Av P, Crofford LJ, Wilder RL, Hla T. Induction of vascular endothelial growth factor expression in synovial fibroblasts by prostaglandin E and interleukin-1; a potential mechanism for inflammatory angiogenesis. FEBS Lett 1995;372:83-7.
52. Tsujii M, Kawano S, Tsuji S, Sawaoka H, Hori M, Dubois RN. Cyclooxygenase regulates angiogenesis induced by colon cancer cells. Cell 1998;93: 705-16.
53. Dannenberg AJ, Altorki NK, Boyle JO, et al. Cyclo-oxygenase 2: a pharmacological target for the prevention of cancer. Lancet Oncol 2001;2:544-51.
54. Gasparini G, Longo R, Sarmiento R, Morabito A. Inhibitors of cyclo-oxygenase 2: a new class of anticancer agents? Lancet Oncol 2003;4:605-15.
55. Mutoh M, Watanabe K, Kitamura T, et al. Involvement of prostaglandin E receptor subtype EP_4 in colon carcinogenesis. Cancer Res 2002;62:28-32.
56. Sonoshita M, Takaku K, Sasaki N, et al: Acceleration of intestinal polyposis through prostaglandin receptor EP2 in Apc (Delta 716) knockout mice. Nat Med 2001;7:1048-51.
57. Amano H, Hayashi I, Endo H, et al. Host prostaglandin E_2-EP3 signaling regulates tumor-associated angiogenesis and tumor growth. J Exp Med 2003; 197:221-32.
58. Sharma S, Stolina M, Yang SC, et al. Tumor cyclooxygenase 2-dependent suppression of dendritic cell function. Clin Cancer Res 2003;9:961-8.
59. Yang L, Yamagata N, Yadav R. Cancer-associated immunodeficiency and dendritic cell abnormalities mediated by the prostaglandin EP_2 receptor. J Clin Invest 2001; 111:727-35.
60. Fujino H, West KA, Regan JW. Phosphorylation of glycogen synthase kinase-3 and stimulation of T-cell factor signaling following activation of EP_2 and EP_4 prostanoid receptors by prostaglandin E2. J Biol Chem 2002;277:2614-9.
61. Zhao Y, Agarwal VR, Mendelson CR, Simpson ER. Estrogen biosynthesis proximal to a breast tumor is stimulated by PGE2 via cyclic AMP, leading to activation of promoter II of the CYP19 (aromatase) gene. Endocrinology 1996;137:5739-42.
62. Daniel TO, Liu H, Morrow JD, Crews BC, Marnett LJ. Thromboxane A2 is a mediator of cyclooxygenase-2 dependent endothelial migration and angiogenesis. Cancer Res 1999;59:4574-7..
63. Liu CH, Chang SH, Narko K, et al. Overexpression of COX-2 is sufficient to induce tumorigenesis in transgenic mice. J Biol Chem 2001;276:18563-9.
64. Neufang G, Furstenberger G, Heidt M, Marks F, Muller –Decker K. Abnormal differentiation of epidermis in transgenic mice constitutively expressing cyclooxygenase-2 in skin. Proc Natl Acad Sci USA 2001;98:7629-34.
65. Muller-Decker K, Furstenberger G, Annan N, et al. Preinvasive duct-derived neoplasms in pancreas of keratin 5-promoter cyclooxygenase-2 transgenic mice. Gastroenterology 2006;130:2165-78.
66. Tiano HF, Loftin CD, Akunda J, et al. Deficiency of either cyclooxygenase (COX)-1 or COX-2 alters epidermal differentiation and reduces mouse skin tumorigenesis. Cancer Res 2002; 62:3395-401..
67. Oshima M, Dinchuk JE, Kargman SL, et al. Suppression of intestinal polyposis in APCD716 knockout mice by inhibition of cyclooxygenase-2 (Cox 2). Cell 1996;87:803 9.
68. Howe LR, Chang SH, Tolle KC, et al. HER2/neu-induced mammary tumorigenesis and angiogenesis are reduced in cyclooxygenase-2 knockout mice. Cancer Res 2005;65:10113-9.
69. Williams CS, Tsujii M, Reese J, Dey. SK, Dubois, RN. Host cyclooxygenase-2 modulates carcinoma growth. J. Clin Invest 2000;105:1589-94.

70. Chulada PC, Thompson MB, Mahler JF, et al. Genetic disruption of Ptgs-1, as well as of Ptgs-2, reduces intestinal tumorigenesis in Min mice. Cancer Res 2000;60:4705-08.
71. Kawamori T, Rao CV, Seibert K, Reddy BS. Chemopreventive activity of celecoxib, a specific cyclooxygenase-2 inhibitor, against colon carcinogenesis. Cancer Res 1998;58:409-12.
72. Jacoby RF, Seibert K, Cole CE, Kelloff G, Lubet, RA. The cyclooxygenase-2 inhibitor celecoxib is a potent preventive and therapeutic agent in the *min* mouse model of adenomatous polyposis. Cancer Res 2000; 60:5040-4.
73. Oshima M, Murai N, Kargman S, et al. Chemoprevention of intestinal polyposis in Apc$^{\Delta 716}$ mouse by rofecoxib, a specific cyclooxygenase-2 inhibitor. Cancer Res 2001;61:1733-40.
74. Harris RE, Alshafie GA, Abou-Issa H, Seibert K. Chemoprevention of breast cancer in rats by celecoxib, a cyclooxygenase 2 inhibitor. Cancer Res 2000;60:2101-03.
75. Howe LR, Subbaramaiah K, Patel J, et al. Celecoxib, a selective cyclooxygenase 2 inhibitor, protects against epidermal growth factor receptor 2 (HER-2)/neu-induced breast cancer. Cancer Res 2002; 62:5405-07.
76. Fischer SM, Lo HH, Gordon GB, et al, Chemopreventive activity of celecoxib, a specific cyclooxygenase-2 inhibitor, and indomethacin against ultraviolet light-induced skin carcinogenesis. Mol Carcinog 1999; 25:231-40.
77. Rioux N, Castonguay A. Prevention of NNK-induced lung tumorigenesis in A/J mice by acetylsalicylic acid and NS-398. Cancer Res 1998; 58:5354-60.
78. Grubbs CJ, Lubet RA, Koki AT, et al. Celecoxib inhibits N-butyl-N-(4-hydroxybutyl)-nitrosamine-induced urinary bladder cancers in male B6D2F1 mice and female Fischer-344 rats. Cancer Res 2000;60:5599-02.
79. Buttar NS, Wang KK, Leontovich O, et al. Chemoprevention of esophageal adenocarcinoma by COX-2 inhibitors in an animal model of Barrett's esophagus. Gastroenterology 2002;122:1101-12.
80. Shiotani H, Denda A, Yamamoto K, et al. Increased expression of cyclooxygenase-2 protein and 4-nitroquinoline-1-oxide-induced rat tongue carcinomas and chemopreventive efficacy of a specific inhibitor, nimesulide. Cancer Res 2001; 61:1451-6.
81. Giardiello FM, Hamilton SR, Krush AJ, et al. Treatment of colonic and rectal adenomas with sulindac in familial adenomatous polyposis. N Engl J Med 1993;328:1313-6.
82. Steinbach, G, Lynch PM, Phillips RKS, et al. The effect of celecoxib, a cyclooxygenase-2 inhibitor, in familial adenomatous polyposis. N Engl J Med 2000; 342:1946-52.
83. Bertagnolli MM, Eagle CJ, Zauber AG, et al. Celecoxib for the prevention of sporadic colorectal adenomas. N Engl J Med 2006;355: 873-84.
84. Arber N, Eagle CJ, Spicak J, et al. Celecoxib for the prevention of colorectal adenomatous polyps. N Engl J Med 2006; 355: 885-95.
85. Baron JA, Sandler RS, Bresalier RS, et al. A randomized trial of rofecoxib for the chemoprevention of colorectal adenomas. Gastroenterology 2006;131: 1674-82.
86. Bresalier RS, Sandler RS, Quan H, et al. Cardiovascular events associated with rofecoxib in a colorectal adenoma chemoprevention trial. N Engl J Med 2005; 352:1092-102.
87. Solomon SC, Pfeffer MA, McMurray JJV, et al. Effect of celecoxib on cardiovascular events and blood pressure in two trials for the prevention of colorectal adenomas. Circulation 2006; 114:1028-35.
88. McAdam BF, Catella-Lawson F, Mardini IA, et al. Systemic biosynthesis of prostacyclin by cyclooxygenase (COX)-2: the human pharmacology of a selective inhibitor of COX-2. Proc Natl Acad Sci USA 1999: 96:272-7.
89. Limburg PJ, Wei W, Ahnen DJ, et al. Randomized, placebo-controlled, esophageal squamous cell cancer chemoprevention trial of selenomethionine and celecoxib. Gastroenterology 2005; 129:863-73.
90. Heath EI, Canto MI, Piantadosi S, et al: Secondary chemoprevention of Barrett's esophagus with celecoxib: results of a randomized trial. J Natl Cancer Inst 2007;99:545-57.
91. Leung WK, Ng EKW, Chan FKL, et al. Effects of long-term rofecoxib on gastric intestinal metaplasia: results of a randomized controlled trial. Clin Cancer Res 2006;12:4766-72.
92. Altorki NK, Keresztes RS, Port JL, et al. Celecoxib, a selective cyclo-oxygenase-2 inhibitor, enhances the response to preoperative paclitaxel and carboplatin in early-stage non-small-cell lung cancer. J Clin Oncol 2003;21:2645-50.

93. Dang CT, Dannenberg AJ, Subbaramaiah K, et al. Phase II study of celecoxib and trastuzumab in metastatic breast cancer patients who have progressed after prior trastuzumab-based treatments. Clin Cancer Res 2004;10:4062-7.
94. Canney PA, Machin MA, Curto J. A feasibility study of the efficacy and tolerability of the combination of Exemestane with the COX-2 inhibitor Celecoxib in post-menopausal patients with advanced breast cancer. Eur J Cancer 2006; 42:2751-6.
95. Pruthi RS, Derksen JE, Moore D et al. Phase II trial of celecoxib in prostate-specific antigen recurrent prostate cancer after definitive radiation therapy or radical prostatectomy. Clin Cancer Res 2006; 12:2172-7.
96. Gogas H, Polyzos A, Stavrinidis I, et al. Temozolomide in combination with celecoxib in patients with advances melanoma. A phase II study of the Hellenic Cooperative Oncology Group. Ann Oncol 2006;12:1835-41.
97. El-Rayes BF, Zalupski MM, Manza SG, et al. Phase-II study of dose attenuated schedule of irinotecan, capecitabine, and celecoxib in advanced colorectal cancer. Cancer Chemother Pharmacol, 2007 (in press).
98. Cohen S. Isolation of a mouse submaxillary gland protein accelerating incisor eruption and eyelid opening in the newborn animal. J Biol Chem 1962; 237:1555-62.
99. Prenzel N, Fischer OM, Streit S, Hart S, Ullrich A. The epidermal growth factor receptor family as a central element for cellular signal transduction and diversification. Endrocr Relat Cancer 2001; 8:11-31.
100. Hirsch FR, Varella-Garcia M, Bunn PA, Jr., et al. Epidermal growth factor receptor in non-small-cell lung carcinomas: correlation between gene copy number and protein expression and impact on prognosis. J Clin Oncol 2003: 21:3798-807.
101. Hirsch FR, Scagliotti GV, Langer CJ, et al. Epidermal growth factor family of receptors in preneoplasia and lung cancer: perspectives for targeted therapies. Lung Cancer 2003;41 Suppl 1:S29-42.
102. Moscatello DK, Holgado-Madruga M, Godwin AK, et al. Frequent expression of a mutant epidermal growth factor receptor in multiple human tumors. Cancer Res 1995;55:5536-9.
103. Prenzel N, Zwick E, Daub H, et al. EGF receptor transactivation by G-protein-coupled receptors requires metalloproteinase cleavage of proHB-EGF. Nature 1999;402:884-8.
104. Liu D, Aguirre Ghiso J, Estrada Y, Ossowski L. EGFR is a transducer of the urokinase receptor initiated signal that is required for in vivo growth of a human carcinoma. Cancer Cell 2002; 1:445-57.
105. Dassonville O, Formento JL, Francoual M, et al. Expression of epidermal growth factor receptor and survival in upper aerodigestive tract cancer. J Clin Oncol 1993;11:1873-8.
106. Lewis TS, Shapiro PS, Ahn NG. Signal transduction through MAP kinase cascades. Adv Cancer Res 1998;74:49-139.
107. Albanell J, Codony-Servat J, Rojo F, et al. Activated extracellular signal-regulated kinases: association with epidermal growth factor receptor/transforming growth factor alpha expression in head and neck squamous carcinoma and inhibition by anti-epidermal growth factor receptor treatments. Cancer Res2001; 61:6500-10.
108. Vivanco I, Sawyers CL. The phosphatidylinositol 3-Kinase AKT pathway in human cancer. Nat Rev Cancer 2002;2:489-501.
109. Chan TO, Rittenhouse SE, Tsichlis PN. AKT/PKB and other D3 phosphoinositide-regulated kinases: kinase activation by phosphoinositide-dependent phosphorylation. Annu Rev Biochem 1999;68:965-1014.
110. Grunwald V, Hidalgo M. Developing inhibitors of the epidermal growth factor receptor for cancer treatment. J Nal Cancer Inst 2003;95:851-67.
111. Bonner JA, Harari PM, Giralt J, et al. Radiotherapy plus cetuximab for squamous cell carcinoma of the head and neck. N Engl J Med 2006;354:567-78.
112. Shepherd FA, Rodrigues Pereira J, Ciuleanu T, et al. Erlotinib in previously treated non-small cell lung cancer. N Engl J Med 2005;353:123-32.
113. Moore MJ, Goldstein D, Hamm J, et al. Erlotinib plus gemcitabine compared with gemcitabine alone in patients with advanced pancreatic cancer: A phase III trial of the National Cancer Institute of Canada Clinical Trials Group. J Clin Oncol 2007; 25:1960-6.
114. Pai R, Soreghan B, Szabo IL, Pavelka M, Baatar D, and Tarnawski AS. Prostaglandin E2 transactivates EGF receptor: a novel mechanism for promoting colon cancer growth and gastrointestinal hypertrophy. Nat Med 2002; 8: 289-93.

115. Shao J, Lee SB, Guo H, Evers BM, Sheng H. Prostaglandin E2 stimulates the growth of colon cancer cells via induction of amphiregulin. Cancer Res 2003;63:5218-23.
116. Buchanan FG, Wang D, Bargiacchi F, DuBois RN. Prostaglandin E2 regulates cell migration via the intracellular activation of the epidermal growth factor receptor. J Biol Chem 2003;278:35451-7.
117. Buchanan FG, Gorden DL, Matta P, Shi Q, Matrisian LM, DuBois RN. Role of β-arrestin 1 in the metastatic progression of colorectal cancer. Proc Natl Acad Sci USA 2006;103:1492-7.
118. Thiery JP. Epithelial-mesenchymal transitions in tumor progression. Nat Rev Cancer 2002;2:442-54.
119. Bremnes RM, Veve R, Gabrielson E, et al. High-throughput tissue microarray analysis used to evaluate biology and prognostic significance of the E-cadherin pathway in non-small cell lung cancer. J Clin Oncol 2002;20:2417-28.
120. Lu Z, Ghosh S, Wang Z, Hunter T. Downregulation of caveolin-1 function by EGF leads to the loss of E-cadherin, increased transcriptional activity of β-catenin, and enhanced tumor cell invasion. Cancer Cell 2003;4:499-515.
121. Tsuji M, DuBois RN. Alterations in cellular adhesion and apoptosis in epithelial cell overexpressing prostaglandin endoperoxide synthase 2. Cell 1995;83:493-501.
122. Dohadwala M, Yang S-C, Luo J,, et al. Cyclooxygenase-2-dependent regulation of E-cadherin: prostaglandin E_2 induces transcriptional repressors ZEB1 and Snail in non-small cell lung cancer. Cancer Res 2006;66:5338-45.
123. Thomson S, Buck E, Petti F, et al. Epithelial to mesenchymal transition is a determinant of sensitivity of non-small-cell lung carcinoma cell lines and xenografts to epidermal growth factor receptor inhibition. Cancer Res 2005;65:9455-62.
124. Krysan K, Reckamp KL, Dalwadi H,et.al.. PGE_2 activates MAPK/Erk pathway signaling and cell proliferation in non-small lung cancer cells in an EGF receptor-independent manner. Cancer Res 2005;65:6275-81.
125. Zhang X, Chen Z, Choe MS, et al. Tumor growth inhibition by simultaneously blocking EGFR and cyclooxygenase-2 in a xenograft model. Clin Cancer Res 2005;11:6261-9.
126. Wirth LJ, Haddad RI, Lindeman NI, et al. Phase I study of gefitinib plus celecoxib in recurrent or metastatic squamous cell carcinoma of the head and neck. J Clin Oncol 2005;23:6976-81.
127. Reckamp KL, Krysan K, Morrow JD, et al. A phase I trial to determine the optimal biological dose of celecoxib when combined with erlotinib in advanced non-small cell lung cancer. Clin Cancer Res 2006;12:3381-8.
128. Backlund MG, Mann JR, Holla VR, et al. 15-hydroxyprostaglandin dehydrogenase is down-regulated in colorectal cancer. J Biol Chem 2005;280:3217-23.

22 Cellular Sensitivity to EGF Receptor Inhibitors

Stuart Thomson, John D. Haley, and Robert Yauch

Contents

Introduction
Development of EGFR-Directed Inhibitors
EGFR Biology as a Predictor of Sensitivity
Epithelial-Mesenchymal Transition (EMT) and its
 Correlation with Insensitivity to EGFR Inhibitors
Alternate Receptor Signaling: Bypassing EGFR
Summary
References

Abstract

The EGFR pathway is a critical signaling pathway regulation cell proliferation and survival. As such, it is frequently deregulated in cancer through over expression of both EGF family ligands and receptors and by mutation of critical components within the pathway. These characteristics have made this signaling axis an attractive target for the development of molecularly targeted therapies in the treatment of cancer. To date there are numerous small molecule inhibitors and antibodies, either already in clinical use or in late stage clinical trials, that specifically target EGFR. These inhibitors have achieved great success in treating cancer patients and have generated a large amount of interest in identifying molecular markers that predict clinical benefit and mechanisms of resistance to such treatments. The first major breakthrough in this line of research was the identification of mutations in the EGFR kinase domain, which rendered the receptor hypersensitive to the actions of small molecule kinase inhibitors. However, the mutation rate was insufficient to explain the overall clinical benefit observed with these inhibitors, suggesting patients with wild-type EGFR also received some benefit. Subsequently, numerous efforts have been made to identify biomarkers of response and resistance other than EGFR mutational status.

Here we will summarize the current literature describing attempts to identify such markers, with particular emphasis on markers of sensitivity and resistance to small molecule EGFR tyrosine kinase inhibitors (TKIs). These approaches have encompassed the analysis of expression levels, both at the protein and genomic level, of EGFR and the closely related family members HER2 and HER3 and the analysis of the mutational status of downstream components of the EGFR pathway. In addition, we will highlight the role of the epithelial to mesenchymal transition (EMT) in sensitivity to small molecule EGFR TKIs and finally the potential role of alternative signaling cascades as a mode of cellular resistance to EGFR inhibition.

From: *Cancer Drug Discovery and Development: EGFR Signaling Networks in Cancer Therapy*
Edited by: J. D. Haley and W. J. Gullick, DOI: 10.1007/978-1-59745-356-1_22
© 2008 Humana Press, a part of Springer Science+Business Media, LLC

Key Words: EGFR, HER2, HER3, erlotinib, gefitinib, epithelial to mesenchymal transition, tyrosine kinase inhibitors

1. INTRODUCTION

The development of small molecule inhibitors selectively targeting critical cellular proteins has recently begun to produce clinically significant results in the treatment of cancer. Although perhaps not living up to the "magic bullet," there are clear advantages of these targeted therapies over more traditional chemotherapy regimes in efficacy and toxicity. One area of molecularly targeted therapies (MTT) that has received a great deal of recent attention concerns agents that target the epidermal growth factor receptor (EGFR). Signaling through EGFR is frequently dysregulated in solid tumors, leading to abnormal activation of intracellular signaling pathways (*1*). Both small molecule inhibitors and humanized antibodies directed against this critical receptor have been developed and have been used clinically in the treatment of cancer for a number of years. The clinical use of such targeted therapies has exposed our limitations in understanding how to best utilize these agents and highlights the need to identify clinical biomarkers of response.

In this chapter we will provide a brief overview of the anti-EGFR inhibitors that have been developed to date, concentrating primarily on the ones in current clinical use. In addition we will provide an overview of the current literature on the identification and use of biomarkers to predict sensitivity to this class of molecularly targeted therapy.

2. DEVELOPMENT OF EGFR-DIRECTED INHIBITORS

Small molecule inhibitors of this trans-membrane tyrosine kinase, such as erlotinib (Tarceva®, OSI Pharmaceuticals/Genentech/Roche) and gefitinib (Iressa®, Astra Zeneca) have been developed and tested clinically. Both erlotinib and gefitinib were approved for the treatment of NSCLC patients who have failed two or three previous rounds of chemotherapy (*2*). In addition, erlotinib was approved in the United States and Europe for the treatment, in combination with gemcitabine (Gemzar, Eli-Lilley), of pancreatic cancer. Two anti-EGFR antibodies approved for the treatment of colorectal cancers include cetuximab (Erbitux, Imclone/Bristol Myers Squibb) and panitumamab (Vectibix, Abgenix/Amgen).

The recent success of these inhibitors has further supported the development of additional antagonists capable of providing potential advantages over these existing therapies. New anti-EGFR therapies have focused on the development of inhibitors with multi-targeted activities, better potency or pharmacokinetic properties and the ability to overcome erlotinib/gefitinib-resistance mutations in EGFR. Preclinical studies have suggested that the dual inhibition of both EGFR and HER2 could result in greater tumor growth inhibition compared to EGFR inhibition alone, which has led to the development of several dual-kinase SMIs. The most advanced molecule in this class, lapatinib (GlaxoSmithKline), was recently shown to delay disease progression in trastuzumab refractory breast cancer (*3*) and is likely to receive FDA approval in this setting. Additional dual-EGFR/HER2 kinase SMIs, capable of providing prolonged target suppression through their irreversible binding properties are in earlier stages of clinical development and include HKI272 (Wyeth), BIBW-2992 (Boehringer-Ingelheim) and CI-1003 (Pfizer) (see Table 22.1). HKI272 provides the additional property of being capable of inhibiting the activity of EGFR in the context of erlotinib/gefitinib-resistance mutations in preclinical models. The development of multi-targeted SMIs has also extended beyond the HER family receptors and includes EGFR antagonists with anti-angiogenic activity through the targeting of VEGF-R2, such

Table 22.1
EGFR Antagonists in Clinical Development

Type	Therapeutic	Company	Target	Stage of development (indications)
SMI (reversible)	Erlotinib	OSI/Genentech/Roche	EGFR	Approved (NSCLC)
	Gefitinib	AstraZeneca	EGFR	Approved (NSCLC)
	Lapatinib	GlaxoSmithKline	EGFR, HER2	phase III (breast)
	ZD6474	AstraZeneca	EGFR, VEGFR2	phase III (NSCLC)
	AEE788	Novartis	EGFR, HER2, VEGFR2	phase I/II (GBM)
SMI (irreversible)	HKI-272	Wyeth	EGFR, HER2	phase II (NSCLC, breast)
	BIBW-2992	Boehringer Ingelheim	EGFR, HER2	phase II (breast)
mAb	Cetuximab	ImClone/Bristol-Myers Squibb	EGFR	Approved (colorectal)
	Panitumamab	Abgenix/Amgen	EGFR	Approved (colorectal)
	Matuzumab	EMD/Merck KgGA	EGFR	phase II (NSCLC, esophageal, gastric)
	Pertuzumab	Genentech/Roche	HER2	phase II (NSCLC, ovarian, breast)

as ZD6474 (AstraZeneca) and AEE788 (Novartis). Finally, the development of additional monoclonal antibodies has not been overlooked, with the humanized anti-EGFR monoclonal antibody, Matuzumab (EMD/Merck KgGA) and an anti-HER2 monoclonal antibody capable of inhibiting the dimerization of HER2 with EGFR (Pertuzumab, Genentech/Roche) both in phase II clinical evaluation.

While the clinical benefit provided by EGFR inhibitors is impressive when compared to current standard of care, it also reveals the current limitations of this MTT approach. For example in the phase III NSCLC erlotinib trial BR.21 (4), overall response rate was only 8.9% and yet the hazard ratio for treatment benefit associated with overall survival was 0.7. In addition to suggesting that response rate, as measured by RECIST criteria, was not a good indicator of potential survival benefit, this data also suggested that although patients clearly benefited from erlotinib treatment, a substantial population did not receive any clinical benefit. This observation has generated research to identify clinical markers predictive of response, as well as to identify the underlying mechanistic explanation for a restricted response.

3. EGFR BIOLOGY AS A PREDICTOR OF SENSITIVITY

While EGFR expression and mutational status have been the most extensively studied mechanisms for sensitization and resistance to EGFR inhibitors, increasing evidence has supported an important role for co-receptors in modifying the response to EGFR antagonists. Here we will touch on the role of each of these predictors of response, as well as two critical signaling pathways, Ras and Akt, that potentially impact on efficacy of EGFR targeted therapies.

3.1. EGFR Mutations

The identification of mutations in the EGFR kinase domain (5-7) and the demonstration that these mutated receptors were more sensitive to erlotinib (8) led to the hypothesis that these inhibitors would only be effective against tumors bearing heterozygous mutations in the EGFR gene. The in vitro demonstration of prolonged ligand-dependent signaling from these mutated receptors and hypersensitivity of cell lines bearing these mutations suggested that these types of tumors would be more addicted to EGFR signaling and thus be more susceptible to inhibition of the pathway. Another key observation was the identification of a second point mutation in tumors (T790M) that had become resistant to EGFR inhibitor treatment, leading to the analogy with the acquired-resistance model proposed for imatinib (Gleevec®) (9). However, there remains some controversy as to the importance of EGFR mutations in the clinical setting. Initial retrospective analyses of gefitinib treated NSCLC tumors for EGFR mutation suggested that those testing positive for mutation received the most benefit from gefitinib treatment as measured by both response rate and survival (10, 11). However, analysis of the only placebo-controlled EGFR inhibitor study completed to date (BR21) concluded that there was no significant difference in survival in patients with mutation in the erlotinib treated arm compared to the placebo arm (12). In addition, data from the BR.21 (12), Talent (13) and Tribute (14, 15) studies suggest that, within the placebo arm, patients with mutation in EGFR survive longer than those with wild type EGFR irrespective of treatment. The concept that EGFR mutations may indicate a more positive prognosis contradicts the widely held belief that EGFR overexpression and activation is a poor prognostic factor. This may explain the longer survival observed in patients with mutation in the non-placebo controlled studies. These mutations and their impact on EGFR biology are described in detail in Chapter 20.

3.2. EGFR Copy Number, IHC, and FISH Analysis

The initial approaches to identifying clinical biomarkers of response focused on quantification of the target within patient biopsy tissue. This has been particularly successful in the case of measurement of HER2 protein levels by IHC in breast cancer tissues as selection criteria for patients receiving trastuzumab (HER2 directed humanized monoclonal antibody, Herceptin®). Patients with elevated ErbB2 expression showed a larger benefit to trastuzumab treatment as compared with those expressing low levels (16). As elevations in EGFR protein expression and gene copy number are frequent in both squamous and non-squamous NSCLC (17), this principle has been applied retrospectively to EGFR-related therapy trials in NSCLC but with less conclusive results.

3.2.1. EGFR Protein Expression

It is clear from a number of studies that protein expression levels of EGFR in cell lines does not correlate with sensitivity to either erlotinib or gefitinib (Fig. 22.1; (18-20)), but rather it is the activation of this pathway through autocrine ligand production that is important in defining sensitivity to these inhibitors in vitro (19, 20).

Extensive efforts by a number of different groups have been undertaken to measure EGFR protein levels in patient tumor tissue by immunohistochemistry (IHC) in order to investigate both its prognostic significance (21) and also its role as a predictive marker of response to EGFR therapy (reviewed in (22)). However, in contrast to the success of the HER2 test, these studies have been controversial, with no clear relationship between EGFR IHC protein levels and survival or response to therapy.

The reasons for this difference between EGFR and HER2 as predictors of response to their respectively targeted therapies remain unclear. Multiple centers have used differing

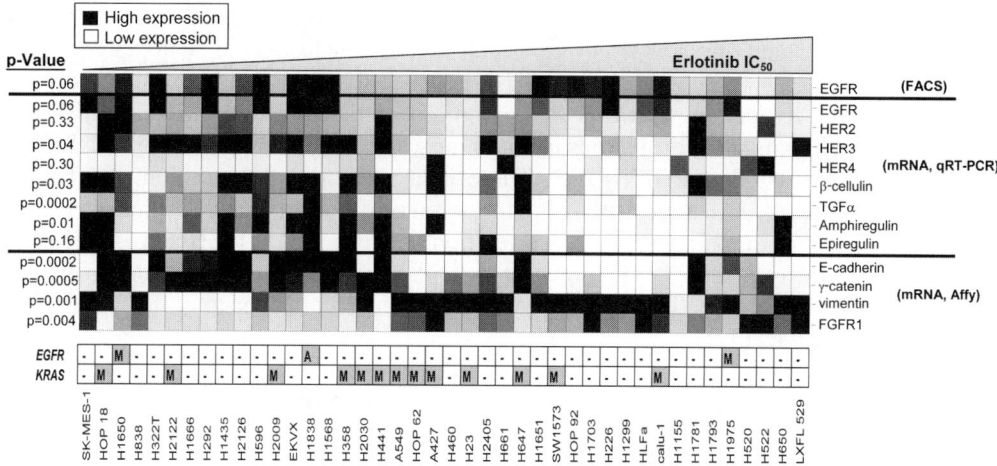

Fig. 22.1. **Characterization of the Relationship of Cellular Sensitivity to Erlotinib with EGFR-pathway Variables and EMT in a Panel of NSCLC Cell Lines.** Inhibition of cell growth in the presence of erlotinib was determined across a panel of NSCLC cell lines. Cell lines are sorted based on ascending IC50 (or decreasing sensitivity to erlotinib). The *EGFR* and *KRAS* gene status are depicted below the heatmap (A, amplification; M, mutation). The heatmap represents either protein expression (FACS-based) or mRNA expression (qRT-PCR or Affymetrix-microarray chip-based) of various HER family receptors/ligands and classical EMT marker genes. The p-value was calculated from a one-sided t-test of the sensitive versus resistant cell lines. Figure was modified from Yauch et al. (*20*).

antibody, assay and scoring systems giving rise to variability in the assay procedures. For example, scoring of intensity of staining (0–3) of EGFR protein levels in erlotinib and gefitinib trials in NSCLC (reviewed (*23*) (*10, 24, 25*)); or a cetuximab trial in colorectal cancer (*26*) failed to show any relationship between EGFR protein levels and response. However, other studies have employed a scoring system that employs both signal intensity (0–4) and percentage of cells stained within the section (0–100%), thus giving a range of scoring from 0–400 (*27*). This study has suggested that high level of EGFR expression does correlate with increased time to progression and survival in erlotinib treated patients. In addition a retrospective analysis of the gefitinib ISEL trial indicated that EGFR protein expression was related to clinical outcome, although the correlation did not reach statistical significance (*28*). Analysis of tumor samples from the BR21 trial, using a similar scoring system, also indicated that high EGFR protein expression was linked to clinical outcome (*12*).

These studies demonstrate the limitations of the currently available IHC EGFR tests and highlight the need for a uniform assay and scoring system in order to evaluate this potential biomarker. For now it seems that the limits of detection may exclude patients capable of response to EGFR TKIs and antibodies (*29*) if selection were based solely upon this criterion.

3.2.2. EGFR FISH

In parallel to measurement of EGFR protein levels by IHC, many groups have successfully attempted to measure EGFR at the genomic level. EGFR copy number has been reported to correlate with response to EGFR TKIs. For example the BR.21 placebo controlled trial of erlotinib in 2nd and 3rd line NSCLC noted a 20% response rate in EGFR amplified patients while only 2.4% in the unamplified subset (p=0.03; reviewed (*30*)). Similarly a study of 102 NSCLC patients receiving the EGFR TKI gefitinib reported a correlation between EGFR FISH score and both time to progression (p<0.001) and survival (p=0.03; (*27*)). These latter studies used different metrics for the scoring of FISH positivity, as compared to an earlier study of (183) NSCLC patients who showed a trend toward EGFR FISH score and survival (*17*). Nevertheless, the conclusions of both studies were similar: that EGFR gene copy number (FISH+) is generally increased in patients benefiting from EGFR TKI therapy. However the lack of concordance between EGFR FISH and EGFR IHC data highlight the difficulties in obtaining a standardized approach to both EGFR immunohistochemistry and EGFR FISH. These data also raise the question of whether EGFR copy number is indicative of EGFR expression or if it more generally detects errors in DNA replication or repair. Recently a correlation between EGFR FISH and EGFR activating mutations was observed (*31*), however patients with increased copies of EGFR but with wild type EGFR showed increased time to progression as compared to FISH⁻/EGFR wild type patients (reviewed (*32*)).

3.3. EGFR Dimerization Partners

3.3.1. HER2

In addition to mutations in downstream effectors of EGFR activity, genetic alterations in the EGFR coreceptor, HER2, have also been reported to modify the activity of EGFR inhibitors. Intragenic somatic mutations in the kinase domain of HER2 have been described in ~4% of lung adenocarcinomas and can result in enhanced HER2 tyrosine kinase activity (*33, 34*). Activating HER2 mutations are expected to be a negative predictor of response to EGFR antagonists, as the ectopic expression of mutant HER2 in cell lines leads to resistance to EGFR inhibition (*34*). Although the data is extremely limited, no patients with HER2 mutations have been reported to respond to gefitinib (*35*). Interestingly, cell lines expressing mutant HER2 remain exquisitely sensitive to the dual ErbB kinase inhibitors, lapatinib and CI-1033, supporting the potential utility of HER2-targeted therapies in this small fraction of NSCLC.

In contrast, HER2 expression itself has been demonstrated to confer increased sensitivity to EGFR antagonists. Cappuzo et al. have reported that increased HER2 copy number in EGFR-positive NSCLC patients treated with gefitinib was associated with a significantly better response rate, a longer time to progression and a trend toward better survival (*27*). Although further clinical studies are warranted, preclinical studies have provided additional support of this concept. Multiple groups have demonstrated that HER2 overexpressing cancer cell lines and xenografts exhibit enhanced sensitivity to the antiproliferative effects of gefitinib (*36, 37*). The off-target activity of gefitinib on HER2 may not be sufficient to explain this effect, as the affinity of gefitinib for receptor HER2 dephosphorylation is 100-fold less compared to EGFR and it is unlikely that concentrations of gefitinib achieved in patients would be effective against HER2. It is possible that the elevated levels of HER2 could preferentially drive EGFR/HER2 heterodimerization over EGFR homodimerization leading to increased EGFR activation (*38*). HER2 is not only the preferred dimerization partner for the ErbB family members, but it's expression has been demonstrated to enhance the recycling rate of EGFR leading to a reduction in receptors that are internalized for degradation (*39, 40*). Interestingly, it has also been suggested that gefitinib can disrupt the formation of HER2/HER3 heterodimers in HER2-overexpressing cells, resulting in the sequestration of the HER2 and HER3 into inactive EGFR heterodimers (*41*)

3.3.2. HER3

Despite the lack of intrinsic tyrosine kinase activity, recent reports have also proposed an intriguing role for HER3 in regulating EGFR TKI activity. Upon heterodimerization with other HER family members, HER3 can be transphosphorylated and subsequently activate the PI3K pathway. In transformed cell types it has been suggested that HER3 is the primary means of coupling EGFR activation to the PI3K/Akt pathway (*42, 43*), and this coupling has been linked to EGFR antagonist sensitivity (*44*). In support of this notion, a correlation between

HER3 expression and EGFR TKI sensitivity has been reported in cell lines by several groups (*19, 20, 44, 45*) and the ability of EGFR inhibition to decrease Akt pathway activity has been associated with EGFR TKI sensitivity. Furthermore, it has recently been reported that the inability of extended EGFR TKI treatment to sustain Akt dephosphorylation through HER3 reactivation may serve as mechanism by which tumors elude EGFR antagonist activity (*46*). Taken together, these studies have implicated a potentially important role for this kinase-inactive dimerization partner in linking the activity of EGFR antagonists to downstream survival pathways and drug efficacy. The clinical significance of HER3 expression and/or transphorylation status remains to be elucidated.

3.4. EGFR Regulated Downstream Signaling Pathways
3.4.1. K-Ras

An additional factor suggested to predict for the efficacy of EGFR inhibitors has been the mutational status of *KRAS* in NSCLC. K-ras is a small GTPase that lies directly downstream of the EGFR and is a key branching point for EGF-related signaling cascades (*1*). *KRAS* is frequently mutated in NSCLC (25%) and it is believed that activating mutations of this signaling component may override any potential benefit of EGFR inhibition. Preclinical studies do not seem to support this hypothesis, as no correlation between *KRAS* mutation status and erlotinib sensitivity has been reported in either NSCLC or pancreatic cancer cell lines (*19, 20, 45, 47, 48*). Furthermore, mutant K-ras is unable to confer resistance to EGFR inhibition in either lung adenocarcinomas derived from $Kras^{LA1}$ transgenic mice or in immortalized human bronchial epithelial cells transfected with mutant *KRAS* (*47*). However, a limited number of clinical studies have suggested that *KRAS* mutations may correlate with a reduction in patient benefit to EGFR inhibitors. Analysis of the TRIBUTE trial suggested that *KRAS* mutations correlated with a reduced time to progression in patients receiving erlotinib in combination with chemotherapy (*14*). Furthermore, an analysis of albeit a small number of patients in several studies suggested that patients harboring tumors with *KRAS* mutations showed no response to either EGFR TKIs or cetuximab administered as a single agent and/or in combination with various chemotherapy regimes (*35, 49, 50*). Nevertheless, larger prospective studies would be necessary to more definitely demonstrate whether *KRAS* mutations would predict for a poorer clinical outcome in the approved, single-agent setting.

As opposed to playing an active role in conferring resistance, *KRAS* mutations may be reflective of a tumor driven by distinctive molecular defects promoting tumorigenesis and progression. In support of this theory, *KRAS* mutations are associated with tumors arising in patients with a history of smoking, whereas response to EGFR TKIs is associated with non-smoking histories (*24*). Furthermore, there have been no reports of *KRAS* mutations arising in patients who progressed on erlotinib treatment, suggesting that it is not a main mechanism of acquired resistance to EGFR therapy. Links between EGFR and K-ras signaling are described in detail in Chapter 7.

3.4.2. Akt pathway

Tumors may utilize the EGFR-independent activation of PKB/Akt as an additional mechanism to resist EGFR antagonists. Genetic aberrations in the PI3K pathway leading to Akt phosphorylation have been reported to occur in subsets of human neoplasms through various mechanisms, including activating mutations in the catalytic and regulatory subunits of PI3K itself and through loss of the negative regulator of PI3K, PTEN (*51*) (see also Chapter 8). Decreased PTEN levels have been shown to be associated with resistance to EGFR inhibitors both in vitro and in vivo (*52, 53*); and conversely, the restoration of PTEN activity in PTEN-deficient cell lines results in increased sensitivity to EGFR TKIs (*53-55*).

Even in the context of EGFR activating mutations, further activation of Akt through the ectopic expression of oncogenic PI3K (p110α^{E545K}) or oncogenic Akt (myristoylated Akt) is sufficient to confer resistance to gefitinib. Clinically, recognition of the underlying mechanisms leading to PKB/Akt activation is imperative to developing biomarkers of response/resistance, as studies evaluating the predictive value of phosphorylated Akt alone in patients treated with EGFR antagonists have led to conflicting results. This is likely due to the fact that activated EGFR could also drive Akt phosphorylation, which is supported by preclinical studies demonstrating higher levels of Akt phosphorylation in EGFR mutant vs. wild-type expressing cells (*7*). Whereas several studies have reported negative associations of high phospho-Akt with patient benefit to EGFR TKIs (*35, 56*), high tumor phospho-Akt has been positively associated with better outcome when assessed in the context of EGFR mutations (*10*) or EGFR FISH positivity (*27*). Thus, identifying the underlying mechanism leading to PKB/Akt activation in a tumor may not only provide a more predictive biomarker of EGFR antagonist activity, but also lead to the rational selection of novel therapeutic combinations capable of overcoming potential resistance.

4. EPITHELIAL-MESENCHYMAL TRANSITION (EMT) AND ITS CORRELATION WITH INSENSITIVITY TO EGFR INHIBITORS

Although mutations in the EGF receptor tyrosine kinase domain have been strongly implicated in predicting clinical response to small molecule kinase inhibitors, it was clear from the phase III clinical trial of erlotinib that patients who expressed wild type EGFR received clear clinical benefit from such therapy (*12*). These observations, coupled with the fact that EGFR mutations have only been reported in approximately 10% of the NSCLC population, prompted a number of groups to investigate what additional markers may predict sensitivity of patients, carrying wild type EGFR, to small molecule tyrosine kinase-inhibitor therapy. A number of independent groups have used genomic and proteomic profiling of NSCLC cell lines to identify molecular markers of response to small molecule EGFR tyrosine kinase inhibitors.

Satisfyingly, three groups independently identified similar groups of genes and encoded proteins in NSCLC cell lines as being predictive of EGFR inhibitor sensitivity in vitro and in xenograft models (*19, 20, 57, 58*). It was apparent that cell lines deemed sensitive to erlotinib in in vitro growth inhibition assays expressed classical epithelial cell markers, such as E-cadherin and γ-catenin, whereas those deemed insensitive to erlotinib treatment had lost such markers and instead gained expression of markers more traditionally associated with mesenchymal cells, such as vimentin, fibronectin and Zeb1/TCF8 (Fig. 22.1; (*19, 20, 58*)). These changes in the protein expression profiles of the cells strongly implied that the erlotinib-insensitive cell lines had undergone an epithelial to mesenchymal transition or EMT. These observations have been extended to other cancer indications such as pancreatic, colorectal, and breast cancer cell lines, strongly suggesting that this is an important and widespread indicator of EGFR inhibitor sensitivity in cancer (*59*).

EMT is a well-established phenotypic transformation in development (*60*), whereby cells originating from an epithelial layer undergo a transition to a more mesenchymal phenotype, resulting in cells with a more motile nature. This process is reversible, suggesting a large degree of plasticity within these cells. It has become apparent in recent years that tumor cells utilize a process very similar to developmental EMT during tumor progression. There is increasing evidence that tumor cells, especially at the invasive front of the tumor mass (*61*), transition from an epithelial phenotype to a mesenchymal-like phenotype allowing the cells to invade the surrounding stromal tissue and migrate into the lymphatic or vasculature and metastasize to distant sites (*60*).

One of the most studied and key markers of EMT is E-cadherin. This is a transmembrane protein involved in Ca^{2+}-dependent cell-cell adhesion (62). Loss of E-cadherin has long been associated with poor prognosis in cancer patients and it has been described as a tumor suppressor gene (63). Indeed, Christofori and collegues reported that the loss of E-cadherin expression promoted the transition from adenoma to carcinoma in a mouse pancreatic cancer model (64). These studies imply that rather than being a marker of a cellular phenotypic change, E-cadherin is actively involved in maintaining an epithelial character. In addition, a retrospective analysis of a phase III trial in NSCLC with erlotinib plus chemotherapy compared to chemotherapy alone (TRIBUTE), showed that E-cadherin expression was a significant predictive marker for increased time to disease progression mediated by erlotinib treatment (20), supporting the previous in vitro studies of E-cadherin positivity correlating with sensitivity to EGFR small molecule inhibitors. Although further clinical evaluation is clearly required, these initial studies suggest that E-cadherin, and EMT as a process, may be excellent biomarkers for the efficacy of EGFR inhibitors in cancer patients.

The physiological cues that initiate EMT are varied and complex. A large number of growth factors (EGF, PDGF, VEGF, TGFb, Wnt, SDF1, PGE2), cytokines (ILE1, IL) and stress stimuli (hypoxia) have been reported to induce EMT in cell-based models (60). In general, all of these stimuli are known to induce tumor progression through proliferative and anti-apoptotic pathways as well as through the induction of EMT. Although these signals are diverse, there are a common set of transcription factors that appear to be the key regulators of this transition and include SNAI1, ZEB1, SLUG, and TWIST. These factors directly bind to the promoter region of a large number of genes, including the E-cadherin gene, shutting off their transcription through recruitment of chromatin modifying complexes (65). Of note overexpression or down-regulation of these factors results in downstream genes being both up- or down-regulated, suggesting that they control a complex gene expression program (66). In addition overexpression of each of these factors in an epithelial cell background has been reported to induce EMT, with the resulting mesenchymal-like cells exhibiting increased motility, invasiveness and tumorigenicity in nude mice. Conversely, silencing of SNAIL in mouse cancer cells reduces their ability to grow in vivo (67). These observations strongly imply a critical role for these transcription factors in regulating EMT and tumor progression and imply that strategies aimed at targeting this transition in cancer patients may have clear clinical benefit.

The reasons why tumor cells that have undergone EMT are now less sensitive to EGFR inhibition than their epithelial counterparts remain unclear. However, it does appear that cells that have undergone EMT express lower levels of EGF-family ligands (Fig. 22.1, (19, 20)), implying a reduced dependency upon the EGFR pathway. There are some reports of a physical interaction between E-cadherin and EGFR (68), suggesting an active role of E-cadherin in regulating EGFR signaling, possibly in a ligand-independent manner. Loss of E-cadherin during EMT may thus render the cells less dependent upon EGFR signaling and so less sensitive to its inhibition. In a similar vain, ErbB3 has been shown to be expressed to high levels in epithelial erlotinib-sensitive cell lines (19, 44, 45) and down regulated in mesenchymal-like cells, suggesting it plays a prominent role in erlotinib sensitivity. ErbB3 is known to couple strongly to the PI3K pathway and as cells transition to a mesenchymal-like state, PI3K signaling may be controlled via alternative routes (Fig. 22.2 and section 5). Interestingly, ErbB3 transcript levels have been shown to decrease upon SNAIL expression, implying a potentially direct role for SNAIL in regulating ErbB3 expression. Therefore, a switch in dependency from EGFR-dependent proliferation and survival to EGFR-independent proliferation and survival during EMT may be one explanation for the reduced sensitivity to EGFR-directed inhibitors.

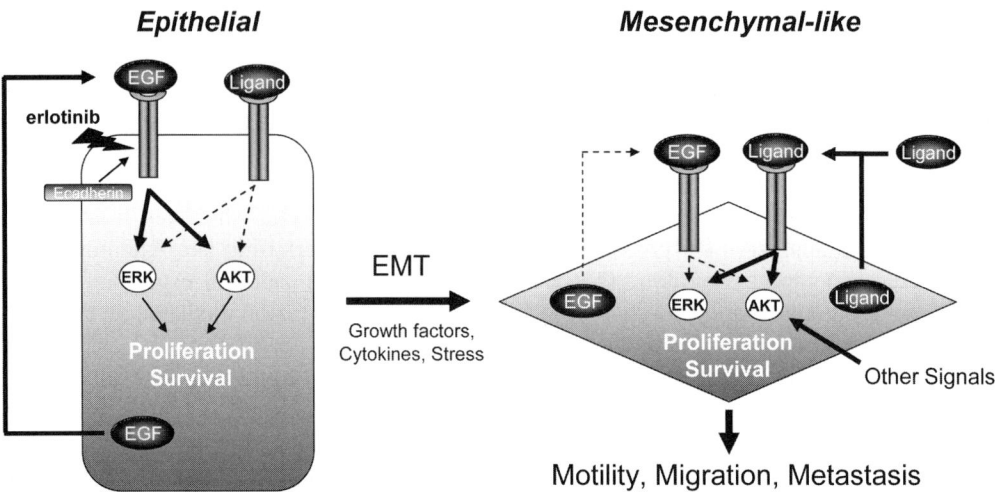

Fig. 22.2 Epithelial and mesenchymal cells switch from EGFR signaling to alternative routes of proliferation and survival

Also of interest is the fact that these critical EMT transcription factors have been described as anti-apoptotic factors (*69-71*), providing cells in which they were expressed with resistance to pro-apoptotic stimuli and chemotherapy agents. Of interest in this regard is a recent elegant study showing that recurrent mammary tumors in a mouse *neu2*-driven model express high levels of SNAIL and that the recurrent tumor cells have undergone EMT (*72*). The implication of this result is that mesenchymal-like cancer cells have the ability to remain dormant until an as yet unknown trigger stimulates their re-growth. These studies suggest that the mesenchymal-like cells resulting from an EMT are very different from their epithelial counterparts and have adapted to survive in different ways. Identifying and targeting these pathways in mesenchymal-like cells will hopefully lead to more effective cancer therapies which can be used alone and in combination with epithelial-directed therapies, such as EGFR TKIs.

5. ALTERNATE RECEPTOR SIGNALING: BYPASSING EGFR

Signal transduction pathways have been researched extensively over the years and linear pathways have been predicted for many receptor tyrosine kinase cascades. However, it is becoming increasingly clear that there is a high degree of crosstalk, parallel signaling, and interdependence among these pathways that leads to the activation of common proliferative and survival pathways. This finding opens up the concept of cells switching dependency upon certain RTK pathways resulting in a resistance mechanism to molecular targeted therapies. Indeed, it is apparent that NSCLC cell lines that are insensitive to EGFR TKIs express lower levels of EGF-family ligands, suggesting that these cells are less dependent upon EGFR signaling than the more sensitive cell lines (Figs. 22.1 and 22.2; (*19, 20*)). In the next section we highlight two different RTK signaling cascades that have been implicated in mediating resistance to anti-EGFR therapy.

5.1. IGF1R

IGF1R signaling is increasingly being seen as a major contributor to malignant progression and a number of approaches to target this receptor are currently underway (*73*).

IGF1R is a transmembrane receptor tyrosine kinase implicated in the transmission of proliferative and survival signals. Its ability to strongly couple to the PI3K/Akt pathway has implicated it as a resistance mechanism to EGFR kinase inhibition. There are a number of lines of evidence that lend support to this hypothesis. High concentrations of IGF1 were shown to block erlotinib-induced apoptosis in DiFi colon cancer cells, presumably through the IGF1-induced activation of the Akt pathway in the presence of EGFR inhibition (74). A different approach was undertaken by Chakravarti and colleagues (75), who identified 2 glioblastoma cell lines that differed in their sensitivity to the EGFR tyrosine kinase inhibitor AG1478. The less sensitive cell line exhibited up-regulation of IGF1R signaling and sustained activation of the PI3K/Akt axis in presence of the inhibitor. A more recent report has indicated that treatment of erlotinib-insensitive NSCLC cell lines, with erlotinib initiated an up regulation of IGF1R signaling, resulting in activation of cell survival pathways, including increased expression of survivan (76). Furthermore the authors presented evidence that a drug-resistant clone of H460 cells showed a higher sensitivity to an IGF1R inhibitor than the parental H460 cells. An additional study indicated increased signaling through IGF1R in both breast and prostate cancer cell lines resistant to gefitinib (77). These and other studies suggest that a combination strategy inhibiting both EGFR and IGF1R signaling would be more effective than inhibition of either pathway alone, and has been shown to be the case in a number of different pre-clinical models. Combination of EGFR and IGF1R inhibition has been reported to be synergistic in cell growth and apoptotic assays in glioblastoma cells (75), hepatocellular carcinoma cell lines (78), and NSCLC cell lines and xenografts (76).

Although the rationale for combination of EGFR and IGF1R inhibitors from pre-clinical models is strong, it will require extensive analysis of human tumor samples to identify biomarkers that predict whether such combinations would be successful in the clinic.

5.2. PDGFR

Activation of another receptor tyrosine kinase, PDGFR, has also been implicated as a potential mechanism for insensitivity to EGFR inhibition. PDGFR α and β have both been shown to be overexpressed in many different cancers, and have a role not only in primary tumor formation but angiogenesis and tumor cell metastasis (79, 80) through their activation of intracellular signaling cascades such as ERK and Akt.

These characteristics, much like IGF1R, suggest that PDGFR may be able to bypass EGFR-signaling and provide continued cell survival signals even in the presence of anti-EGFR therapies. Support for this idea was recently published by Adam and colleagues, who presented evidence of a dependency on PDGFR signaling in bladder cancer cell lines that were insensitive to gefitinib (81). PDGFR-dependency has also been reported in ovarian cancer cell lines (82). In addition, our group has shown that PDGF receptors are up-regulated in many NSCLC cell lines insensitive to erlotinib treatment that have undergone an EMT (Thomson et al., unpublished). This is particularly interesting as it suggests that as tumor cells undergo EMT they begin to become EGFR-independent and acquire alternative mechanisms of survival signaling (Fig 22.2). Furthermore, Jechlinger and colleagues have provided evidence that autocrine PDGFR signaling is required to maintain breast cancer cells in a mesenchymal-like state, and this promotes breast cancer metastasis (83). Indeed, PDGFR has been reported to be a good marker of more aggressive, metastatic cancer (82-84). These data then suggest that as tumors progress and become more highly invasive and metastatic they potentially lose their EGFR-dependency and acquire a dependency on PDGFR signaling. It would therefore be of interest to determine whether this is a wide spread phenomenon in patients who progress while on anti-EGFR therapy and if so whether a subsequent anti-PDGFR therapy would be of benefit.

6. SUMMARY

The development of molecularly targeted therapies has been a very successful approach in the ongoing battle against cancer however there are many unsolved problems. A more detailed understanding of which patients may benefit from treatment and in which ways tumor cells are able to escape from inhibition of a particular target are required to allow more effective next generation inhibitors to be developed.

We have begun to understand some of the issues associated with EGFR-directed therapies. The identification of EGFR kinase domain mutations was a big step forward in being able to predict which patients may be most susceptible to small molecule inhibitors. Equally, the observation that patients with wild type EGFR may still receive clinical benefit from these agents and the pre-clinical identification of EMT as an excellent correlate with EGFR-directed small molecule inhibitor sensitivity suggest both a way of selecting patients and of identifying additional ways of attacking tumor cells. Taken together it is tempting to speculate that as EGFR-dependent epithelial tumor cells progress they undergo an EMT to become more migratory and invasive. In doing so they also lose dependency upon EGFR signaling and use alternative pathways to activate critical signaling nodes (Fig. 22.2). As discussed here some of these alternative methods could include signaling through the IGF1R or PDGFR pathways, but could also encompass any of the many ways in which these signaling nodes can be activated. The ways in which these tumor cells adapt and progress may be dictated by the cues they receive from the microenvironment. It remains a major challenge to unravel the relevance of these different stimuli to allow the rational design of future molecular targeted therapies that will replace and augment those that are already available.

REFERENCES

1. Yarden Y, Sliwkowski MX. Untangling the ErbB signalling network. Nature reviews 2001;2:127-37.
2. Siegel-Lakhai WS, Beijnen JH, Schellens JH. Current knowledge and future directions of the selective epidermal growth factor receptor inhibitors erlotinib (Tarceva) and gefitinib (Iressa). The oncologist 2005;10:579-89.
3. Konecny GE, Pegram MD, Venkatesan N, et al. Activity of the dual kinase inhibitor lapatinib (GW572016) against HER-2-overexpressing and trastuzumab-treated breast cancer cells. Cancer research 2006;66:1630-9.
4. Shepherd FA, Rodrigues Pereira J, Ciuleanu T, et al. Erlotinib in previously treated non-small-cell lung cancer. The New England journal of medicine 2005;353:123-32.
5. Lynch TJ, Bell DW, Sordella R, et al. Activating mutations in the epidermal growth factor receptor underlying responsiveness of non-small-cell lung cancer to gefitinib. The New England journal of medicine 2004;350:2129-39.
6. Pao W, Miller V, Zakowski M, et al. EGF receptor gene mutations are common in lung cancers from "never smokers" and are associated with sensitivity of tumors to gefitinib and erlotinib. Proceedings of the National Academy of Sciences of the United States of America 2004;101:13306-11.
7. Sordella R, Bell DW, Haber DA, Settleman J. Gefitinib-sensitizing EGFR mutations in lung cancer activate anti-apoptotic pathways. Science 2004;305:1163-7.
8. Carey KD, Garton AJ, Romero MS, et al. Kinetic analysis of epidermal growth factor receptor somatic mutant proteins shows increased sensitivity to the epidermal growth factor receptor tyrosine kinase inhibitor, erlotinib. Cancer research 2006;66:8163-71.
9. Ritchie E, Nichols G. Mechanisms of resistance to imatinib in CML patients: a paradigm for the advantages and pitfalls of molecularly targeted therapy. Current cancer drug targets 2006;6:645-57.
10. Han SW, Kim TY, Hwang PG, et al. Predictive and prognostic impact of epidermal growth factor receptor mutation in non-small-cell lung cancer patients treated with gefitinib. J Clin Oncol 2005;23:2493-501.
11. Tokumo M, Toyooka S, Kiura K, et al. The relationship between epidermal growth factor receptor mutations and clinicopathologic features in non-small cell lung cancers. Clin Cancer Res 2005;11:1167-73.

12. Tsao MS, Sakurada A, Cutz JC, et al. Erlotinib in lung cancer - molecular and clinical predictors of outcome. The New England journal of medicine 2005;353:133-44.
13. Fuster LM, Sandler AB. Select clinical trials of erlotinib (OSI-774) in non-small-cell lung cancer with emphasis on phase III outcomes. Clinical lung cancer 2004;6 Suppl 1:S24-9.
14. Eberhard DA, Johnson BE, Amler LC, et al. Mutations in the epidermal growth factor receptor and in KRAS are predictive and prognostic indicators in patients with non-small-cell lung cancer treated with chemotherapy alone and in combination with erlotinib. J Clin Oncol 2005;23:5900-9.
15. Herbst RS, Prager D, Hermann R, et al. TRIBUTE: a phase III trial of erlotinib hydrochloride (OSI-774) combined with carboplatin and paclitaxel chemotherapy in advanced non-small-cell lung cancer. J Clin Oncol 2005;23:5892-9.
16. Fornier M, Risio M, Van Poznak C, Seidman A. HER2 testing and correlation with efficacy of trastuzumab therapy. Oncology (Williston Park, NY 2002;16:1340-8, 51-2; discussion 52, 55-8.
17. Hirsch FR, Varella-Garcia M, Bunn PA, Jr., et al. Epidermal growth factor receptor in non-small-cell lung carcinomas: correlation between gene copy number and protein expression and impact on prognosis. J Clin Oncol 2003;21:3798-807.
18. Ono M, Hirata A, Kometani T, et al. Sensitivity to gefitinib (Iressa, ZD1839) in non-small cell lung cancer cell lines correlates with dependence on the epidermal growth factor (EGF) receptor/extracellular signal-regulated kinase 1/2 and EGF receptor/Akt pathway for proliferation. Molecular cancer therapeutics 2004;3:465-72.
19. Thomson S, Buck E, Petti F, et al. Epithelial to mesenchymal transition is a determinant of sensitivity of non-small-cell lung carcinoma cell lines and xenografts to epidermal growth factor receptor inhibition. Cancer research 2005;65:9455-62.
20. Yauch RL, Januario T, Eberhard DA, et al. Epithelial versus mesenchymal phenotype determines in vitro sensitivity and predicts clinical activity of erlotinib in lung cancer patients. Clin Cancer Res 2005;11:8686-98.
21. Meert AP, Martin B, Delmotte P, et al. The role of EGF-R expression on patient survival in lung cancer: a systematic review with meta-analysis. Eur Respir J 2002;20:975-81.
22. Bunn PA, Jr., Dziadziuszko R, Varella-Garcia M, et al. Biological markers for non-small cell lung cancer patient selection for epidermal growth factor receptor tyrosine kinase inhibitor therapy. Clin Cancer Res 2006;12:3652-6.
23. Toschi L, Cappuzzo F. Understanding the new genetics of responsiveness to epidermal growth factor receptor tyrosine kinase inhibitors. The oncologist 2007;12:211-20.
24. Clark GM, Zborowski DM, Santabarbara P, et al. Smoking history and epidermal growth factor receptor expression as predictors of survival benefit from erlotinib for patients with non-small-cell lung cancer in the National Cancer Institute of Canada Clinical Trials Group study BR.21. Clinical lung cancer 2006;7:389-94.
25. Perez-Soler R, Chachoua A, Hammond LA, et al. Determinants of tumor response and survival with erlotinib in patients with non--small-cell lung cancer. J Clin Oncol 2004;22:3238-47.
26. Chung KY, Shia J, Kemeny NE, et al. Cetuximab shows activity in colorectal cancer patients with tumors that do not express the epidermal growth factor receptor by immunohistochemistry. J Clin Oncol 2005;23:1803-10.
27. Cappuzzo F, Hirsch FR, Rossi E, et al. Epidermal growth factor receptor gene and protein and gefitinib sensitivity in non-small-cell lung cancer. Journal of the National Cancer Institute 2005;97:643-55.
28. Hirsch FR, Varella-Garcia M, Bunn PA, Jr., et al. Molecular predictors of outcome with gefitinib in a phase III placebo-controlled study in advanced non-small-cell lung cancer. J Clin Oncol 2006;24:5034-42.
29. Hirsch FR, Witta S. Biomarkers for prediction of sensitivity to EGFR inhibitors in non-small cell lung cancer. Current opinion in oncology 2005;17:118-22.
30. Comis RL. The current situation: erlotinib (Tarceva) and gefitinib (Iressa) in non-small cell lung cancer. The oncologist 2005;10:467-70.
31. Takano T, Ohe Y, Sakamoto H, et al. Epidermal growth factor receptor gene mutations and increased copy numbers predict gefitinib sensitivity in patients with recurrent non-small-cell lung cancer. J Clin Oncol 2005;23:6829-37.
32. Johnson BE, Janne PA. Selecting patients for epidermal growth factor receptor inhibitor treatment: A FISH story or a tale of mutations? J Clin Oncol 2005;23:6813-6.

33. Shigematsu H, Takahashi T, Nomura M, et al. Somatic mutations of the HER2 kinase domain in lung adenocarcinomas. Cancer research 2005;65:1642-6.
34. Wang SE, Narasanna A, Perez-Torres M, et al. HER2 kinase domain mutation results in constitutive phosphorylation and activation of HER2 and EGFR and resistance to EGFR tyrosine kinase inhibitors. Cancer cell 2006;10:25-38.
35. Han SW, Kim TY, Jeon YK, et al. Optimization of patient selection for gefitinib in non-small cell lung cancer by combined analysis of epidermal growth factor receptor mutation, K-ras mutation, and Akt phosphorylation. Clin Cancer Res 2006;12:2538-44.
36. Moasser MM, Basso A, Averbuch SD, Rosen N. The tyrosine kinase inhibitor ZD1839 ("Iressa") inhibits HER2-driven signaling and suppresses the growth of HER2-overexpressing tumor cells. Cancer research 2001;61:7184-8.
37. Moulder SL, Yakes FM, Muthuswamy SK, Bianco R, Simpson JF, Arteaga CL. Epidermal growth factor receptor (HER1) tyrosine kinase inhibitor ZD1839 (Iressa) inhibits HER2/neu (erbB2)-overexpressing breast cancer cells in vitro and in vivo. Cancer research 2001;61:8887-95.
38. Hendriks BS, Opresko LK, Wiley HS, Lauffenburger D. Coregulation of epidermal growth factor receptor/human epidermal growth factor receptor 2 (HER2) levels and locations: quantitative analysis of HER2 overexpression effects. Cancer research 2003;63:1130-7.
39. Graus-Porta D, Beerli RR, Daly JM, Hynes NE. ErbB-2, the preferred heterodimerization partner of all ErbB receptors, is a mediator of lateral signaling. The EMBO journal 1997;16:1647-55.
40. Hendriks BS, Opresko LK, Wiley HS, Lauffenburger D. Quantitative analysis of HER2-mediated effects on HER2 and epidermal growth factor receptor endocytosis: distribution of homo- and heterodimers depends on relative HER2 levels. The Journal of biological chemistry 2003;278:23343-51.
41. Anido J, Matar P, Albanell J, et al. ZD1839, a specific epidermal growth factor receptor (EGFR) tyrosine kinase inhibitor, induces the formation of inactive EGFR/HER2 and EGFR/HER3 heterodimers and prevents heregulin signaling in HER2-overexpressing breast cancer cells. Clin Cancer Res 2003;9:1274-83.
42. Kim HH, Sierke SL, Koland JG. Epidermal growth factor-dependent association of phosphatidylinositol 3-kinase with the erbB3 gene product. The Journal of biological chemistry 1994;269:24747-55.
43. Soltoff SP, Carraway KL, 3rd, Prigent SA, Gullick WG, Cantley LC. ErbB3 is involved in activation of phosphatidylinositol 3-kinase by epidermal growth factor. Molecular and cellular biology 1994;14:3550-8.
44. Engelman JA, Janne PA, Mermel C, et al. ErbB-3 mediates phosphoinositide 3-kinase activity in gefitinib-sensitive non-small cell lung cancer cell lines. Proceedings of the National Academy of Sciences of the United States of America 2005;102:3788-93.
45. Buck E, Eyzaguirre A, Haley JD, Gibson NW, Cagnoni P, Iwata KK. Inactivation of Akt by the epidermal growth factor receptor inhibitor erlotinib is mediated by HER-3 in pancreatic and colorectal tumor cell lines and contributes to erlotinib sensitivity. Molecular cancer therapeutics 2006;5:2051-9.
46. Sergina NV, Rausch M, Wang D, et al. Escape from HER-family tyrosine kinase inhibitor therapy by the kinase-inactive HER3. Nature 2007;445:437-41.
47. Fujimoto N, Wislez M, Zhang J, et al. High expression of ErbB family members and their ligands in lung adenocarcinomas that are sensitive to inhibition of epidermal growth factor receptor. Cancer research 2005;65:11478-85.
48. Suzuki M, Shigematsu H, Hiroshima K, et al. Epidermal growth factor receptor expression status in lung cancer correlates with its mutation. Human pathology 2005;36:1127-34.
49. Lievre A, Bachet JB, Le Corre D, et al. KRAS mutation status is predictive of response to cetuximab therapy in colorectal cancer. Cancer research 2006;66:3992-5.
50. Pao W, Wang TY, Riely GJ, et al. KRAS mutations and primary resistance of lung adenocarcinomas to gefitinib or erlotinib. PLoS medicine 2005;2:e17.
51. Cully M, You H, Levine AJ, Mak TW. Beyond PTEN mutations: the PI3K pathway as an integrator of multiple inputs during tumorigenesis. Nat Rev Cancer 2006;6:184-92.
52. Kokubo Y, Gemma A, Noro R, et al. Reduction of PTEN protein and loss of epidermal growth factor receptor gene mutation in lung cancer with natural resistance to gefitinib (IRESSA). British journal of cancer 2005;92:1711-9.
53. Mellinghoff IK, Wang MY, Vivanco I, et al. Molecular determinants of the response of glioblastomas to EGFR kinase inhibitors. The New England journal of medicine 2005;353:2012-24.

54. Bianco R, Shin I, Ritter CA, et al. Loss of PTEN/MMAC1/TEP in EGF receptor-expressing tumor cells counteracts the antitumor action of EGFR tyrosine kinase inhibitors. Oncogene 2003;22:2812-22.
55. She QB, Solit D, Basso A, Moasser MM. Resistance to gefitinib in PTEN-null HER-overexpressing tumor cells can be overcome through restoration of PTEN function or pharmacologic modulation of constitutive phosphatidylinositol 3Î-kinase/Akt pathway signaling. Clin Cancer Res 2003;9:4340-6.
56. Haas-Kogan DA, Prados MD, Tihan T, et al. Epidermal growth factor receptor, protein kinase B/Akt, and glioma response to erlotinib. Journal of the National Cancer Institute 2005;97:880-7.
57. Coldren CD, Helfrich BA, Witta SE, et al. Baseline gene expression predicts sensitivity to gefitinib in non-small cell lung cancer cell lines. Mol Cancer Res 2006;4:521-8.
58. Witta SE, Gemmill RM, Hirsch FR, et al. Restoring E-cadherin expression increases sensitivity to epidermal growth factor receptor inhibitors in lung cancer cell lines. Cancer research 2006;66:944-50.
59. Buck E, Eyzaguirre A, Barr S, et al. Loss of homotypic cell adhesion by epithelial-mesenchymal transition or mutation limits sensitivity to epidermal growth factor receptor inhibition. Molecular cancer therapeutics 2007;6:532-41.
60. Thiery JP. Epithelial-mesenchymal transitions in tumour progression. Nat Rev Cancer 2002;2:442-54.
61. Brabletz T, Jung A, Spaderna S, Hlubek F, Kirchner T. Opinion: migrating cancer stem cells - an integrated concept of malignant tumour progression. Nat Rev Cancer 2005;5:744-9.
62. Halbleib JM, Nelson WJ. Cadherins in development: cell adhesion, sorting, and tissue morphogenesis. Genes & development 2006;20:3199-214.
63. Christofori G, Semb H. The role of the cell-adhesion molecule E-cadherin as a tumour-suppressor gene. Trends in biochemical sciences 1999;24:73-6.
64. Perl AK, Wilgenbus P, Dahl U, Semb H, Christofori G. A causal role for E-cadherin in the transition from adenoma to carcinoma. Nature 1998;392:190-3.
65. Peinado H, Ballestar E, Esteller M, Cano A. Snail mediates E-cadherin repression by the recruitment of the Sin3A/histone deacetylase 1 (HDAC1)/HDAC2 complex. Molecular and cellular biology 2004;24:306-19.
66. Moreno-Bueno G, Cubillo E, Sarrio D, et al. Genetic profiling of epithelial cells expressing e-cadherin repressors reveals a distinct role for snail, slug, and e47 factors in epithelial-mesenchymal transition. Cancer research 2006;66:9543-56.
67. Olmeda D, Jorda M, Peinado H, Fabra A, Cano A. Snail silencing effectively suppresses tumour growth and invasiveness. Oncogene 2006.
68. Qian X, Karpova T, Sheppard AM, McNally J, Lowy DR. E-cadherin-mediated adhesion inhibits ligand-dependent activation of diverse receptor tyrosine kinases. The EMBO journal 2004;23:1739-48.
69. Barrallo-Gimeno A, Nieto MA. The Snail genes as inducers of cell movement and survival: implications in development and cancer. Development (Cambridge, England) 2005;132:3151-61.
70. Maestro R, Dei Tos AP, Hamamori Y, et al. Twist is a potential oncogene that inhibits apoptosis. Genes & development 1999;13:2207-17.
71. Vega F, Medeiros LJ, Leventaki V, et al. Activation of mammalian target of rapamycin signaling pathway contributes to tumor cell survival in anaplastic lymphoma kinase-positive anaplastic large cell lymphoma. Cancer research 2006;66:6589-97.
72. Moody SE, Perez D, Pan TC, et al. The transcriptional repressor Snail promotes mammary tumor recurrence. Cancer cell 2005;8:197-209.
73. Samani AA, Yakar S, LeRoith D, Brodt P. The role of the IGF system in cancer growth and metastasis: overview and recent insights. Endocrine reviews 2007;28:20-47.
74. Moyer JD, Barbacci EG, Iwata KK, et al. Induction of apoptosis and cell cycle arrest by CP-358,774, an inhibitor of epidermal growth factor receptor tyrosine kinase. Cancer research 1997;57:4838-48.
75. Chakravarti A, Loeffler JS, Dyson NJ. Insulin-like growth factor receptor I mediates resistance to anti-epidermal growth factor receptor therapy in primary human glioblastoma cells through continued activation of phosphoinositide 3-kinase signaling. Cancer research 2002;62:200-7.
76. Morgillo F, Woo JK, Kim ES, Hong WK, Lee HY. Heterodimerization of insulin-like growth factor receptor/epidermal growth factor receptor and induction of survivin expression counteract the antitumor action of erlotinib. Cancer research 2006;66:10100-11.
77. Jones HE, Goddard L, Gee JM, et al. Insulin-like growth factor-I receptor signalling and acquired resistance to gefitinib (ZD1839; Iressa) in human breast and prostate cancer cells. Endocrine-related cancer 2004;11:793-814.

78. Desbois-Mouthon C, Cacheux W, Blivet-Van Eggelpoel MJ, et al. Impact of IGF-1R/EGFR crosstalks on hepatoma cell sensitivity to gefitinib. International journal of cancer 2006;119:2557-66.
79. Pietras K, Sjoblom T, Rubin K, Heldin CH, Ostman A. PDGF receptors as cancer drug targets. Cancer cell 2003;3:439-43.
80. Yu Y, Sweeney M, Zhang S, et al. PDGF stimulates pulmonary vascular smooth muscle cell proliferation by upregulating TRPC6 expression. American journal of physiology 2003;284:C316-30.
81. Kassouf W, Dinney CP, Brown G, et al. Uncoupling between epidermal growth factor receptor and downstream signals defines resistance to the antiproliferative effect of Gefitinib in bladder cancer cells. Cancer research 2005;65:10524-35.
82. Matei D, Emerson RE, Lai YC, et al. Autocrine activation of PDGFRalpha promotes the progression of ovarian cancer. Oncogene 2006;25:2060-9.
83. Jechlinger M, Sommer A, Moriggl R, et al. Autocrine PDGFR signaling promotes mammary cancer metastasis. The Journal of clinical investigation 2006;116:1561-70.
84. Carvalho I, Milanezi F, Martins A, Reis RM, Schmitt F. Overexpression of platelet-derived growth factor receptor alpha in breast cancer is associated with tumour progression. Breast Cancer Res 2005;7: R788-95.

23 Utilizing Combinations of Molecular Targeted Agents to Sensitize Tumor Cells to EGFR Inhibitors

Elizabeth Buck, Alexandra Eyzaguirre, and Kenneth K. Iwata

CONTENTS

INTRODUCTION
REDIRECTING AKT SIGNALING TO EGFR CONTROL
AFFECTING EMT STATUS
CONCLUSION
REFERENCES

Abstract

EGFR inhibitors have achieved clinical antitumor activity as single agents. The specific inhibition of EGFR and associated pathways provides a mechanism for efficacious inhibition of tumor cell growth while minimizing toxicities often associated with chemotherapeutic drugs. The challenge of using targeted cancer drugs as single agents is the potential for de novo or acquired resistance due to established or adapted alternate signal transduction pathways. In this chapter, we will describe how cancer drug combinations with EGFR inhibitors can be rationally identified by utilizing our understanding of the molecular mechanism and related biomarkers of EGFR inhibitor sensitivity. Such combinations may ultimately provide better efficacy and reduced toxicity for patients.

Key Words: EMT, epithelial mesenchymal transition, erlotinib, EGFR, IGF-1R, ER, HER3, mTOR, HDAC, src, COX-2.

1. INTRODUCTION

Proteins related to the epithelial-mesenchymal-transition (EMT) have been used to resolve differential sensitivity to EGFR antagonists for a wide array of solid tumor types including NSCLC, pancreatic, colorectal, and breast. Epithelial-like tumor cells are comparatively more sensitive to growth inhibition by EGFR inhibitors, such as erlotinib (Tarceva, OSI Pharmaceuticals), than those tumor cells that have undergone EMT and acquired a mesenchymal-like phenotype ((*1-4*) and reviewed by Thomson et al, this edition). Recent efforts have focused on the molecular mechanisms responsible for rendering EGFR-directed cell growth for epithelial tumor cells. The ability of EGFR antagonists to inhibit Akt activity

From: *Cancer Drug Discovery and Development: EGFR Signaling Networks in Cancer Therapy*
Edited by: J. D. Haley and W. J. Gullick, DOI: 10.1007/978-1-59745-356-1_23
© 2008 Humana Press, a part of Springer Science+Business Media, LLC

correlates with their sensitivity, and inhibition of Akt by EGFR antagonists occurs predominantly in epithelial-like tumor cells (5-7). Specifically, EGFR transactivation of HER3 has been shown to confer activity to Akt, and EGFR appears to be co-expressed with HER3 principally in epithelial tumor cells. HER3 expression has been reported to be regulated by a similar transcriptional control mechanism as other epithelial-specific proteins such as the junctional protein E-cadherin. One transcriptional repressor of such proteins, snail, which is activated in cells undergoing EMT, also represses the expression of HER3 (8). In addition to its association with HER3 expression, evidence suggests that E-cadherin might be involved directly in mediating EGFR signal transduction important for regulation of HER3 and Akt. E-cadherin can activate EGFR in a ligand-independent manner, and this has been shown to confer activation to downstream machinery within the EGFR signaling cascade including Erk and Akt (9-12).

For mesenchymal-like tumor cell lines that are insensitive to growth inhibition by EGFR antagonists, Akt appears to be regulated by an EGFR-independent mechanism. This may include activation due to mutations in the PI3K-PDK1-Akt cascade such as those that affect PI3K or PTEN (13-16). Alternatively, other receptor tyrosine kinases such as the insulin like growth factor receptor-1 (IGF-1R) or the platelet derived growth factor receptor (PDGFR) may preferentially regulate Akt in mesenchymal tumor cells.

Collectively these data demonstrate that EMT is, at least in part, responsible for the inherent heterogeneity of tumors (e.g., epithelial and mesenchymal phenotypes). This tumor heterogeneity as well as the plasticity that exists between different cell states (e.g., EMT and MET) results in a collection of tumor cells utilizing differential signal transduction pathways and relying upon diverse survival requirements. This likely underlies the differential efficacy observed for using anticancer drugs, such as EGFR inhibitors, as single agents for a broad group of unselected patients. More effective cancer treatment may be achieved by combining cancer drugs against multiple, but specific, targets to maximize the diversity of tumor cells that will be effectively targeted. Understanding the molecular pathways used by the tumor cells would allow the rational selection of molecular targeted drugs to inhibit multiple and overlapping signaling pathways to allow for maximum efficacy.

Combination therapy represents a strategy to both maintain the sensitivity to EGFR inhibitors for epithelial tumors that have acquired resistance due to long term treatment as well as to impart sensitivity to mesenchymal tumors that exhibit de novo resistance to EGFR inhibition. Such strategies could include combinations with agents exploit the plasticity of tumor cells by affecting the EMT status of mesenchymal tumor cells as well as agents that directly interfere with cell signaling cascades specifically to restore signal flow from EGFR to Akt. Several recent reports have highlighted the utility of combination strategies and will be discussed herein.

2. REDIRECTING Akt SIGNALING TO EGFR CONTROL

2.1. Exploiting Cell Surface Receptor Crosstalk

Tumor cells harbor multiple cell surface receptors that can act in a redundant manner to translate external signals to a common set of intracellular machinery in order to regulate cell growth and survival. Cooperation among cell surface receptors toward regulation of the Akt pathway has been described, and this crosstalk has been exploited by combining EGFR antagonists with inhibitors of alternate cell surface receptors to redirect Akt activity to the EGFR signal transduction cascade (17, 18). Studies illustrating the success of this approach have involved combinations of EGFR inhibitors with antagonists of the estrogen receptor (ER) (17), HER2 (19), or the insulin-like growth factor receptor (IGF-1R) (18). Herein, the rationale for the combined targeting of the EGFR with either ER or IGF-1R antagonists will be discussed.

2.1.1. COMBINED TARGETING OF THE EGFR AND IGF-1R

Two signal transduction cascades that lie downstream of EGFR and are important for regulating cell growth and survival for tumor cells are the MAPK and Akt pathways. Blockade of signaling through EGFR can cause selection pressure that results in compensation by alternative receptor tyrosine kinases (RTKs) for the regulation of these pathways. Such receptor crosstalk is well documented between the EGFR and IGF-1R. Signaling through the IGF-1R promotes cell proliferation and survival for a wide range of tumor types (20-22), and both antibody-based and low molecular weight inhibitors of IGF-1R signaling have demonstrated antitumor activity in both the in vitro and in vivo settings. The IGF-1R has been shown to be a strong transducer of activity to the PI3K pathway in order to maintain cell survival in response to a variety of cancer therapeutics including cytotoxic chemotherapeutics, radiation, and molecular targeted therapeutics (23-27).

Enhanced signaling through IGF-1R has been shown to mediate resistance to EGFR inhibitors through sustained activation of the PI3K-Akt pathway. Both breast and prostate tumor cells that lose sensitivity to the EGFR inhibitor gefitinib gain an increase in IGF-1R phosphorylation and IGF-driven Akt activity that is accompanied by enhanced sensitivity to IGF-1R inhibitors (28, 29). For mesenchymal NSCLC cell lines, treatment with an EGFR antagonist or engineered expression of a dominant negative IGF-1R generated an increase in the phosphorylation of the reciprocal receptor (30). Here the combined targeting of EGFR and IGF-1R demonstrated synergistic antitumor activity. Glioblastoma cells resistant to growth inhibition by an EGFR antagonist exhibit a high expression level of IGF-1R, and treatment of these cells with an inhibitor of the EGFR results in both augmented overall expression of IGF-1R and an increase in phosphorylated IGF-1R. Cotreatment of tumor cells with both an EGFR and IGF-1R inhibitor resulted in a reduction in Akt phosphorylation that was greater than that achieved by either inhibitor as a single agent. Moreover, the combination achieved a greater than additive induction in apoptosis along with an inhibition of cell invasion (31). The success for the EGFR and IGF-1R inhibitor combination has translated to *in vivo* models. In mice bearing A549 or MCF-7 tumors, treatment with either an EGFR or IGF-1R neutralizing antibody as a single agent led to short term tumor regression, however only co-treatment with both neutralizing antibodies led to sustained tumor regression as long as 60 days (32). For in vitro models the combination of EGFR and IGF-1R antagonists has demonstrated synergy for a broad panel of tumor types including breast (26, 28, 29), glioblastoma (31), pancreatic, and NSCLC (30). For breast tumor cell lines overexpression of the IGF-1R reduced sensitivity to the EGFR inhibitor gefitinib, and the combination of gefitinib with the IGF-1R inhibitor AG1024 generated synergistic growth inhibition as well as a promotion of apoptosis. The combination of EGFR and IGF-1R antagonists are able to reduce phosphorylated Akt levels below that obtained by either single agent, and, although EGFR antagonists generally cause tumor cell growth stasis and not growth regression, EGFR antagonists can inhibit cell survival in combination with IGF-1R antagonists.

An additional rationale for combining an EGFR inhibitor with an IGF-1R inhibitor stems from observations that IGF driven signaling appears to be involved in triggering EMT and also for the maintenance of the invasive phenotype for mesenchymal cells (33, 34). IGF-1R inhibitors have been shown to suppress cell migration and invasion (28). Prolonged exposure to IGF has been shown to trigger EMT for breast epithelial cells (33). The engineered expression of a constitutively active version of IGF-1R is transforming for MCF-10A mammary epithelial cells, and this is concomitant with EMT as the MCF-10A cells lose the expression of E-cadherin and gain the expression of mesenchymal protein markers including vimentin and snail (Adrian Lee, SABC, 2006). Treatment of MCF-10A cells with a low molecular weight inhibitor of the IGF-1R blocks transformation and EMT. Therefore, in addition to the direct effects on the Akt signaling cascade, an IGF-1R inhibitor may be able to block

EMT to maintain sensitivity to EGFR inhibition. A further understanding of the signaling networks that mediate IGF-driven EMT as well as the molecular basis for the reciprocal relationship that exists for EGFR and IGF-1R signaling may provide us with a biomarker signature to allow our identification of specific tumor settings where combining inhibitors of these specific receptors may be most important.

2.1.2. COMBINED TARGETING OF THE EGFR AND ER

The estrogen receptor is expressed in a variety of tumor types including NSCLC and pancreatic tumors in addition to breast tumors, and the ability of ER signaling to drive tumorigenesis for these various tumors is well documented (*35-37*). Traditionally, ligand binding to the ER promotes an active nuclear receptor that can bind to estrogen response elements and promote the transcription of target genes. More recently, the ability of a cytoplasmic pool of ER to participate directly in the activation of kinases has been realized (*38, 39*). Bidirectional communication between the ER and EGFR has been well documented. For example, estradiol promotes the autocrine production of EGF by breast tumor cells (*40*), and the EGFR may transactivate ER to relay signals to downstream pathways including the MAPK pathway. Recent data for NSCLC studies further expanded our understanding for the crosstalk between ER and EGFR. Estradiol was found to impose a down-regulation of EGFR expression, and treatment of tumor cells with the anti-estrogen fulvestrant generated an increase in EGFR signaling (*37*). The reciprocal was also observed, where treatment with the EGFR inhibitor gefitinib evoked an increase in ER expression. The combination of both EGF and estradiol generated a synergistic induction in the activity for the MAPK pathway, and the combined blockade of ER and EGFR with fulvestrant and gefitinib achieved synergistic cell growth inhibition in vitro, and heightened tumor growth inhibition in vivo.

Data for breast tumors cell suggests that EGFR signaling may also mediate resistance to ER blockade. The expression of EGFR and ER inversely correlate in breast tumors, and increased expression of EGFR is associated with decreased sensitivity to endocrine therapy (*41, 42*). The engineered overexpression of EGFR in the hormone-dependent breast tumor cell line ZR-75-1 conferred decreased sensitivity to anti-hormonal therapies (*43*). Long-term culture of ER-expressing MCF-7 cells with fulvestrant genereated hormone resistance, and this was accompanied by an increase in EGFR expression and enhanced sensitivity to gefitinib (*44*). Molecularly, the fulvestrant-resistant MCF-7 cells gained the capacity for autocrine activation of EGFR through the increased expression of ligands such as TGF-α, and this correlated with augmented signaling within EGFR-mediated signaling cascades such as the MAPK pathway. More specifically, the growth of these cells appeared to be driven by EGFR-HER2 heterodimerization (*18*). Collectively, these data indicate that the reciprocal relationship between EGFR and ER signaling can confer resistance to single agent inhibitors during prolonged treatment for both breast and other types of solid tumors. This highlights the need for either concurrent or sequential combination strategies for sustained therapeutic benefit.

2.2. Exploiting Intracellular Feedback Loops
2.2.1. COMBINED TARGETING OF EGFR AND MTOR

Intracellular feedback loops can cause redirection of signaling cascades that regulate Akt activity, providing a mechanism for potential resistance to molecular targeted therapeutics that affect Akt activity through a single pathway. Combination strategies that exploit this resistance mechanism have demonstrated success in redirecting Akt signaling to EGFR control. One such illustration of this is the combination of an EGFR inhibitor with the mTOR inhibitor Rapamycin. Rapamycin is a high molecular weight polyketide that effectively inhibits signals downstream of mTOR that are important for control of cell cycle progression and proliferation. However, Rapamycin treatment can result in an increase in Akt phosphorylation that is accompanied by a promotion of cell survival, and as a single agent Rapamycin has shown limited utility to inhibit cell growth (*45-50*). Here, rapamycin's ability to inhibit tumor cell proliferation is likely offset by its ability to inhibit apoptosis. Several mechanisms have been proposed to account for Rapamycin's pro-survival activity. First, Rapamycin, which inhibits only the mTOR-raptor complex, may lead to a shift in equilibrium from the mTOR-raptor to the mTOR-rictor complex. Akt activity has been shown to be activated by mTOR-rictor (*47*). Second, by inhibiting signals downstream of mTOR, including p70S6K, rapamycin circumvents a negative regulatory feedback loop involving the p70S6K-IRS1-PI3K-Atk pathway (*51-53*). Here serine phosphorylation of IRS-1 by p70S6K inhibits its ability to act as a conduit for transferring signals from IGF-1R to PI3K. Activated IGF-1R does not interact with PI3K directly, but rather phosphorylates IRS-1 at select tyrosine residues that serve as docking nodes for PI3K. Only PI3K docked to IRS-1 can be activated by IGF-1R (*54-57*). Rapamycin promotes IRS-1-PI3K coupling by blocking p70S6K activity, which is inhibitory to IRS-1 function. This provides a strong mechanistic rationale for combining Rapamycin with an inhibitor of the IGF-1R, and this combination has demonstrated success (*58*). However, the combination of Rapamycin with an EGFR inhibitor has also achieved success in preclinical models (*59-61*). For both renal cell carcinoma and glioblastoma tumors that carry mutations that activate Akt in a ligand-independent manner, synergistic growth inhibition has been achieved by combining an EGFR and mTOR inhibitor (*60, 61*), and this combination has shown early clinical utility (*59*). We have recently reported that the EGFR inhibitor erlotinib can synergize with rapamycin for other types of cancer cells including those derived from NSCLC, breast, pancreatic, and colorectal tumors (*62*). Here we showed that for mesenchymal-like tumor cells such as H460, although erlotinib has no effect on basal Akt activity, it can inhibit Akt activity that is Rapamycin-driven (Fig. 23.1).

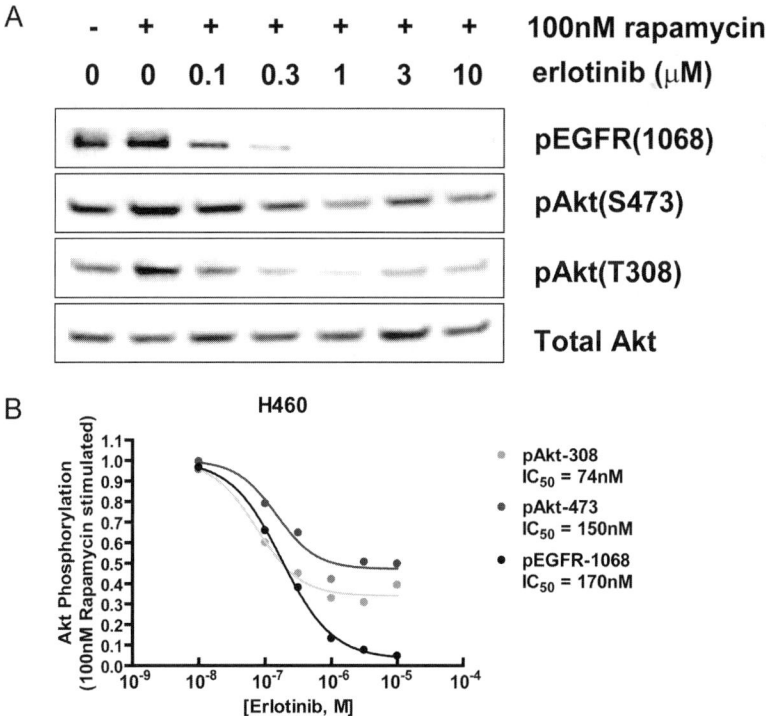

Fig. 23.1 Erlotinib Inhibits Rapamycin-induced Akt Phosphorylation. Effect of varying concentrations of erlotinib on Akt phosphorylation in the presence of rapamycin by immunoblot (A) with quantitation of band intensity (B).

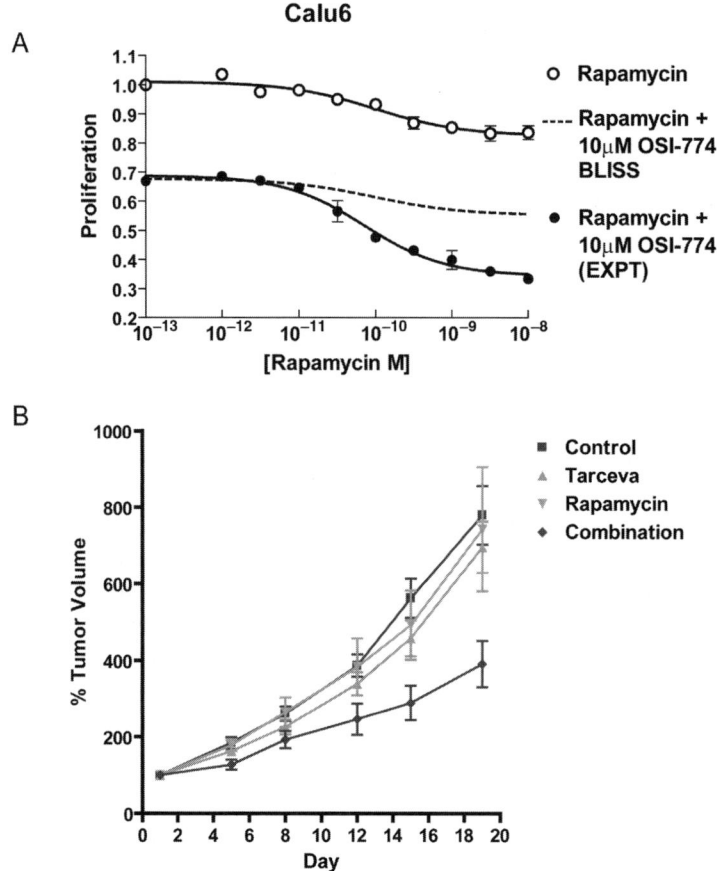

Fig. 23.2. Rapamycin synergizes with erlotinib to inhibit cell growth in both in vitro and in vivo models. A. Effect of varying concentrations of erlotinib, alone or in the presence of rapamycin, on the growth of Calu6 tumor cells. The BLISS curve represents the theoretical expectation for additivity. B. Effect of erlotinib, rapamycin, or the combination on the growth of Clau6 tumors in vivo.

This is accompanied by synergistic growth inhibition and induction of apoptosis in vitro and also synergistic tumor growth inhibition in vivo, (Fig. 23.2). The mechanism whereby erlotinib might affect Rapamycin-driven Akt activity but not basal Akt activity is not yet completely understood, however this observation highlights the necessity for combination therapies and the need to identify biomarkers indicative of patients likely to receive the most benefit from specific combination regimens.

3. AFFECTING EMT STATUS

Epithelial tumor cells have been shown to be substantially more sensitive to EGFR inhibitor therapeutics than tumor cells that have undergone EMT and acquired a mesenchymal-like behavior, therefore, combining EGFR antagonists with agents that either block EMT or promote a mesenchymal-epithelial-transition (MET) could likely have therapeutic benefit. The drivers of EMT as well as the signaling pathways that maintain the mesenchymal-like cell state are multiple and complex. Many drivers of EMT have been proposed and include: inflammatory signals such as those evoked by COX-II; the capacity of growth factors such as TGF-β, EGF,

FGF, and IGF to evoke elevated Akt activity; hormones such as human growth hormone (HGH); signaling by non-receptor kinases such as src; and elevated integrin signaling (*34, 63-66*). Signals that drive EMT could emanate from either the tumor cells themselves, such as autocrine production of TGF-β, or from stromal cells that infiltrate the tumor and provide signals that stimulate EMT in a paracrine manner. Therefore, there exists a strong rationale for both targeting EMT in tumor cells directly or by blocking the ability of tumor stromal cells to promote EMT. Several recently reported studies that address EMT in the context of sensitivity to EGFR inhibitors provide evidence of success for this strategy.

3.1. Combinations of EGFR and HDAC Inhibitors

Histone deacetylases (HDACs) are involved in chromatin remodeling and modification of non-histone transcription regulatory proteins, and thus they modulate the expression of genes important for complex biological events. HDAC activity has been shown to be associated with the enhanced proliferation and survival of tumor cells for both hematologic and solid malignancies, and inhibitors of HDACs attenuate the growth of tumor cells. In addition to activity in vitro, inhibitors of HDACs have achieved antitumor activity in animal models (*67*).

Preclinical data have demonstrated that HDAC inhibitors can enhance the activity of EGFR antagonists. HDAC inhibition has been reported to lead to the down-modulation of both EGFR and ErbB2 expression, and the combination of HDAC inhibition with ErbB blockade has demonstrated enhanced proliferative inhibition, apoptosis induction and signaling inhibition for prostate and breast cell lines (*68, 69*). The mechanism by which HDAC inhibitors affect the expression of members of the ErbB family likely involves the molecular chaperone Hsp90. The expression of the molecular chaperone Hsp90 is down-regulated by HDACs, and, since multiple RTKs including those within the ErbB family require Hsp90 for proper folding, there is a concomitant decrease in the expression of properly folded EGFR.

Mutations in EGFR the give rise to acquired resistance to EGFR inhibitors have been reported. Specifically, the T790M mutation has been shown to mediate resistance to low molecular weight inhibitors of the EGFR such as erlotinib or gefitinib by blocking their ability to bind at the ATP binding site (*70*). Mutant RTKs are reported to be substantially more dependent on Hsp90 for proper folding than wild-type proteins. Given the observation for the control of Hsp90 expression by HDACs, an HDAC inhibitor may be able to restore sensitivity to EGFR inhibition for resistance mutants such as T790M.

More recently, inhibitors of Histone deacetylases (HDACs) have been shown to promote an MET transition that is associated with enhanced sensitivity to EGFR inhibition. EMT, as well as the maintenance of the mesenchymal state, is controlled, at least in part, by a family of transcription factors that include ZEB1, Slug, Snail and SIP1(*65*). This group acts to transcriptionally repress genes important for the epithelial phenotype including E-cadherin, and the ability of transcription factors to repress these genes is dependent on their interaction with both the transcriptional co-repressor CtBP and HDACs. Here the recruitment of HDACs leads to chromatin condensation and gene silencing (*71*). Recent work supports the hypothesis that the combination of EGFR inhibitors with HDAC inhibitors is a promising strategy to overcome resistance to EGFR TKIs. For example, it has been shown that the HDAC inhibitor trichostatin A (TSA) prevents TGF-β1 induced EMT in human renal epithelial cells (*72*). Pretreating gefitinib-resistant cell lines with the HDAC inhibitor MS-275 induces the expression of E-cadherin and EGFR and leads to a synergistic growth-inhibitory and apoptotic effect of gefitinib in gefitinib resistant cell lines similar to that in gefitinib-sensitive NSCLC cell lines (*2*). In the same way, E-cadherin transfection into a gefitinib-resistant cell line induced E-cadherin expression and augmented EGFR activation by EGF as compared to untransfected resistant cell lines. Increase in E-cadherin expression by transfection also increased sensitivity to gefitinib of the resistant cell line to levels observed in sensitive NSCLC cell lines (2). This data has suggested that expression of E-cadherin in cell lines might increase dependence on EGFR for growth and survival.

In summary, the combination of HDAC inhibitors with EGFR inhibitors offer evident advantages: by down-regulating EGFR or HER2, HDAC inhibitors potentiate the effects of EGFR TKIs and by inhibiting Zeb1 from repressing E-cadherin expression, the use of HDAC inhibitors in combination with EGFR inhibitors could prevent EMT and circumventing TKI resistance. In addition, the effect of HDAC inhibitors on Hsp90 could also have a potential effect against EGFR inhibitor resistant mutants.

3.2. Combination with Src Inhibitors

The ability of the non-receptor tyrosine kinase src to promote tumorigenesis and drive metastatic potential has been extensively described (73, 74), and increased activity for src is linked to enhanced metastatic potential (75). Consistent with its correlation with metastasis, recent data suggests that src activity is an important driver for EMT as well as for the maintenance of the mesenchymal phenotype. The ability of mesenchymal tumor cells to migrate from a primary tumor and extravasate to the blood stream is a hallmark event in metastasis, and src activity has been shown to be an important driver of both motility and invasion for mesenchymal tumor cell lines. Through activation of focal adhesion kinase (FAK), src is involved in regulating the formation and disemenation of focal contacts that is required for cell mobility (76). Cells harboring a kinase-deficient src exibit impaired cell migration, and low molecular weight inhibitors of src family kinases can inhibit cell migration (77).

Src activity has also been shown to play a role in the signaling events that mediate the transition from the epithelial to the mesenchymal phenotype. The engineered overexpression of activated src in epithelial tumor cells can drive EMT, and a dominant negative src can reverse the mesenchymal phenotype (78, 79). For colorectal tumor cells, enhanced src activity leads to disruption of E-cadherin mediated cell adhesion, a hallmark of the mesenchymal phenotype (80). Preclinical studies have shown that while inhibition of src does not affect the overall growth for primary tumors, blockade of src activity does attenuate cell migration as well as limit metastasis. Tumors harboring dominant negative mutants of src exhibited a high degree of epithelial differentiation compared with parental counterparts (81). Specifically, inhibition of src activity was associated with increased homotypic cell adhesion as well as the loss of markers of the mesenchymal phenotype including vimentin. Cells treated with low molecular weight inhibitors of src demonstrate increased E-cadherin expression and enhanced homotypic cell adhesion. In vivo, treatment of xenograft tumors with an inhibitor of src achieved a reduced rate of metastasis, consistent with the potential of src inhibitors to block EMT (82, 83). Collectively, these data suggest that although src inhibitors demonstrate weak anti-proliferative activity as single agents, tumors treated with the combination of a src inhibitor with an EGFR inhibitor are likely to achieve substantial growth inhibition for the primary tumor as well as a reduction in metastatic potential.

3.3. Combination with COX-2 Blockade

Cyclooxygenase 2 (COX-2), the enzyme that catalyzes the conversion of arachidonic acid to the prostaglandins, plays a role in carcinogenesis and is expressed in many premalignant and malignant tissues (84-86). Cooperative signaling between COX-2 and the EGFR has been described. PGE2, a major product of COX-2, confers transactivation of EGFR by stimulating the synthesis and secretion of ligands for activation of the EGFR. This enhanced EGFR activity promotes activation of the MAPK pathway, which in turn drives the transcription of the gene encoding COX-2. This observation for reciprocal amplification of EGFR and COX-2 activity as a driver of tumor cell growth highlights the potential for successfully combining an inhibitor of the EGFR and COX-2. In addition to the established crosstalk between these two enzymes, COX-2 signaling is associated with signaling events that mediate EMT (87). The overexpression of COX-2 or its product PGE2 results in a decrease in E-cadherin levels and homotypic cell adhesion. Treatment of cells with PGE2 generates an induction in the activity for transcriptional repressors that evoke EMT such as snail, along with an enhanced mesenchymal-like phenotype. The COX-2 inhibitor sulindac sulfide can reverse the gain of this mesenchymal phenotype. These observations provide a strong rationale for combining COX-2 and EGFR antagonists, in terms of blocking both enzymatic crosstalk and EMT, to achieve augmented growth inhibition compared with a single agent EGFR inhibitor.

Recently, synergistic tumor cell growth inhibition for SCCHN has been reported by combining the EGFR inhibitor gefitinib with the COX-2 antagonist celecoxib (88). This synergy for growth inhibition was associated by a greater than additive decrease in the phosphorylated levels of EGFR, Erk, and Akt. In vivo, although celexocib administration failed to achieve significant tumor growth inhibition as a single agent it did further augment the growth inhibition in response to gefitinib. In APCmin/+ mice, the combination of the COX-2 inhibitor sulindac with an EGFR inhibitor led to a significant reduction in polyps, providing evidence for the success of this combination in chemoprevention.

4. CONCLUSION

Although the new generation of molecular targeted therapies, such as the EGFR inhibitor erlotinib, is showing promise in the clinic as single agents against tumors that were previously untreatable, not all tumors respond and not all patients are receiving maximal benefit. As described in this chapter, tumors are comprised of a heterogeneous population of cells that exhibit distinct morphologies and can harbor discrete mechanisms responsible for tumor cell growth and survival. In addition, even within the same tumor cell there may be plural and redundant signal transduction pathways to regulate the aberrant behavior of the tumor cell. This overlap among signal transduction pathways has been shown to be responsible for not only the de novo resistance of select tumor cells to EGFR inhibitor therapeutics but also to contribute to the acquired resistance to such therapeutics after prolonged treatment. These observations highlight the necessity for utilizing drug combinations to improve the therapeutic efficacy against a broad range of tumors and to maintain long-term sensitivity. The multipronged attack of mechanisms that drive a disease state through combinations of therapeutics has been extensively described for treating viral disease. Cocktails of anti-retroviral inhibitors of HIV have exhibited synergy and have achieved a profound clinical success over the past decade. For cancer, the ability of combinations of molecular targeted agents to achieve synergistic effects in the clinic is currently being realized. Cytotoxic chemotherapies and radiation have routinely been used in combination, however these therapies often exhibit overlapping toxicities, limiting the potential to use these treatments optimally in combination. Additionally, given the extent in overlap in mechanisms of action for these therapies, the resistance mechanisms to such agents also are apparently convergent. Molecular targeted agents can specifically block different signaling networks, and typically exhibit fewer and independent toxicities, enabling these agents to be used quite effectively in combination. Synergies have been observed for various combinations, inviting the potential for lowering the dose of specific agents when used in combination.

Our expanding understanding of the differential mechanisms that drive cell signaling for epithelial and mesenchymal tumor cells as well as the signaling events that regulate tumor cell plasticity such as EMT and MET provides us the knowledge to effectively and rationally design cocktails of molecular targeted therapeutics for the treatment of tumors. Such understanding also equips us with the ability to use combinations either concurrently or sequentially to maintain sustained therapeutic benefit from therapeutics such as EGFR inhibitors. Such combinations have demonstrated success in preclinical models, and currently, clinical trials are underway to measure their clinical efficacy. Moving forward, efforts to obtain an understanding of the molecular mechanism responsible for response to a combination may provide us with predictive biomarkers such that patients most likely to respond to a specific combination may be selected. Such a process brings us closer to "individually tailored" therapies for cancer patients.

REFERENCES

1. Thomson S, Buck E, Petti F, et al. Epithelial to mesenchymal transition is a determinant of sensitivity of non-small-cell lung carcinoma cell lines and xenografts to epidermal growth factor receptor inhibition. Cancer Res 2005;65:9455-62.
2. Witta SE, Gemmill RM, Hirsch FR, et al. Restoring E-cadherin expression increases sensitivity to epidermal growth factor receptor inhibitors in lung cancer cell lines. Cancer Res 2006;66:944-50.
3. Yauch RL, Januario T, Eberhard DA, et al. Epithelial versus mesenchymal phenotype determines in vitro sensitivity and predicts clinical activity of erlotinib in lung cancer patients. Clin Cancer Res 2005;11:8686-98.
4. Buck E, Eyzaguirre A, Barr S, et al. Loss of homotypic cell adhesion by epithelial-mesenchymal transition or mutation limits sensitivity to epidermal growth factor receptor inhibition. Mol Cancer Ther 2007;6:532-41.
5. Buck E, Eyzaguirre A, Haley JD, Gibson NW, Cagnoni P, Iwata KK. Inactivation of Akt by the epidermal growth factor receptor inhibitor erlotinib is mediated by HER-3 in pancreatic and colorectal tumor cell lines and contributes to erlotinib sensitivity. Mol Cancer Ther 2006;5:2051-9.
6. Engelman JA, Janne PA, Mermel C, et al. ErbB-3 mediates phosphoinositide 3-kinase activity in gefitinib-sensitive non-small cell lung cancer cell lines. Proc Natl Acad Sci U S A 2005;102:3788-93.
7. Moasser MM, Basso A, Averbuch SD, Rosen N. The tyrosine kinase inhibitor ZD1839 ("Iressa") inhibits HER2-driven signaling and suppresses the growth of HER2-overexpressing tumor cells. Cancer Res 2001;61:7184-8.
8. De Craene B, Gilbert B, Stove C, Bruyneel E, van Roy F, Berx G. The transcription factor snail induces tumor cell invasion through modulation of the epithelial cell differentiation program. Cancer Res 2005;65:6237-44.
9. Andl CD, Rustgi AK. No one-way street: cross-talk between e-cadherin and receptor tyrosine kinase (RTK) signaling: a mechanism to regulate RTK activity. Cancer Biol Ther 2005;4:28-31.
10. Comoglio PM, Boccaccio C, Trusolino L. Interactions between growth factor receptors and adhesion molecules: breaking the rules. Curr Opin Cell Biol 2003;15:565-71.
11. Fedor-Chaiken M, Hein PW, Stewart JC, Brackenbury R, Kinch MS. E-cadherin binding modulates EGF receptor activation. Cell Commun Adhes 2003;10:105-18.
12. Pece S, Chiariello M, Murga C, Gutkind JS. Activation of the protein kinase Akt/PKB by the formation of E-cadherin-mediated cell-cell junctions. Evidence for the association of phosphatidylinositol 3-kinase with the E-cadherin adhesion complex. J Biol Chem 1999;274:19347-51.
13. Bachman KE, Argani P, Samuels Y, et al. The PIK3CA gene is mutated with high frequency in human breast cancers. Cancer Biol Ther 2004;3:772-5.
14. Bianco R, Shin I, Ritter CA, et al. Loss of PTEN/MMAC1/TEP in EGF receptor-expressing tumor cells counteracts the antitumor action of EGFR tyrosine kinase inhibitors. Oncogene 2003;22:2812-22.
15. Levine DA, Bogomolniy F, Yee CJ, et al. Frequent mutation of the PIK3CA gene in ovarian and breast cancers. Clin Cancer Res 2005;11:2875-8.
16. She QB, Solit D, Basso A, Moasser MM. Resistance to gefitinib in PTEN-null HER-overexpressing tumor cells can be overcome through restoration of PTEN function or pharmacologic modulation of constitutive phosphatidylinositol 3Î-kinase/Akt pathway signaling. Clin Cancer Res 2003;9:4340-6.
17. Bianco R, Troiani T, Tortora G, Ciardiello F. Intrinsic and acquired resistance to EGFR inhibitors in human cancer therapy. Endocr Relat Cancer 2005;12 Suppl 1:S159-71.

18. Jones HE, Gee JM, Taylor KM, et al. Development of strategies for the use of anti-growth factor treatments. Endocr Relat Cancer 2005;12 Suppl 1:S173-82.
19. Miller KD. The role of ErbB inhibitors in trastuzumab resistance. Oncologist 2004;9 Suppl 3:16-9.
20. Kaiser U, Schardt C, Brandscheidt D, Wollmer E, Havemann K. Expression of insulin-like growth factor receptors I and II in normal human lung and in lung cancer. J Cancer Res Clin Oncol 1993;119:665-8.
21. LeRoith D, Roberts CT, Jr. The insulin-like growth factor system and cancer. Cancer Lett 2003;195:127-37.
22. Rubin R, Baserga R. Insulin-like growth factor-I receptor. Its role in cell proliferation, apoptosis, and tumorigenicity. Lab Invest 1995;73:311-31.
23. Adams TE, McKern NM, Ward CW. Signalling by the type 1 insulin-like growth factor receptor: interplay with the epidermal growth factor receptor. Growth Factors 2004;22:89-95.
24. Gooch JL, Van Den Berg CL, Yee D. Insulin-like growth factor (IGF)-I rescues breast cancer cells from chemotherapy-induced cell death--proliferative and anti-apoptotic effects. Breast Cancer Res Treat 1999;56:1-10.
25. Lu Y, Zi X, Zhao Y, Mascarenhas D, Pollak M. Insulin-like growth factor-I receptor signaling and resistance to trastuzumab (Herceptin). Journal of the National Cancer Institute 2001;93:1852-7.
26. Nahta R, Yuan LX, Zhang B, Kobayashi R, Esteva FJ. Insulin-like growth factor-I receptor/human epidermal growth factor receptor 2 heterodimerization contributes to trastuzumab resistance of breast cancer cells. Cancer research 2005;65:11118-28.
27. Turner BC, Haffty BG, Narayanan L, et al. Insulin-like growth factor-I receptor overexpression mediates cellular radioresistance and local breast cancer recurrence after lumpectomy and radiation. Cancer research 1997;57:3079-83.
28. Jones HE, Goddard L, Gee JM, et al. Insulin-like growth factor-I receptor signalling and acquired resistance to gefitinib (ZD1839; Iressa) in human breast and prostate cancer cells. Endocr Relat Cancer 2004;11:793-814.
29. Knowlden JM, Hutcheson IR, Barrow D, Gee JM, Nicholson RI. Insulin-like growth factor-I receptor signaling in tamoxifen-resistant breast cancer: a supporting role to the epidermal growth factor receptor. Endocrinology 2005;146:4609-18.
30. Morgillo F, Woo JK, Kim ES, Hong WK, Lee HY. Heterodimerization of insulin-like growth factor receptor/epidermal growth factor receptor and induction of survivin expression counteract the antitumor action of erlotinib. Cancer research 2006;66:10100-11.
31. Chakravarti A, Loeffler JS, Dyson NJ. Insulin-like growth factor receptor I mediates resistance to anti-epidermal growth factor receptor therapy in primary human glioblastoma cells through continued activation of phosphoinositide 3-kinase signaling. Cancer research 2002;62:200-7.
32. Goetsch L, Gonzalez A, Leger O, et al. A recombinant humanized anti-insulin-like growth factor receptor type I antibody (h7C10) enhances the antitumor activity of vinorelbine and anti-epidermal growth factor receptor therapy against human cancer xenografts. Int J Cancer 2005;113:316-28.
33. Irie HY, Pearline RV, Grueneberg D, et al. Distinct roles of Akt1 and Akt2 in regulating cell migration and epithelial-mesenchymal transition. The Journal of cell biology 2005;171:1023-34.
34. Morali OG, Delmas V, Moore R, Jeanney C, Thiery JP, Larue L. IGF-II induces rapid beta-catenin relocation to the nucleus during epithelium to mesenchyme transition. Oncogene 2001;20:4942-50.
35. Iwao K, Miyoshi Y, Ooka M, et al. Quantitative analysis of estrogen receptor-alpha and -beta messenger RNA expression in human pancreatic cancers by real-time polymerase chain reaction. Cancer Lett 2001;170:91-7.
36. Stabile LP, Davis AL, Gubish CT, et al. Human non-small cell lung tumors and cells derived from normal lung express both estrogen receptor alpha and beta and show biological responses to estrogen. Cancer research 2002;62:2141-50.
37. Stabile LP, Lyker JS, Gubish CT, Zhang W, Grandis JR, Siegfried JM. Combined targeting of the estrogen receptor and the epidermal growth factor receptor in non-small cell lung cancer shows enhanced antiproliferative effects. Cancer research 2005;65:1459-70.
38. Levin ER. Bidirectional signaling between the estrogen receptor and the epidermal growth factor receptor. Mol Endocrinol 2003;17:309-17.
39. Zhang Z, Maier B, Santen RJ, Song RX. Membrane association of estrogen receptor alpha mediates estrogen effect on MAPK activation. Biochemical and biophysical research communications 2002;294:926-33.

40. Dickson RB, Huff KK, Spencer EM, Lippman ME. Induction of epidermal growth factor-related polypeptides by 17 beta-estradiol in MCF-7 human breast cancer cells. Endocrinology 1986;118:138-42.
41. Nicholson RI, McClelland RA, Finlay P, et al. Relationship between EGF-R, c-erbB-2 protein expression and Ki67 immunostaining in breast cancer and hormone sensitivity. European journal of cancer (Oxford, England 1993;29A:1018-23.
42. Nicholson RI, McClelland RA, Gee JM, et al. Epidermal growth factor receptor expression in breast cancer: association with response to endocrine therapy. Breast Cancer Res Treat 1994;29:117-25.
43. van Agthoven T, van Agthoven TL, Portengen H, Foekens JA, Dorssers LC. Ectopic expression of epidermal growth factor receptors induces hormone independence in ZR-75-1 human breast cancer cells. Cancer research 1992;52:5082-8.
44. McClelland RA, Barrow D, Madden TA, et al. Enhanced epidermal growth factor receptor signaling in MCF7 breast cancer cells after long-term culture in the presence of the pure antiestrogen ICI 182,780 (Faslodex). Endocrinology 2001;142:2776-88.
45. Dutcher JP. Mammalian target of rapamycin inhibition. Clin Cancer Res 2004;10:6382S-7S.
46. Kim DH, Sarbassov DD, Ali SM, et al. mTOR interacts with raptor to form a nutrient-sensitive complex that signals to the cell growth machinery. Cell 2002;110:163-75.
47. Sarbassov DD, Guertin, D. A., Ali, S. M., and Sabatini, D. M. Phosphorylation and Regulation of Akt/PKB by the Rictor-mTOR Complex. Science 2005;307:1098-101.
48. Sarbassov DD, Ali SM, Kim DH, et al. Rictor, a novel binding partner of mTOR, defines a rapamycin-insensitive and raptor-independent pathway that regulates the cytoskeleton. Curr Biol 2004;14:1296-302.
49. Sarbassov DD, Ali SM, Sabatini DM. Growing roles for the mTOR pathway. Curr Opin Cell Biol 2005..
50. Yonezawa K, Tokunaga C, Oshiro N, Yoshino K. Raptor, a binding partner of target of rapamycin. Biochem Biophys Res Commun 2004;313:437-41.
51. Harrington LS, Findlay GM, Gray A, et al. The TSC1-2 tumor suppressor controls insulin-PI3K signaling via regulation of IRS proteins. The Journal of cell biology 2004;166:213-23.
52. Tremblay F, Marette A. Amino acid and insulin signaling via the mTOR/p70 S6 kinase pathway. A negative feedback mechanism leading to insulin resistance in skeletal muscle cells. The Journal of biological chemistry 2001;276:38052-60.
53. Wan X, Harkavy B, Shen N, Grohar P, Helman LJ. Rapamycin induces feedback activation of Akt signaling through an IGF-1R-dependent mechanism. 2006.
54. Gual P, Le Marchand-Brustel Y, Tanti JF. Positive and negative regulation of insulin signaling through IRS-1 phosphorylation. Biochimie 2005;87:99-109.
55. Lee AV, Gooch JL, Oesterreich S, Guler RL, Yee D. Insulin-like growth factor I-induced degradation of insulin receptor substrate 1 is mediated by the 26S proteasome and blocked by phosphatidylinositol 3Î-kinase inhibition. Molecular and cellular biology 2000;20:1489-96.
56. Liu YF, Herschkovitz A, Boura-Halfon S, et al. Serine phosphorylation proximal to its phosphotyrosine binding domain inhibits insulin receptor substrate 1 function and promotes insulin resistance. Molecular and cellular biology 2004;24:9668-81.
57. Paz K, Hemi R, LeRoith D, et al. A molecular basis for insulin resistance. Elevated serine/threonine phosphorylation of IRS-1 and IRS-2 inhibits their binding to the juxtamembrane region of the insulin receptor and impairs their ability to undergo insulin-induced tyrosine phosphorylation. The Journal of biological chemistry 1997;272:29911-8.
58. O'Reilly KE, Rojo F, She QB, et al. mTOR inhibition induces upstream receptor tyrosine kinase signaling and activates Akt. Cancer Res 2006;66:1500-8.
59. Atkins MB, Hidalgo M, Stadler WM, et al. Randomized phase II study of multiple dose levels of CCI-779, a novel mammalian target of rapamycin kinase inhibitor, in patients with advanced refractory renal cell carcinoma. J Clin Oncol 2004;22:909-18.
60. Gemmill RM, Zhou M, Costa L, Korch C, Bukowski RM, Drabkin HA. Synergistic growth inhibition by Iressa and Rapamycin is modulated by VHL mutations in renal cell carcinoma. Br J Cancer 2005;92:2266-77.
61. Goudar RK, Shi Q, Hjelmeland MD, et al. Combination therapy of inhibitors of epidermal growth factor receptor/vascular endothelial growth factor receptor 2 (AEE788) and the mammalian target of rapamycin (RAD001) offers improved glioblastoma tumor growth inhibition. Mol Cancer Ther 2005;4:101-12.

62. Buck E, Eyzaguirre A, Brown E, et al. Rapamycin synergizes with the epidermal growth factor receptor inhibitor erlotinib in non-small-cell lung, pancreatic, colon, and breast tumors. Mol Cancer Ther 2006;5:2676-84.
63. Huber MA, Kraut N, Beug H. Molecular requirements for epithelial-mesenchymal transition during tumor progression. Curr Opin Cell Biol 2005;17:548-58.
64. Kang Y, Massague J. Epithelial-mesenchymal transitions: twist in development and metastasis. Cell 2004;118:277-9.
65. Thiery JP. Epithelial-mesenchymal transitions in development and pathologies. Curr Opin Cell Biol 2003;15:740-6.
66. Vincent-Salomon A, Thiery JP. Host microenvironment in breast cancer development: epithelial-mesenchymal transition in breast cancer development. Breast Cancer Res 2003;5:101-6.
67. Saito A, Yamashita T, Mariko Y, et al. A synthetic inhibitor of histone deacetylase, MS-27-275, with marked in vivo antitumor activity against human tumors. Proceedings of the National Academy of Sciences of the United States of America 1999;96:4592-7.
68. Chinnaiyan P, Varambally S, Tomlins SA, et al. Enhancing the antitumor activity of ErbB blockade with histone deacetylase (HDAC) inhibition. International journal of cancer 2006;118:1041-50.
69. Nimmanapalli R, Fuino L, Bali P, et al. Histone deacetylase inhibitor LAQ824 both lowers expression and promotes proteasomal degradation of Bcr-Abl and induces apoptosis of imatinib mesylate-sensitive or -refractory chronic myelogenous leukemia-blast crisis cells. Cancer research 2003;63:5126-35.
70. Pao W, Miller VA, Politi KA, et al. Acquired resistance of lung adenocarcinomas to gefitinib or erlotinib is associated with a second mutation in the EGFR kinase domain. PLoS Med 2005;2:e73.
71. Marks PA, Richon VM, Rifkind RA. Histone deacetylase inhibitors: inducers of differentiation or apoptosis of transformed cells. Journal of the National Cancer Institute 2000;92:1210-6.
72. Yoshikawa M, Hishikawa K, Marumo T, Fujita T. Inhibition of histone deacetylase activity suppresses epithelial-to-mesenchymal transition induced by TGF-beta1 in human renal epithelial cells. J Am Soc Nephrol 2007;18:58-65.
73. Bolen JB. Nonreceptor tyrosine protein kinases. Oncogene 1993;8:2025-31.
74. Yeatman TJ. A renaissance for SRC. Nat Rev Cancer 2004;4:470-80.
75. Frame MC. Src in cancer: deregulation and consequences for cell behaviour. Biochim Biophys Acta 2002;1602:114-30.
76. Schlaepfer DD, Mitra SK, Ilic D. Control of motile and invasive cell phenotypes by focal adhesion kinase. Biochim Biophys Acta 2004;1692:77-102.
77. Fincham VJ, Frame MC. The catalytic activity of Src is dispensable for translocation to focal adhesions but controls the turnover of these structures during cell motility. The EMBO journal 1998;17:81-92.
78. Behrens J, Vakaet L, Friis R, et al. Loss of epithelial differentiation and gain of invasiveness correlates with tyrosine phosphorylation of the E-cadherin/beta-catenin complex in cells transformed with a temperature-sensitive v-SRC gene. The Journal of cell biology 1993;120:757-66.
79. Rodier JM, Valles AM, Denoyelle M, Thiery JP, Boyer B. pp60c-src is a positive regulator of growth factor-induced cell scattering in a rat bladder carcinoma cell line. The Journal of cell biology 1995;131:761-73.
80. Avizienyte E, Wyke AW, Jones RJ, et al. Src-induced de-regulation of E-cadherin in colon cancer cells requires integrin signalling. Nature cell biology 2002;4:632-8.
81. Boyer B, Bourgeois Y, Poupon MF. Src kinase contributes to the metastatic spread of carcinoma cells. Oncogene 2002;21:2347-56.
82. Nam JS, Ino Y, Sakamoto M, Hirohashi S. Src family kinase inhibitor PP2 restores the E-cadherin/catenin cell adhesion system in human cancer cells and reduces cancer metastasis. Clinical cancer research 2002;8:2430-6.
83. Calcagno AM, Fostel JM, Orchekowski RP, et al. Modulation of cell adhesion molecules in various epithelial cell lines after treatment with PP2. Mol Pharm 2005;2:170-84.
84. Dannenberg AJ, Lippman SM, Mann JR, Subbaramaiah K, DuBois RN. Cyclooxygenase-2 and epidermal growth factor receptor: pharmacologic targets for chemoprevention. Journal of clinical oncology 2005;23:254-66.
85. Dannenberg AJ, Subbaramaiah K. Targeting cyclooxygenase-2 in human neoplasia: rationale and promise. Cancer cell 2003;4:431-6.

86. Dubinett SM, Sharma S, Huang M, Dohadwala M, Pold M, Mao JT. Cyclooxygenase-2 in lung cancer. Prog Exp Tumor Res 2003;37:138-62.
87. Dohadwala M, Yang SC, Luo J, et al. Cyclooxygenase-2-dependent regulation of E-cadherin: prostaglandin E(2) induces transcriptional repressors ZEB1 and snail in non-small cell lung cancer. Cancer Res 2006;66:5338-45.
88. Chen Z, Zhang X, Li M, et al. Simultaneously targeting epidermal growth factor receptor tyrosine kinase and cyclooxygenase-2, an efficient approach to inhibition of squamous cell carcinoma of the head and neck. Clinical cancer research 2004;10:5930-9.

Index

A

Abelson tyrosine kinase (Abl), 33–34, 37–40
    activated downstream of deregulated EGFR and, 76
    CML and forms of target, 37
    complex with imatinib and sites of mutations, 38
    imatinib resistance mutations and, 300
Abl kinase SMI imatinib (STI571), 34
c-Abl tyrosine kinase, 56
Actin-related protein (Arp)2/3 complex, 247
Activated Cdc42-associated kinase-1 (Ack-1), 243
Activated EGFR, accelerated internalization and degradation of, 48
Activation loop (A-loop), 33–34, 36–37, 40–41
Activator protein-1 (AP-1), 90, 339–340, 344
Acute promyelocytic-like leukemias (APLL), 81
AG1478, EGFR kinase inhibitor, 8, 80, 131–132, 161, 282, 284, 287, 363
AKT phosphorylation, 316, 360, 371–373
Akt (protein kinase B), 104. *See also* Phosphoinositide 3-kinase (PI3K)
    cell viabilty, maintenance of, 106
    phosphorylation of FOXO proteins by, 106
    in regulation of metabolism, 107
    targets, 106
    transcription, regulation of, 106–107
Akt signaling
    EGFR-independent activation of, 316
    link between EGFR and, 298
    redirecting to EGFR control, 370–374
    transactivation of EGFR and increased, 344
Alix protein, 56
Alternate receptor signaling
    IGF1R signaling, 362–363
    PDGFR signaling, 363
Amphiregulin (AR), 16, 74, 77, 90, 132, 223, 227, 244, 268, 342, 344
Androgen receptor, 22, 64, 124, 130
Angiogenesis, 74, 78–79, 90, 155, 157, 238, 264–266, 268, 341, 363
Angiogenic cytokines, EGFR-mediated regulation of, 264–266
4-Anilinoquinazoline, 32, 36, 40, 299–300
Anti-angiogenic effects, of EGFR antagonists, 267–268
Antibody-dependent cellular cytotoxicity (ADCC), 10, 163
Anti-EGFR antibodies, 8, 92, 268, 295, 354
Anti-EGFR therapies, 8, 222, 354, 363
Anti-ErbB2 antibodies, 8
Arachidonic acid. *See also* Prostaglandins
    cyclooxygenase 2 (COX-2), role of, 376
    importance of metabolism in tumorigenesis, 341
    metabolism of, 338
ARF nucleotide binding site opener (ARNO), 107
Argos protein, 171
Ataxia-telangiectasia mutant (ATM), 105
ATP competitors, for EGFR, 130
AU-rich elements (AREs), 339–340
Autophosphorylation
    of Akt, 105
    of EGFR for c-Src binding, 122
    of EGFR for motile phenotype, 261
    of EGFRvIII, 282–284
    FAK at tyrosine 397, 258
    increased levels of, 298
    and MIG-6 domain, 243
    of p110 γ on serine 1101, 100
    on tyrosine 1045, 69
    of tyrosine residues in carboxyl terminal of EGFR, 74
    on tyrosine residue Tyr216 in the activation loop, 64
    of Y416, 120–121
AZD0530 inhibitor, 131, 238

B

Back-to-back EGFR-ECD untethered dimer, 7
BAD phosphorylation, by MAPK, 159
BAD protein, 75, 106, 159, 241
Betacellulin (BTC), 16, 74, 90, 223, 263–264, 266
Bispecific (BsAb)/multispecific antibodies, 163
Breast cancer
    Abl kinases and, 76
    activity of trastuzumab in treatment of, 297
    altered ErbB2 expression in, 18
    autocrine PDGFR signaling in, 363
    AZD0530 and gefitinib role in, 238
    cadherin-11 expression in, 146–147
    C4HD proliferation and IGF-IR antisense message in, 160
    co-expression ErbB2 and ErbB3 in, 228
    COX-2 in, 339

Breast cancer (*continued*)
   c-Src activation in, 238
   cytokines bFGF and PDGF-BB in, 267
   EGFR, prognostic role of, 224
   ErbB3 expression in, 226
   ErbB4 ICD and Eto2 interaction in, 194
   ErbB receptors and, 172–173
   ErbB2 role in, 225
   ErbB2 transgenic model of, 173–174
   expression of EGFR in, 224
   expression of Syk in, 238
   Gab2 overexpression in, 239
   gefitinib and anti-ErbB2 monoclonal antibody herceptin for, 229
   HER2-positive and HER2-negative, 25
   HRG family proteins role in, 227
   IGF-IR expression and, 158
   LRIG1 and Met receptor tyrosine kinase in, 179
   measurement of HER2 protein levels by IHC in, 356
   missense EGFR TKD mutations in, 305
   overexpress ErbB2 respond to, 8
   p95^{HER2} produced in, 23
   prognostic role of ErbB2 in, 225–226
   Raf-MEK-ERK signaling pathway and, 106
   RALT expression in, 178
   Rho family GTPase Cdc42 and, 246
   suppression of Cdc42 in, 246
   tamoxifen-resistant, 125, 130
   trastuzumab to HER2-positive patients, 20
   TSG101 transcripts detection in, 247
   Y845 phosphorylation and, 124
Bronchioloalveolar carcinomas (BAC), 295, 303–304

C

Cadherin-catenin signaling, 259
Cadherins
   adhesion initiates cell signaling, 144
   adhesive properties of, 140
      extracellular domain, 140–141
      intracellular domain, 141–143
   cadherin/catenin complexes, destabilization of, 147–148
   in cancer
      cell cycle control, 146
      contact inhibition, 145–146
      EMT and, 144–145
      inappropriate profile and pro-migratory effects, 147
      loss of adhesion, 145
      loss of expression, 145
      endocytosis, 148
      and tyrosine kinase receptors, 147
C225 antibody, 5, 7–8, 11, 195, 265
Caspase 9, pro-apoptotic protease, 106
α-Catenin, 143–144
β-Catenin, 107, 143, 261
Caveolin, 129, 131, 261, 280, 282
Cbl, E3-ligase, 129
Cbl proteins, 55–56
   as E3-ligase, 129, 179
   in mammalian cells, 50
   mediating ErbB2 ubiquitination, 66
   somatically mutated EGFRs induce phosphorylation of, 69
   and tyrosine 1045 of EGF receptor, 175, 298
c-Cbl protein, 50, 236, 243
   inhibition of function, 246–247
   phosphorylation of, 281
Cell migration, regulation of, 107. *See also* Phosphoinositide 3-kinase (PI3K); Phosphatidylinositol (PtdIns)
Cell surface proteins, translocation and functions, 190
Cellular kinase CDK2, 17–18, 22, 36–37, 41
Centaurins, 107
Cetuximab, 5, 7–8, 16, 23–24, 92, 239, 295, 301, 308, 315, 354, 359
Cholangicarcinomas, EGFR TKD mutations in, 304
Cholera toxin, 192
Chromosomal genomic hybridization (CGH), 308
Chronic myelogenous leukemia (CML), 37, 81, 131, 294
Clathrin
   as adaptor for class II PIK enzymes and, 108
   coated pits, 48–52, 69, 129, 175, 188, 245
   phosphorylation by c-Src, 129
   vesicle, 49
Clathrin-dependent internalization, 49–50. *See also* EGFR internalization
   activation of tyrosine kinase, 49
   mutational analysis, of EGFR endocytosis, 49–50
   p38, role in, 50
   serine/threonine phosphorylation, of EGFR, 50
Clathrin-independent internalization. *See* EGFR internalization
Cofilin, 261–262
Colony stimulating factor-1 (CSF-1), 191, 258
Colorectal adenocarcinomas (CRC), EGFR TKD mutations in, 304
Conserved amino acids in EGF, 6
Cortactin, 129, 247
Cowden syndrome, 241
CREB binding protein (CBP), 106

Index

CR1 loop, 6–7
  for EGFR and ErbB2, 9
  human EGFR and ErbB4, structural homology between, 10
CR2 pocket, between EGFR, ErbB3, and ErbB4, 9
cyclic-AMP dependent kinase, 33
Cyclic nucleotide response element binding (CREB), 106
CyclinA, 41
Cyclin/Cdk complexes, 106
Cyclooxygenase-2 (COX-2)
  affecting EMT status, 374–375
  and COX-1, 338, 342, 345
  and EGFR, in cancer treatment, 337, 344–346
  expression in cancers, regulation of, 340
  inhibiting carcinogenesis, 341–343
  overexpressed in premalignant and malignant tissues, 339
  and prostaglandins, 264
  regulation of expression, 338–339
  3'-untranslated region (UTR), of mRNA, 339–340
CYP19 gene, 341
Cystine-rich domain (CR1), 5
Cytohesin-1, 107

D

Dasatanib (BMS-354825), 131–132
Dbl homology (DH), 107
Deubiquitination enzymes (DUBs), 56
Diacylglycerol (DAG), 75–76, 240
Dictyostelium, 262
Dimerization, 7
Drosophila LRR/Ig protein Kekkon-1. *See* LRR-containing proteins
Drosophila melanogaster, 171
Dual specificity phosphatases (DUSPs), 171, 244
Dynamin, 49, 52, 129, 191

E

E-cadherin, 82, 92. *See also* Cadherins
  and apoptotic effect of gefitinib in, 375
  and γ-catenin, 360
  and CD44, cleavage of, 263
  and cell-cell interactions, 260–261
  determining EGFR TKI sensitivity, role in, 317
  and EGFR role in cancer, 140–148
  histone deacetylase (HDAC) inhibition and, 318
  levels and homotypic cell adhesion, 377
  loss of, 361
  regulation of cell growth by, 145–146
  for regulation of HER3 and Akt, 370
  regulation of migration by, 147
  regulator β-catenin, 267
  role in epithelial intercellular adhesion and, 344
  signaling to EGFR, 148–150
    activation of signaling, 148–149
    regulation, E-cadherin/EGFR axis, 149–150
    src and cell adhesion, 376
  as tumor-suppressor and metastasis-suppressor gene, 144–145
EGF. *See* Epidermal growth factor
EGF:EGFR complexes, 48
EGF endocytosis, 47–48, 50. *See also* EGFR internalization
EGF-induced down-regulation, of EGFR, 48
EGF internalization. *See* EGFR internalization
EGF-like growth factors, 222, 226–228
EGFR. *See* Epidermal growth factor receptor
EGFR antagonists, 355
EGFR biology, as predictor of sensitivity, 355
  EGFR copy number, IHC, and FISH analysis, 356–358
  EGFR dimerization partners, 358–359
  EGFR mutations, 356
  EGFR-regulated downstream signaling pathways, 359–360
EGFR-dimer configuration, 6
EGFR-directed inhibitors, 354
EGFR down-regulation, 48
  modulators of, 56
EGFR and integrin signaling, 259
EGFR and SFK inhibitors. *See also* C-Src protein
  ATP competitive inhibitors, for SFK, 131–132
  dominant negative c-Src, expression of, 132
  Src homozygous null mice, 132
EGFR/E-cadherin axis, 150
EGFR-ECD:ErbB2-ECD heterodimers, 9
EGFR-ECD-Fc fusion protein, 7
EGFR β-solenoid domains, 4
EGF receptor system
  modeling and simulation
    differential equation methods, 211
    individual based methods, 211–213
    modeling behavior on cell surface in, 215
EGF receptor ubiquitination and degradation, 174–175
EGFR-EGF crystals, 6
EGFR-ErbB2 heterodimers, 6, 11
EGFR expression, in cancer, 76
EGFR family members, antibody binding to, 10–11
  2C4 (pertuzumab), ErbB2 antibody, 10–11
  herceptin antibody, toward CR2 domain of ErbB2, 10
  mab806 vs. mab528 antibody, 11
EGFR FISH score, 357
EGFR gene, 8, 35, 278
  amplification, 223
  copy number, 298, 313–314
  heterozygous mutations in, 356

EGFR/IGF-IR inhibition, 161
EGFR/IGFR monoclonal antibodies, 162–163
EGFR/IGFR small molecule inhibitors, 161–162
EGFR SMI research, 40–42
EGFR in non-tumor cells, of neoplastic environment, 228–229
EGFR internalization, 7
  clathrin-independent mechanisms of, 48–49, 52
  c-Src substrates, regulating degradation and, 129
  deubiquitination enzymes (DUBs), regulating degradation and, 56
  gefitinib resistance and, 247
  Grb2-and tyrosine phosphorylation-independent, 50
  non-receptor tyrosine kinase, c-Abl, in inhibition of, 246
  pathways through endosomal compartment, 53
  proteins implicating in regulation of, 56
  and targeting receptor to lysosomes for, 69
  through clathrin-coated pits, 50–52
  ubiquitination activity and, 56
EGFR intron 1 and single-nucleotide polymorphisms, 316
EGFR kinase, 6–7. *See also* EGFR kinase domain
  activation, 7
  allosteric influence, on activity, 32, 40
  anilinoquinazolines and, 300
  ATP-binding cleft, nature of inhibition in, 34
  complex with erlotinib and sites of mutations, 38
  gefitinib and activation of Akt and Erk, 238
  GPR30-mediated transcription and, 124
  inactive state, 7, 40
  inhibitor AG1478 and, 8
  inhibitor PKI-166 and apoptosis, 242
  inhibitors targeting PI3K in gliomas, 287
  kinase/SMI interactions, 35
    tyrosine residue (Tyr845 and Tyr869), 35–36
  L858R/L861Q mutations and activity of, 39
  phosphorylation of Y845 by c-Src, 122, 124–125
  PI3K/Akt pathway and inhibition of, 363
  potent inhibitors of, 35
  for rapid receptor endocytosis and phosphorylation, 49
  signaling, activation of, 6
  structurally characterized SMIs and ATP for, 34
  T790M, in treatment with erlotinib/gefitinib, 38–39
  tyrosine phosphorylation of Gab1 and, 281
  tyrosine residue, as Tyr845, 35–36
  X-ray structures, wild-type, 36–37
    DFG tripeptide and αc helix, 36
    erlotinib and gefitinib, orientations, 36–37
    lapatinib-bound A-loop, 37
    lapatinib quinazoline core H-bonds, 37
EGFR kinase domain
  activation loop and phosphorylation, 68
  deletions in lung cancer, 278
  identification of mutations in, 356, 364
  mechanism of activation of, 41
  somatic mutations in, 68–69, 91
  ubiquitination sites, mapping, 51
EGFR, KRAS and p53 mutation, in smokers, 302–303
EGFR-ligand complex, 6
EGFR-mediated downstream signaling pathways
  MAPK pathway, 74–75
  PI3k/Akt pathway, 75
  PLC γ pathway, 75–76
EGFR-mediated regulation, of angiogenic cytokines, 264–266
2-7EGFR mutation, 8. *See also* EGFRvIII, receptor system
EGFR mutations. *See* EGFR-TKD mutations; Non-small-cell lung cancer (NSCLC)
EGFR overexpression
  in absence of growth factor, 175
  and activation as poor prognostic factor, 356
  downstream effects and in cancer, 76
  IGF-IR and, 159
  MMPs correlations with, 263
EGFR-related peptide (ERRP), 178, 265
EGFR signaling, 280
  and cancer, 343
    EGFR and COX-2, combined targeting of, 344–345
    cascades
      site-specific phosphorylation dynamics, 204–205
  in endothelial cells (EC), 266
  pertubation of feedback control of, 242 (*see also* Human carcinomas)
    feedback loops, 242–244
  in tumor cells, 265
EGFR sorting in MVB, molecular mechanisms, 53–55
  ESCRTI and ESCRTIII complexes, TSG101 and hVps24 for, 54–55
  fusion of MVBs with primary lysosomal vesicles, 55
  Hrs microdomains, formation of, 54
  inhibitors, blocking degradation, 55
  ubiquitination, for lysosomal targeting, 54
EGFR, tethered and untethered forms, 7
EGFR-TKD mutations
  in cholangicarcinomas, 304
  in colorectal adenocarcinomas (CRC), 304

Index

esophageal adenocarcinomas, 304
gastric adenocarcinomas, 305
glioblastomas, 305–306
of ovarian cancers, 305
pancreatic adenocarcinomas, 305
prostate adenocarcinomas, 305
of renal cell carcinoma, 305
in squamous cell carcinomas of the head and neck (SCCHN), 304
synovial sarcoma, 306
tumor cytogenetics, in NSCLC, 297
EGFR transactivation. *See also* C-Src protein
GPCR-mediated EGFR transactivation, 123–124
nuclear steroid hormone receptor-mediated, 124–125
other receptors and molecules for, 125–126
EGFR tyrosine kinase inhibitors, 92, 222, 224
migration of microvascular endothelial cells, effect on, 228
in NSCLC treatment, 295, 306–311
EGFR tyrosine phosphoproteome
temporal dynamics, 203–204
EGFR ubiquitination, 51–52, 54. *See also* EGFR internalization
Cbl mediates, 69, 129
and ESCRT complexes, 55
ligand-induced, 66
EGFRvIII, receptor system. *See also* Glioma-associated EGFRvIII signaling
detection in cancers, 74
expression in tumors, 279
FLAG-tagged, 65
as immunotherapeutic target, 285–287
Mab L8A4 and expression on U87MG-EGFRvIII cells, 282
mutation, 8
in NSCLC, 296–297
peptide as tumor vaccine, 286
as signaling target, 286
signal transduction, 281–285
cell membrane localization, 282
ligand binding, dimerization and autophosphorylation, 282–283
signaling pathways, 283
transfection of, 260
EGFRwt gene amplification, 278
EGFRwt receptor system, 280
signal transduction, pathways of, 280–281
EGF system, role of, 156
EMP-1 expression, 317
Endogenous EGFR ligand, 7
Endosomal sorting complex required for transport (ESCRT-I), 245, 247
Epigen (EPG), 90
Epiregulin (EPR), 16, 74, 90, 223

Epithelial-mesenchymal transition (EMT), 144, 146, 317, 344–345, 357, 369–372
affecting status, 374–375
COX-2 blockade, combination with, 376–377
EGFR and HDAC inhibitors, combinations of, 375–376
Src inhibitors, combination with, 376
and EGFR inhibitors insensitivity, 360–362
Epithelial *vs.* mesenchymal differentiation, 317
ErbB3 and ErbB4 expressions, human carcinomas, 226
ErbB2 CR1 loop, conformation, 9
ErbB degradation mechanisms, 175–177
chaperone-mediated stability, 176
E3 ubiquitin ligases, role in, 176–177
Nrdp1 protein levels, regulation of, 177
ErbB dimers
diversity of, 18–19
dimers potent at stimulating proliferation, 18
downstream pathways
ErbB receptor expression, differential level of, 18–19
PI3K, MAPK, PKC, and JNK pathways, 18
proximity-based assay, to determine level of interaction, 19
ErbB2-ECD, 3D-structure of, 6, 10
ErbB2-ECD fragments, crystal structures of, 9
ErbB2/ErbB3 expression. *See also* Breast cancer
in ErbB2-induced mouse mammary tumors, 174
ErbB2/ErbB3 oncogenic unit, 173
ErbB2 expression, in human carcinoma, 225–226
ErbB family kinase domains, 40
ErbB family members
dimerization and activation, 16–17
ligands for induction, 16
extracellular portion domains, 17–18
ErbB family, of receptor tyrosine kinases (RTKs), 90
ErbB2 gene, 16, 172–173, 225
amplification, 174, 226
ErbB heterodimers, 19–20
cancer therapy, inhibition in
direct inhibition of tyrosine kinase activity, 23
by monoclonal antibody therapeutics, 23–25
ErbB1/ErbB2, in cancer, 20–21
ErbB2/ErbB3, in cancer, 21–23
ErbB2 heteromers, 8
ErbB3 kinase, 8
ErbB4 ligand-binding domain, 3D-structure of, 9
ErbB, negative regulatory pathways, 174–177
ErbB, nuclear functions for, 194–195

ErbB2 on Hsp90, determinants for stability, 66–68.
   See also Hsp90 (heat shock protein)
   GA sensitivity and electrostatic nature of M5
      loop, 67
   homology in amino acid sequences and
      phosphorylation, 68
   Hsp90 binding motif, localization, 66–67
   post-translational modification, 68
ErbB pathways, conventional, 188
   ErbB receptor signaling, 188
   ErbB receptor trafficking, 188–189
ErbB receptors
   and cognate ligands, 223
   family interactome
      quantitative characterization of, 200–202
      SILAC approach, for temporal
         analysis, 201–202
   in human carcinomas, expression of, 222
   and ligands in tumors, co-expression of,
      227–228
ErbB splice variants, 178
ErbB translocation to nucleus, mechanism, 189
   ErbB fragments and protease-dependent route,
      189–191
   holoreceptors, 191–192
   Sec61 pathway, 192–194
Erlotinib. *See also* Non-small-cell lung cancer
      (NSCLC)
   in cancer treatment, 295
   EGFR TKD mutations and, 299–301
   structures of, 35
   susceptibility and EGFR mutants, 39–40
Esophageal adenocarcinomas, EGFR TKD
      mutations in, 304–305
Estrogen receptor (ER), 76, 79, 124, 130, 159,
      226–227, 241, 370
   and EGFR, antitumor activity of, 372
E3 ubiquitin ligases, 50, 174, 176
   feedback negative regulation, of EGFR and
      ErbB3, 177
Eukaryotic protein kinases, 32
Exon 2-7 deletion mutation, 8
Extracellular domains (ECDs)
   ECD-directed monoclonal antibody cetuximab,
      301
   EGFR-ECD, 6–11
      deletions, 305
   homophilic interactions
      within, 141
   of human EGFR and ErbB2, 5
   of IGF-1R, 4
   N-terminal, in lumen of ER, 67
   regulation of EGFR kinase (signaling) and, 4
Extracellular matrix (ECM), 258–259
   cell-ECM adhesive interactions, 263
   composition and EGF-induced signaling, 260
   degradation, 262

F

F-actin polymerization, 107
Factor 4E-binding protein 1 (4E-BP1), 107
Familial adenomatous polyposis (FAP), 264,
      341–343
Fc fusion proteins, 7
Ferguson EGFR-ECD structures, 6
Fibronectin, 258, 260, 263, 360
Fluorescence in situ hybridization (FISH), 297,
      313–314
   EGFR FISH, 313, 316, 318–321, 357–358, 360
5-Fluorouracil, 8
Focal adhesion kinase (FAK), 128–130, 203, 238,
      246, 258–260, 265, 376
Forkhead box O (FOXO) family, of transcription
      factors, 106

G

GAB1 and *GAB2* gene, 239
GA-induced ErbB2 degradation, 65
Gastric adenocarcinomas, EGFR TKD mutations
      in, 305
Gastrointestinal stromal tumors (GIST), 131
Gefitinib. *See also* EGFR/IGFR small molecule
         inhibitors; EGFR tyrosine kinase inhibitors
   in cancer treatment, 295
   EGFR TKD mutations and, 299–301
   structures of, 35
   susceptibility and EGFR mutants, 39–40
Geldanamycin (GA), 64–68. *See also* EGFR kinase
      domain; Hsp90
General receptor for phosphoinositides (GRP1),
      107
Glioblastoma, EGFR TKD mutations in, 305–306
Glioma-associated EGFRvIII signaling
   for therapeutic targeting
      EGFRvIII as localizing target, 285
      EGFRvIII as signaling target, 286
      EGFRvIII peptide as tumor
         vaccine, 286
      TKIs (tyrosine kinase inhibitors), 286–287
Glycogen synthase kinase 3 (GSK3), 107
Grb2-associated binder-1 (Gab-1), 102, 239, 281
Grb2-dependent mechanisms, 49
Growth factor-induced cell migration, 259
GTPase activating proteins (GAPs), 89, 91, 107
GTP/GDP exchange factors (GEFs), 89–90, 107
   RHO family, 240, 262

H

Hdm2 ubiquitination, 194
Head and neck cancer cell lines (HNSCC), 122, 132

Index

Heparin binding-EGF (HB-EGF), 16, 90, 124, 223, 227, 266–268
Hepatocellular carcinoma related protein (HCRP), 247
Herceptin, 10, 162, 172, 178, 244, 356
HER3-ECD 3D-structure, 5
Heregulin (HRG), 16, 24–25, 90, 173, 190–191, 194, 227, 264
HER-2 gene, 284. *See also* Breast cancer
HER2, HER3 and EGFR ligands, co-expression of, 316–317
HER2/neu receptors, 159
Herstatin, 178, 284–285
Heterodimerization, 6, 18
 of activated EGFR with Her3, 298, 317
 cetuximab binding within domain III of ErbB, inhibiting, 24
 EGFR-HER2, 372
 EGFR/IGFR contribute to resistance, 159–160
 of EGFR with ErbB2, 246
 ErbB3 dependent on kinase-intact family for, 16
 HER2 lacking functional ligand-binding domain and, 90
 inhibitor, 318
 proximity-based assay, for level of interaction, 19
Hip1 protein, 104, 247
Histidine-alanine-valine (HAV) sequence, 141–142
Histone deacetylases (HDACs), 318, 375
 and EGFR, in cancer treatment, 375–376
Homodimerization, 18. *See also* Heterodimerization
 EGFRvIII with EGFRwt/ErbB family members, 282
 of EGFRwt, 281
 equilibrium toward ErbB2, 20
Hsp90 (heat shock protein)
 association and GA, 68–69, 298
 to check and enable folding of nascent polypeptides and, 176
 down-regulated by HDACs and, 375
 to maintain stability of mature ErbB2, 65–66
 for maturation of nascent EGFR and ErbB2, 65
Human carcinomas
 attenuation of, EGFR down-regulation and role of, 245
  c-Cbl function, inhibition of, 246–247
  endocytic down-regulation, pertubation of, 247
  receptor down-regulation and, 247
 EGF-like growth factors expression, 226–227
 EGF-like peptides, expression of, 227
 EGFR expression in, 222–225
 EGFR signaling pathways
  amplification of, 236
  decrease in down-regulation of, 245–247
  feedback loops, pertubations in, 237, 242–244
  future perspectives of, 247–248
 ErbB3 and ErbB4 expression, 226
 ErbB2 expression of, 225–226
 ErbB receptors and ligands, co-expression in, 227–228
 feedback loops, role of, 242–244
 non tumor cells, EGFR expression and function, 228–229
Human epidermal growth factor receptor (HER or ErbB), 15
Human growth hormone (HGH), 375
Human papillomavirus type 16 (HPV 16), 246–247
Hypoxia inducible factor (HIF), 63, 266–267
Hypoxia response elements (HRE), 266

I

ICD-EGFR kinase, 7
IGF/EGF ligands, 156–157
IGF/EGF receptors, 158–159
IGFR-1 expression, 316
IkB kinase (IKK), 106
Imatinib, 34, 36, 38, 40, 131, 300
 point mutation in T790M and acquired-resistance model for, 356
 resistance and mutations in c-kit and, 294
 second generation (AMN107, nilotinib), 37
Inducible nitric oxide synthase (iNOS), 74, 195
Inositol 1,4,5 trisphosphate (IP3), 75–76, 240
Insulin like growth factor-1 (IGF-1), 157, 160, 227
 and EGFR, antitumor activity of, 371–372
Insulin-like growth factor receptor ECD (IGF-IR), 4, 156–163
 suppression by ASODNs, 159
Insulin like growth factor receptor-1 (IGF-1R), 4, 158, 162, 287, 316, 370–373
Insulin receptor kinase domain, 33
Insulin receptor substrate isoforms, 156
Integrin-linked kinase (ILK), 105
Intracellular domain (ICD), 7, 16, 18, 21, 23
 actin link, 141–143
 antibody P2, recognizing epitope in EGFRwt, 283
 of E-cadherin, as regulatory function, 149
 of ErbB2, 16, 23 (*see also* Heterodimerization)
 ErbB4 intracellular domain fragment, production of, 188
 folding cadherin (*see* β-Catenin)
Intracellular feedback loops. *See also* EGFR signaling
 categories of, 242–244
 exploitation of, 372–374

Intracellular signaling cascades. *See also* EGF receptor system
 differential equation models of, 213–214
 higher level models for, 215–216
 larger system biology software systems, 216
 modeling methods for, 214–215
  BioGenNet system, 214
  parallel distributed processing, 215
  synthetic biology approach, 215

J
c-Jun NH(2)-terminal kinase (JNK), 160, 283

K
Kekkon-1 (Kek1), transmembrane protein, 171
Kekkon proteins, 243. *See also* LRIG1 protein
Kinase domain from EGFR, 33
KRAS mutations, 91, 302–304, 315, 359
K-ras mutations, 92, 239

L
Lapatinib, 16, 23, 32–33, 35, 37–41, 130, 294, 354, 358. *See also* EGFR antagonists
Lazarus effect, 295
Ligand affinity, on EGFR-ECD truncated, 7
Ligand-binding, pH sensitive histidine in, 9–10
Ligand-induced activation, 8, 178
LIM kinase, 262
Loss of heterozygosity (LOH), 241, 297
lrig1 gene, 179, 243
LRIG1 protein, 56, 179–180, 243
LR2 pocket, in vertebrate orthologs of EGFR, ErbB3, and ErbB4, 9
L858R proteins, 39
 e19del and L858R mutants, 298
 exon 19 deletion *vs.* L858R *vs.* other mutations, in tumors, 307–308
LRR-containing proteins, 179
Lymphangiogenesis, 264–266

M
mab806 antibody, 8, 11
Macrophage colony stimulating factor (M-CSF), 81, 229
Mammalian ErbB negative regulation, 171
 mediated by E3 ubiquitin ligases, 174–177
 suppression of receptor activity, 178–179
Mammalian target of rapamycin (mTOR), 75, 105, 107, 160, 241–242, 266, 373. *See also* Rapamycin
MAPK-and PI3K-induced inhibition, of proapoptotic BH3, 159
MAP kinases (MAPKs), 240, 244, 281
MAPK pathway, inhibition of, 284

MAPK phosphatases (MKPs), 244
Matrix metalloproteinases (MMPs), 123–124, 259–260, 263, 267
Mesenchymal-epithelial-transition (MET), 317, 370, 374
 amplification, 316–317
Metastasis, 267
Microvessel density (MVD), 267
MIG-6 gene, 244
Mitogen-activated protein kinase (MAPK), 50, 156, 261
 pathway inhibition, 284
Molecular chaperone HSP90, 63–64
 client proteins and, 63
 co-chaperone p23 and Aha1, interaction with, 64
 forming complex with, 64
 ternary complex of Hsp90 ·p50^{cdc37}·kinase, 64
Molecularly targeted therapies (MTT), 354–355
Multivesicular bodies (MVBs), 48, 53–55
Murine mammary tumor virus (MMTV), 173–174

N
N-cadherin, 140, 146–147
Neuregulin (NRG), 9, 16–17, 90, 173, 194, 223, 227
Neuregulin receptor degradation protein-1 (Nrdp1), 176
Nilotinib, 37–38
Non-erbB-family protein kinase domains, 40
Non-receptor tyrosine kinases, 75, 79, 145, 147, 236, 238, 246
Non-small-cell lung cancer (NSCLC), 224, 239, 264
 EGFR and ER expression, in treating, 372
 EGFR and IGF-1R expression, in treating, 371–372
 EGFR expression and gene copy number in, 311–315
  EGFR expression in, 312–313
  EGFR gene copy number, 313–314
  relationship of, 314–315
 and EGFR inhibitors sensitivity, molecular features of, 315–318
 EGFR TKD mutations and inhibitors in vitro
  EGFR inhibitors, various classes of, 300–301
  Exon 19 deletion/L858R, 299
  gefitinib and erlotinib, sensitivity/resistance to, 299–300
 EGFR TKD mutations, clinical-pathological relationships of, 301
  demographic associations, 301
  EGFR, KRAS and p53 mutations and smoking, 302–303

ethnicity, 303
histopathologic types, of NSCLC, 303–304
EGFR TKD mutations, molecular and mechanistic aspects
  cytogenetics of, 297
  EGFRvIII in NSCLC, 296–297
  oncogenic signaling, by mutant EGFRs, 297–298
  spectrum and prevalence of, 296
EGFR TKD mutations to EGFR TKI sensitivity, relationship of, 306–311
erlotinib with EGFR pathway variables and EMT, relationship, 357
histopathologic types of, 303–304
KRAS mutations and primary resistance to EGFR TKIS, 315
molecular testing in clinical trials in, 318
pathology sample and molecular assay in, 318–322
treatment of, 295–296
tumor cytogenetics, of EGFR TKD mutations in, 297
Nuclear Factor kB (NFkB), 106
Nuclear receptor corepressor (NCoR), 339

O

Oncogene mutations, in tumor, 294
Oncogene (neu), 8, 73, 158, 222, 339. See also Breast cancer
Ovarian carcinoma, EGFR TKD mutations in, 305
Overall survival (OS), 224, 307

P

Pancreatic adenocarcinomas, EGFR TKD mutations in, 305
Panitumumab, 16, 23–25
p130 Cas, adapter protein, 130
p120 Catenin, 144
Peptide nucleic acid-locked nucleic acid (PNA-LNA), 321
Periostin, secretory protein, 260
Pertuzumab, 10, 24–25, 160, 294, 318, 355
p95 ^{HER2} heterodimers, 23. See also ErbB heterodimers
Phosphatidylinositol 4,5 bisphosphate (PIP2), 75, 240
Phosphatidylinositol (PtdIns), 98
  GAP1^m and GAP1IP4BP, regulation by PtdIns($3,4,5$)P3, 107
  PtdIns($3,4,5$)P3 and PtdIns($3,4$)P2, downstream targets of, 103–104
Phosphatidylinositol 3,4,5 trisphosphate (PIP3), 240, 262
Phosphoinositide-dependent kinase (PDK-1)

downstream targets of, 105
Phosphoinositide 3-kinase (PI3K), 258, 262, 281, 343
  class III PI3K enzyme, 101
  class II PI3K enzymes, 100–101
  class I PI3K
    adaptor subunits, 100
    catalytic subunits, 99–100
    and EGFR enhancing IGF-IR signaling, 160
    ERBB receptor-mediated recruitment of, 102–103
    isoforms and relationship between, 98–99
    options for recruitment, to activated EGF receptor, 103
  pathway, inhibition of, 284–285
  PI3K-C2α, affecting clathrin-mediated endocytosis and, 108
  and regulation of vesicle transport, 107–108
  signaling, in human cancers, 240–241
  substrate specificity of, 101–102
Phospholipase C γ (PLC γ), 237, 258, 261
Phospholipid hydrolysis and signaling, 240–242
Phosphotyrosine binding (PTB), 100, 175, 200, 236
PIK3CA gene, 241
PIK3CA mutation, 316
Platelet-derived growth factor (PDGF), 78, 90, 98, 130, 202–203, 361
Platelet derived growth factor receptor (PDGFR), 77, 131, 203, 363, 370
Pleckstrin homology (PH), 240
Porcine aortic endothelial (PAE) cells, 49
p65 PAK protein, 262
PP1 and PP2, ATP competitive inhibitors for SFK, 131
Presenilin-dependent cleavage of ErbB4, 194
p160 ROCK protein, 262
Progression-free survival (PFS), 24, 244, 278, 306–307, 322
Prolactin (PRL) activated mammary gland transcription factor, 81. See also STAT signaling pathways
Proliferating cell nuclear antigen (PCNA), 195
Prostaglandins
  biosynthesis of, 337–343
  PGE 2 activating signal transduction pathways and carcinogenesis, 342
  prostaglandin E2 (PGE2), 264
  receptors, signaling and carcinogenesis, 340–341
Prostate adenocarcinomas, EGFR TKD mutations in, 305
Protein kinase A (PKA), 33, 104–105, 344
Protein kinase catalytic domains, 33

Protein kinase C (PKC), 76, 99, 104–105, 125, 162, 190, 240, 261, 281, 339
  dependent phosphorylation, of Thr654, 50
Protein phosphorylation, in cell signaling, 33
Protein tyrosine phosphatase (PTP), 125, 180, 239
Proteolysis, 55, 258, 263
Proteomic profiling signatures, 317–318. *See also* Non-small-cell lung cancer (NSCLC)
PTEN loss, 242, 287, 316
PTEN, mutations of, 241

Q
Quantitative PCR (qPCR), 313–314
Quantitative proteomics, 200–201, 204. *See also* EGFR tyrosine phosphoproteome
Quantitative reverse-transcriptase PCR (qRT-PCR), 312–313

R
Raf family of proteins, 90
RalB-Sec5 effector pathway, in human cancer, 240
RalGDS, in human cancer, 240
Rapamycin
  activity of p70S6K in situ, inhibited by, 105
  and Akt phosphorylation, 372
  binding to FKBP, 21
  enhancing effect of HK-272 in, 318
  enhancing sensitivity of PTEN-deficient glioblastoma cells to, 242
  with inhibitor of IGF-1R, 373
  synergizes with erlotinib to, 374
RAS activation
  and cancer, 91
  by EGFR pathway
    activation by RTKs, 90
    ErbB activation by, 90–91
  by mutant EGFR in cancer, 91–92
Ras effector pathways, in human cancer, 240
Ras GTPases pathways, in EGFR signaling, 238–240
Ras guanine nucleotide exchange factor (GEF), 238
Ras protein family, 89
R-cadherin, 146–147
Receptor activator of NF-kB ligand (RANKL), 229
Receptor-associated late transducer (RALT), 178
Receptor tyrosine kinases (RTKs), 16, 32, 48, 73, 79, 90, 192, 258, 294, 370–371
Recombinant human IGF binding protein 3 (rhIGFBP-3), 162
Relapse free survival (RFS), 76, 224
Renal cell carcinoma, EGFR TKD mutations in, 305
Rheb GTPase, 107, 241

Rho GTPases, 144, 262
Ribosomal protein S6 (RPS6), 161
RNA interference (RNAi), 22, 49–50, 52, 55

S
Saccharomyces cerevisiae, 98
Sec61 β protein, 194
Serine/threonine phosphorylation, of EGFR, 50
Serum response element (SRE), 107
Signal transducers, oncogenic changes in, 235–237
  non-receptor tyrosine kinases, 238
  phospholipid hydrolysis and signaling, 240–242
  Ras GTPases, role of, 238–240
Signal transduction, via EGFRWT. *See also* EGFRvIII, receptor system
  cell membrane localization, 280
  endosomal localization and signaling pathways, 281
Site-specific phosphorylation dynamics. *See* EGFR signaling
Skp2 ubiquitin ligase, 159
Small molecule inhibitors (SMI), 32, 34–36, 38, 40. *See also* EGFR antagonists
Small RNA interference (siRNA), 50–51, 53, 56, 105, 108, 191
SOCS4/5 protein, 56
β-Solenoid domains, 4
Sprouty 2 protein, 55
Squamous cell carcinomas of the head and neck (SCCHN), 76, 80, 82, 126, 258, 264, 304, 377
Squamous cell carcinomas (SCC), 260, 296, 304, 314
c-Src expression, in EGFR signaling, 238
Src family kinases (SFKs), 123, 130, 246, 376
Src homology (SH), 74, 100, 120, 157, 235, 281
Src-homology 4 (SH4) domain, 120
Src inhibitors and EGFR, in cancer treatment, 376
Src kinase substrate. *See* p120 Catenin
c-Src-/-knock-out mice, 132
C-Src protein
  and EFGR, synergism in oncogenesis, 122
  interactions with EGFR, 121–122
  signaling downstream of EGFR, mechanism, 126, 128
    cytochrome c oxidase II (Cox II), 127
    EGFR effectors phosphorylated and regulated by, 128–129
    Map kinase and PLCγ, 128
    PI-3 kinase, 127–128
    STATs, 126
    steroid hormone receptors for, 130
    substrates for regulation, 129–130

Index

signaling upstream of EGFR (see EGFR transactivation)
structure and autoregulation, 120
Src-related kinase Lck, 64
STAT (signal transducers and activators of transcription) signaling pathways, 76
  nuclear translocation and downstream effects, 78
  STAT3 activation, 79–80
    EGFR independent activation of, 80
  STAT5 activation, in cancer, 81–82
    EGFR independent activation, 82
  STAT activation in signal transduction, 77–78
    serine residues, phosphorylation of, 78
  STAT family members, 77
  STAT1 in cancer, 78–79
Sts1/TULA2 protein, 56
Syk expression, in EGFR signaling, 238
Systems biology markup language (SBML), 216

T

Tamoxifen, 121, 125, 130, 159, 238
  MCF-7-derived resistace, 162
T-cell protein tyrosine phosphatase (TCPTP), 260
Terminal respiratory unit (TRU), 308
Thromboxane A2 (TxA2), 338. *See also* Prostaglandin
Tiam1, in human cancer, 107, 240
Time to progression (TTP), 307, 312, 315, 317, 357–359
T790M escape mutation, 40, 42
T790M mutation, 299–301, 305, 311, 318, 375
Transferrin receptor, 48, 52–53
Transforming growth factor (TGF), 53, 74, 90, 124, 222–223, 244, 277
  TGF-α expression, in human carcinomas, 226–227
  TGF-α, for activation and internalization EGFR, 7
Trans-phosphorylation, 16, 18

Trastuzumab, 10, 16, 23, 159
TSC1 and TSC2, germline mutations in, 241
TSC1/TSC2 protein complex, 107
Tuberous sclerosis complex-2 (TSC2), 107, 241
Tumor cell invasion
  adhesion of cells, 258–261
  cell motility, 261–262
  cell proteolysis, 263
  COX-2 and prostaglandins, 264
Tumor heterogeneity, 319–320, 370
Tumor susceptibility gene 101 (Tsg101), 247
Tumor vaccination, EGFRvIII peptide in, 286
Type I IGF receptor (IGF-IR), 156
Type II IGF receptor (IGF-IIR), 156
Tyrosine kinase domain (TKD), 32, 90, 189, 224–225, 295
  in EGFR, mutations in NSCLC, 296–304
  in EGFR, mutations in tumor other than NSCLC, 304–306
Tyrosine kinase inhibitor (TKI), 16, 21, 222, 259, 279, 286–287, 294, 345, 360, 363

U

Urokinase plasminogen activator (uPA), 263

V

Vascular endothelial growth factor (VEGF), 132, 267, 340–341, 361
Vimentin, 260, 317, 360, 371, 376

W

WASP/SCAR/WAVE, family of proteins, 262

Y

Yme1, inhibitory effect on EGFR down-regulation, 56

Z

ZD6474 inhibitor, 268, 355